Manual of
School Health

Second Edition

Manual of
School Health

KEETA DESTEFANO LEWIS, RN, MSN, PhD, FNASN
School Nurse Specialist
Napa County Office of Education
Health Consultant
Napa, California

BONNIE J. BEAR, RN, BSN, MA
School Nurse Specialist
San Diego City Schools
San Diego, California

SAUNDERS
An Imprint of Elsevier Science
Philadelphia   London   New York   St. Louis   Sydney   Toronto

SAUNDERS
An Imprint of Elsevier Science

11830 Westline Industrial Drive
St. Louis, Missouri 63146

MANUAL OF SCHOOL HEALTH, 2E   ISBN 0-7216-8521-8
Copyright © 2002, Elsevier Science (USA). All rights reserved.

NOTICES

Previous edition copyrighted 1986.

Library of Congress Cataloging-in-Publication Data
Lewis, Keeta DeStefano.
   Manual of school health / Keeta DeStefano Lewis, Bonnie J. Bear.—2nd ed.
     p. ; cm.
   Includes bibliographical references and index.
   ISBN 0-7216-8521-8
     1. School nursing—Handbooks, manuals, etc. I. Bear, Bonnie J. II. Title
   [DNLM: 1. School Nursing—Handbooks. WY 49 L674m 2002]
   RJ247 .L48 2002
   371.7'12—dc21

                                                          2002066839

Acquisitions Editor: Darlene Como
Developmental Editor: Laura Selkirk
Publishing Services Manager: Pat Joiner
Project Manager: Maureen Niebruegge
Designer: Mark Oberkrom
Cover Art: Mark Oberkrom

TG/MVY

Printed in the United States of America.

Last digit is print number: 9   8   7   6   5   4   3   2   1

REVIEWERS

Howard S. Adelman, PhD
Professor of Psychology
University of California–Los Angeles
Co-Director, UCLA Center for
  Mental Health in Schools
Los Angeles, California

Jeffrey Anshel, OD
Optometrist
President, Corporate Vision
  Consulting
Carlsbad, California

Virginia Armstrong, RN, PhD
Content Manager
Medschool Web Site
Culver City, California

Gordon R. Bear, LCSW, BCD
Psychotherapist, Consultant
San Diego, California

Martha Dewey Bergen, RN, MS, DNSc, FNASN
Senior Teaching Specialist
University of Minnesota School of
  Nursing
Minneapolis, Minnesota

Bonnie Rose Bernstein, PhD
Psychologist
San Diego Unified School District
San Diego, California

Lynda Boyer-Chuanroong, RN, MPH
School Health Programs
San Francisco Unified School District
San Francisco, California

Beverly J. Bradley, RN, PhD, FNASN
Assistant Clinical Professor
Division of Community Pediatrics
University of California–San Diego
San Diego, California

Robert E. Clark, PhD
Fellow
Department of Psychiatry
University of California–San Diego
San Diego, California

Janice Doyle, RN, MSN
Consultant Nurse, Bethel School
  District
Affiliate Faculty, Pacific Lutheran
  University
Tacoma, Washington

Joshua D. Feder, MD
Child and Family Psychiatrist
Neurobehavioral Institute, Inc.
Del Mar, California

Kimberly Goodman, RN, BSN
Staff Nurse, Intermediate Care
  Unit/Trauma
Sharp Memorial Hospital
San Diego, California

Joan L. Havard, MED, CCC/A
Clinical Audiologist
Speech, Language, and Hearing
  Specialist
Santa Clara County Office of
  Education
Santa Clara, California

Sheila M. Holcomb, RN, MSN
School Nurse
Folsom Cordova Unified School
    District
Faculty, Division of Nursing
California State University–
    Sacramento
Sacramento, California

Meri Jackson, RN, CNP
Nurse Practitioner
San Diego Unified School District
San Diego, California

Lisa Lewis Javar, RN
Sexual Assault Nurse Examiner
Sexual Assault Response Team
    (SART)
Napa, California ·

Richard A. Kaplan, MD
Pediatric Neurologist
Department of Neurology
Southern California Kaiser
    Permanente Medical Group
San Diego, California

Peter M. Keenan, RN, MS, CPNP
Clinical Coordinator
Pediatric Health Associates and the
    Young Parent's Program
Children's Hospital
Boston, Massachusetts

**Patsy L. Mahoney, RNC, CEN,
MSN, EdD**
Associate Professor and Director of
    Continuing Nursing Education
Pacific Lutheran University School of
    Nursing
Tacoma, Washington

Maureen Ward Moffatt, RN, MN
School Nurse Specialist
San Diego City Schools Infant-
    Toddler Development Program
San Diego, California

Paul Oga, PharmD
Managing Pharmacist
Napa, California

Stephanie M. Porter, RN, MSN
Director of Clinical Services Institute
    for Community Inclusion
Children's Hospital
Boston, Massachusetts

**Susan Proctor, RN, MPH, DNS,
FNASN**
Professor and Coordinator
School Nurse Program—Division of
    Nursing
California State University–
    Sacramento
Sacramento, California

**Dorothy J. Reilly, RN, MSN,
NCSN**
School Nurse
Pinon Elementary School
Los Alamos, New Mexico

Larry Schellenberg, RRT, CPFT
Pulmonary Division
Children's Hospital and Health
    Center
San Diego, California

Rodney Skager, PhD
Professor Emeritus
Graduate School of Education and
    Information Studies
University of California–Los Angeles
Los Angeles, California

Nancy Skager, RN, BSN, MSN
School Nurse, Family Case Manager
Monterey Unified Peninsula School
    District
Monterey, California

Kay Stuckhardt, RDH, MPH
Oral Health Specialist
Anderson Center for Dental Care
Children's Hospital and Health
  Center
San Diego, California

Linda Taylor, PhD
Clinical Psychologist, Los Angeles
  Unified School District
Co-Director, UCLA Center for
  Mental Health in Schools
University of California–Los Angeles
Los Angeles, California

Joan Thackaberry, RN, MSN, CS
School Nurse Practitioner
The Out of Door Academy
Sarasota, Florida

Sue Will, RN, MPH, FNASN
School Nurse
Central High School
Saint Paul, Minnesota

Patricia Wolfe, PhD
Private Educational Consultant
Napa, California

Conquer your dreams
with knowledge
Heal your inner fears
with hope
Pursue the love of learning
and share
the spirit of true health
Che

FOREWORD

—He who has health has hope, and he who has hope has everything.—Arabic proverb

If a social anthropologist were to visit this country and seek my recommendation for one location to best study our culture, it would be somewhere within hearing distance of a school health office. Standing there, he or she would learn the common acute and chronic ailments of our time and witness examples of modern medical technology and pharmacology. More interesting is that he or she would hear young voices unabashedly describing the pressures of modern home life. The most popular abuses of illicit substances, the myriad of favorite risk-taking behaviors, as well as other maladaptive responses to modern stresses, would soon become apparent. Many positive conversations would also be audible. It would be a great place to learn about many community resources, which help families flourish in the modern environment. Also, there would be words of counseling and the glee of success among youth. Our eavesdropper would learn of our educational, social and health systems (things like managed health care, the plight of those without health insurance, and our focus on literacy and science), and bear witness to society's prevalent attitudes to those who are different (by virtue of a disability, a sexual orientation, or a racial characteristic).

The school's health office is a microcosm of modern society. Not only its ailments and signs of despair, but its genius, compassion, and hope. It is not surprising, therefore, that this edition of the *Manual of School Health* needed to be so much larger and comprehensive than its predecessor. As a physician working concomitantly in the public education and the private health sectors, I can easily attest to the vast changes and complexities affecting both health and education in the past 15 years. It is difficult to pinpoint how the span of a few years has so magnified the importance of school nurses, school counselors, and other health professionals (the audience likely to use this *Manual*). Perhaps employed parents have become increasingly busy and require the assistance of schools to help monitor nonacademic factors in students' lives. The introduction of rare but well-publicized school shootings may have accentuated the acuity on which we see the potential bad—and good—of our nation's children. It is also possible that those who argue vehemently on both sides of the spectrum—that schools need to provide all support services and that schools should provide nothing other than academics—have thrown schools' health offices squarely in the cross-fire of societal pressures without too much assurance that help is on the way.

This *Manual* is a great step towards the help that school health offices need. It is a first resource for traditional school health matters, such as first-aid and vision screening. It also offers clear and insightful tips on the health ramifications of the most contemporary school health issues, such as commercialization of schools, students' feelings of isolation, the newest management strategies for chronic diseases, computer ergonomics and heavy backpacks. After all, it is expected that school health professionals have enough knowledge for each of these (and more) to offer guidance on the matter.

School nurses and others in their positions are often the first to detect symptoms of health problems in our nation's school-age population—symptoms that represent any one of hundreds of medical diagnoses. School nurses are also often the first to detect public health trends when problems arise repeatedly in a student population. They may be among the first in the school, for example, to act on the truth that a student's violent behavior or substance abuse is a health matter and a public health concern, not simply an offense. As the prime interface between physicians and educators, school nurses require succinct descriptions of diseases and syndromes that can enhance their ability to correctly identify dozens of potential diagnoses and to communicate authoritatively with physicians and public health authorities.

The breadth of topics in this *Manual* is testimony to the full meaning of the word "health." As such, chapters on child and adolescent development, the environment, and the effects of a chronic disease on one's education are bound to be helpful to many professionals beyond traditional health care providers. Hopefully, many will refer to it and benefit. Topics that are inherently difficult to discuss, such as domestic violence, date rape, and sexuality, are dealt with using candor and plain facts. By reading and then relaying information, not judgment, users of this manual are likely to bring a level of openness about such topics to those students, parents, school administrators, and fellow staff with whom they work.

Howard L. Taras, MD
Professor of Clinical Pediatrics
University of California–San Diego
Chair, Committee on School Health
American Academy of Pediatrics
San Diego, California

FOREWORD

You are in for a treat. This book, a wonderful addition to the school nursing and school health literature, is the second edition of its earlier cousin. It will be a vital handbook and ready resource for nurses, teachers, administrators, parents, and others who are faced daily with a growing array of health concerns affecting the contemporary pediatric population. It is with a sense of honor that I offer some introductory words to this excellent sourcebook for schools.

I have known the authors for many years. Both are expert school nurses and are particularly knowledgeable about the young child population, having had extensive experience with infant, toddler, and preschool special education children. Keeta conducted research for both her master's and doctoral degrees in the area of prenatally drug-exposed infants. Both have become nationally recognized experts in the management of the infant and child in the special education environment.

Before their sojourn into the world of the very young child, however, Keeta and Bonnie were nurses in the K-12 setting, where they garnered valuable experience in managing the health problems of children in regular education and special education. Keeta collaborated with her now-retired colleague, Helen Thomson, to author the first edition of the *Manual of School Health* (1986). As the twenty-first century approached, however, the first edition, an important resource for schools, was in need of revision.

Keeta and Bonnie's mutual practice interest spawned a desire to work together in planning and producing the second edition. As expert and seasoned school nurses, they had ready access to sources of new knowledge in the field of school nursing. Both had been long-time members of the California School Nurses Organization and the National Association of School Nurses and could draw upon the expertise of colleagues as well.

This edition is especially unique. It incorporates some of the same important dimensions included in the first edition and augments those with some valuable contemporary perspectives. All earlier chapters have been revised, and some have been renamed. Revised chapters in the new edition include *Growth and Development Characteristics, Vision and Hearing, Acute Conditions, Chronic Conditions, Substance Abuse, Special Education,* and *Emergency Disaster Preparedness and First Aid.* Four new chapters are added: *Affective and Behavioral Disorders, Violence, Adolescent and Gender-Specific Issues,* and a unique addition, *Twenty-first Century Health Challenges.* Particularly useful to the reader are a bibliography and a list of pertinent Web sites that follow each chapter.

In Chapter 1, *Growth and Development Characteristics,* those readers familiar with the first edition will note some additional nuances, such as a focus on the newborn and the presentation of discrete developmental stages for school-age children and adolescents.

Chapter 2, *Vision and Hearing,* is expanded to include tables of drugs affecting the development of the eyes and the ears, and testing procedures for the young or difficult-to-test-child. The *Acute Conditions* chapter, Chapter 3, retains all of the health issues of the early edition and provides updated information on conditions such as Lyme disease, bacterial skin infections, and the common cold. Similarly, Chapter 4, which addresses *Chronic Conditions,* captures much of the first work, reframes other conditions in light of current research and parlance (e.g., juvenile diabetes mellitus is now diabetes mellitus, types 1 and 2), and adds other chronic disorders (hepatitis and Turner's syndrome). A table is included titled, "Peak Flow Interpretation System," which is especially useful in the management of asthma as a chronic condition.

Chapter 5, new to the book, speaks to the burgeoning problem of *Affective and Behavioral Disorders.* Herein, the authors address disorders of attention and behavior such as autism, Tourette's syndrome, and attention deficit-hyperactivity disorder (ADHD), as well as pervasive developmental disorders (PDD). Highlights of this chapter are tables of many psychopharmacologic agents for the treatment of ADHD and PDD. *Substance Abuse* is revisited in Chapter 6, and many of the newer substances, such as Ecstasy, GHB, and MDA, are examined. The chapter features the signs and symptoms of both use and toxicity and the school nursing role in the management and treatment of substance disorders in the school setting. Chapter 7 is also new in this volume and addresses *Violence*—to self, to others, and by others. The reader will find information on self-mutilation, date rape, and gangs in addition to that regarding child and domestic violence and suicide. Particularly noteworthy in this chapter is recent research on brain findings related to violent behavior.

Chapter 8, a new offering, reflects on *Adolescent and Gender-Specific Issues.* Here, such traditional subjects as pregnancy and STIs are discussed together with consideration of emergent issues such as tattooing, body piercing, and steroid use. Useful guides are included for the professional teaching of breast self-examinations (BSE) and testicular self-examinations (TSE), and a contraceptive table is provided that compares and contrasts methods and their efficacy. Assessment tools for use with the child in *Special Education* are a highlight of Chapter 9. The most recent editions of many widely-used assessment instruments are overviewed and the names of their publishers provided. Unique problems such as latex allergies are also discussed.

A cornerstone of this book is the chapter titled *Twenty-first Century Health Challenges.* Chapter 10 touches upon a wide variety of contemporary behaviors, which have health implications or are dominant health issues in themselves. Examples are the use of heavy backpacks, computer-workstation concerns, the exploitation of schools by corporations for commercial purposes, and conditions such as major depression and bipolar illness. The chapter also addresses social trends and their implications for physical and mental health; topics included are as diverse as gambling and home schooling. Incorporated in this chapter are a discussion of terrorism and bioterrorism and the need to recognize infectious agents such as anthrax and smallpox, as well as the signs and symptoms of infectious processes from several likely agents. Finally, the chapter speaks to the use of the school as a community-based health care center, a notion espoused in the early 1990s and deserving of reexamination. In the final chapter, Chapter 11, the authors present a fine overview of contemporary perspectives on *Emergency Disaster Preparedness and First Aid,* subjects which are of interest to both school professionals and parents. This chapter is sure to be of value to every school.

The book concludes with a series of wonderful appendices, which are valuable resources in themselves. If you are a nurse, consider keeping a copy of this text at each work site so that you and others will have ready access to its use. It will provide valuable and pertinent information every day.

It is a privilege to present this book to its many potential readers.

Susan E. Proctor, RN, MPH, DNS, FNASN
Professor and Coordinator
School Nurse Program—Division of Nursing
California State University–Sacramento
Sacramento, California

PREFACE

*T*his new second edition of the *Manual of School Health* is a gift to all of the nurses, health professionals, and parents who supported the first edition published in 1986. This manual is widely used by school nurses and numerous other professionals who work with infants, toddlers, and children of all ages and in all educational grades. It is a unique fast reference book regarding the school-age child.

School nurses are often the first to detect current trends in the pediatric population and behaviors of students that may lead to violence both to one's self and to others, to be aware of substance abuse, and to advocate for health care and not punitive action. Hundreds of diagnoses and treatment modalities are necessary for the school nurse to be current and proactive in providing a full range of services. This book provides data for determining early signs and symptoms and for timely referral to primary care providers or public health agencies for management and follow-up. Biotechnology has provided information and new treatments on a grand scale, saving and treating individuals who in the past would have been deprived of or escaped this support. The book addresses trends occurring in the school realm such as commercialism of schools, computer ergonomics, and heavy backpack use.

Now, with the encouragement and support from school nurses, administrators, and professionals working with the school-age population, we have developed and organized this more comprehensive and inclusive edition. With unconditional support, constructive comments, and continuous encouragement, we realize the incredible responsibility and accountability that follows as we provide this revision.

SPECIAL FEATURES

This manual continues to be a summary of information found most relevant to the needs of the child and young adult in the school setting. We have included conditions and concerns suggested by nurses who participated in focus groups across the United States. We continue to define *school-age* as those students from birth through age 21, thus including children in infant and toddler programs and childcare and those in special education programs.

- The *technologies,* including the use of the electron microscope, computed tomography (CT), positron emission tomography (PET), and functional magnetic resonance imaging (fMRI) scans, and genome project identifying genes in the body and their functioning, are influencing factors throughout the manual.
- The *Brain Findings* subsections are related to growth, development, behaviors, learning, and health.
- *Growth and Development Characteristics* include prenatal, psychosexual, moral, and spiritual development.
- *Affective and Behavioral Disorders* discusses primarily DSM-IV disorders.
- *Violence* is included as associated to school, home, others, and self.

- *Substance Abuse* includes club drugs, date rape drugs, and inhalants, with the major contribution being the "Neurobiology of Addiction."
- *Twenty-first Century Health Challenges* are the contemporary issues facing students, staff, parents and the nurse.
- Chapter 11, the last chapter, discusses *Emergency Disaster Preparedness and First Aid.*
- *Web Sites and Resources* provide access to additional data and related agencies/organizations.

Numerous learning methodologies are included to enhance and expedite the use of critical information by the nurse.
- The *School Nursing Role* is focused in several chapters.
- *Alerts* for emergency interventions such as toxic effects of drugs, diabetes, and status epilepticus.
- *Guidelines* summarize important information necessary for well-planned, comprehensive health care.
- *Key points* provide a summary of pertinent health care elements to be addressed at the school site and/or for individualized health/educational plan (IHP, IEP) development.
- Numerous *Tables and Boxes* are diverse and provide additional concise information applicable to specific situations and assessment procedures.
- School *Exclusion and Readmission* policies provide appropriate suggestions for those without current guidelines.
- *60 Illustrations* are easy to follow and offer a visual component.
- The *Glossary* defines concepts and key terms for a quick, accurate understanding.
- *Appendixes* are valuable elements for school health assessments, interventions and management.
- *End Sheets* on the inside front and back covers provide another avenue of fast reference information.

It is our philosophy that the family remains the unit of care and is an integral part of all health care, intervention, and academic planning that occurs in the school setting. All school staff and teaching faculty need to be encouraged to include the parent(s) in their child's school experience.

ACKNOWLEDGMENTS

With this revised second edition of *The Manual of School Health,* the opportunity is available for us to express our gratitude for the support of the original book and the encouragement and eager applause provided for this, our revised, more comprehensive edition. The first book, published in 1986, was uniquely accepted by school nurses, community nurses, educators, other professionals, and staff working with all ages of school children and not the least, but excitingly, by parents and grandparents. This acceptance and support of the manual makes us aware of our incredible responsibility and accountability, which we take very seriously.

Our dear friend and colleague, *Helen Thomson,* coauthored the first edition of the book. We sincerely appreciate her contribution to the original work. Her expertise and nursing experience were missed during the long preparation of this revised manual.

A very special appreciation to *Thomas Eoyang,* who has been a support for this book from its inception in 1984 and continues as the hero of the manual; to *Laura Selkirk,* associate developmental editor of this new-millennium book and her eager dedication and continued support throughout all phases of the manual. Our thanks to *Jeanne Robertson* for her excellence in the world of illustrations.

Profound gratitude and thanks to *Gordon Bear,* husband to Bonnie, dear friend to Keeta, and colleague to both, for his extreme attentiveness, helpfulness, sensitivity, support, and mentoring throughout this exciting endeavor.

A special appreciation to *Maureen Moffatt* for her thoughtful, clarifying, and challenging review of all of the chapters. Our thanks to *BJ Albright* and *Mary Laughton* for their helpful assistance with the manuscript technology and preparation and to *Virginia Means* for her reviews and organizational support.

And deep gratitude and love to all of our colleagues who reviewed the manuscript, made suggestions, and encouraged us throughout this process, to Susan Proctor, who remains the "shero" of the manual and last but not least, to the parents who made suggestions and provided their personal stories and experiences about their children's physical and emotional health, which may be neglected or often forgotten.

Finally, we wish to express our deepest gratitude and love to our *families* and *dear friends.* The time and energy spent in the writing has demanded many changes in their lifestyle, which they accepted unconditionally. They continue to be a source of inspiration.

Keeta DeStefano Lewis
Bonnie J. Bear

CONTENTS

Manual of
School Health

CHAPTER 1

Growth and Development Characteristics

*T*he nurse often encounters concerns regarding the development of a child, adolescent, or young adult. These concerns frequently center around intelligence, speech, motor problems, emotional/social skills, psychosocial status, morality or spirituality, and physical needs. To adequately assess, evaluate, treat, seek consultation, or make referral, the nurse needs knowledge of normal growth and development in all domains. This chapter is a guide for facilitating such assessment. Characteristics such as physical traits; gross and fine psychomotor skills; emotional, social, and sexual development; and developmental tasks related to morality and spirituality for individual age groups are presented in a systematic and sequential form for easy reference.

This chapter covers the life cycle from the time of conception through young adulthood. School nurses increasingly are employed to serve this population throughout the United States; many states currently offer school nurse services to students throughout this life cycle.

The human growth and development section summarizes embryonic growth (conception to 6 weeks) and fetal development (7 weeks to 9 months). The period of infancy through early childhood (birth to 5 years) is of utmost importance to the nurse because children develop and grow rapidly during this critical time. Any deviation from the norm must be detected at this time so that early intervention and remediation can begin.

By elementary age (6 to 12 years), most major developmental problems have been identified. However, many problems are so subtle that they remain undetected until later developmental stages. As children enter the school environment, they face increased physical and mental demands. Numerous health, emotional, and developmental problems can occur during this age span. The nurse plays an important role in early detection, appropriate nursing care, and referral.

Adolescents (13 to 18 years) are in transition from childhood to adulthood. This period is characterized by many rapid physical, emotional, and sexual changes. In addition, it is imperative that this age group successfully meets numerous developmental tasks. These challenging tasks and rapid succession of changes contribute to stress-related illness, dysfunctional family life, interpersonal conflicts, and possibly antisocial behavior. The risk-taking adolescent too often becomes identified with an unhealthy lifestyle and a myriad of teenage issues and concerns that are well known to the school nurse. Young adult development (19 through 21 years) is summarized in this chapter, concluding with the reaching of maturity and achievement of developmental tasks of the young adult.

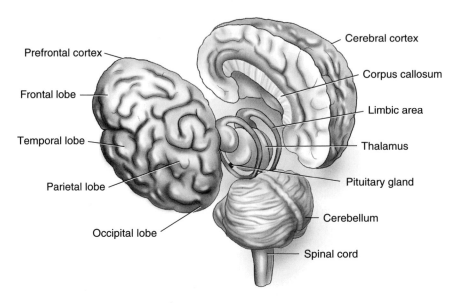

Figure 1-1 Structure of the brain.

EMBRYONIC AND FETAL DEVELOPMENT

Brain Findings

The ectoderm, endoderm, and mesoderm layers separate at approximately day 10 to 13 of gestation. The neural plate forms from the ectoderm and eventually becomes the brain and spinal cord.

Differentiation of the hindbrain, the midbrain, and the forebrain, the three major divisions of the brain, begins by the third week of gestation.

STRUCTURES OF THE BRAIN

The *cerebral cortex,* also called the *neocortex,* is the outer covering of the brain. The brain has *two hemispheres,* and each hemisphere has four major lobes that can be further subdivided into many specialty areas. The *four lobes* are frontal, occipital, parietal, and temporal.

- The *frontal lobes* are responsible for thinking, conceptualizing, planning, emotional regulation and planning, social interaction, abstract thinking, decision, and memory.
- The *occipital lobes* are the primary centers for visual processing.
- The *parietal lobes* are concerned with functions of calculation, orientation, movement, and particular types of recognition, somatic interpretation, and integration.
- The *temporal lobes* are responsible primarily for sound, hearing, speech comprehension (left side generally), and the formation of long-term memory.

The *fibrous corpus callosum* connects the two hemispheres and allows them to pass information back and forth.

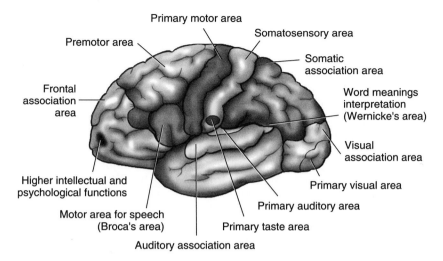

FIGURE 1-2 Mapping of the brain, including thought, movement, and sensory functions.

At 7 months' gestation, *convolutions* begin to form in the outer layer of the brain to accommodate for the restricted space; this formation is one of the factors responsible for the eventual power of the brain. These convolutions allow the cortex to increase its surface area (and computing power) without an increase in skull size.

During the first 7 months, an average of 250,000 neurons per minute migrate to designated places; approximately 50% are pruned away before birth. This process is also called *apoptosis,* programmed cell death.

Language areas for general processing are located in the left hemisphere in approximately 96% of the population. There are two major language areas:

- *Wernicke's area* is located in the frontal lobe near the junction of the temporal lobe and is associated with comprehension of speech. This area is also near the auditory cortex, which receives sound signals from the ears.
- *Broca's area* is located at the posterior of the frontal lobe in the left hemisphere and is associated with generating speech. It also is near the motor cortex area that controls muscles of the lips and mouth.

OTHER CORTICAL AREAS

The *angular gyrus* is located on the margins of the temporal, parietal, and occipital lobes, up and behind Wernicke's area. This area is associated with vision, spatial skills, and language and is believed to act as a bridge between the language process and visual word recognition (meaning).

The *motor cortex* is located at the junction of the frontal and parietal lobes, below the area where a set of headphones might sit across the top of the head. The motor cortex plays a critical role in controlling muscle movements (as do the cerebellum and basal ganglia). All movement areas of the body have a corresponding area in the motor cortex. The right side controls muscles on the left side of the body, and the left side controls those on the right side.

The *premotor cortex* is dedicated to initiation and sequencing of movements and is part of the frontal lobe.

The *somatosensory cortex,* a strip across the top of each hemisphere, is adjacent and posterior to the motor cortex and is associated with the processing of incoming sensory stimulation: pain sensation, touch, pressure, temperature, and proprioception (body position in space).

The *thalamus* lies beneath the cortex and acts as a relay station that transmits incoming sensory signals to the appropriate part of the cortex for further processing (e.g., pain). All sensory systems except the sense of smell send signals to the thalamus (e.g., touch, sight, hearing).

The *hypothalamus,* a small organ, lies below the thalamus. The hypothalamus, together with the *pituitary gland,* is involved in activities vital to survival (e.g., maintenance of blood glucose levels, body temperature, body rhythms [heart rate, thirst, activity and rest, sexual desire, reproductive and menstrual cycles]). The hypothalamus integrates the autonomic nervous system between the sympathetic and parasympathetic branches.

The *cortex* controls the hypothalamus, which is a subcortical brain structure. In turn, the hypothalamus controls the pituitary gland, which is often referred to as the "head gland" because it controls the other glands of the body by changing the chemicals that flow through the bloodstream.

The *hippocampus,* a structure shaped like a ram's horn, is located deep within the temporal lobe near the amygdala and hypothalamus. It is associated with conscious long-term memory, spatial ability, emotional behavior, learning, and motivation. Damage to the hippocampus causes severe memory problems.

The *amygdala* consists of two almond-shaped structures located at the anterior end of each hippocampus. They coordinate autonomic and endocrine responses with states of emotions (e.g., anger, fear) and are involved in the regulation and storage of emotional memory.

The *nucleus accumbens* is a small, hooklike structure linked to pleasure, cravings, and reward.

The *ventral tegmental area (VTA),* located at the top of the brainstem, relays messages of pleasure from their nerve cells to nerve cells in the nucleus accumbens through the neurotransmitter dopamine. This pleasure circuit also includes the prefrontal cortex and is called the *mesolimbic dopamine system.* It is associated with acts of pleasure (e.g., eating, sexual activity, addiction).

To understand the brain, scientists delineate it by shape and function and name its structures and areas; however, the purpose of particular structures of the brain or which areas are involved in any given brain activity are not always clearly understood.

OTHER FETAL DEVELOPMENT

Until approximately 6 weeks, the embryo is basically gender neutral. Genetic predetermination and the absence or presence of male hormones begin the sexual design for development.

At *6 weeks* a male embryo begins to convert gonadal lumps into testes, which produce testosterone; at *12 weeks* a female embryo begins to develop ovaries. External genitalia are present at *8 weeks'* gestation. At *25 weeks* the fetus weighs approximately 1 lb and has 100 billion neurons. The fetus responds to the maternal voice, light, and smells in utero, suggesting learning occurs in utero.

Human deoxyribonucleic acid (DNA) contains approximately 30,000 to 40,000 genes. Genetic endowment and the environment have a decisive role in development. *Genes* either determine development, such as eye color, hair color, and body size, or predispose an individual to certain diseases, disorders, or traits (e.g., temperament).

The *intrauterine environment* can influence development (e.g., early and significant exposure to alcohol, nicotine, cocaine, poor nutrition, and stress).

EARLY CHILDHOOD: BIRTH TO 5 YEARS

NEWBORN: BIRTH TO 1 MONTH

I. *Brain Findings*
  A. Brain weight at birth is approximately 1 lb.
  B. The cortex is approximately one half of adult thickness at birth and 1 mm thick.
  C. The brain has approximately 100 billion neurons and more than 50 trillion synapses at birth.
  D. Some apoptosis or pruning of overgrowth of neurons continues after birth.
  E. Synapses form in the newborn's brain at the rate of approximately 3 billion per second at given times.
  F. Most of the brain's neurons are not yet formed into networks. The brain's early developmental task is that of forming and reinforcing connections/networks of neurons and pruning of others. This process is a function of genetic control of development and experience with the outside environment.
  G. Each neuron can be connected to as many as 15,000 other neurons but averages approximately 6000 connections.
  H. The brain's capacity is not fixed at birth and is most plastic during infancy; however, synapses can be formed at any age.
  I. Brain development is nonlinear. It does not grow at a steady rate but has peaks for learning of various skills.
  J. The brain appears to be programmed to search for rules and order in experiences.
  K. The brain constitutes approximately 12% of body weight at birth and approximately 2% to 3% of body weight at adulthood.
  L. Brain growth is reflected in the head circumference; growth charts (see Appendix A) indicate that brain growth occurs more rapidly in the first year of life than any other subsequent age. The brain reaches ½ its eventual size by 12 months.
  M. The newborn's head is approximately ¼ of total body length.
  N. The brain is active, growing, and enduringly dynamic.

II. **Physical and Anatomical Traits**
NOTE: Child should continue to follow own growth curve, which is more important than conformity to averages.
  A. Undifferentiated, almost immobile at birth with many primitive reflexes (e.g., sucking, grasping, rooting, squinting).
  B. Weight gain 5-7 oz weekly (150-210 g).
  C. Height growth 1 in (2.5 cm) monthly.

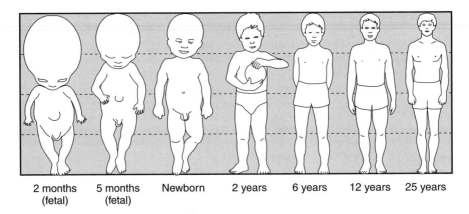

2 months   5 months   Newborn   2 years   6 years   12 years   25 years
(fetal)   (fetal)

FIGURE 1-3 Head and body proportions from prenatal development to 25 years.

D. Head circumference larger than chest circumference; median head circumference at birth 13.5 in (35 cm), chest 13 in (33 cm). Head circumference increases over 3 in (8 cm) during first 6 months of life.
E. Chubby appearance. At 1 month muscles firmer than at birth.
F. Posterior fontanel often closed at birth; if open, will close between 2-3 months.
G. Anterior fontanel is open until 14 months.
H. Obligatory nose breathing.
I. Visual acuity approaches 20/100.

III. **Gross and Fine Psychomotor Traits**
A. Asymmetric posture with head to one side, one arm extended, and the other flexed toward the shoulder (asymmetric tonic-neck reflex [ATNR] posture).
B. Extremities extend and abduct with fanning of fingers, followed by flexion and adduction of the extremities. Results from a sudden horizontal lowering of infant (Moro/startle reflex).
C. Head is unsteady when infant is pulled to sitting position.
D. Movement of arms and legs is symmetrical bilaterally and generally smooth.
E. Both hands clenched, grasp reflex strong.
F. Momentarily grasps rattle placed in hand, grasp reflex.
G. Follows object to midline, but focuses best on objects 8-15 in away.
H. Prefers black-and-white geometric designs.

IV. **Cognitive and Language Traits**
A. Involuntary reflexive behavior.
B. Makes comfort sounds during feeding.
C. Gurgling or crying sounds of baby.
D. Alerts to high-pitched voices.
E. Cries when unhappy. Small, throaty noises may turn into cooing by the end of first month.
F. Arms flex and fists clench after sudden loud noise (Moro/startle reflex). Head turns toward voice or other soft auditory stimuli in alert state.

V. Emotional and Social Traits
  A. Inward and autistic-like orientation, asocial but symbiotic; newborn feels joined to the mother as in utero.
  B. Unable to discern self, non-self, and others.
  C. Detectable temperament differences: active, irritable, quiet, alert.
  D. May recognize parent's voice, especially the mother's voice.
  E. Derives simple physical pleasure from being held, cuddled, and rocked.
  F. Regards face intently while being engaged verbally.
  G. Reacts to social overtures by reducing general activity.
  H. Social smile begins at 2 months.
VI. Psychosexual Traits
  A. Orality: primary source of pleasure centered on mouth, lips, and tongue.
  B. Male babies have penile erections before birth (ultrasound) and after birth.
  C. Sensual feeling triggered by kicking, rocking, or rubbing genitals gives sensory pleasure that may not be erotic as in later stage of sexuality.
  D. Sucking and rooting reflexes during breast feeding or bottle feeding are the precursors of sexual pleasures.
VII. Moral and Spiritual Traits
  A. Premoral, amoral, primordial.
  B. Egocentric, narcissistic.

INFANCY: 2 TO 12 MONTHS
3 Months (12 Weeks)

I. *Brain Findings*
  A. Visual cortex synaptic formation peaks while brain is enhancing the connections that allow eyes to focus on objects. Allows level of depth perception.
  B. In the motor cortex at approximately 2 months of age, the infant begins to lose startle and rooting reflexes and the mastering of purposeful movements begins for more coordinated movements.
  C. Expression of genetic predisposition is influenced by environmental factors, including physical, mental, social, and emotional.
  D. Development of subcortical and limbic areas is influenced by early experiences of trauma or ongoing abuse and may result in extreme depression, anxiety and/or inability to develop empathy or form appropriate attachments.
  E. Brain development is highly susceptible to chemical, structural, hormonal, and environmental influences (e.g., drugs, poor nutrition, physical trauma, radiation, poverty).
II. Physical and Anatomical Traits
  A. Posterior fontanel closed.
  B. Has gained approximately 5 lb (2.3 kg).
  C. Length increased 3.75 in (9-10 cm).
  D. Head circumference has grown approximately 2 in (5 cm).

    E. Chest circumference has increased 2.75 in (7 cm).

    F. Establishes sleep-wake cycles.

III. Gross and Fine Psychomotor Traits

    A. ATNR begins to disappear, and head usually is held in the midline.

    B. On abdomen, can lift head 90 degrees with weight supported on forearms.

    C. Tightens muscles when pulled to a sitting position in an attempt to control head.

    D. Turns head and eyes to a moving object within visual range.

    E. Puts hands and objects in mouth.

    F. Grasp reflex is inactive.

    G. Hands generally open or loosely closed.

    H. Holds rattle for a short time if placed in hand.

    I. Regards one or both hands.

    J. With contact, actively pulls on clothing and blanket.

    K. Follows object with eyes to 180 degrees.

    L. Can sit with head erect for short periods with support.

    M. Lifts head while lying in supine position.

    N. Makes precrawling attempts.

    O. Attempts to grasp objects but misses.

IV. Cognitive and Language Traits

    A. Reflexive behavior generally replaced by voluntary movements.

    B. Most have recognition for common objects: bottle, mobiles, toys.

    C. Babbling.

    D. Responds to a familiar face by cooing, chuckling noise, or laughter.

    E. Vocalizing accompanies smiling.

    F. Crying is more related to specific needs or wants; crying becoming differentiated.

    G. Vocal responses are reflexive in display: yawn, gurgle, sneeze, coo, cry, laughter, squealing.

    H. Single vowel sounds are predominant: "aaah," "ooooo."

    I. Actively interested in environment, curious, visually searches to locate sounds.

V. Emotional and Social Traits

    A. Beginning separation of self from others.

    B. Can be attentive, calm, and alert.

    C. Displays recognition signs at sight of mother.

    D. Longer period of wakefulness without crying.

    E. Stops crying at sight of parent.

    F. Smiles often to others, may laugh.

    G. Demands attention by fussing, enjoys attention.

    H. Freezes in the presence of strangers.

VI. Psychosexual Traits

    A. Remains the same as newborn.

VII. Moral and Spiritual Traits

    A. Remains the same as newborn.

6 Months (24 Weeks)

I. Physical and Anatomical Traits

    A. Since birth, weight has doubled and has grown an average of 6 in.

NOTE: Between 6 and 12 months, average weight gain is 3-5 oz weekly (90-150 g) and height growth is ½ in (1.25 cm) monthly.

    B. Head circumference has increased 3 in (8 cm).

    C. Beginning of tooth eruption, generally lower central incisors.

    D. Growth rate slower than first 6 months.

    E. By 4 to 7 months has full color vision.

II. Gross and Fine Psychomotor Traits

    A. Raises chest and upper part of abdomen off surface with weight on hands.

    B. Rolls over from stomach to back (supine) and, in another month, from back to stomach (prone).

    C. Sits alone but may need to lean forward on hands.

    D. Holds onto feet and pulls to mouth.

    E. Begins weight bearing when held.

    F. Rocks on hands and knees.

    G. Palmar grasp.

    H. Will drop one cube if another presented.

    I. Can transfer cube from hand to hand and manipulate objects.

    J. Holds own bottle.

    K. Grasps and explores small objects.

    L. Begins pincer grasp and self-feeding.

    M. Drinks from a cup when cup held to lips.

III. Cognitive and Language Traits

    A. May look in response to name.

    B. Response may vary to angry or happy voices.

    C. Responds and imitates differences in intonation (melody pattern).

    D. Imitates simple actions or movements; hands on head, waves or responds to "bye-bye."

    E. Babbling sounds are one-syllable utterances, consonants, and vowels: "da," "ma," "di."

    F. Recognizes vowel sounds basic to speech.

    G. Responds to voice by turning head or vocalization.

    H. Variety of vocal responses to show feeling. May squeal to show pleasure.

    I. Talks to people as well as to own toys.

    J. Smiles and laughs aloud.

    K. Experiments with own voice.

IV. Emotional and Social Traits

    A. May withdraw from strangers.

    B. Shows displeasure at removal of toy.

    C. Holds arms out to be picked up.

    D. Smiles at mirror images.

    E. Laughs aloud when stimulated, such as person hiding head in towel.

    F. Begins to show distress if mother leaves.

    G. Other family members, beyond mother, become important or trusted.

V. **Psychosexual Traits**
   A. Can wean infant from pleasures derived from the breast or bottle.
   B. Biting and oral aggression, exploration begin.
VI. **Moral and Spiritual Traits**
   A. Beginning to value caregiver over others and to show likes and dislikes based on voluntary choices associated with less distress or discomfort.
   B. Definite ability to delay personal gratification to get beyond primary narcissism.

9 Months (36 Weeks)

I. *Brain Findings*
   A. Between 7 and 12 months, linkage occurs among concepts, feelings, and language.
   B. At approximately 8 or 9 months the hippocampus becomes more functional in forming, storing, and recalling some types of memories. This is the beginning of cause-and-effect behavior. Infants can be taught that their behavior (e.g., touching an object) will result in a certain outcome (e.g., hearing a pleasant sound).
   C. In certain time periods (nonlinear brain development), various types of learning are more efficient, such as at 1 month, increased activity in subcortical and cortical regions makes visual and auditory stimulation important because regions are associated with control of sensorimotor functions; at 8 months, frontal lobe shows increased metabolic activity, and this is an important time for strengthening or weakening caregiver attachment and self-regulation because this cortex is associated with the ability to think, plan, regulate, and express emotion.
II. **Physical and Anatomical Traits**
   A. Rapid weight gains begin to decrease, with a gain of 3.3 lb (1.5 kg) between 6 and 9 months.
   B. Gains 3-5 oz per week; grows 1 cm a month.
   C. Eruption of upper lateral incisor.
III. **Gross and Fine Psychomotor Traits**
   A. Sits well without supports.
   B. Pulls self to standing position.
   C. Stands holding onto furniture.
   D. Cruises.
   E. Bounces actively when held in standing position.
   F. Gets to sitting position alone.
   G. Pivots while seated.
   H. Crawls on hands and knees, purposefully creeping; can crawl backward.
   I. Drinks from a cup.
   J. Pincer grasp is developing; bangs two blocks together.
   K. Attempts to grasp third cube.
   L. Hand preference may be noticeable.
   M. Mouthing is prominent.
IV. **Cognitive and Language Traits**
   A. Produces four or more sounds.
   B. Combines two or more syllables but without specific meaning: "da-da," "ba-ba."

    C. Will imitate sounds such as clicking of tongue or a cough but does not form words.

    D. Responds to own name.

    E. Understands "bye."

    F. Comprehends "no-no."

    G. Understands simple commands.

    H. Has one word with specific reference.

    I. Imitates animal sounds.

    J. All vowels, many consonants present.

    K. More adept with nonverbal communication, gestures.

    L. Listens intently to conversations.

V. Emotional and Social Traits

    A. Can maintain object constancy, internalizing caring and familiar family members.

    B. Able to trust others; increasing interest in pleasing others.

    C. Interacts in a purposeful, reciprocal manner.

    D. Can ascertain moods and imitate them (e.g., crying when someone cries).

    E. Separation anxiety issues; fear of going to bed and being alone; nighttime rituals important.

    F. Distressed by new and strange situations and people.

    G. Powerful urge toward independence in feeding and locomotion.

    H. Responds to simple requests.

    I. Plays peek-a-boo and pat-a-cake.

    J. Shows displeasure if activity is inhibited.

VI. Psychosexual Traits

    A. No change from 6-month infant.

VII. Moral and Spiritual Traits

    A. May show signs of inhibition or suppression when admonished for inappropriate conduct.

    B. Has sense of awe for the caretakers as powerful or preferred people.

TODDLER: 1 YEAR TO 3 YEARS

Brain Findings

Neurons remain relatively stable while synapses increase during the first 3 years. The brain's neuroplasticity is reflected by change in response to experience.

    The brain can compensate or alter itself after insults dependent on timing, intensive intervention, and the nature of the insult. The plasticity of the young brain is more acute than the adult brain.

    Animal research supports the fact that more synaptic growth occurs when living in enriched environments versus thinning of neuron networks, which occurs in impoverished environments.

12 Months (48 Weeks)

I. Physical and Anatomical Traits

    A. Weight has tripled since birth.

    B. Head circumference has increased approximately 5 in (12 cm) since birth.

    C. Anterior fontanel almost closed.
    D. Has grown an average of 10 in (25 cm) since birth.
    E. Chest is equal to or slightly greater in circumference than the head.
    F. Has total of six to eight deciduous teeth.

II. Gross and Fine Psychomotor Traits
    A. Stands without support.
    B. Walks holding onto furniture and when both hands are held.
    C. Most children walk alone between 12 and 15 months.
    D. When sitting, can twist around to pick up an object.
    E. Begins to throw things on floor.
    F. Neat pincer grasp.
    G. Finger feeds self.
    H. Beginning to use spoon with assistance, much spilling.
    I. Can hold crayon.
    J. Starts sequential play by separately placing several cubes into container.
    K. Waves with wrist.
    L. Turns pages of a book, many at a time.

III. Cognitive and Language Traits
    A. Recognition of personal name.
    B. Begins to look where parent points, recognizes objects by name.
    C. Understands simple requests (e.g., "give it to me").
    D. Discriminates simple geometric forms (e.g., circle).
    E. Egocentric pretend play.
    F. Actively searches for a hidden object.
    G. Generally has several other words in addition to "mama" and "dada."
    H. Most words are nouns.
    I. Squeals and makes noise for attention and pleasure.
    J. Can wave bye-bye and plays pat-a-cake.
    K. Vocalizes when spoken to.
    L. Expressive jargon: imitates animal sounds, shakes head for no, 25% of language intelligible to an unfamiliar person.

IV. Emotional and Social Traits
    A. Reacts to restrictions with frustration.
    B. Able to show emotions of fear, anger, affection, and jealousy.
    C. May develop attachments to security blanket or favorite toy.
    D. Smiles at, pats, or even kisses mirror image.
    E. Differences between boys and girls are seen in the way they assert themselves; boys are more assertive.
    F. Gives toy to person on request.
    G. Plays peek-a-boo by covering face.
    H. Crying usually indicates distress.
    I. Rolls ball to another.

V. Psychosexual Traits
    A. Gender-specific stereotyped play begins as part of parents' socialization process.

VI. Moral and Spiritual Traits
    A. Parents and caretakers are the primary role models for conduct.
    B. Infant conforms behavior to approval and disapproval of caring and supervising adults.

18 Months (72 Weeks)

I. Physical and Anatomical Traits
    A. Anterior fontanel closed.
    B. Gains 4.4-6.6 lb/year.
    C. For girls, 5 times their current weight is approximately their future adult weight.
    D. For girls, 2 times their current height is approximately their future adult height.
    E. Decreased growth rate results in reduced food intake.
    F. Body proportions change: arms and legs grow at faster rate than head.
    G. Trunk long and legs short.
    H. First four molars have erupted.
    I. Some girls physiologically able to control urinary and anal sphincters.

II. Gross and Fine Psychomotor Traits
    A. Runs clumsily, falls often.
    B. Walks backward.
    C. Walks up stairs with one hand held.
    D. Creeps downstairs.
    E. Seats self on chair.
    F. Beginning to jump with both feet.
    G. Pulls and pushes toys.
    H. Throws ball overhand.
    I. Proficient with finger foods.
    J. Takes off some garments occasionally (e.g., shoes, socks, pants).
    K. Builds tower of three or four cubes.
    L. Uses spoon to feed self without rotation.
    M. Turns pages of a book (two or three at a time).
    N. Scribbles spontaneously.
    O. Makes strokes imitatively.
    P. Picks up small bead and puts in receptacle.

III. Cognitive and Language Traits
    A. Vocabulary increases rapidly, may learn as many as 12 words a day. Correlation reported between highly verbal parent/caregiver and development of language.
    B. Uses words to make needs known.
    C. May combine two words spontaneously for elementary sentences: "All gone," "Big boy."
    D. May repeat end of adult sentences.
    E. Remains in jargon phase.
    F. Can follow two-directional commands.
    G. Favorite words may be "no" and "mine."

IV. Emotional and Social Traits
    A. Solitary play declines and parallel begins, but still possessive of own toys.

    B. Increases pretend play.
    C. Frustration may trigger temper tantrums.
    D. Siblings and peers become more important for bonding.
    E. Beginning to test limits.
  V. Psychosexual Traits
    A. Stereotypical gender dress and play is usually promoted by parents.
    B. Aware of being wet or dry and will sit on the toilet to imitate adults.
  VI. Moral and Spiritual Traits
    A. Comprehension for adult's moral code consists of simple good/bad distinctions.
    B. Verbal sanctions and corporal punishment does inhibit nonconformity or oppositional behavior.

24 Months (2 Years)

  I. Physical and Anatomical Traits
    A. For boys, 5 times current weight is approximately their future adult weight.
    B. Boys, 2 times current height is approximately their future adult height.
    C. Weight gain 4-6 lb (1.8 to 2.7 kg)/year.
    D. Height gain of 4-5 in (10-12.5 cm)/year.
    E. Chest circumference now exceeds head circumference.
NOTE: Head circumference approximately 19 in (48.5 cm). Little growth takes place after this time, since average adult size is only 19.6 in (50 cm).
    F. Protuberance of abdomen with slight lordosis of the spine.
    G. Wide-spaced gait.
    H. Dry at night, 50% of children.
    I. Usually bowel trained but still occasional accidents.
    J. Most toddlers have 20/60 vision.
    K. Primary dentition of 20 teeth.
  II. Gross and Fine Psychomotor Traits
    A. Throws overhand.
    B. Picks up objects from floor without falling.
    C. Walks up and down stairs alone, 2 feet per step.
    D. Runs without falling.
    E. Kicks ball.
    F. Puts on coat with assistance; washes and dries hands.
    G. Uses a straw.
    H. Holds small glass in one hand and drinks with moderate spilling.
    I. Inserts spoon in mouth and does not turn upside down.
    J. Helps remove clothes.
    K. Puts on shoes, socks, and pants.
    L. Builds a tower of six to seven cubes.
    M. Aligns two or more cubes for a train.
    N. Turns book pages one at a time.
    O. Imitates vertical and circular pencil strokes.

P. Cuts crudely with scissors.

Q. Unscrews lids and can turn doorknob.

III. **Cognitive and Language Traits**

  A. Uses more words than jargon.

  B. Vocabulary consists of 300 words or more, talks incessantly.

  C. Sentence length is two- to three-word combination.

  D. May form plurals by adding "s" (doll-dolls).

  E. Uses negative two-word phrases: "no go."

  F. Uses pronouns: "I," "me," "you," "mine."

  G. Speech emerges as a way to communicate ideas, needs, and wants (e.g., toilet, food, drink).

  H. Can follow four-directional command.

  I. Refers to self by given name.

  J. Jargon decreases.

  K. Language 65% intelligible.

  L. Difficulty discerning reality and fantasy.

  M. Trial-and-error learning, but can comprehend simple designs.

  N. Knows five body parts, including mouth, nose, tongue, eye, and ear.

IV. **Emotional and Social Traits**

  A. Fear of dark, ghosts and monsters, and bodily injury.

  B. Greater autonomy and independence.

  C. Initiates activity rather than just imitating.

  D. Time of discovery, curiosity, and social interactions.

  E. May become bossy, self-willed, and manipulative.

  F. Able to explain feelings and desires using gestures and simple phrases.

  G. Generally trusts adults; can be very affectionate.

  H. Plays more with siblings and peers, learning simple rules.

  I. Shows signs of possessiveness and jealousy.

  J. Can regress to more infantile ways with distress or insecurity.

  K. Occasionally seeks solitude and quiet when emotionally confused or upset.

  L. Parallel play.

  M. Reacts strongly to separation from parents.

  N. Resists going to bed.

  O. Extreme use of "no."

  P. World revolves around self.

V. **Psychosexual Traits**

  A. With toilet training, more touching and play with genitalia/anus.

  B. Interest in urine and feces.

  C. Adults caring for and supervising toddler should teach modesty and model privacy relating to body parts.

  D. Beginning self-control of urination and defecation.

VI. **Moral and Spiritual Traits**

  A. Behavior viewed by adults as both very immature/naive and stubborn/willful defiance.

  B. Parents begin socializing toddler in basic rules of conduct, imposing restrictions to teach simple right and wrong.

30 Months (2½ Years)

I. Physical and Anatomical Traits
   A. Birth weight quadruples.
   B. Has complete set of primary teeth (20).
   C. Daytime bladder control with occasional accidents when absorbed in play.

II. Gross and Fine Psychomotor Traits
   A. Jumps in place with both feet off floor.
   B. Walks on tiptoes.
   C. Balances on one foot for 1 second.
   D. Walks backward.
   E. Builds tower of eight cubes.
   F. Adds chimney to train alignment.
   G. Imitates horizontal and vertical pencil strokes.
   H. Holds pencil/crayon with thumb and fingers.
   I. Uses fork held in fist.
   J. Unbuttons large buttons.
   K. Removes pull-down clothing.
   L. Dresses and undresses with help.

III. Cognitive and Language Traits
   A. Increased curiosity and simple questions (i.e., why? how come?).
   B. Very one-sided reasoning, cannot understand an issue from two angles.
   C. Conversational with parent, communicates with sentences using two or more ideas.
   D. Vocabulary consists of 450 words or more.
   E. Can understand simple time concepts.
   F. Refers to self by use of pronoun "I."
   G. Knows first and last name.
   H. Dysfluencies are common (i.e., stuttering).
   I. Uses prepositions.

IV. Emotional and Social Traits
   A. Parallel play increases.
   B. Shows sympathy or pity to familiar people.
   C. Tends to be impetuous, contrary.
   D. Dawdling, defiant, or ritualistic.

V. Psychosexual Traits
   A. Knows own sex and begins to notice sex difference.
   B. Self-regulation of bowel and bladder continues.
   C. Pleasure can be associated with excretory function.

VI. Moral and Spiritual Traits
   A. Concept of right and wrong, good and bad, is limited.
   B. Obedience is based on fear of sanction or punishment and desire to please.

YOUNG CHILD: 3 TO 5 YEARS
Brain Findings

Normal brain development and learning is a process of making or eliminating synapses (i.e., primarily a building of new cells or clearing away of unused brain cells). Repeated activation of the cells strengthens neuronal pathways, whereas inactive cells are likely to be pruned.

The 3-year-old brain has approximately 1000 trillion synapses (more than an adult brain) and is 2½ times more active than an adult's brain; remaining that way throughout approximately the first decade of life (Shore, 1997).

Prime times for growth occur in particular areas of the brain (e.g., cataracts impair visual acuity if not detected and removed early in life).

3 Years (36 Months)

I. Physical and Anatomical Traits
   A. Protuberant abdomen and lordosis disappear, and child grows thinner.
   B. Develops individual body characteristics as result of genetics and lifestyle.
   C. Average weight gain 4-6 lb (1.8-2.7 kg).
   D. Average height gain 2-2.5 in (5-6.25 cm).
   E. Eruption of deciduous teeth complete.

II. Gross and Fine Psychomotor Traits
   A. Walks and runs without looking at feet.
   B. Jumps off bottom step.
   C. Pedals tricycle.
   D. Catches and kicks a ball.
   E. Broad jumps.
   F. Hangs by hands.
   G. Balances on one foot momentarily.
   H. Goes up stairs, alternating feet, and down two feet per step.
   I. Eats with fork held in fingers, feeding self well.
   J. Minimal spilling when using cup, glass, or spoon.
   K. Pours from pitcher or bottle.
   L. Prepares simple meals, such as cold cereal.
   M. Snips with scissors.
   N. Builds tower of 9-10 cubes.
   O. Imitates a bridge with cubes.
   P. Copies a circle, cross.
   Q. Makes a circle with facial features.

III. Cognitive and Language Traits
   A. Understands cold, hungry, and tired.
   B. May correctly name colors.
   C. Starts the "why," "what," "where" questions.
   D. Continues to talk, even when no one is listening.
   E. Sense of quantity (big or little) emerging.
   F. Vocabulary of 900 words, understands 1200-2000.
   G. Language 90%-100% intelligible.
   H. Uses consonants "m," "n," "ng," "p," "f," "h," "w."
   I. Speech is simple three- to four-word sentences.
   J. Uses plurals.
   K. Sentences may not be syntactically correct.
   L. Uses past tense and personal pronouns (I, you, me, she) and most prepositions (under, on, in front of).
   M. Hesitation and repetitions may be common.

    N. Refers to self as "I."

    O. Knows first and last name, sex, and often name of own street.

    P. May recite favorite nursery rhyme, begins to sing songs.

IV. Emotional and Social Traits

    A. Less jealous of younger sibling(s).

    B. More interest in playing with others, associative play.

    C. Common coping skills are temper tantrums, crying, negativism, affection seeking, and regression.

V. Psychosexual Traits

    A. Recognizes appropriate sex of others.

    B. Learns gender roles and has more sense of privacy of body parts with modesty.

    C. Boys identify more with father and male figures.

    D. Has a generalized conception of birth, baby comes out of mommy's stomach.

VI. Moral and Spiritual Traits

    A. Capable of being ashamed and feeling guilty in specific situations, not yet generalized.

    B. Will pray with simple words and gestures as imitative behavior.

    C. Aware of dangers regarding body safety and pets being disabled or dying.

4 Years (48 Months)

I. Physical and Anatomical Traits

    A. Growth rate is similar to previous year.

    B. Birth length doubled.

    C. Legs make up 44% of body length.

    D. In past year has gained approximately 4-6 lb (1.8-2.7 kg) and 2-2.5 in (5-6.25 cm).

II. Gross and Fine Psychomotor Traits

    A. Goes down stairs one foot per step.

    B. Skips on one foot.

    C. Catches a ball with extended arms and hands.

    D. Hops on one foot.

    E. Enjoys stunts or aerobatics.

    F. Puts on shoes and socks without help.

    G. Imitates square and diamond with pencil.

    H. Draws three parts of a stick man.

    I. Laces shoes but may not tie bow.

    J. Washes and dries hands and face.

    K. Buttons and unbuttons.

    L. Manages front snaps and belts.

    M. Removes and puts on pullover garments.

    N. Knows front from back of clothing.

III. Cognitive and Language Traits

    A. Recalls recent past.

    B. Comprehends big and little.

    C. Points to body parts.

    D. Follows three-directional commands.

   E. Names one or two colors but recognizes others.
   F. Asking of "why" questions at peak level.
   G. Confuses fact with fiction while telling a story, exaggerates.
   H. Vocabulary of 1500 words or more.
   I. Uses consonants, sentence length four-five words.
   J. Language almost complete in structure and form. Sentences include adjectives, adverbs, conjunctives, nouns, verbs, and prepositions.
   K. Often uses boastful, bossy, and sometimes profane language.
   L. May count correctly.
   M. Speech should be totally intelligible; however, some sounds may not be complete.

IV. Emotional and Social Traits
   A. Very independent, may run away from home.
   B. Mood swings.
   C. More aggressive physically and verbally with family members.
   D. Enjoys associative play (e.g., simple board games).
   E. Can make and honor an agreement.
   F. Able to control emotions (e.g., crying, laughing).
   G. Converses with imaginary playmate or companion.
   H. Emotional reaction to dreams, scary or happy.

V. Psychosexual Traits
   A. Stronger identification with parent of opposite sex.
   B. More curiosity and interest in genital area.

VI. Moral and Spiritual Traits
   A. Less egocentrism and more social awareness, but still egocentric and wishful thinking.
   B. Obeys out of fear of punishment and desire to please.
   C. Concrete sense of justice about possessions or personal hurt, simple fairness constructs.
   D. Animistic beliefs: objects have feelings, consciousness, and thoughts as humans.
   E. Primitive sense of bad or good (e.g., monsters, ghosts, angels).

5 Years (60 Months)

I. Physical and Anatomical Traits
   A. Girls are slightly ahead of boys in skeletal growth.
   B. Hand dominance is developed; about 90% are right-handed.

II. Gross and Fine Psychomotor Traits
   A. Skips on alternate feet.
   B. Jumps rope and over objects.
   C. Tandem walks forward.
   D. Can walk balance beam.
   E. Catches a ball with hands.
   F. Hops two or more times on each foot.
   G. Prints some numbers, letters, and possibly name.
   H. When appropriate, chooses fork over spoon.
   I. Washes and dries self without supervision.
   J. Needs occasional supervision in dress and hygiene.
   K. Manages zipper in back.

    L. Ties shoelaces.

    M. Combs hair with help.

    N. Brushes and rinses teeth.

    O. Wipes self independently, flushes toilet after use.

III. Cognitive and Language Traits

    A. Draws six or more parts of a stick figure.

    B. Knows the names of coins (penny, nickel, etc.).

    C. Follows a three-directional activity.

    D. Knows opposites (large, small, etc.).

    E. Understands concept of same and different.

    F. Knows time-associated words (days of week, month).

    G. May know own right and left hand, but cannot identify on others.

    H. Vocabulary consists of 2200 words.

    I. Consonants "t," "v," "l," and "th."

    J. Uses sentences consisting of five to eight words.

    K. Language is generally complete in terms of structure and form.

    L. Uses different forms of sentences, including complex sentences and conditional clauses.

    M. Recognizes object pronouns (her, him, them).

IV. Emotional and Social Traits

    A. Less rebellious and quarrelsome than at age 4.

    B. Takes increased responsibility for actions, more trustworthy.

    C. Eager to please.

    D. Capable of expressing emotions through drawings, drama, game playing.

    E. Able to verbalize motivation and meaning of different emotions.

    F. Expresses sorrow or hurt if encouraged or instructed.

    G. Preference for specific playmates and fondness for certain family members.

V. Psychosexual Traits

    A. Strongly identifies with interests and activities of same-sex parent.

    B. Dramatic play enacting parent role in same sex behavior (e.g., playing house).

    C. Transition of negative feelings toward parent of opposite sex to positive feelings.

    D. Sexual fantasies on occasion by pretend play (e.g., being married or having babies).

    E. Greater interest in sexual body parts and questions about birth.

    F. Aware of adult sexual organs.

VI. Moral and Spiritual Traits

    A. Able to tell right from wrong, knows when behavior is good or bad according to adult standards.

    B. Internalizing adult standards and values, beginning of social conscience.

    C. Begins to question parents' thinking and principles.

    D. Can play games by rules but may cheat to avoid losing.

    E. May notice prejudice and bias in outside world.

    F. May have been trained to express spirituality through rituals of singing, reciting sacred words, or praying.

   G. Increased questions and imagination about ultimate life concerns (e.g., death, suffering, higher power, creation, wonders of nature).

ELEMENTARY/LATENCY CHILD: 6 TO 12 YEARS

Brain Findings

The brain forms trillions of synapses, organizing them into networks of neural pathways or maps. When continuously used, these networks become a relatively permanent part of the brain's circuitry; however, if not repeatedly used, they can be eliminated. The critical period to learn a first language is lost at approximately 6 to 13 years if a child is profoundly deaf with no intervention or is living in a linguistically secluded environment. The prefrontal cortex has a growth spurt and makes an overabundance of new synapses. Pruning of these synapses occurs in different parts of the brain at varying times and is part of the maturational process. The relatively short attention span during prepubescent years is related to the fact that the *reticular activating system (RAS)* only becomes fully myelinated at or after puberty. This structure is found in the *medulla oblongata* and is involved in maintaining attention and overall level of arousal.

The *hypothalamus* activates, controls, and integrates the endocrine system. The cerebral centers trigger the endocrine system to initiate major body changes from puberty through adulthood. The endocrine system includes the pituitary, thyroid, parathyroid and adrenal glands, ovaries, testes, and islets of Langerhans in the pancreas.

EARLY ELEMENTARY: 6 TO 8 YEARS

   I. **Physical and Anatomical Traits**
      A. Binocular vision well developed.
      B. Begins to lose primary teeth.
      C. Permanent teeth appear at the rate of four per year.
      D. Considerable variation in height and weight.
   NOTE: From 6-12 years, height and weight growth shows a sex-related difference. Girls tend to gain slightly less weight each year than boys. Growth in height is similar for both sexes; however, boys tend to be a little taller until approximately age 12.
      E. Larger and stronger muscles, good coordination related to posture, locomotion, and activity.
   II. **Gross and Fine Psychomotor Traits**
      A. Constant activity, difficulty sitting still.
      B. Balances on one leg for 10 seconds.
      C. Roller skates.
      D. Hops on alternating feet.
      E. Clumsy and awkward movements.
      F. Tandem walks backward.
      G. Dexterity increases, still has imprecise small-muscle coordination.
      H. Clumsy pencil manipulation.
      I. Cuts, folds, pastes, colors, draws, paints, and uses clay.
      J. Some reversals of letters.
      K. Knows right from left.

III. Cognitive and Language Traits
  A. Person drawing includes neck, hands, and clothes.
  B. Speech sound errors almost gone.
  C. Corrects own grammar.
IV. Emotional and Social Traits
  A. Capable of a wide range of emotional states, ideas, and thinking.
  B. Identified with a primary temperament style of relating.
  C. Capable of emotional self-regulation and control appropriate to different situations.
  D. Understands family group in terms of birth order, parental pair, and sibling group.
  E. Definite acceptance of an affinity to a racial, ethnic, and religious group.
  F. Tattles on others.
  G. Shares and cooperates more.
  H. Often jealous of younger siblings.
  I. Imitates adults.
  J. Behavior is unpredictable, agreeable, and loving one minute, disliking everything and everyone the next.
  K. Demanding of others.
  L. Compulsive about winning and does not lose gracefully.
  M. Needs and enjoys company of peers.
  N. Likes active games and rough play.
  O. Difficulty making decisions.
  P. Tells tales.
V. Psychosexual Traits
  A. Knows gender differences, identifies with sex roles, and has a primary sexual orientation as to preference and affinity.
  B. Experiences sensual pleasure and sexual arousal through masturbation or manipulation of genitals.
  C. Capable of discerning socially acceptable mores or customs regarding toileting, physical touch, and dress codes.
VI. Moral and Spiritual Traits
  A. Parents viewed as the ultimate or primary authorities for good conduct.
  B. Internalized hierarchy of values about reality enabling simple moral decisions.
  C. Greater respect for law rather than mere fear of law.
  D. Able to find personal security with simple faith in higher power and to associate a personal worth in the care of the higher power for self and others.

MIDDLE ELEMENTARY: 8 YEARS

I. Physical and Anatomical Traits
  A. Growth rate approximately 2 in (5 cm) per year.
  B. Arms grow longer in proportion to body.
  C. More limber, bones grow faster than ligaments.
  D. Continues to lose baby teeth, has 10-11 permanent teeth.

II. Gross and Fine Psychomotor Traits

A. Gradual increase in rhythm and smoothness of movements, strength and endurance increase.

B. Constantly on the go: jumping, skipping, chasing, and so on.

C. Long-distance throwing.

D. Fine motor control smoother and speed increased.

E. Uses common tools (e.g., hammer and saw).

F. Helps with household tasks, assumes responsibility for certain household chores.

G. Likely to overdo, hard to quiet down after recess.

H. Writes cursive.

I. Uses knife for cutting.

J. Prepares for bathing and can carry out when reminded.

K. Clips, cuts, and files fingernails and toenails.

L. Styles hair with a comb.

III. Cognitive and Language Traits

A. Concentration, memory, and recall are substantial, allowing for learning and academic gains.

B. Understands abstract vocabulary; uses compound and complex sentences.

C. Ability increases for developing creative aptitudes (e.g., art, sewing, playing instruments).

D. Special interests (e.g., stamp collecting, baseball cards) become emerging hobbies.

E. Reads for enjoyment, likes pictorial magazine.

IV. Emotional and Social Traits

A. Relationships with parents and family are strengthened with domestic life (e.g., chores, games, leisure activities, camping, organized sports).

B. Involved with peers in group activities but has one or two best friends at school or in neighborhood.

C. Dramatic and emotionally expressive.

D. Likes to compete and play games, enjoys school.

E. Prefers certain friends and groups.

F. More critical of self.

G. Likes to select own clothes.

H. Still likes to be tucked in at bedtime.

I. Social manners are better but still need improvement.

J. Dislikes doing things alone.

K. Friendly, gregarious.

L. Argues, wheels and deals.

M. Concerned with parental approval and disapproval.

N. Prefers immediate reward for work (preferably money).

O. Sensitive to criticism.

V. Psychosexual Traits

A. Prefers same-sex friends and companions.

B. Girls may begin puberty with release of sex hormones, boys may have a later onset of 2 or 3 years.

C. Usually both boys and girls are self-conscious about bodies (e.g., modesty) but curious about sex differences; body image issues emerge.

VI. **Moral and Spiritual Traits**
   A. More critical of self, sensitive to criticism, and can be ashamed of bad grades.
   B. Sense of morality determined by family value system and rules.
   C. Likes reward systems and seeks recognition for good behavior.
   D. Influenced by authority figures and seeks role models, heroes, and so on.
   E. Learning to distinguish natural from supernatural (e.g., can see cause and effect in a natural realm, fantasy and reality, wishing and faith).
   F. Receptive to religious training, understanding dogma and performing rituals.

MIDDLE ELEMENTARY: 10 YEARS

I. **Physical and Anatomical Traits**
   A. Because of decrease in height growth and an increase in weight gain, tendency toward obesity at this age.
   B. High energy level and active lifestyle.

II. **Gross and Fine Psychomotor Traits**
   A. Able to engage in complex physical activities, can excel in competitive/organized sports.
   B. Almost equal to fine motor skills of an adult.

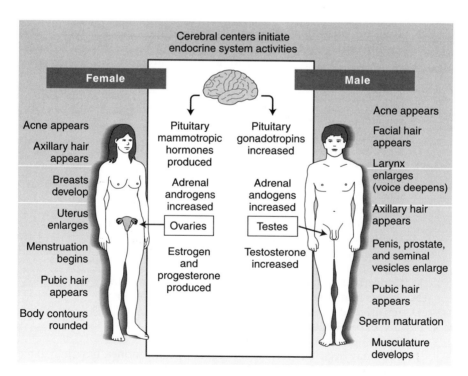

FIGURE 1-4 The endocrine system and developing characteristics of puberty.

    C. Makes things and does small repair work.

    D. Limited cooking and sewing.

    E. Does simple paintings and drawings.

    F. Takes responsibility for care of hair but may need reminding.

    G. Can wink alternately.

III. Cognitive and Language Traits

    A. Good reality testing with distinct boundaries from fantasy and wishful thinking.

    B. Seeks to be logical, able to engage in elementary levels of inductive and deductive reasoning.

    C. Can be multilingual or proficient in several languages.

IV. Emotional and Social Traits

    A. Parents and siblings remain as primary reference groups but peers become more significant.

    B. Other adults at school, church, temple, and youth organizations become role models, mentors, and ego ideals.

    C. Demonstrates affection.

    D. Respects parents; tends to idolize both and enjoys their company.

    E. Sharp outbursts of anger, which are brief and explosive, but does not bear grudges.

    F. Can tolerate frustration.

    G. Tends to be "cliquey," especially girls.

    H. Likes belonging to clubs (scouts) and forms own.

    I. Girls have "best friends" and like small, intimate groups.

    J. Hero worship.

    K. Still separates into like-sex groups for games and activities.

    L. Cries when angry.

V. Psychosexual Traits

    A. Masculine and feminine roles learned with more confidence and mastery.

    B. Most girls are either preparing for menstruation or have developed secondary sex characteristics (e.g., breast enlargement).

    C. Boys are conscious of body build and are more interested in the opposite sex, especially the more mature girls.

    D. See Appendix D for Tanner growth charts for girls and boys.

VI. Moral and Spiritual Traits

    A. Opposed to cheating.

    B. More aware of different value systems and ethical orientations given the wider exposure to neighbors, school, and other community organizations.

    C. Maintains law-and-order approach to morality.

    D. Generally concerned about being good, obeying authorities, and treating others with fairness and kindness.

LATE ELEMENTARY: 12 YEARS

I. Physical and Anatomical Traits

    A. Onset of puberty or sex hormonal activation, somewhat determines body size, energy level, and somatic integrity.

    B. Menarche 9-15 years in girls. Usually cannot reproduce for 1-2 years after menarche because of anovulation.

    C. Boys attain puberty between 12 and 16 years.

    D. Girls tend to be larger than boys.

    E. Body lines begin to soften and round out in girls.

    F. Posture more similar to an adult.

    G. Between 12 and 14 years, all permanent teeth have erupted, except for third molars, wisdom teeth.

II. Gross and Fine Psychomotor Traits

    A. Participates intensely in activity then suddenly reaches saturation point and collapses.

    B. Enjoys gross motor activities, but now capable of more refined motor activities.

III. Cognitive and Language Traits

    A. Vocabulary and speech patterns more conforming to peer terminology and slang.

    B. Enjoys conversation, especially with peers and friends.

IV. Emotional and Social Traits

    A. Hormonal changes influence emotionality, leading to mixed feelings, moodiness, or outbursts.

    B. More independence from parents; even challenging authority and testing limits.

    C. Concerned about peer acceptance, having close peer relationships, may have best friend.

    D. Girls are prone to segregate into twosomes; like talking about boys.

    E. Earning money is a good motivator.

V. Psychosexual Traits

    A. More intense curiosity about sexual anatomy, reproduction, and gender behavior.

    B. Secondary sex characteristics become apparent (e.g., increased size of genitals, coarseness of pubic hair).

    C. Usually more self-conscious with need for privacy and desire for modesty.

    D. Enjoys group activities that involve both sexes; may show interest in opposite sex.

VI. Moral and Spiritual Traits

    A. Interpersonal issues regarding privacy, dress, speech, public manners or etiquette, and respect for adults have an ethical meaning in terms of right or wrong, good or bad.

    B. Beginning of doubt or questioning about the family's religious practices, relevance of spirituality, and general philosophical outlook on life.

ADOLESCENCE: 13 TO 18 YEARS

Brain Findings

Early adolescent elimination of synapses seems to be the dominant process. The overabundance of connections appears to make room for a complex system of neural pathways. Repeated experiences strengthen synaptic networks, which tend to become permanent.

Prefrontal cortex is not fully developed, whereas the emotional area is actively developing, which may be described as the emotional area overriding the prefrontal area (emotional response versus logic and reasoning). This may help explain why adolescents are more emotional and impulsive than adults.

Parietal lobes continue to mature through the middle teen years and are believed to integrate information from sensory signals (e.g., visual, auditory, tactile). Tendencies to act impulsively and misjudge dangerous situations also may be related to a genetic predisposition or may be the result of brain chemical differences found in individuals. These tendencies are strongly influenced by environmental factors (e.g., drugs, alcohol, watching television violence, romanticizing gunplay) and are a function of the prefrontal cortex.

Sex hormones change the brain's structural arrangement, including emotional centers and thoughts about sex. Testosterone production increases during puberty, which influences the activity of the amygdala, producing feelings of fear and anger. This is more pronounced in the male but may account for increased aggressiveness and irritability in both sexes during this age. Increased levels of estrogen influence growth of the hippocampus (e.g., the female structure develops proportionally larger than the male structure). Estrogen and testosterone surges may have a profound influence on moodiness and the sex drive.

Myelination (regulation of emotion, judgment, impulse control) occurs earlier in females than male adolescents. Male myelination may not be equal until about age 30. In late adolescence, approximately half of all synapses have been discarded. This makes the brain more efficient.

EARLY ADOLESCENCE: 13 TO 15 YEARS

I. **Physical and Anatomical Traits**
   A. Height and weight vary according to genetic endowment, nutrition, sleep patterns, and exercise.
   B. Growth decelerating in girls, stature reaches 95% of adult height.
   C. Marked increase in muscle mass in boys related to androgen.
   D. Self-conscious about deformities, disabilities, or disease.
   E. Personal hygiene practices governed by adult exhortations and peer pressure.

II. **Gross and Fine Psychomotor Traits**
   A. Capable of wide range of endurance; coordination of body mastery dependent on temperament, physical aptitudes for sports, and adult expectations (parents, teachers, youth workers).

III. **Cognitive and Language Traits**
   A. Usually has an identifiable level of learning and academic achievement as low, average, or high.
   B. Most of the intellectual growth influence is centered at school or associated with teacher(s) as an ego ideal.
   C. Concern with philosophical, political, and social problems.
   D. Idealistic and rich fantasy life.

IV. **Emotional and Social Traits**
   A. More push for independence and disengagement from parents.
   B. Capable of emotional intensity and wide range of feelings yet marked by insecurity and less than predictable self-control.

    C. Social orientation to the peer group, usually relating upward to older youth and very aware of degree of popularity or acceptance with fear of rejection.

    D. Beginning to take initiative toward establishing a stable boyfriend/girlfriend relationship.

V. **Psychosexual Traits**

    A. Most youth will come into puberty and seek an acceptable feminine or masculine orientation.

    B. Some youth experiment with their sexual self, whereas most youth cope with sexual impulses, fantasies, and genital gratification through masturbation.

    C. Learning about the facts of life and sexual knowledge is accelerated with peer information most influential.

    D. Exploration of body appeal and physical attraction to opposite sex.

VI. **Moral and Spiritual Traits**

    A. More inward and introspective about life. Generally concerned about being a responsible youth with care, tolerance, honesty, and industry.

    B. Able to foresee future implications of current behavior.

    C. Able to project a persona of goodness and critical about being phony or hypocritical about values and beliefs.

MIDDLE ADOLESCENCE: 15 TO 17 YEARS

I. **Physical and Anatomical Traits**

    A. Most growth spurts have occurred and physical maturation is completed.

    B. Height growth usually ceases at 16-17 years for females.

    C. Adult cardiovascular rhythms by age 16.

    D. By age 17, muscle mass is two times greater in boys than girls, resulting in strength two to four times greater in boys.

II. **Gross and Fine Psychomotor Traits**

    A. Similar to the 13- to 15-year-old youth.

III. **Cognitive and Language Traits**

    A. Increase in abstract thinking.

    B. Capacity for hypothetical reasoning.

    C. Able to make decisions with conceptual ability to foresee long-term consequences.

    D. Idealistic and rich fantasy life.

IV. **Emotional and Social Traits**

    A. Capable of the emotional intensity and wide range of feelings as an adult.

    B. Distinctive feelings of omnipotence and exceptionality promote greater risk-taking behavior.

    C. Views self from the standards of an adult in terms of maturity and responsibility.

    D. Greatest need is to distinguish oneself from parents having one's own identity or degree of separateness.

    E. Usually relates upward for a reference group and friendship.

V. Psychosexual Traits
  A. Generally pursuing close, affectionate, and sexual relationships with the opposite sex.
  B. Adult pressures to be sexually conservative, yet engage in safe sex, when there is erotic and romantic behavior in relationships.
  C. Sexual feelings may be felt toward the same-sex and opposite-sex peers, causing the youth to have gender orientation confusion and concern.
  D. Very secretive about sexual behavior and great need to present a sophisticated persona of sexual adequacy.

VI. Moral and Spiritual Traits
  A. Capable of wise moral judgment about self-care, relationships, and lifestyle.
  B. Formal operational thinking allows for exploring deeper meaning of religious symbols and rituals.
  C. Sensitive to issues of fairness, justice, charity, and authority or power.
  D. May become very religious and invested in transcendental spirituality or reject religion and be indifferent to spiritual reality.
  E. Can identify passionately with religious leaders such as Moses, Jesus, Malcolm X, and Mother Theresa.

LATE ADOLESCENCE: 17 TO 19 YEARS

I. Physical and Anatomical Traits
  A. Physically mature with reproductive growth almost complete.
  B. Height growth usually ceases at 18-20 years for males.

II. Gross and Fine Psychomotor Traits
  A. Well-developed with coordination and agility.
  B. Possesses the dexterity and the precision movements similar to an adult.

III. Cognitive and Language Traits
  A. Capable of formal cognitive operations, including abstract thinking, complex problem solving, and prepositional reasoning.
  B. Advanced reasoning skills, capable of rigorous thinking and can communicate in complex sentences with adult vocabulary.
  C. Can articulate ideologies and engage in philosophical discourse.
  D. Aware of intellectual strengths and usually has a realistic perspective on success at higher learning beyond high school.

IV. Emotional and Social Traits
  A. Physical and emotional separation from parents more complete.
  B. Generally can distinguish emotional states and has acceptable emotional self-regulation.
  C. Emotional disturbances or disorders may be diagnosed and treated similar to an adult.
  D. Peer orientation has become at least equally significant as relating to adult family members and other adults.
  E. Usually has close association with a peer group with common ethnic, civic, occupational, or religious interests.

   F. Concerned about having special friendships and being in an intimate relationship.
V. **Psychosexual Traits**
   A. Strong erotic and affectionate feelings are being integrated for loving relationship with the opposite sex or same sex. Capable of forming intimate relationships.
   B. Conscious of sexual maturity and experience, with personal need to enjoy adult sexuality according to legal and social norms.
VI. **Moral and Spiritual Traits**
   A. More social pressures to go beyond an egocentric orientation to life with a caring and tolerant code of ethics.
   B. Development of a personal value system with evidence that value autonomy occurs.
   C. More emphasis on subjective and internal aspects of religious life and less active participation in organized and institutional religion.
   D. Membership in a religious cult often associated with psychosocial stress and identity diffusion.
   E. Interpersonal and personal wrongdoing capable of being adjudicated as an adult criminal.
   F. Capable of having a credo for life that conforms to the highest universal and transcendent principles/precepts known to mankind.

YOUNG ADULT: 19 TO 21 YEARS

Brain Findings

The brain has tripled in weight from that at birth. The increase in weight is primarily a function of the increase in support cells (glia, non-neurons) and is not related to network activity. Maturation continues throughout the twenties, and learning takes place throughout life.

NOTE: With all maturational growth completed, young adults must find personal success and social support with the developmental tasks listed below:

- Acceptance of the physical/biological endowment, temperamental style, and gender identity that represents their unique, personal self.
- Emancipation from family dependence to become emotionally, financially, and legally self-responsible as an adult.
- Completion of the necessary educational and training processes to secure a meaningful occupational position.
- Establishment of caring and committed peer relationships for the fulfillment of sexual, affectionate, companionate, and love needs.
- Accomplishment of lifestyle decisions about marriage, parenthood, and family life.
- Adoption of a personal system of values for social, moral, and legal well-being.
- Maintenance of a realistic yet fulfilling philosophy of life and spiritual frame of reference to cope with the ultimate issues of aging, disease, existential anxiety, suffering, death, and immortality.

ADOLESCENT GENDER DEVELOPMENTAL CHARACTERISTICS

MALE

- Facial hair.
- Fuller eyebrows.
- Voice deepens.
- Muscle development and strength increase steadily.
- Face elongates, mouth and jaw become fuller.
- Shoulders rapidly increase in breadth.
- Axillary, body, and pubic hair.
- Increased growth of penis, testes, and testicles.
- Color of skin on scrotum darkens.
- Erections increase.
- Production of spermatozoa.
- Nocturnal emissions.
- Androgen hormone produced.
- Maturation of reproductive organs is 12-18 years.
- Between ages of 12 and 16 years, gains 4-12 in (10-30 cm) in height and 15-65 lb (7-30 kg) in weight.
- Height growth usually ceases at 18-20 years.

FEMALE

- Voice becomes fuller and slightly deeper.
- More subcutaneous fat.
- Axillary and perineal hair.
- Breast development: nipples enlarge and protrude, areolas enlarge, rounded shape.
- External genitalia enlarge.
- Pelvis enlarges.
- Hips widen.
- Ovulation.
- Menstruation.
- Estrogen hormone produced.
- Maturation of reproductive organs average 10-16 years.
- Between age 10 and 14 years, gains 1-7.9 in (5-20 cm) in height and 15-55 lb (7-25 kg) in weight.
- Height growth usually ceases at 16-17 years.

GENDER DEVELOPMENT

FEMALE AND MALE

- Accelerated growth, beginning earlier in females.
- Skeletal system growth exceeds growth of supporting muscles.
- Large muscles develop faster than small muscles.
- Body odor.
- Sebaceous glands become more active and cause acne.
- Attain maximum growth and ossification takes place.
- Skin texture coarsens, pores enlarge, acne.

- Rapid growth of neck, arms, legs, hands, and feet in comparison to trunk.
- Extremities reach adult size before trunk.
- Jaw becomes fuller as adult size reached; however, mandible in males is wider and lower.
- Gonadotropic hormones present in urine.

WEB SITES

Dana Foundation and the Dana Alliance
    http://www.dana.org
Families and Work Institute
    212-465-2044
    http://www.familiesandwork.org
Society of Neuroscience
    202-462-6688
    http://www.sfn.org

BIBLIOGRAPHY

Blum D: *Sex on the brain: the biological differences between men and women,* New York, 1997, Penguin Putnam.

Carper J: *Your miracle brain,* New York, 2000, HarperCollins.

Carter R: *Mapping the mind,* Los Angeles, 1998, University of California Press.

Chess S, Thomas A: *Temperament and development,* New York, 1986, Brunner/Mazel.

Coles R: *The moral intelligence of children,* New York, 1997, Random House.

Coles R: *The spiritual life of children,* Boston, 1990, Houghton Mifflin.

Damon W: The moral development of children, *Sci Am* 281:72-78, 1999.

Damon W: *The moral child: nurturing children's natural moral growth,* New York, 1988, Free Press.

Diamond MC: *Enriching heredity: the impact of the environment on the anatomy of the brain,* New York, 1988, Free Press.

Diamond MC, Hopson J: *Magic trees of the mind: how to nurture your child's intelligence, creativity, and healthy emotions from birth through adolescence,* New York, 1998, Penguin Putnam.

Duvall E: *Family development,* ed 4, Philadelphia, 1971, Lippincott.

Elkind D: *The development of the child,* New York, 1978, Wiley.

Erikson E: *The life cycle completed,* New York, 1985, WW Norton.

Fowler JW: *Stages of faith: the psychology of human development and the quest for meaning,* San Francisco, 1981, Harper & Row.

Freud A: *Normality and pathology in childhood: assessment of development,* New York, 1965, International Universities Press.

Gardner H: *Multiple intelligences: the theory in practice,* New York, 1993, Basic Books.

Gesell A, Armatruda CS: *Developmental diagnosis,* New York, 1947, Haber.

Greenfield SA: *The human brain: a guided tour,* New York, 1997, Basic Books.

Greenspan SI: *First feelings: milestones in the development of your baby and child,* New York, 1985, Viking Press.

Havighurst RJ: *Human development and education,* New York, 1953, David McKay.

Havighurst RJ: *Developmental tasks and education,* ed 3, New York, 1952, Longman Publishers.

Hooper J, Teresi D: *The 3-pound universe,* New York, 1986, Dell.

Kagan J: *The nature of the child,* New York, 1984, Basic Books.

Kohlberg L: *The philosophy of moral development,* San Francisco, 1981, Harper & Row.

Kotulak R: *Inside the brain: revolutionary discoveries of how the mind works,* Kansas City, Mo, 1996, Andrews and McMeel.

LeDoux J: *The emotional brain,* New York, 1996, Simon & Schuster.

Maslow AH: *Motivation and personality,* ed 2, New York, 1970, Harper & Row.

Moir A, Jessel D: *Brain sex: the real difference between men and women,* New York, 1991, Dell.

Pert C: *Molecules of emotion,* New York, 1997, Scribner.

Piaget J: *The origins of intelligence in children,* New York, 1952, International Universities Press.

Schaefer CE, DiGeronimo TF: *Ages & stages: a parent's guide to normal child development,* New York, 2000, John Wiley & Sons.

Siegel D: *The developing mind: toward a neurobiology of interpersonal experience,* New York, 1991, Guilford Press.

Shore R: *Rethinking the brain: new insights into early development,* New York, 1997, Families and Work Institute.

Swedo S, Leonard HL: *Is it just a phase? How to tell common childhood phases from more serious disorders,* New York, 1998, Golden Books.

Sylwester R: *A celebration of neurons: an educator's guide to the human brain,* Alexandria, Va, 1995, Association for Supervision and Curriculum Development.

Wolfe P: *Brain matters: translating research into classroom practice,* Alexander, Va, 2001, Association for Supervision and Curriculum Development.

CHAPTER 2

Vision and Hearing

Vision and hearing problems are the "quiet debilitators." Often defects in these two important senses are so subtle that they are unnoticed until educational or significant medical implications emerge. Because vision and hearing problems generally begin in a child's critical years of development, early detection and diagnosis are vital so that medical treatment and rehabilitation can begin sooner, physical or behavioral complications can be avoided or minimized, and long-term educational implications can be eliminated or reduced. Such measures ensure that the child will have a fuller and more productive life.

Ideally the first visual and hearing screening should occur when the newborn is in the nursery. Tests for the infant and very young child do not obtain acuities or thresholds; testing relies on elicitation of responses from various forms of stimuli. The younger the child, the more general the screening procedure.

Any nurse who works with infants and young children can play a major role in early detection of a vision or hearing deficit. The nurse has the opportunity to observe behavior, listen to parental concerns, and, in many instances, perform developmental, hearing, and vision screening. The school nurse is often the first person to observe and screen an older child with a vision and hearing problem.

Once the nurse suspects a vision or hearing problem, an appropriate referral should be initiated. Depending on the circumstances the referral is made to the attending physician or one or more specialists, such as an ophthalmologist, optometrist, otolaryngologist, or audiologist.

Various vision and hearing problems occur in children and young adults. This chapter addresses the more common problems and presents major characteristics of vision and hearing development, a list of high-risk conditions that impair infants, screening methods, and certain testing procedures. Useful glossaries and acronyms of vision and hearing terms are listed at the end of their respective sections.

Information regarding vision, hearing, and brain development has been added to this chapter. Technology and research have prompted a new awareness of the importance of early vision and hearing deprivations. Wiesel and Hubel won the Nobel Prize for two very significant discoveries. First, they found that even with an intact brain, if an individual does not process visual experiences by age 2, he or she will not be able to see. Second, if words are not heard by age 10, the individual will never totally learn his or her native language (Kotulak, 1996). The fetal and developing brain differs from that of an adult; thus this period of early experiences is essential for brain development in these sensory systems.

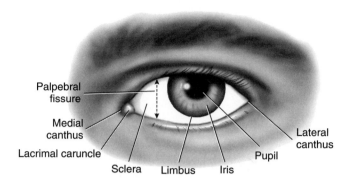

Palpebral fissure
Medial canthus
Lacrimal caruncle
Lateral canthus
Sclera   Limbus   Iris
Pupil

A

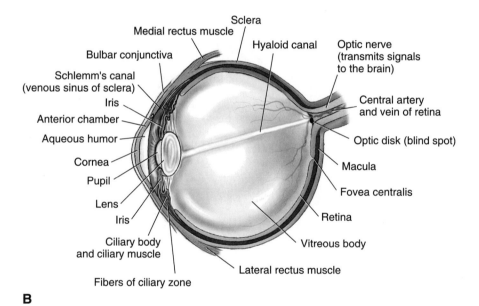

Sclera
Medial rectus muscle
Hyaloid canal
Bulbar conjunctiva
Optic nerve (transmits signals to the brain)
Schlemm's canal (venous sinus of sclera)
Iris
Central artery and vein of retina
Anterior chamber
Aqueous humor
Optic disk (blind spot)
Cornea
Macula
Pupil
Fovea centralis
Lens
Iris
Retina
Ciliary body and ciliary muscle
Vitreous body
Lateral rectus muscle
Fibers of ciliary zone

B

FIGURE 2-1 Normal structure of the eye. **A,** Anterior view. **B,** Cross-sectional view.

Figures 2-1 to 2-4 illustrate the basic structures of the eye and ear and the pathways and mechanics that enable vision, hearing, and the understanding of a language.

The cross-section depicts the lens in each eye, focusing light on the retina and turning the image upside down. Receptors in the retina convert the image into nerve impulses that travel along the optic nerve to the optic chiasm, where half of the nerves from each eye cross over to the other side of the brain, continuing on alternate pathways to the visual cortex. What is seen in the right half of the visual field is transmitted to the left hemisphere of the brain,

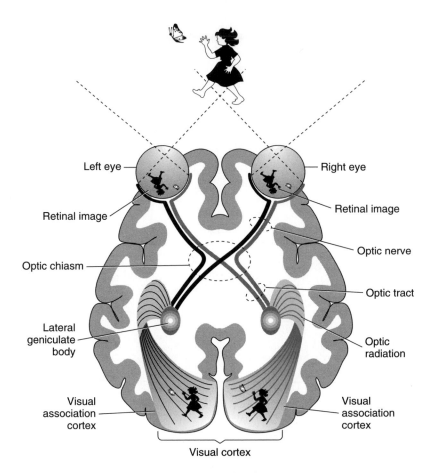

FIGURE 2-2 Visual pathway.

and what is seen in the left half of the visual field is transmitted to the right hemisphere. Each hemisphere is aware of what the other perceives as visual information flows back and forth.

The visual cortex lies within the occipital lobes. Other visual association areas are located in various areas of the cerebral hemispheres; these areas interpret visual images. See Figures 1-1 and 1-2.

Sound is perceived in both the left and right sides of the auditory cortex in the brain from impulses received by both ears. The left hemisphere translates sound impulses into meaning and is the language-processing center of the brain. The auditory cortex receives incoming impulses; the angular gyrus links vision to Wernicke's area, whereas Wernicke's area supplies the meanings of words, and Broca's area controls the mechanics of speech.

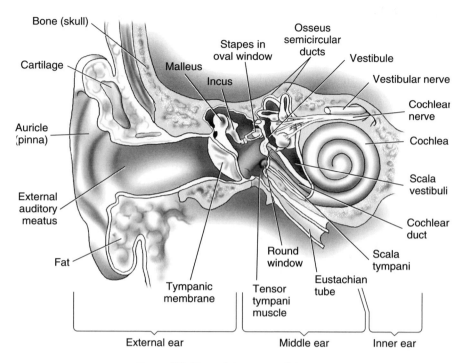

FIGURE 2-3 Normal structures of the ear.

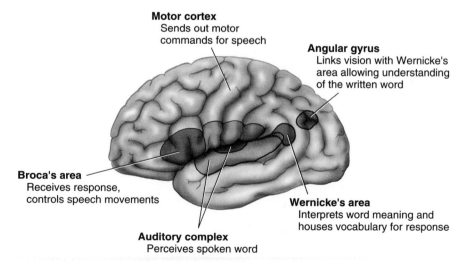

FIGURE 2-4 Auditory processing of sounds in the brain.

MAJOR CHARACTERISTICS OF VISUAL DEVELOPMENT

Cortical neuronal dendritic growth and synaptic information begins in the twenty-fifth week of gestation. This growth is extremely active around birth and continues into the first 2 years of life. In human infants the maturity of the visually evoked potential has been correlated with the degree of dendrite information (Hoyt, Jastrzebski, and Marg, 1983). Vision depends on human experiences to strengthen the neurons.

The visual development for the full-term, healthy infant is described in the following text.

I. **Prenatal**
  A. The lens of the eye begins to develop about the twenty-seventh day of fetal growth with differentiation of the lens capsule.
  B. Eyes are completely formed by the fifteenth week of gestation.
  C. Cortical neuron dendrite growth and synaptic information begins in the twenty-fifth week of gestation.
  D. Eyelids are fused with a thin membrane until the end of the twenty-eighth week.
  E. Pupils respond to light between the twenty-ninth and thirty-first weeks.
  F. Premature infants are normally myopic because of the elongated anterior-posterior diameter of the orbit.

NOTE: Some techniques devised for assessing visual acuity in infants use the evoking of optokinetic nystagmus, visually evoked potentials (VEPs), and preferential looking. These methods often indicate an infant's visual acuity to be much better than previously reported.

II. **Birth to 4 Weeks**
  A. Cortical neuronal dendrite growth and synaptic information is remarkably active around birth.
  B. Some neural pathways that relay information from the retina to the brain may be immature.
  C. Pupils usually are constricted for several weeks.
  D. Measurable color discrimination by 2 weeks but needs brighter colors and larger objects than do adults.
  E. Visual acuity is generally 20/400 to 20/600, regardless of type of visual testing, because of the short diameter of newborn eye, retinal immaturity, and incomplete myelination of optic nerve.
  F. The eye's size is approximately ½ to ¾ the size of an adult eye; however, the cornea is almost adult size at birth, thus babies appear to have "huge" eyes.
  G. Can fixate on moving object in range of 45 degrees.
  H. Eyes move independently.
  I. Sees and responds to illumination; after exposure to bright light will refuse to open eye.
  J. Blinks, squints, or may sneeze when exposed to bright lights.
  K. Fixates on contrasts (e.g., black and white).
  L. Eye and head movements not coordinated (doll's-eye reflex present).
  M. Newborn is generally hyperopic or farsighted because of immaturity of the lens of the eye and spherical nature of the orbit.

N. Large-angle or severe strabismus at birth should be evaluated immediately.

III. **1 Month (4 Weeks)**
   A. Fixates on face and objects about 8 to 12 in (acuity 20/100 to 20/200) and can follow object.
   B. Vision is hyperopic or farsighted.
   C. Can fixate on large moving object in range of 90 degrees.
   D. Tear glands start to function.
   E. Intermittent strabismus may be present.
   F. Watches parents intently when they speak.

IV. **2 Months (8 Weeks)**
   A. Visual acuity is 20/60 to 20/200, depending on type of visual testing.
   B. Peripheral vision of 180 degrees.
   C. Myelination completed around 2½ months.
   D. Blinking, protective reflex, present between 2 and 5 months.
   E. Binocular vision and convergence on near objects begins at 6 weeks.
   F. Follows moving object with eyes; movement may be jerky.

V. **3 Months (12 Weeks)**
   A. Critical period for visual development is somewhat controversial but is probably between 1 week and 3 months of age. In general, if visual defects are not found and treated by 3 months of age, then optimal vision may not be achieved.
   B. Regards hand; however, legally blind infants do the same.
   C. Convergence should be well established.
   D. Saccades are well developed.
   E. Doll's-eye reflex has disappeared.
   F. Can follow moving object from side to side (range of 180 degrees).
   G. Smooth pursuit well developed.
   H. Briefly able to fixate on near objects.
   I. Reaches toward toy.
   J. Charmed with bright objects, color preference for bright yellows and reds.
   K. Visuomotor coordination emerges.
   L. Eyes parallel most of the time.

VI. **4 Months (16 Weeks)**
   A. Visual acuity 20/60 to 20/200, depending on type of testing.
   B. Binocular vision fairly well established.
   C. Differentiation of fovea complete.
   D. Color vision closer to that of an adult.
   E. Tears are present.
   F. Fixates on 1-in cube.
   G. Recognizes familiar objects (e.g., feeding bottle).
   H. Observes mirror images.
   I. If strabismic, referral should be made by 4-6 months of age.

VII. **6 Months (24 Weeks)**
   A. Visual acuity 20/20 to 20/150, depending on type of testing.
   B. Stereoscopic vision well developed by 3-7 months.
   C. Color of iris can be determined.

      D. Adjusts position to view objects.

      E. Watches falling toy.

      F. Eye-hand coordination is developing.

      G. Smooth eye movements in all directions.

      H. Color preference for bright reds and yellows is developing.

      I. No deviation from parallelism should exist.

VIII. 9 Months (36 Weeks)

      A. Ability to discern fine details is at adult level by age 6-9 months.

      B. Depth perception development begins between the seventh and ninth month.

      C. Ability to fuse two retinal images begins to mature.

      D. Can fixate on and follow object in all directions.

      E. Attentive to environment.

      F. Observes activities of people and animals with sustained interest within distance of 10-12 ft.

IX. 1 Year (12 Months)

      A. Visual acuity 20/20 to 20/60, depending on type of testing.

      B. Cornea is adult in size (12 mm), and eye muscles are reaching adult level of functioning; can fixate and follow object in all directions.

      C. Macula will mature by the end of first year.

      D. Tracks rapidly moving objects.

      E. Recognizes familiar people at 20 ft or more.

      F. Can place peg into small hole and stack blocks.

X. 1½ Years (18 Months)

      A. Convergence well established.

      B. Fixates on small objects.

      C. Sees and points to distant interesting object outdoors.

XI. 2 Years (24 Months)

      A. Potential for 20/20 acuity.

      B. Optic nerve myelination completed by 7 months to 2 years.

      C. Eye is 85% of adult size.

      D. Accommodation well developed.

      E. Fixates on small object for 60 seconds.

      F. Recognizes fine details in picture books.

XII. 3 Years (36 Months)

      A. Visual acuity is 20/20 as measured by VEPs.

      B. Convergence smooth.

      C. Copies geometric designs: circle, cross.

XIII. 4 Years (48 Months)

      A. Visual acuity 20/20.

      B. Tear (lacrimal) glands are completely developed.

      C. Can distinguish shapes and letters.

XIV. 5 Years

      A. Visual acuity 20/20.

      B. Depth perception developed.

XV. 7 to 10 Years

      A. Eye achieves full globe size or full size of orbit between 5 and 7 years.

      B. Hyperopia continues until approximately age 7 years.

Box 2-1	*High-Risk Conditions for Visual Impairment of the Newborn*
Prenatal	**Postnatal**
Family history	Premature or low birth weight
Maternal rubella	Oxygen toxicity (retrolental fibroplasia)
Syphilis, gonococci	Meningitis/encephalitis
Chlamydia	Herpes infections
Toxoplasmosis	Histoplasmosis
Cytomegalovirus	Syphilis, human immunodeficiency virus (HIV)
Herpes infections	Disorders: albinism, cataracts, hydrocephalus, retinoblastoma, septo-optic dysplasia, sickle cell disease
	Trauma: birth, shaken baby syndrome

  C. By 9 years the visual system is mature enough to resist effects of abnormal visual stimulation.

  D. Continuation of synapse development in visual cortex to approximately 10 years.

  E. Implications for amblyopia because immaturity in cellular development in occipital lobe contributes to amblyopia.

XVI. **12 Years**

  A. Eye growth is completed between 10 and 12 years.

REFRACTIVE ERRORS

ASTIGMATISM

 I. **Definition**

  A. Astigmatism is a refractive error in which light rays are bent in different directions because of the irregularity of the cornea, producing a blurred image. May occur along with myopia or hyperopia.

 II. **Etiology**

  A. Astigmatism may be caused by an irregularly shaped or defective curvature of the cornea or lens, which creates unequal refraction of light rays by the dioptic system, in different meridians. This prevents the eye from focusing clearly on an image. Astigmatism may be congenital or acquired.

 III. **Signs, Symptoms, and History**

Dependent on severity of refractive error in each eye:

  A. Higher astigmatism.

   1. Blurred vision.

   2. Squinting.

   3. Tilting or turning of the head.

   4. Reading material held close to eyes.

  B. Lower astigmatism.

   1. Tired eyes.

   2. Blurred vision.

   3. Frontal headache.

  C. Mild astigmatism.

   1. May have no symptoms.

Table 2-1 **Central Nervous System Drugs That Produce Adverse Effects on the Visual System**

Drug	Significant Adverse Symptoms and Effects	Pertinent Examinations	Follow-Up Examination Frequency
Barbiturates	Ptosis, ocular hypotony, color vision disturbance, diplopia, nystagmus, dermatitis of eyelids, conjunctivitis, mydriasis, miosis, optic atrophy, papillitis	Visual acuity, color vision, eye movement, pupil	6-12 mo
Chloral hydrate	Miosis, ptosis, tearing, diplopia, conjunctivitis	Visual acuity, eye movement	3-6 mo
Chlorpromazine (Thorazine)	Miosis, oculogyric crises, elevation of IOP, pigment deposit on lens, hyperpigmentation of eyelids, conjunctiva, cornea and retina; optic atrophy	Visual acuity, eye movement	3-6 mo
Phenytoin (Dilantin)	Blurred vision, conjunctivitis, nystagmus, ptosis	Visual acuity, eye movement	Annually
Haloperidol (Haldol)	Blurred vision from mydriasis, decreased IOP, lens opacities	Visual acuity, near vision, eye movement	If symptoms occur
Morphine	Miosis, blurred vision, transient myopia, weakness of convergence	Pupil examination, visual acuity, refraction, eye movement	If symptoms occur, every 6 mo
Thioridazine (Mellaril)	Reduced vision, pigmentary retinopathy	Visual acuity, color vision, visual field	Complete examination by ophthalmologist; if taking 800 mg daily, assess 2-6 mo
Tricyclic antidepressants (Elavil)	Mydriasis, cycloplegia	Visual acuity, refraction, pupil	If symptoms occur, check every 6 mo with ophthalmologist
Trimethadione (anticonvulsant)	Sensitivity to bright lights, faded colors, conjunctivitis	Visual acuity, color vision	6-12 mo if symptoms
Diazepam (Valium)	Blurred vision, blink suppression, diplopia, nystagmus if overdose	Visual acuity, pupil, refraction, eye movement	6-12 mo

Drug	Effects	Examination	Frequency
Amphetamines	Mydriasis, blurring of vision, increased IOP, widened lid fissures	Visual acuity, pupil, refraction, eye movement	6-12 mo
Cannabis (Marijuana)	Visual disturbances, color perception, decreased IOP, diplopia	Visual acuity, pressure check	Glaucoma examination every 12 mo
Chloroquine (Aralen) (antimalarial, systemic lupus, rheumatoid arthritis)	Retinal pigment epithelial damage, corneal deposits, whitening of eyelashes, ptosis, corneal edema, decreased corneal sensitivity, optic atrophy	Visual acuity, ophthalmoscopy	Eye examination by physician, acuity checks every 3-6 mo
Isoniazid	Optic neuritis, keratitis	Visual acuity, ophthalmoscopy, visual fields	Complete eye examination; visual acuity and color vision every 3-6 mo
Streptomycin	Optic neuritis	Visual acuity, color vision/visual fields, ophthalmoscopy	Complete eye examination; every 6-12 mo
Sulfonamides	Exudative conjunctivitis, transient myopia, ocular palsies, iritis, optic neuritis, retinal hemorrhage, edema	Visual acuity, eye movement, color vision, ophthalmoscopy	Monthly if symptoms
Tetracycline	Blurred vision, papilledema	Visual acuity, refraction, ophthalmoscopy	3-6 mo during long-term therapy
Tryparsamide (syphilis)	Optic neuritis, constriction of fields	Visual acuity, color vision, visual fields, ophthalmoscopy	Total eye examination, every 6 mo
Furosemide (Lasix)	Color vision disturbance, decreased IOP	Visual acuity, color vision, pressure check	Annually
Ibuprofen	Color vision disturbance, blurred vision	Visual acuity, color vision, ophthalmoscopy	If symptoms occur
Salicylates	Retinal hemorrhages, mydriasis, ocular hypotony, nystagmus, conjunctivitis, optic neuritis	Visual acuity, color vision, ophthalmoscopy, pressure check, visual fields	Every 6 mo

Continued

Modified from Payan-Langston D: *Manual of ocular diagnosis and therapy,* ed 3, Boston, 1991, Little, Brown.
IOP, Intraocular pressure.

Table 2-1   *Central Nervous System Drugs That Produce Adverse Effects on the Visual System—cont'd*

Drug	Significant Adverse Symptoms and Effects	Pertinent Examinations	Follow-up Examination Frequency
Corticosteroids	Transient myopia, exophthalmus, ptosis, mydriasis, cataracts, retinopathy	Visual acuity, ophthalmoscopy	Every 2-3 mo
Oral contraceptives	Optic neuritis, scotomas, central retinal vein and artery occlusion, papillitis	Visual acuity, color vision, visual fields, ophthalmoscopy	Complete eye examination; every 3 mo or sooner if symptoms
Vitamin A	Ocular palsies, retinal hemorrhages, nystagmus, diplopia, loss of eyebrows and eyelashes, papilledema	Eye movement, ophthalmoscopy	When symptoms; long duration or overdose
Vitamin D	Conjunctival and corneal calcium deposits	Visual acuity	Follow up every 6-12 mo for calcification

Modified from Payan-Langston D: *Manual of ocular diagnosis and therapy,* ed 3, Boston, 1991, Little, Brown.

IV. **Effects on Individual**
   A. Safety, susceptibility to accidents because of blurry vision.
   B. Difficulty with close schoolwork and chalkboard activities, depending on associated visual error. May tire quickly with reading assignments and seem easily distracted.
   C. May have same clinical manifestations as myopia.
V. **Management/Treatment**
   A. Corrective lenses for refractive errors that compensate for the irregular and abnormal curvature of the cornea.
   B. Rescreen at appropriate intervals.
   C. Be cautious of a child who does not like to wear the new glasses. Astigmatism corrections usually require an adaptation period. Check with prescribing doctor if doubt exists.
VI. **Additional Information**
   A. Most people's eyes are not perfectly symmetrical; thus they may have small amounts of astigmatism. Astigmatism is common in infants. Condition can result in amblyopia.

MYOPIA

I. **Definition**
   A. Commonly called *nearsightedness*, myopia is the ability to see objects clearly within close range. Myopia is a refractive error in which parallel light rays from a distant object focus in front of the retina, causing images at a distance from the individual to appear blurred.
II. **Etiology**
   A. Myopia may be caused by a long anterior-posterior diameter of the eyeball or a cornea curve that is too severe, thereby refracting the light rays too much. Heredity plays a role in myopia.
III. **Signs, Symptoms, and History**
   A. Blurred distance vision.
   B. Safety; may walk into objects.
   C. Unusual posturing.
   D. Squints at distant object to sharpen vision.
   E. Rubs eyes frequently.
   F. Headache, but rare.
   G. Dizziness.
   H. Nausea after close work, but rare.
   I. Holds book close to face (severe or high myopia); however, this behavior is normal behavior between 4 and 7 years. It is also a first sign of a problem.
   J. Depending on classroom seating, unable to see chalkboard or at home, television.
   K. Fails distance acuity screening.
IV. **Effects on Individual**
   A. Difficulty participating in sports or playground activities.
   B. Safety in jeopardy (e.g., unable to read road signs).
   C. May miss chalkboard instructions if not sitting at front of classroom.
   D. Academic performance may be affected.

V. Management/Treatment

A. Refraction, if indicated, with concave (minus) lens to focus rays on retina. Either fitted glasses or contact lens may be used.

B. Recheck periodically with and without prescribed glasses to see if error remains corrected.

C. Surgery: laser techniques to reduce curvature of the cornea. These surgeries can be performed as early as 18 years, but typically should not be done before the eye has stopped growing.

VI. Additional Information

A. Growth produces visual changes, so child may need new eyeglasses every 1 or 2 years. Generally stabilizes around the mid-teen years.

HYPEROPIA

I. Definition

A. Commonly called *farsightedness,* hyperopia is the ability to see objects better at a distance. Hyperopia, also termed *hypermetropia,* is a refractive error in which parallel light rays focus behind the retina, causing images close to the individual to appear blurred. In middle age, hyperopia is called *presbyopia* and is caused by the decreased elasticity of the crystalline lens.

II. Etiology

A. Hyperopia may be caused by a shortness of the eyeball or by a lens that is too flat (unresponsive) to bend light rays adequately, thereby causing image to focus beyond the retina.

III. Signs, Symptoms, and History

A. Blurred vision at close range.

B. Tired eyes when focusing for prolonged periods of time.

C. Pain.

D. Frontal headaches.

E. Eye strain after long periods of reading or writing.

F. Lines run together while reading.

G. Symptoms A to F intensified when individual is tired or ill.

H. Light sensitivity.

I. Fails visual screening.

J. Esotropia or an inward (medial) deviation of one or both eyes from parallelism.

K. Children often hyperopic until about 5 to 7 years old.

L. Fails testing on distance acuity charts as on a stereoscope with plus lenses.

IV. Effects on Individual

A. Schoolwork may suffer, and child may be unable to keep up with classmates.

B. Teachers may expect only poor academic achievement.

C. Student is more easily irritated because of constant eyestrain.

D. Nervous during school visual tasks (e.g., reading).

E. May develop poor self-esteem if vision is affecting academic achievement or performance in playground activities and sports.

V. Management/Treatment
A. Refraction with use of convex (plus) lens to focus rays on retina.
B. Correction may be necessary in children with only a moderate degree of hyperopia and no other symptoms or a strabismus.
C. Recheck periodically, with and without prescribed glasses, to determine whether error remains corrected.

VI. Additional Information
A. Most infants are hyperopic, and children continue to be until they reach about 5 to 7 years, when the condition starts to decrease. These children can accommodate to objects at close range. If the child is truly hyperopic, the continual muscular effort of accommodation may cause eyestrain to result in strabismus (esotropia). Hyperopia is measured in diopters rather than Snellen "fractions."

ANISOMETROPIA

I. Definition
A. Anisometropia is present when a different refractive power occurs in each eye. A difference in visual acuity of two or more lines exists following distance or near-point acuity testing. This makes the two eyes unable to function together.

II. Etiology
A. When refractive errors in the eyes differ, the muscle relaxation or contraction of one eye corrects the vision for that eye but worsens the vision in the other eye. The condition may be congenital or acquired as a result of disease or asymmetrical changes that occur with age.

III. Signs, Symptoms, and History
A. Dependent on severity of the refractive error in each eye.
B. Clinical manifestations may be the same as those of myopia.

IV. Effects on Individual
A. The brain learns to ignore the visual image from the weaker eye (suppression); if the condition is severe, amblyopia can result.
B. Eyes generally appear normal and remain straight; screening is necessary to detect amblyopia.

V. Management/Treatment
A. Any deviation in parallelism (eye muscle imbalance) should be identified and corrected.
B. Corrective lenses, preferably contact lenses, improve the vision in each eye, allowing them to function as a unit.

VI. Additional Information
A. This condition should be identified and treated as soon as possible because it can lead to amblyopia and loss of vision in children younger than 7 years.

COLOR DEFICIENCIES

COLOR DEFICIENCY/CONFUSION

I. Definition
A. Color deficiency or confusion is the inability to distinguish between the primary colors red, green, and blue. Color vision is a function of

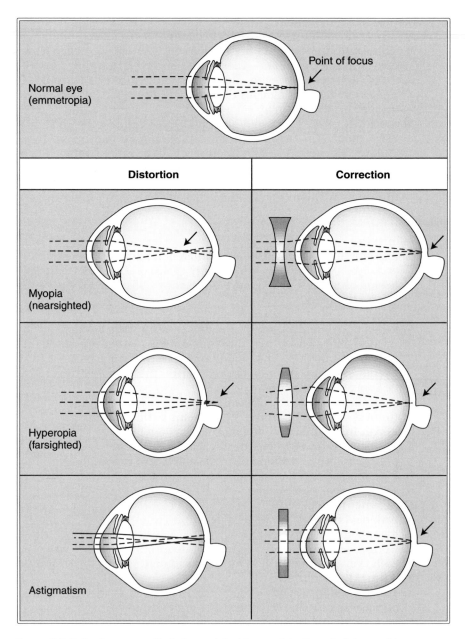

FIGURE 2-5 Refractive errors displaying point of focus, distortion of globe, and lens correction. *Arrow* indicates point of focus, or fovea.

the cones in the fovea centralis of the eye. When stimulated by light, the cones transmit impulses to the brain. The cones facilitate discernment of color, and the rods help adjustment to light and dark. Deficiencies range from mild to severe. Color blindness, or the complete absence of photochemical receptors in the cones, is rare but limits vision to black, white, and gray shades.

II. **Etiology**

    A. Color deficiency is a defect inherited as an X-linked recessive trait that primarily affects the male population. The gene for color vision may not be faulty, but the gene that chemically triggers the color vision gene to function may be defective. Occasionally, color deficiency may be acquired from injury, disease (sickle cell anemia, diabetes), or certain drugs (antibiotics, chlorpromazine [Thorazine]); however, most incidences are hereditary. In any given classroom, 5% of the students may have color deficiencies. Approximately 8% of males and 0.5% of females are affected. Deficiencies in the green photochemical receptors are the most common; blue deficiencies are the least common. Color deficiency can affect many areas of life, including education, safety, and occupational choices. Few occupations are dependent on color.

III. **Signs, Symptoms, and History**

    A. Unable to discriminate colors.

    B. Difficulty learning primary colors.

    C. Family history of color deficiency.

    D. Fails pseudoisochromatic screening or other color vision testing.

IV. **Effects on Individual**

    A. At early age unable to follow directions about coloring materials.

    B. Teacher and student may become frustrated because of student's inability to learn colors and perform other color-related tasks.

    C. May become frustrated and be identified as nonachiever in classroom.

    D. May be teased by other children.

    E. Difficulty matching and coordinating colors for personal dress.

    F. May be perceived as a difficult student or not intelligent.

    G. Student must seek guidance and counseling regarding career goals in relationship to color confusion.

V. **Management/Treatment**

    A. No known complete correction. However, a variety of treatments are available: use of light and filters; red or green overlay on colored text; X-Chrom lens (X-Chrom Corp, Ft Lauderdale, Florida) (one red contact in one eye), ColorMax lenses, (Color Vision Technologies, Justin, California) (lens coated to filter certain colors). The efficacy of these methods needs further investigation.

    B. Parents, teachers, and other professionals must be aware of the color deficiency; understand that the student could say that grass is green and a tree trunk is brown but does not perceive color and is only repeating what he or she is told, thus compensating the degree of deficiency by masking the problem.

    C. Student usually learns to distinguish colors by own system of assigning brightness or location. Teacher and parent can help student to articulate this process for the child to maximize learning.

    D. Provide guidance for adolescents regarding driving issues and color difficulties that may be related to high school and college course work, vocational plans, and possible military goals.

    E. Career plan limitations depend on degree of deficiency.

    F. Color difficulties that could affect college education and career plans include interior decorator, commercial pilot, law enforcement, firefighter, some electrical and chemical engineering, cosmetology.

VI. **Additional Information**

    A. All cases of color deficiency/confusion differ; some individuals see all colors if shown one at a time but are unable to identify colors when they are mingled. Still others (e.g., green color confusion) may see gray, white, or yellow in daylight, and others report the green traffic light at night looks the same as street lights, rendering this a useless traffic cue.

    B. The color-defective male inherits the deficiency from his mother. Heterozygous females (carriers) have one recessive gene for color deficiency and one dominant gene for normal color vision. The male Y chromosome does not carry a color discrimination gene. Color deficiency results when genes cross over during meiosis, causing an alteration in the red or green cone pigments. The crossover may result in a hybrid, the loss of a gene, or duplication of the gene (does not cause problem). If a female has X genes for color blindness from her father and normal X genes from her mother, she is a carrier and can transmit the condition to her sons. If the chromosome inherited from her mother is defective for color vision and she also inherits a defective X chromosome from her father, she will be color-blind.

CLASSIFICATIONS OF COLOR BLINDNESS

Three basic groups of anomalous trichromatism or dichromatism exist; monochromatism is rare.

1. *Deuteranomaly/deuteranopia:* Difficulty with green; deuteranomaly is the most common form of color blindness (5%). Often have problems with red-green discrimination. Can identify color if contrasted with another color in good light. Can choose red and green from package of colored papers, but if handed a red or green crayon and asked for the color, they may be puzzled. Red-green weakness produces trouble along the "tomato line" in the white light spectrum.

2. *Protanomaly/protanopia:* Bold red is seen as black or as nonexistent. Affected individuals seem to need abnormal amount of red or have no sense of red color vision. Red-orange and yellow-green may be seen as brown. May say red and green are the same color but will see two different browns.

3. *Tritanomaly/tritanopia:* Problems with blue, yellow, or both colors. Often acquired but not inherited. May see blue and yellow as white; see mint green or pink as equal to light blue.

Traffic lights in most areas in the United States are not a problem because of the consistent placement of colors. Also, the red and green in the traffic lights are not pure colors.

The Farnsworth-Munsell 100 Hue Test consists of different shades of colored disks or pegs that are lined up. The order selected by the student provides information on the specific color cone deficiency.

Color names are used to represent human feeling, moods, and thoughts, such as "I feel blue," "she is white as a ghost," or "draw the colors of the rainbow." Colors also signal danger, such as red or yellow in nature. Human beings use colors for verbal communications, to learn from color-coded materials, as adjectives or nouns in language, or to enjoy and remember their environment and joy in nature.

DISORDERS OF BINOCULARITY

AMBLYOPIA

I. **Definition**
 A. Amblyopia is a visual condition associated with reduced visual acuity in one eye in the presence or absence of organic eye disease. Vision is suppressed in one eye to avoid seeing double. Unfortunately, it often is called *lazy eye.*

II. **Etiology**
 A. The three main causes of amblyopia are (1) uncorrected strabismus (usually esotropia), (2) anisometropia or unequal refractive errors of each eye, and (3) physical occlusion, such as ptosis or cataract. Heredity plays a role; can be functional or organic. Organic causes can include optic atrophy, macular scar, or *anoxic occipital brain damage.* Amblyopia is usually a result of changes in the occipital lobe and less likely from specific damage to the eye (e.g., deterioration of fovea/macular degeneration). Functional amblyopia is referred to as those conditions in which the visual acuity deficit may be reversible with occlusion therapy (patching of unaffected eye) and treatment of refractive errors. Classifications include strabismic amblyopia, unilateral distortion of form caused by amblyopia (usually anisometropia), ametropic amblyopia (significant bilateral refractive errors), deprivation amblyopia (impaired clarity of image formed on retina in infancy), and occlusion amblyopia (prolonged occlusion of normal eye) (Kushner, 1998).

III. **Signs, Symptoms, and History**
 A. Eyes may cross or wander.
 B. Child shuts or covers one eye.
 C. Avoids close work.
 D. Squints.
 E. Two-line difference or more between eyes in acuity testing at near or far distance.
 F. May have no symptoms, making adequate screening critical.

IV. **Effects on Individual**
 A. If condition remains untreated, loss of vision in weaker eye.
 B. Child may be considered clumsy or lacking in motor development because of poor depth perception.

C. During correction, child may become upset when good eye is patched. Patching may cause skin irritation caused by adhesive materials.

V. **Management/Treatment**
   A. Refractive amblyopia needs early correction of visual acuity.
   B. With strabismic amblyopia, force use of the weaker eye by covering the better eye (occlusive therapy). Later in treatment, patching may be alternated because amblyopia may be induced in the better eye if eye is covered for too long. Patching is part of a total vision therapy program.
   C. Other strabismus corrections include eye drops to blur vision in the good eye as an alternative to patching, or as a last resort, surgical correction of occlusion.

VI. **Additional Information**
   A. Disease or damage of the remaining good eye will cause low vision or lateral blindness. Refractive amblyopia should be corrected during the first 5 to 6 years of life; thereafter treatment becomes more difficult. If left untreated, the condition can cause profound and irreversible visual loss in the affected eye. Success depends on compliance to treatment and degree of condition. Close follow-up by preschool nurse or personnel and vision specialist is critical. Amblyopia is the most frequent cause of visual loss in childhood.

OTHER VISUAL CONDITIONS

ALBINISM

I. **Definition**
   A. Albinism refers to a group of genetic conditions that affect the pigment cell system (melanocyte) causing reduction or absence of normal pigmentation of the eye, hair, and skin. The altered gene does not allow the production of normal amounts of pigment, called *melanin.*

II. **Etiology**
   A. Several different types of albinism exist and are caused by alterations at six different genes. The two main categories of albinism are (1) oculocutaneous albinism (OCA), in which the degree of melanotic pigment of the eyes, skin, and hair, photophobia, nystagmus, hypoplastic foveae, and decreased visual acuity varies and (2) ocular albinism (OA), in which the melanin pigment is normal or only slightly diluted in the skin and hair. OCA is more common than OA. Albinism can be inherited as autosomal recessive and X-linked OA; rarer forms are associated with a variety of other anomalies. The list of alterations, their genes, and chromosomal locations are listed in "Additional Information."

III. **Signs, Symptoms, and History**
   A. Decreased visual acuity, farsightedness, nearsightedness, and astigmatism common.
   B. Nystagmus, strabismus, and photophobia may be present.
   C. Iris color usually blue-gray or light brown.

    D. The altered gene prevents normal melanin pigment development. Melanin pigment absorbs ultraviolet light to protect the skin and other areas from sunlight. Melanin is present in the retina and the fovea of the retina, and if it is not present, these structures do not develop appropriately.

    E. The nerve connections between the retina and certain parts of the brain are altered if melanin is not present during development.

    F. Iris pigment is reduced; iris is translucent to light but develops and functions normally in these children.

  IV. **Effects on Individual**

    A. Children with albinism can function well in a mainstream classroom environment with specific attention to their special visual needs.

    B. Preschool services (birth to age 5) are available through federally mandated services, Individuals with Disabilities Education Act (IDEA).

    C. May use a head tilt and commonly hold the written page close to eyes while reading.

    D. Often hyperactive with short attention span; personal safety at risk.

    E. Psychosocial and self-esteem are issues of concern.

  V. **Management/Treatment**

    A. Symptomatic with routine ophthalmological care.

    B. Usually do not tan but burn easily in the sun.

    C. Need sunscreen, hats, dark glasses to prevent overexposure to sun and other special clothing for outdoor play.

    D. Benefit from written materials that have a black-on-white high contrast, large-type textbooks, audiotapes, computers, and various optic devices.

    E. Optic devices can include handheld monocular, video enlargement machine (closed circuit television), telescopic lenses mounted over eyeglasses, and other types of magnifiers.

    F. Copies of the teacher's board notes are helpful for older children.

Box 2-2	***Alterations, Their Genes, and Chromosomal Locations***
OCA1	Tyrosinase-related OCA, chromosome 11
OCA1A	Classic tyrosinase-negative OCA
	Legally blind range 20/200-20/400
	Visual acuity range 20/90-20/400
OCA2P	Gene-related OCA, chromosome 15
	Visual acuity range 20/60-20/150
OCA3	Tyrosinase-related OCA, chromosome 9
HPS1	Hermansky-Pudlak syndrome, chromosome 10
	Common in Puerto Rican population; visual acuity range 20/60-20/400
CHS1	Chédiak-Higashi syndrome, chromosome 1
OA1	X-linked ocular albinism, chromosome X
	Occurs primarily in males; visual acuity range 20/50-20/400

OCA, Oculocutaneous albinism.

VI. Additional Information
  A. Approximately 1 in 17,000 people has a type of albinism. In the United States, approximately 18,000 people are affected.

CATARACTS
I. Definition
  A. In a cataract, the crystalline lens located behind the pupil becomes opaque. Cataracts may be monocular, binocular, complete, or partial and can be on or in the lens or capsule. Cataracts impair vision and may cause blindness.

II. Etiology
  A. Cataracts may be congenital, hereditary, or caused by an infectious process or metabolic condition. They also can result from trauma, inflammation, radiation, degeneration, and long-term administration of corticosteroids. The many types of cataracts are classified by morphology (size, shape, location) or etiology (cause or time of appearance).

III. Signs, Symptoms, and History
  A. Blurred vision.
  B. Absence of red reflex.
  C. Gradual, progressive, painless loss of vision.
  D. Occasional double vision in affected eye.
  E. Gray opacity in lens.
  F. Nystagmus (late symptom).
  G. Amblyopia may result from uncorrected congenital and infantile cataracts.
  H. Strabismus.

IV. Effects on Individual
  A. May need frequent change of prescriptive lenses.
  B. Fear of blindness.
  C. Apprehension regarding hospitalization and surgery.
  D. Hinders normal school activities.

V. Management/Treatment
  A. For child with congenital monocular cataract, surgery is necessary as soon as possible after birth and before 2 months if vision is to be normal.
  B. Surgical removal of lens (aphakia).
  C. Intraocular lens implants are most common.
  D. Sometimes eyeglasses or soft contact lens are prescribed to compensate for refractive power loss after lens has been removed.

VI. Additional Information
  A. *Aphakia* is the term used when the lens has been removed during surgery. The absence of the lens causes an increase in the size of the image with glasses; however, this abnormal magnification is less with contact lenses. Contact lenses are the treatment of choice for congenital cataract in infants younger than 1 year of age. After 2 years of age, intraocular lens implantation (IOL) should be considered. The visual field is also considerably affected.

CONGENITAL BLINDNESS

I. **Definition**
   A. Congenital blindness is a visual acuity for distance of 20/200 (6/60 m) or less in the better eye or peripheral vision of less than 200 in the better eye; also known as *legal blindness.*

II. **Etiology**
   A. The following factors may contribute to blindness:
      1. Familial factors such as a genetic disease.
      2. Intrauterine insult (e.g., rubella or toxoplasmosis).
      3. Perinatal factors such as prematurity or oxygen toxicity.
      4. Postnatal factors such as trauma or infection (e.g., measles).
      5. Inflammatory disorders (e.g., juvenile arthritis).

III. **Signs, Symptoms, and History**
   A. No eye-to-eye contact with caregiver.
   B. Inability to follow large moving objects.
   C. Abnormal eye movements.
   D. Unresponsiveness to visual stimuli.
   E. Does not move around.
   F. Fixed pupils.
   G. Strabismus.
   H. Constant nystagmus.

IV. **Effects on Individual**
   A. Blindisms develop to compensate for inadequate stimulation (e.g., body rocking, finger flicking, arm twirling).
   B. May have continuous falls, bumps, and bruises if environment is not made safe.
   C. Motor and speech skills delayed.
   D. Social play curtailed because of child's fear of falling or running into unknown obstacles.
   E. Inability to observe others who may be role models.
   F. Delayed development of social behaviors.
   G. Misses important visual cues.
   H. General delay in all developmental milestones because they are in some way related to sight (e.g., crawling is guided in movement by sight, social smile is learned by observation, development of eating skills and use of utensils rely heavily on sight).
   I. Older child's self-concept may be harmed because peers may laugh if dress is inappropriately matched; facial expression is lacking, which may be misunderstood as lack of interest or sullenness.

V. **Management/Treatment**
   A. Early diagnosis important.
   B. Surgical repair if indicated.
   C. Eyeglasses.
   D. Special training for parents and child.
   E. Early orientation and mobility instruction.
   F. Speech and language development.
   G. Early stimulation program.
   H. Referral to available resources and counseling services.

VI. Additional Information
  A. For education purposes, a child who loses vision before the age of 5 or 6 is classified as having a congenital vision defect. These children have difficulty with visual imagery and memory of color. The child who becomes blind at an older age retains concepts of reading, writing, and colors and may easily transfer this knowledge to learning the Braille system. Educational implications differ greatly for both groups. Technology has opened new and challenging avenues for individual or group learning.

GLAUCOMA
I. Definition
  A. Glaucoma is defined as increased intraocular pressure that may cause atrophy of the optic nerve, damage to the retina, and eventual blindness. Several types of glaucoma exist; however, congenital glaucoma is most often associated with infants and young children.
II. Etiology
  A. Glaucoma is a congenital defect resulting from inadequate development of the filtering mechanism of the eyes anterior chamber angle. It also can be acquired by an injury resulting in scar tissue blocking the drainage of aqueous humor or a disease process.
III. Signs, Symptoms, and History
  A. Earliest symptoms are epiphora, photophobia, and redness of eye.
  B. Pupil large and fixed.
  C. Eyeball enlarges because young eye is distensible.
  D. Sclera is blue tinged.
  E. Cornea is thinned, cloudy, and bulging.
  F. Usually bilateral.
  G. Congenital glaucoma symptoms are visible early in life.
IV. Effects on Individual
  A. Limited peripheral vision causes clumsiness and bumping into objects.
  B. Discomfort affects general well-being and behavior when intraocular pressure increases.
  C. Limited vision affects motor skills.
  D. Parents overindulge and overprotect child, thus stunting child's physical, social, and emotional growth.
V. Management/Treatment
  A. Surgery is necessary to increase the outflow of fluids to the eye. A second surgery may be necessary, but pressure reducing medications are used first; surgery is reserved as a last option.
VI. Additional Information
  A. In early stages, corneal haziness is reversible once the ocular pressure has been reduced. Juvenile glaucoma, sometimes called *open-angle glaucoma,* occurs between 3 and 20 years of age and follows a course similar to that of adult glaucoma. It is usually related to another disease process. The "puff test" for measuring intraocular pressure may be used as early as 4 years of age. This test is administered as play, instructing the child to keep eyes open wide until the puff comes.

NYSTAGMUS

I. Definition

    A. Nystagmus is an involuntary repetitive movement of one or both eyeballs. It can be a rhythmic oscillation in any direction and at any speed or frequency. Nystagmus often is associated with defective vision.

II. Etiology

    A. Nystagmus is congenital or acquired. It may be ocular or systemic (neurological). Congenital nystagmus may be caused by organic eye disease. Corneal opacity, congenital cataract, albinism, total color blindness, or congenital anomalies of the optic nerve may cause ocular nystagmus. Neurological nystagmus is secondary to lesions in the brain.

III. Signs, Symptoms, and History

    A. Eyes move repetitively in any direction at different speeds with no purpose.

    B. In congenital nystagmus, eye movement can be in all directions of gaze.

    C. In ocular nystagmus, searching movement is pendular of equal speed and amplitude.

    D. In neurological nystagmus, movements are horizontal, rotary, or jerky.

IV. Effects on Individual

    A. May become self-conscious or embarrassed by response of others to condition.

    B. May avoid eye contact.

    C. Head posturing to obtain null point (eye position that stabilizes nystagmus, such as face turn, chin elevation or depression, and head tilt that minimizes nystagmoid eye movements).

V. Management/Treatment

    A. Complete assessment necessary.

    B. Treatment of underlying cause.

VI. Additional Information

    A. Intermittent nystagmus in an infant until approximately age 3 months is normal. Continuous nystagmus from birth is not normal and should be evaluated. Congenital nystagmus generally is not diagnosed until the child is 2 or 3 months old.

STRABISMUS

I. Definition

    A. Strabismus is an abnormal deviation of ocular alignment. When the optic axes are not directed simultaneously to the same object, the eyes appear to be gazing in two directions.

II. Etiology

    A. Numerous causes of strabismus exist; the most common is eye incoordination. With disorders of binocularity, the eyes do not function equally either in tandem or in perception of images. The underlying causes are variations in refractive deviations of alignment or organic disease. Amblyopia may develop when the child attempts to suppress vision in the deviating eye.

III. **Signs, Symptoms, and History**
   A. Parents of a newborn state that the child's eyes cross.
   B. Diplopia (double vision) if no suppression; young children do not express this symptom.
   C. Tilts head when reading.
   D. Closes one eye to see or rubs eyes.
   E. Frequently blinks or squints eye.

IV. **Effects on Individual**
   A. May appear clumsy and awkward because of unequal vision and poor depth perception.
   B. Poor self-esteem for cosmetic reasons.
   C. Awkward writing skills.
   D. Young child has difficulty doing puzzles, block building, and other fine motor tasks that affect development of preacademic skills.
   E. Unable to see moving objects or prints easily.

V. **Management/Treatment**
   A. Restore normal visual acuity in each eye by patching, glasses, or pleoptics.
   B. Eyeglasses, surgery, or a combination of surgery and eyeglasses.
   C. Provide binocular vision by orthoptics with or without refractive lenses (however, binocular vision may be unobtainable) or surgery.
   D. Botulinum toxin injections temporarily weaken the stronger muscle, which allows the weaker muscle to strengthen. May need to be repeated to achieve orthotopia (absence of strabismus).

VI. **Additional Information**
   A. Strabismus has four separate classifications: (1) *esotropia,* an inward or medial deviation of one or both eyes; (2) *exotropia,* an outward or lateral deviation of one or both eyes; (3) *hypertropia,* an upward or superior deviation of one or both eyes; and (4) *hypotropia,* which is uncommon. Esotropia, convergent strabismus, may be nonparalytic or paralytic. Nonparalytic (comitant) esotropia is the most common type in infants and children. The angle of deviation in the deviating eye is constant in all areas of gaze. The two types of nonparalytic esotropia are nonaccommodative and accommodative.
   B. Nonaccommodative esotropia manifests early in life, often at birth but generally by the first year. The condition can be congenital or acquired. The cause is related to abnormalities of the eye or its development rather than refractive error. Treatment is vision therapy, orthoptics, or surgery.
   C. The onset of accommodative esotropia is usually between 18 months and 4 years of age. The deviation is often monocular but may be alternating, and the child is hyperopic. If treatment is delayed, amblyopia develops. Treatment includes eyeglasses followed by a vision therapy program.
   D. Paralytic (noncomitant) esotropia results from birth injury or congenital anomaly and is seen much less frequently than comitant es-

otropia. The angle of deviation in the deviating eye varies in all directions of gaze.

E. *Exotropia* (divergent strabismus) is less common in infants and children than esotropia. The prevalence increases with age. Exotropia is intermittent or constant. The onset of intermittent exotropia generally is not noted before the age of 2 or 3 years. There is usually a greater exotropia for distance; fusion occurs for near vision. Intermittent exotropia may progress to constant exotropia. Treatment consists of vision therapy programming. Constant exotropia is less common than intermittent exotropia. The condition may be present at birth or progress from intermittent to constant exotropia. The onset may occur later in life if the condition is related to loss of vision in one eye. Constant exotropia is usually monocular but may be alternating. Myopia of varying degrees of severity is often associated with constant exotropia. The treatment is surgery.

F. *Hypertropia* is a vertical deviation of one eye and may be paralytic or nonparalytic. In paralytic hypertropia the amount of deviation varies according to the direction of the gaze. Hypertropia is treated with prismatic lenses. In nonparalytic hypertropia, the angle of deviation is always the same and does not depend on the direction of the gaze. The treatment is eyeglasses or surgery.

G. *Pseudostrabismus* is the appearance of strabismus as a result of prominent epicanthal folds or a wide-bridged nose. A small portion of the medial aspect of the eye is covered, creating an illusion of strabismus. The cover/uncover and corneal light reflex tests (Hirschberg test) differentiate between true and pseudostrabismus. As children grow, the flat nasal bridge develops, lifting the excessive epicanthal skin, which corrects the condition.

H. *Hypertelorism* is a disproportionate growth of the facial bones. As a primary deformity, it may cause wide-spaced separation of the eyes. The eyes appear exotropic even though they are perfectly straight. Testing for deviations determines whether the eyes are normal.

TESTING PROCEDURES

Vision is the main sensory modality for educational activities. Therefore consistent visual assessment during the school age years is important. Early detection and correction of visual problems may prevent deficits in academic performance and permanent vision loss. The screening and testing methods presented in this section can be used for a comprehensive school vision screening program.

DISTANCE ACUITY

I. **Snellen, Sloan, LEA, or Illiterate E**
   A. Screening criteria.
      1. These tests are used for preschool (ages 3-4 years), kindergarten or first grade (age 5 or 6 years), second grade (age 7 years), and children with special needs as required. Some children may be

Table 2-2	*Classifications of Visual Function for Distance and Near Point Acuity*

Acuity Effects	Educational Implications
Normal Vision	
20/12, 20/15, 20/20, 20/25	No educational implications
	20/20 is Snellen notation for normal vision; healthy people generally average better than 20/20
Near Normal Vision	
20/30	Discriminates print used in classified ads
20/40	Minimum acuity required by many states for driver's license
20/50, 20/60	Can read newsprint
	Children with 20/50 can easily read telephone book
Moderate Low Vision	
20/70, 20/80	Considered partially sighted in United States after best correction; meets eligibility requirements for some services
20/100, 20/125, 20/160	20/100 able to read print of children's books, has problems seeing details, and reads at distance less than 10 ft
	Reading aids or magnifier generally provide adequate reading speed
Severe Low Vision	
20/200, 20/250	In United States, arbitrary delineation for legal blindness after correction in better eye or visual field no larger than 200
20/300	Gross orientation and mobility are usually adequate
	Difficulty seeing traffic signs and numbers on buses
20/400	Requires high-power magnifiers for reading and/or short reading distance (4 in-2 ft)
CF 10 ft	Reading speed and endurance reduced
	Qualifies for tax deduction, rehabilitation services, and numerous other types of assistance
Profound Low Vision	
20/400 (CF 8 ft)	Numerous problems with visual orientation and mobility
20/1000 (CF 4 ft)	White cane useful
	If motivated and persistent, can read visually with high-power magnifiers; others rely on nonvisual methods such as Braille, radio, talking books
Near Blindness	
CF 3 ft	Has light perception but vision unreliable
LP	Relies on nonvisual aids
Total Blindness	
NLP	NLP; relies totally on other sensory input

CF, Count fingers; *LP,* light perception; *NLP,* no light perception.

Box 2-3   *Distance Acuity*

Preschool Children
- Illiterate E charts
- Allen cards
- Blackbird test
- LEA symbols
- Denver test
- Camera systems

Special Education Children
- Camera systems
- Faye symbol chart

- HOTV
- STYCAR tests

School-Age Children
- Snellen, Sloan, LEA symbols, or Illiterate E charts
- Stereoscope

Table 2-3   *Visual Screening Recommendations*

Age	Screening
Birth-3 mo	Inspection and observation Red reflex Corneal light reflex (Hirschberg test)
6 mo-1 yr	Inspection and observation Red reflex Corneal light reflex Blink reflex Fixate and follow bilaterally Alternate occlusion
Toddler (1-3 yr)	Inspection and observation Visual acuity Red reflex Corneal light reflex Blink reflex Cover-uncover and alternate cover
Preschool (3-5 yr)	Inspection and observation Visual acuity Red reflex Blink reflex Corneal light reflex Cover-uncover and alternate cover
School-age-adolescent	Inspection and observation Visual acuity Peripheral vision/visual fields Fixation Cover-uncover and alternate cover

difficult to test at these ages with a distance acuity chart because of developmental level rather than a visual problem.

B. Equipment and preparation.

1. Self-illuminating 10- or 20-ft (3- or 6-m) distance chart. Illiterate E or other similar optotypes preferable to picture symbols (e.g., house, apple) charts. Single optotypes on a line should be avoided unless the child is unable to test with a line of multiple optotypes.
2. Window cards for occluding background figures for younger children only when exposed to multiple optotypes first and unable to succeed.
3. Eye occluder.
4. Rescreening and referral forms.
5. Eliminate shadows and glare in testing room.
6. Position chart at eye level.

C. Screening procedure.

1. Have student stand or sit at recommended distance from chart (10 or 20 ft). If student is standing, the toe of the foot should be on the line and, if student is sitting, place back legs of chair on marked line.
2. Give screening instructions and how student is to respond; demonstrate if necessary with single large E.
3. Show student how to use occluder to cover one eye or have assistant occlude one eye. Tell student to keep both eyes open while using occluder. This is an important concept.
4. If student wears glasses, screen with glasses in place to determine baseline acuity. Then repeat testing without glasses.
5. Evaluate each eye separately, right eye first and then left eye.
6. Begin at 20/40 line and proceed downward. If visual acuity difficulties are suspected, begin screening at 20/200 line and proceed downward. Continue until student is able to read correctly three of four symbols on the short line or four of six symbols on the longer line.

NOTE: Check individual state criteria, since each state varies.

7. Observe for blinking, tilting of head, squinting, rubbing of eyes, or complaints of blurring.
8. When screening young children, attempt full line first; if unsuccessful, use window cards to expose only one symbol at a time.

D. Failure criteria.

1. The failure criteria in 3-year-olds is a visual acuity in either eye of 20/50 or poorer. This indicates inability to correctly identify one more than half the symbols on the 40-ft line on the chart at a distance of 20 ft (6 m).
2. Any 3-year-old with a two-line difference in visual acuity between the eyes in the passing range, (e.g., 20/20 in one eye, 20/40 in the other eye) fails the distance acuity examination.
3. In all other ages and grades, visual acuity of 20/40 or poorer indicates inability to identify correctly one more than half the symbols on the 30-ft line of the chart at a distance of 20 ft (recommendation of the National Society to Prevent Blindness).

4. Each state generally has its own standards and criteria, and the National Association of School Nurses provides vision guidelines.
5. The accepted standard for normal acuity is 20/20 (Neff, 1991). For acuity of 20/20, at a distance of 20 feet (numerator) letters 7 mm in height (denominator) can be seen (20/20 line). If the individual can only read the 20/100 line, that indicates he or she sees at 20 feet what an individual with normal visual acuity would see at 100 feet.

E. Rescreening.
1. All students/children who fail initial screening must be re-screened (use the same screening procedure).

NOTE: Check codes in own state, since this varies.

F. Action.
1. If a child fails the second screening, notify parents and send a written referral for a complete professional eye examination by an oph-thalmologist or optometrist.

NOTE: Check state criteria before referral, since the criteria vary. The referral should indicate test results, screening dates, observations of the child, and any teacher comments. Follow up with parents regarding results of the professional examination and implications for the school setting. Any other visual testing should be considered and referral made if deviations from the norm even when visual acuity is normal, especially if the student is having academic/school difficulty.

G. Additional procedures.
1. Near-point: Focusing lenses, near-point convergence, amplitude of accommodation (provide paragraph of small letters bringing to nose until it blurs, should be 4- to 6-in range, depending on age). Hyperopia screening.
2. Strabismus testing: Cover-uncover test, alternate cover test, corneal light reflex test (Hirschberg test).

II. Color Perception Screening
A. Screening criteria; color plates.
1. All males before age 6 or according to individual state mandates.
B. Screening information.
1. See individual test instructions. Various pseudoisochromatic plate tests are available, such as Ishihara, Dvorine, AO, and American Optical Hardy Rand Rittler (AO HRR) plates. Pseudoisochromatic plates consist of printed plates of letters, numbers, and winding paths composed of colored dots of different sizes that differ systematically in hue from background dots. The student must identify the designs. Each figure color and background dot is so similar that the test figure does not stand out plainly enough for the color-deficient person to identify. These screening tests can be used with children as young as 4 years.
2. All these tests are easy to administer; the manufacturer's instructions should be followed exactly, especially with regard to illumination (e.g., daylight, fluorescent lighting). The most common error is administering the test under incorrect illumination. Proper illumination is as important as the ink used in printing the plates. The tests are designed for use under average daylight, which can be provided by a daylight lamp. If plates are displayed

under ordinary (incandescent) light, a color deficiency may not be identified.

NOTE: Be aware of state standards, since some color perception tests are illegal to use in particular states. Use of slide with incandescent light distorts accurate assessment of color perception.

3. Of the tests mentioned, only the AO HRR is diagnostic, identifying the type and degree of the defect. The others are screening tests that determine whether the child has normal color vision. The Ishihara test frequently is used in schools and is similar to other plates; it consists of numbers imbedded in circles of colored dots. In screening, the number of plates missed does *not* indicate the severity of the defect. Test plates should be protected from unnecessary light exposure and handling. Ink fades with time, and fading is increased by exposure to light. Keep plates clean and untouched. A soft, dry paintbrush or cotton-tipped swab should be used for tracing the symbols on the plates, and plates should not be touched by hands or fingers.

C. Failure criteria.
   1. According to test instructions.
D. Rescreening.
   1. No rescreening is necessary. Rescreen young children to rule out other factors (e.g., illness, fatigue, fear).
E. Action.
   1. Notify parents if a deficiency exists and educate staff about the deficiency.

BINOCULAR VISION: NEAR AND FAR

I. **Cover/Uncover Test (Unilateral Cover Test)**
   A. This test determines the presence or absence of a heterotropia or strabismus. Heterotropia is a misalignment of the eyes that is manifest during binocularity and may be unilateral, alternating, or intermittent depending on the vision. The test should be done at near and far distances.
   B. Screening procedure.
      1. Observe for refixation movement of the uncovered eye while uncovering the covered eye.
      2. As student fixates on target at near (13 in [33 cm]) and far (20 ft [6 m]) distances, cover left eye and observe right eye. If right eye shows no fixation movement, no deviation is present.
      3. If right eye moves to fixate, deviation is present.
      4. Repeat procedure, covering right eye and observing left eye.
   C. Screening results.
      1. When one eye is covered and there is no movement of uncovered eye, no deviation is present.
      2. When one eye is covered and other eye moves inward, exotropia is indicated.
      3. When one eye is covered and other eye moves outward, esotropia is indicated.
      4. When one eye is covered and other moves downward, hypertropia is indicated.

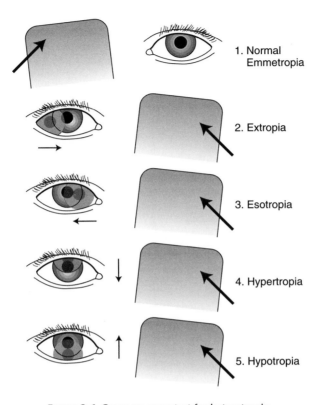

1. Normal
   Emmetropia

2. Extropia

3. Esotropia

4. Hypertropia

5. Hypotropia

FIGURE 2-6 Cover-uncover test for heterotropia.

    5. When one eye covered and other eye moves upward, hypotropia is indicated.

II. Alternate Cover Test

  A. This test can determine the presence or absence of heterophoria or strabismus. Heterophobia is a latent tendency for the eyes to deviate during conditions of monocularity and is normally controlled by fusional mechanisms providing binocular vision and avoidance of diplopia. The eye can deviate under stress, fatigue, illness, or when normal fusion is interfered with, such as covering the eye.

  B. Screening procedure.

    1. Observe for a refixation shift of the covered eye as it is being uncovered. Leave an occluder over one eye for several seconds to dissociate fusion. Move the occluder rapidly over the bridge of the nose to the other eye keeping one eye covered at all times.

    2. Both the student's eyes should be open; student screening should be done at near (13 in [33 cm]) and far (20 ft [6 m]) distances. Heterophorias are controlled by fusion mechanism only when both eyes are open; fusion is disrupted when one eye is covered.

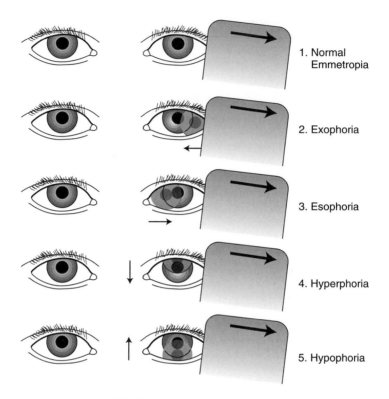

1. Normal
   Emmetropia

2. Exophoria

3. Esophoria

4. Hyperphoria

5. Hypophoria

FIGURE 2-7 Alternate cover test for heterophoria.

3. As the student fixates on a distant object, cover one eye with the occluder and then quickly uncover the eye.
4. As occluder is removed, observe whether the eye under cover has deviated. Perform this procedure on both eyes.
5. If covered eye moves in any direction to fixate when occluder is removed, a heterophoria is present.

C. Screening results.
   1. When eye is uncovered and there is no movement, no deviation is present.
   2. When eye is uncovered and moves inward to fixate, exophoria is indicated.
   3. When eye is uncovered and moves outward to fixate, esophoria is indicated.
   4. When eye is uncovered and moves downward to fixate, hyperphoria is indicated.
   5. When eye is uncovered and moves upward to fixate, hypophoria is indicated.

III. Corneal Light Reflex Test (Hirschberg Test)
This test is used to detect malalignment of the eyes.
  A. Screening procedure.
    1. Direct a penlight toward student's eyes from distance of 13 in (33 cm). Student's eyes should be focused on examiner's face.
    2. Observe images penlight makes on pupils.
    3. If images are equally placed on both eyes, test result is negative.
    4. If penlight images are not equally placed, eyes are malaligned.
  B. Screening results.
    1. Symmetrical light reflection in each pupil indicates normal alignment.
    2. Asymmetrical light reflection in each pupil indicates malalignment.
    3. Light reflection on outer aspect of pupil indicates esotropia.
    4. Light reflection on inner aspect of pupil indicates exotropia.
    5. Notify parents and make a referral for formal evaluation.
    6. Students with epicanthal folds may give false impression of malalignment (pseudostrabismus); however, light reflex test should be equal.

NEAR ACUITY

I. Hyperopia Screening
Hyperopia screening determines farsightedness with use of a plus sphere lens or other methods.
  A. Screening procedure.
    1. Place appropriate strength plus lens glasses on student (+2.25D for younger children; +2.0D or less strength for older children and adults). Ask student to look at Snellen chart for approximately 1 minute.
NOTE: Check state screening recommendations.
    2. Direct student to read 20/30 line of chart.
    3. Test one eye at a time.
    4. The following materials are used to test for near acuity.
      a. Plus lenses.
      b. Near point acuity cards.
      c. Stereoscope.
      d. Young child tests.
  B. Screening results.
    1. If student reads at least four of seven lines correctly, screening has been failed and should be repeated about 2 weeks later.
NOTE: Criteria may vary by state.
    2. Student should be *unable* to read 20/20 or 20/30 line.
    3. If student fails rescreening (e.g., can successfully read 20/30 line), then refer if results still suggest failure.

INFANT, PRESCHOOL, AND SPECIAL EDUCATION SCREENING

Vision is the most important modality for learning. The learning process is not restricted to the traditional school-age years; thus detection and treatment of

| Table 2-4 | *Visual Assessment Techniques for Infants and Young Children* |

Variable	Assessment Techniques
Testing site	Be aware of intensity and location of light source; the source should be behind the children. Darken the room or use colored lights if infant makes no visual responses in normal lighting.
Distractions	Be aware of visual and auditory distractions; minimize to prevent overstimulation (e.g., shadows, light through windows, colorful objects in room, radio, television noise, adults in conversation, children playing nearby).
Positioning	Child should be in secure position; on parent's shoulder or lap; on back or stomach, or in infant seat.
Physiological state	Observe and note if alert, sleepy, fussy, hungry state; ill or recently ill.
Social state	If infant is wary of stranger, caregiver is better person to work with child to elicit behaviors. If infant likes faces, then examiner can use own face as visual stimulus for testing.
Attention	Combine auditory and visual stimulation for attention (voice and face; shake rattle). Then elicit responses with familiar nonaudible object. If unable to try, repeat with shiny/bright objects (tin foil, tinsel, costume jewelry) or high-contrast object, or use filtered light by placing pop bead over penlight. Some colors are seen easier than others, so vary colors of toys and objects for testing.
Observations	Observe carefully; cues are often subtle (e.g., quieting, widening of eyes, moving fingers, reaching for objects). Document all observations and history.
Reward	End with activity infant can do with ease and provide verbal praise and smile.

Modified from Chen D, Friedman C, Cavello G: *Parents and visually impaired infants: identifying visual impairment in infants (PAVII),* Louisville, Ky, 1990, American Printing House for the Blind.

visual problems in the early years is critical to a child's overall optimal development. The Prevent Blindness America organization estimates that 1 in every 20 preschool children in the United States has a vision problem, and if uncorrected, it can lead to needless decrease of vision or loss of sight. New technology and information allows newborns to be screened and tested for visual estimates and impairments. Even with this ability, almost 80% of preschool children have not had an eye examination according to Prevent Blindness America.

AMBLYOPIA SCREENING PROCEDURE FOR INFANTS

The following screening procedure can be used on children younger than 1 year to detect amblyopia.

    I. **Screening Procedure**

        A. Try to occlude one of the infants eyes. Notice infant's behavior.

        B. Occlude other eye.

        C. If infant cries or tries to push away occluder from eye, suspect reduced visual acuity in uncovered eye.

II. Screening Results

A. If visual acuity is normal or near normal, infant will not react strongly to either eye being covered.

B. Make referral for formal testing if you suspect reduced visual function in either eye.

ALLEN CARD TEST

I. Appropriate Age

A. This test for visual acuity may be used on cooperating children 24 months and older.

II. Summary of Test

A. The test consists of seven picture cards (tree, birthday cake, horse and rider, telephone, car, house, and teddy bear) that are presented at a distance of 15 ft. The cards are first shown to the child at a close distance to determine whether the child can identify the pictures correctly. The child is given three to five trials and must identify correctly three of seven pictures to pass this screening. The test does not allow testing of acuity better than 20/30.

BLACKBIRD PRESCHOOL VISION SCREENING SYSTEM

I. Appropriate Age

A. This screening tool can be used to assess the visual acuity in 3- to 6-year-old children, children with special needs, and other children whose eye-hand coordination has not fully developed.

II. Summary of Test

A. The test involves the story of a blackbird in flight, which is in the shape of a modified E, to engage attention. The story can be adapted according to the needs of the child being screened. A wall-mounted chart or flash cards are available. Six individual cards are used; each card has a blackbird picture of varying size on one side and a visual acuity fraction on the reverse side. The cards are presented to the child from a distance of 20 ft (6 m). The child indicates, with her or his arms, the direction of the blackbird's flight. Vision screening guidelines are included for uncommunicative, non-readers, or non-English speaking children, and other difficult-to-test populations. Disposable cardboard eye occluders are available. The blackbird system is now available in Spanish. The system has not been tested for efficacy when compared with these techniques. The *Blackbird Storybook Home Eye Test* is available for parents who choose to prescreen their young children at home. The pass-fail criteria are included.

III. Available Information

A. The kit is available from Blackbird, PO Box 277424, Sacramento, California, 95827. Web address: www.blackbirdvision.com.

DENVER EYE SCREENING TEST

I. Appropriate Age

A. The Denver Eye Screening Test (DEST) is suitable for children 2 years (24 months) and older.

II. Summary of Test
    A. The test uses a single E card (20/30, 6/9 m) that is to be used 15 ft (4.5 m) from the child. A large E (20/100, 6/30 m) is used for demonstration and teaching techniques. The DEST screens children at risk for visual problems from 6 to 30 months by testing for fixation, squinting, and strabismus. Because this test uses a single optotype rather than several on a line, it is not considered as reliable as other tests.

III. Available Information
    A. The instructional material is available from Denver Developmental Materials, Inc., PO Box 6919, Denver, CO 90206-0919; 1-800-419-4729.

CAMERA VISION SCREENING SYSTEMS

I. Appropriate Age
    A. These camera systems can be used with infants as young as 6 months. The systems are especially useful with young children or children with special needs because they are objective and require no response from the child.

II. Summary of Tests
    A. Several camera systems are available. All use a similar process. A photograph is taken of the eyes, and the flash of light induces a red reflex. The resulting photograph of some of the systems provides information regarding visual impairments. Some systems provide pass-fail results by computer interpretation; some provide a diagnosis and objective refraction information; and another requires nurse interpretation of the Polaroid photo. These screening systems test for a variety of conditions, including myopia, hyperopia, strabismus, astigmatism, anisometropia, cataracts, and other media opacities.

III. Available Information
    A. The Welch Allyn SureSight Vision Screener information can be seen at the company Web site: www.welchallyn.com; 1-800-535-6663. The PhotoScreener system Web site address is www.photoscreener.com; 1-800-277-1710. Other screeners are in the developmental stage.

FAYE SYMBOL CHART

I. Appropriate Age
    A. This test can be used with children as young as 27 to 30 months.

II. Summary of Test
    A. This test includes pictures of an apple, house, or umbrella on either a chart or flash cards that are shown to the child at 10 ft (3 m). When compared with other tests, the use of pictures is not as accurate for assessment of acuity as the use of other optotypes.

III. Available Information
    A. The test can be ordered from school health supply companies.

HOTV OR MATCHING SYMBOL

I. Appropriate Age
    A. This test can be used with children from 3 years of age. It avoids the issues of eye-hand coordination and image reversal that can occur with the traditional letter chart.

II. Summary of Test

A. The test uses four letters, H, O, T, and V in a chart that is shown to the child at 10 or 20 ft (3-6 m). The child matches the letters with demonstration cards or names the letters. This avoids eye-hand co-ordination and image reversal concerns that can occur with E vision charts, but because the letters are few and not in a line, the test is less accurate.

III. Available Information

A. These tests can be ordered from school health supply companies.

ILLITERATE ε VISION SCREENING

I. Appropriate Age

A. This test can determine visual acuity in cooperating children as young as 2½ to 3 years using the E game and is one of the most accurate.

II. Summary of Test

A. The child's parent is instructed to teach the test to the child at home using the E game method. The child plays the game by pointing with his or her hand the direction the legs of the E letter are facing. Once the child understands the test and is able to point consistently to the direction of the big E, then a nurse, physician, or other examiner can perform efficient and appropriate screening. This test can be incorporated into day care programs as a group activity. A free home eye test kit in English and Spanish is available through the Prevent Blindness America organization, http://www.preventblindness.org.

STYCAR VISION TESTS

I. Appropriate Age

A. The STYCAR test can be used to determine visual acuity in children 2 years and older. It also may be used with children with developmental delays.

II. Summary of Test

A. The STYCAR test is based on developmental knowledge of the child. An average child copies a vertical line at 2 years, a horizontal line at 2½ years, a circle at 3 years, a cross at 4 years, and a square and triangle at 5 years. The test uses the letters H, L, C, T, O, X, A, V, and U. The number of letters used is determined by the age group to be screened. Children who do not know the letters are given cards to match.

WEB SITES

Vision Service Plan (VSP) Sight for Students
    http://www.sightforstudents.org
American Academy of Ophthalmology
    http://www.aao.org
Better Vision for Children Foundation
    http://www.bvcnow.org/

GLOSSARY OF VISION TERMS

Accommodation The shape of the eye's lens increases through contraction of the ciliary muscle to focus on objects at near distances.

Acquired Not innate or hereditary.

Acuity Ability to discriminate details, as in reading. Measurements indicate the smallest figure or symbol recognizable in central vision. Acuity is a measure of the function of the cones in the fovea centralis.

Amblyopia Reduced vision in one eye; not caused by refractive errors or organic defect. Contributing factors cause developmental lag in occipital lobe and retinal cones; often called *lazy eye*.

Aniridia Lack of iris tissue, usually bilateral with reduced visual acuity and photophobia.

Anisometropia Refractive errors of the two eyes are unequal, usually two or more lines' difference as measured by acuity assessments.

Aphakia Absence of the lens.

Astigmatism Vision defect usually caused by uneven curvature of the cornea.

Binocular vision Ability of the brain to fuse a retinal image from each eye into one single image resulting from clear images on both foveae and parallel alignment of the eyes.

Cataract Any partial or complete clouding of the lens.

Central visual acuity Ability of the eye and brain to discriminate form and shape in the direct line of vision when elicited by stimuli impinging directly on the fovea centralis area of the macula retinae.

Certified ophthalmic registered nurse Nurse with specialized knowledge, experience, and skills to perform assessments, eye examinations, education, and assistance in eye surgeries. Services provided in ambulatory clinics, private offices, operating rooms, and hospitals.

Coloboma Congenital notch or defect of the iris; may also involve retina, macula, or optic nerve. Visual function varies from normal to severely impaired, depending on structures involved.

Cones Photoreceptor cells in the retina that provide detail and color sensitivity.

Congenital Present at birth.

Cornea A clear, transparent structure covering over the iris and pupil; part of the eye's refracting system.

Cortical visual impairment Cortical visual impairment (CVI) is permanent or temporary visual impairment caused by disturbance of the posterior visual pathways, the occipital lobes of the brain, or both. Ranges from severe impairment to total blindness depending on the time of onset, location, and intensity of the insult. Caused by perinatal hypoxia, metabolic disturbances, hydrocephalus, head trauma, infection, and brain defects.

Cycloplegia Paralysis of ciliary muscle, resulting in paralysis of accommodation; usually intentionally induced by an eye examiner to facilitate examination of the structure and function of the eye.

Depth perception Ability to perceive spatial (distance) relationships (stereopsis).

Dichromatis Ability to perceive only 2 of the 160 colors the normal eye discriminates.

Diopter   Unit of measurement that expresses a lens' refractive power. Also a measure of the degree of refractive error. Myopia is measured in minus prism diopters, whereas hyperopia is measured in plus prism diopters.

Diplopia   Perception of two images of a single object; double vision.

Distensible   Capable of being enlarged.

Doll's-eye reflex   Eyes remain stationary when head is moved. Normal reflex for first 10 days of life. Detects paresis of the abducens nerve and weakness of the lateral rectus muscle. May be localized or the result of damage to the central nervous system.

Electron microscopy   Microscopic examination that uses a beam of electrons to form an enlarged image.

Emmetropia   Parallel light rays coming to exact focus on the retina; ideal optical condition.

Epiphora   Tearing of eye.

Esophoria   Deviation of the visual axis of an eye toward the other eye after the visual fusion stimuli has been eliminated.

Esotropia   Strabismus that manifests deviation of a visual axis toward that of the other eye resulting in diplopia, also called *cross-eye* and *convergent* or *internal strabismus.*

Exophoria   Deviation of the visual axis of one eye away from the other eye when the visual fusional stimuli is absent.

Exotropia   Strabismus that manifests permanent deviation of the visual axis of one eye away from the other, resulting in diplopia; also called *wall-eye* and *divergent* or *external strabismus.*

Fixation   The act of holding or staying in a fixed position.

Fovea centralis   A small depression in the center of the macula lutea that contains elongated cones. This is the area of clearest vision because the layers of the retina spread aside, permitting light to fall directly on the cones.

Glaucoma   Eye disorder characterized by increased intraocular pressure and loss of vision.

Hyperopia   A refractive error in which parallel light rays focus behind the retina. Frequently called *farsightedness;* also called *hypermetropia.*

Hyperphoria   Upward deviation of the visual axis of an eye after elimination of the visual fusional stimulus; form of heterophoria.

Hypertropia   Strabismus that displays permanent upward deviation of the visual axis of an eye.

Hypophoria   Downward deviation of the visual axis of an eye after elimination of the visual fusional stimulus; form of heterophoria.

Hypotropia   Strabismus that displays permanent downward deviation of the visual axis of an eye.

Intermittent   Activity is suspended at intervals.

Iris   Eye tissue behind the cornea, which contracts or dilates to regulate the amount of light entering the eye.

Legal blindness   Correction of 20/200 or less with or without a visual field of 20 degrees or less in the better eye.

Lens   Transparent, oval, and colorless structure of the eye that undergoes accommodation to focus rays so that a perfect image is formed on the retina; sometimes called the *crystalline lens.*

Low vision   See Partially sighted.

Macula lutea   A part of the retina behind the lens that is responsible for central vision. The central area of the macula is called the *fovea centralis.*

Miosis   Contraction of the pupil.

Monochromatism   Total color blindness, inability to discriminate hues, all colors of the spectrum, which appear as neutral grays varying in shades of light and dark.

Monocular   Involving only one eye.

Mydriasis   Physiological dilatation of the pupil.

Myopia   A refractive error in which parallel light rays from a distant object focus in front of the retina; often called *nearsightedness.*

Nystagmus   Involuntary repetitive movement of the eyeball. Movement can be horizontal, vertical, rotary, or mixed.

Occlusive therapy   An attempt to straighten or strengthen an eye by patching the other eye.

Ocular hypotony   Low intraocular pressure.

Oculogyric crisis   Eyeballs become fixed in one position for minutes or hours.

Opaque   Unable to be penetrated by light rays or other forms of radiant energy.

Ophthalmologist   Medical doctor who specializes in the treatment of eye diseases and disorders; performs surgery and prescribes treatment.

Optic axis   A straight line through the center of the eye joining the central points of curvature of the anterior and posterior spheres.

Optic nerve   A bundle of nerve fibers that carry light-generated impulses from the eye to the brain.

Optic nerve atrophy   Optic nerve atrophy (ONA) is permanent visual impairment caused by damage to the optic nerve. May be progressive depending on etiology and cause.

Optic nerve hypoplasia   Optic nerve hypoplasia (ONH) is underdevelopment of optic nerve in utero. Visual function can range from near normal to no light perception. One of the three most common causes of visual impairment in children.

Optician   A person trained in the grinding of lenses and fitting of glasses.

Optokinetic   Movement of the eyes, as in optokinetic nystagmus.

Optometrist   Professional degree is Doctor of Optometry (O.D.). Optometrists are independent primary health care providers who examine, diagnose, treat, and manage diseases and disorders of the visual system, the eyes, and associated structures and diagnose related structures. Examines the eyes for the presence of a vision problem, disease, or other abnormality; prescribes lenses and other optical aids and exercises.

Optotype   Test type used for determination of visual acuity, defined by Snellen.

Orientation and mobility specialist   Teacher trained to teach individuals who are visually impaired how to move safely in their environment.

Orthoptics   Technique of eye exercises for correcting defects in binocular vision.

Orthotropia   Alignment of the eyes. The normal condition when the visual axes remain parallel when the visual fusional stimuli has been eliminated either entirely or partially.

Oscillation   Pendulum-like movement, fluctuation, or vibration.

Papillitis   Inflammation of the optic disc (papilla).

Parallelism   Equal distance at every point, having comparable parts.

Partially sighted   Visual acuity better than 20/200 but worse than 20/70 in the better eye after correction.

Peripheral vision   Ability to perceive images and motion outside the direct line of vision.

Phoria   Deviation of the eyes from normal when fusion is prevented; latent; during condition of monocularity.

Photophobia   Varying degrees of intolerance to light.

Pleoptics   Eye exercises for training and stimulating an amblyopic eye.

Ptosis   Drooping of the upper eyelid. May affect vision development.

Pupil   Opening in the center of the iris that determines the amount of light that will pass to the interior of the eye. The iris controls the size of the opening.

Refraction   Bending of a light ray as it passes from one transparent medium into one of a different density.

Refractive error   Ocular condition in which images focus either in front of or behind the retina because of the size of the orbit or inappropriate refraction.

Retina   Innermost layer of the eye that contains the light- and movement-sensitive rods and the color- and detail-sensitive cones.

Retinoblastoma   A malignant intraocular tumor that usually occurs before age 5; generally a congenital condition.

Retinopathy of prematurity   Retinopathy of prematurity (ROP) is an eye disorder in the premature infant. ROP affects immature blood vessels of the retina and is caused by conditions that stop the orderly growth of retinal blood vessels and stimulate their wild overgrowth (e.g., excessive oxygen, infection, excessive exposure to light).

Saccade   Series of abrupt, rapid, jerky movements of both eyes simultaneously when changing the point of fixation on a visualized object; this is normal functioning.

Sclera   The white outer coating of the eyeball.

Scotoma   Area of lost vision in the visual field surrounded by an area of less compromised vision or normal vision.

Snellen chart   Series of letters, symbols, or numbers of decreasing size used for testing distance central vision acuity.

Snellen notion   Ratio that expresses visual acuity. The numerator is the distance at which the test was given; the denominator is the distance at which a person with normal vision can see the chart symbols or the smallest line read on the chart.

Stereopsis   Vision in which the visual field is perceived in three dimensions through a fusion of images from each eye.

Strabismus   Misalignment of the eyes; the two eyes are not focused on the same target. Condition is often called *squint,* which is an English term infrequently used in the United States.

Trichromatism   Ability to distinguish the three primary colors: red, yellow, and blue and mixtures; normal color vision.

Tropia   Deviation of an eye or eyes from the normal position when eyes are open and uncovered.

Uvea   Vascular or second coat of the eye that lies beneath the sclera; consists of the iris, ciliary body, and choroid.

Uveitis   Inflammation of the iris, ciliary body, choroid, or uvea.

Visual evoked potential   Visual evoked potential (VEP) is a test used to gather data about the visual system. A flashing light stimulates the eye; information to the visual cortical pathways in the brain then is measured and documented in electrical activity through scalp electrodes.

ABBREVIATIONS OF VISION TERMS

A/C Anterior chamber
ACTH Adrenocorticotropic hormone
AMB Amblyopia
Ang Angles, drainage system of the eye
BRVO Branch retinal vein occlusion
CAG Closed-angle glaucoma
CD Cup to disc ratio, indication of glaucoma
CF Count fingers
CL Contact lenses
CRVO Central retinal vein occlusion
CT Cover test for strabismus
CVI Cortical visual impairment
Cyclo Cycloplegic drugs to paralyze muscles used
DFE Dilated fundus examination to see the retina
DR Diabetic retinopathy
DUCT Eye muscle test
DVA Distance visual acuity
EOM Extraocular muscle or test for eye movements
EP Esophoria
ERG Electroretinogram
ERRLA Equal, round, reactive to light and accommodation, pupils
ET Esotropia; eye deviates inward, toward the nose
EUA Examination under anesthesia
F Fixation, the ability to keep eye steady on a target
HM Hand motion
IOL Intraocular lens
IOP Intraocular pressure
Lens Crystalline lens
LP Light perception
MAO Monoamine oxidase
NLP No light perception
NPC Near point of convergence
NVA Near visual acuity
O No
OA Optic atrophy
O.D. Optometrist
OD Right eye (oculus dexter)

OKN Optokinetic nystagmus; rhythmic eye movement from moving striped target
OS Left eye (oculus sinister)
OU Both eyes (oculi uterque)
pd Prism diopter
PD Pupillary distance from the center of one to the center of the other
PERRLA Pupils, equal, round, reactive to light and accommodation
POAG Primary open-angle glaucoma
PSC Posterior subcapsular cataract
RD Retinal detachment
Refr Refraction for farsightedness/nearsightedness
RLP Retrolental fibroplasia
ROP Retinopathy of prematurity
RPE Retinal pigment epithelium; layer of cells that nourishes the retina
S Saccade; tracking or shifting eye movement
SLE Slit lamp evaluation; instrument used for eye examination
SRX Spectacle prescription
V Version, following eye movement
VA Visual acuity
VEP Visual evoked potential; tests the central 10 degrees
VF Visual fields, peripheral vision test
WNL Within normal limits
XP Exophoria
XT Exotropia; eye deviates outward
+ Indicates possibility of farsightedness
− Indicates possibility of nearsightedness

MAJOR CHARACTERISTICS OF HEARING DEVELOPMENT

I. **Prenatal**
  A. After the twentieth week of gestation, the fetus may respond to sound by startle, generalized body movement, quieting of activity, and/or autopalpebral reflex (involuntary eye blink).
  B. Cochlea has normal functioning by twentieth week.
  C. Environmental sounds have the greatest impact on auditory ability from the time the inner ear and the eighth cranial nerve become functional to central nervous system maturation; approximately 5 months' gestation to 18 to 28 months of age.
  D. Inner ear reaches adult shape and size by the twentieth to twenty-second week of gestation.
  E. The ears develop simultaneously with kidney formation; thus an anomaly or dysfunction in one system may be indicative of problems in the other.
  F. Tympanic membrane changes relative position during first 2 years of life.

II. **Birth to 1 Month**
  A. Hearing is more developed than vision at birth.
  B. Infant distinguishes between familiar and unfamiliar sounds by 3 days of age.
  C. Responds to sudden sound by crying, blinking eyes, or opening eyes widely.

   D. Extends limbs and fans out fingers and toes; has startle reflex (Moro).
   E. May become still if active at time of stimulation.
   F. Responds to voice more than any other sound.
III. **3 Months (12 Weeks)**
   A. Begins to turn head to the side in attempt to locate sound source.
   B. May smile in response to speech.
   C. Stirs from sleep when there is a loud sound.
IV. **6 Months (24 Weeks)**
   A. Turns head directly to the side, then downward to locate sound made below eye level.
   B. Learns to control and adjust response to sound (e.g., may delay response and listen for sound again or may not attempt localization).
   C. Babbling sounds increase from birth to 32 weeks in infants with normal hearing but decrease in infants who are deaf.
   D. Comprehends "no-no" and "bye-bye."
   E. Imitates sounds.
   F. Discriminates vowel sounds of language or languages to which they are continually exposed.
   G. Hears variances in vowel and consonant sounds that establish neural connections for future speech development. Tested in laboratories by changes in sucking.
 V. **12 Months (52 Weeks)**
   A. Locates sound in any direction and turns toward it.
   B. Understands simple instructions when they are accompanied by gestures (e.g., "Give it to Mommy," "Say bye-bye.").
   C. Says two or three words with meaning by 1 year.
VI. **1½ Years (18 Months)**
   A. Responds to verbal commands.
VII. **2 Years (24 Months)**
   A. Brainstem reaches maturity in the first 2 to 3 years of age.
   B. Auditory cortex reaches near maturity by 2 to 3 years of age.
   C. Directly locates a sound signal of 25 dB at all angles.
   D. Joins words together spontaneously.
   E. Developmental progression of speech and language are good indicators of normal hearing.
VIII. **36 Months and Older**
   A. The critical period for learning language is the first 36 months of life. The brain is developing rapidly during the first 3 years. If the auditory system is not stimulated, neural tracks and clusters do not develop, and language acquisition is negatively affected. Early detection of hearing loss is important for language development; babies can be fitted with hearing aids or assistive hearing devices as early as 4 weeks of age.
   B. Nearly 100% of all children experience some period of hearing loss related to otitis media (OM) in the first 11 years of life. Approximately 15% of children ages 6 to 19 years have a low- or high-frequency hearing loss in one or both ears (Niskar, 1998).

HIGH-RISK CONDITIONS FOR HEARING IMPAIRMENT OF THE NEWBORN

The incidence of significant hearing loss in newborns in the well-baby nursery population is approximately 1 to 3 per 1000 and 2 to 4 per 100 infants in the intensive care unit (ICU) population (American Academy of Pediatrics, 1999). Currently the average age of detection of significant hearing loss is 14 months. This delay in detection should diminish with wider implementation of universal newborn hearing screening (UNHS), but presently only 20% of babies are born in hospitals with UNHS.

Normal hearing at birth does not preclude delayed-onset hearing loss; 50% of children who ultimately are identified with a sensorineural hearing loss (SNHL) do not exhibit any risk factors at birth. Ninety percent of deaf children are born to hearing parents. The Joint Commission on Infant Hearing (JCIH, 2000) recommends infants with the risk factors identified in Table 2-5 should receive audiological monitoring every 6 months until age 3 years.

Table 2-5	*Risk Factors for Hearing Loss*
Neonates (Birth-28 Days)	**Infants (29 Days-2 Years)**
Illness or condition requiring admission of ≥48 hr to NICU	Parental or caregiver concern regarding hearing, speech, language, and/or developmental delay
Stigmata of other findings associated with syndrome known to include SNHL and/or CHL	Family history of permanent SNHL
	Stigmata or other findings associated with syndrome known to include SNHL and/or CHL or eustachian tube dysfunction
Family history of permanent childhood SNHL	Postnatal infections associated with SNHL, including bacterial meningitis
Craniofacial anomalies, including those with morphological abnormalities of pinna and ear canal	In-utero infections, such as CMV, herpes, rubella, syphilis, and toxoplasmosis
In-utero infections, such as CMV, herpes, rubella, syphilis, and toxoplasmosis	Neonatal indicators, specifically hyperbilirubinemia at serum level requiring transfusion, persistent pulmonary hypertension of newborn associated with mechanical ventilation, and conditions requiring use of ECMO
	Syndromes associated with progressive hearing loss, such as neurofibromatosis, osteopetrosis, and Usher's syndrome
	Neurodegenerative disorders, such as Hunter's syndrome, or sensory motor neuropathies, such as Friedreich's ataxia and Charcot-Marie-Tooth syndrome
	Head trauma
	Recurrent or persistent OM with effusion for at least 3 mo

ECMO, Extracorporeal membrane oxygenation; *NICU,* neonatal intensive care unit.

HEARING CONDITIONS

CONDUCTIVE HEARING LOSS

I. Definition
   A. A conductive hearing loss (CHL) is any type of interference in the transmission of sound from the external auditory canal to the inner ear; the inner ear is normal. In CHL, sounds are softer but not distorted.

II. Etiology
   A. Conductive impairments are caused by conditions of the outer or middle ear and may be congenital or acquired (see "Additional Information"). The most common nongenetic cause of CHL in infants and children is OM in its various forms. Young children have more horizontal, flaccid, shorter eustachian tubes, which increases their susceptibility to OM.

III. Signs, Symptoms, and History
   A. About same loss of sensitivity for sounds in all frequencies.
   B. Head noises localized in one or in both ears or unlocalized (tinnitus).
   C. Recurring OM, frequent earaches, or draining ears.
   D. Hearing loss may be intermittent if related to OM.
   E. Others must speak louder than normal.
   F. Individual may speak in relatively quiet voice because he or she is able to hear own voice through bone conduction; because of the air-conduction loss, person is unaware of environmental noise sounds that make hearing difficult for others.
   G. Turns one ear toward speaker.
   H. Frequently needs words or sentences repeated.
   I. Seems unable to follow directions well.
   J. Compensates by using environmental cues.

IV. Effects on Individual
   A. May cause significantly delayed language and speech development when occurring in early learning period.
   B. Vocabulary develops more slowly.
   C. Language deficit can cause learning problems.
   D. Parents may become frustrated and irritated from having to repeat and may interpret inappropriate responses as signs of slowness.
   E. Individual may develop emotional and acting-out behavior secondary to frustration and responses from others.
   F. Individual subjected to parents'/teachers' discipline and anger because he or she appears to be inattentive or responses are inappropriate.
   G. Peer relationships suffer.
   H. Personal safety of individual may become an issue.
   I. English as a second language, vision impairment, or other physical impairment compounds the effects of the hearing loss.

V. Management/Treatment
   A. Removal of impacted cerumen by irrigation or use of wax softeners.
   B. Medications include antibiotics, antifungals, and rarely oral steroids.

C. Surgery (e.g., myringotomy with insertion of pressure-equalizing [PE] tubes or tympanomastoidectomy).
D. Hearing aids.
E. Speech therapy.
F. Plastic surgery (otoplasty).

VI. **Additional Information**

A. OM causes hearing loss between mild and moderate levels. OM is one of the most common chronic conditions of early childhood; affected children may have between 14 and 28 weeks of hearing loss annually in the first 3 years of life, which is the most critical period for language development. A new Food and Drug Administration (FDA)-approved vaccine (pneumococcal 7-valent conjugate vaccine [Prevnar]) is given at 2, 4, and 6 months of age, with a booster during the second year of life. Prevnar prevents pneumococcal bacterial infections, which cause 40% of pediatric ear infections.

B. The CHL that results from middle ear problems such as OM can cause significantly delayed speech, language, and academic skills because the loss most often occurs during a child's critical early learning period. Early identification, referral, and treatment of middle ear disease are extremely important. Most conductive losses can be corrected through medical treatment or surgery.

C. Outer ear conditions that cause CHL include the following:
   1. Occlusion of the outer ear, from cerumen, foreign objects, tumors or malformation (e.g., mouse ear) of the pinna.
   2. Atresia of the external canal, either alone or in combination with other anomalies.
   3. Infection of the external canal (otitis externa), which may cause a mild conductive loss because of edema of the canal walls or accumulation of infectious debris.
   4. Perforation of the tympanic membrane from excessive pressure, necrosed (dead) tissue, trauma, or sudden pressure.
   5. Thickening of the tympanic membrane from middle ear infection.

D. Middle ear conditions that may cause CHL include the following:
   1. OM with effusion.
   2. Otosclerosis, a hereditary disease process of the inner ear that causes a growth of spongy bone in the middle ear and produces a progressive hearing loss when interference with the stapedial vibrations occurs; females are affected twice as often as males. Otosclerosis usually manifests between 11 and 30 years of age.
   3. Tympanosclerosis, new calcium plaques in the middle ear or on the tympanic membrane that occur as a result of OM and cause the conductive mechanism to lose mobility.
   4. Osteogenesis imperfecta (also called *brittle bone disease*), a hereditary condition whose major characteristics are multiple fractures, weak joints, blue sclera, thin translucent skin, and deafness. In a large percentage of cases, CHL occurs from otosclerotic changes; SNHL also has been identified.

SENSORINEURAL HEARING LOSS

I. Definition

    A. SNHL is a loss of hearing caused by a pathological condition in the inner ear (cochlear) or along the nerve pathway (neural) from the inner ear to the brainstem. Differentiation between sensory (cochlear) and neural (eighth cranial nerve abnormality) loss now is possible through new technology (e.g., otoacoustic emissions test), but the term *sensorineural hearing loss* still is widely used. In SNHL, sounds (pitch or timing) are distorted, in contrast to conductive loss, in which the sounds are softer but not distorted; 10% to 20% of SNHLs are progressive (Ruben, 1993).

II. Etiology

    A. SNHL may be caused by congenital defects or acquired at any time during or after birth. Postnatal causes include autoimmune or anatomical factors, trauma, ototoxic medications, infections, exposure to loud sounds, or the loss may be idiopathic (see "Additional Information"). In sensory loss, the cochlea is damaged. In neural loss, the cochlea is normal, but auditory neuropathy, an eight cranial nerve abnormality, is present so that sounds do not reach the brain in a normal fashion.

    B. The congenital defects are hereditary (genetic) or nonhereditary (acquired). A gene responsible for nonsyndromic recessive deafness (loss of hearing with no other medical complications) has been found on chromosome 17. The mutation creates a protein that prevents the hair cells in the inner ear from transmitting sound. The exact mechanism is not yet understood.

    C. Congenital cytomegalovirus (CMV) is the most common infectious, acquired cause of SNHL. CMV generally produces no symptoms, but a small number of infants (6000 to 8000 per year) have clinical symptoms, including 75% with SNHL, which may have delayed onset and may be progressive.

III. Signs, Symptoms, and History

    A. Individual may speak with excessive loudness because of loss of bone conduction.

    B. Some difficulty in speech discrimination.

    C. Better hearing in lower than in high frequencies, resulting in inability to differentiate many words that contain high-frequency consonants (e.g., fake, cake, sake).

    D. Recruitment (abnormal increase in loudness).

    E. Tinnitus—generally constant ringing or buzzing noise, localized in either ear or not localized; pitch tends to be higher in SNHL than in CHL.

    F. Air and bone conduction are nearly the same

IV. Effects on Individual

    A. Delay in speech and language development.

    B. Language deficit can cause learning problems.

    C. Vocabulary develops more slowly.

    D. Parents can become frustrated at lack of communication and child's inability to respond appropriately.

    E. May avoid social interaction with peers because of the reduced ability to understand what others are saying and poor articulation.

   F. Temper tantrums or other behavior patterns may develop out of frustration.
   G. Generally more aggressive than peers.
   H. Tends to have more physical complaints.
   I. Poor self-concept, resulting in emotional problems.
   J. Feels "different" than peers because of necessity of frequent visits to numerous helping professionals, placement in special education class, or small-group tutoring.
   K. Personal safety may become an issue.
   L. English as a second language, vision impairment, or other physical impairment compounds the effects of the hearing loss.
   M. May affect vocational choices, although new technologies are breaking down most barriers.
V. **Management/Treatment**
   A. Hearing aids or amplification (may be used as early as 4 weeks of age).
   B. Prompt treatment of OM because conductive loss compounds SNHL.
   C. Speech and language therapy.
   D. Auditory training.
   E. May be limited to prevention of further loss.
   F. Cochlear implant (electronic device surgically implanted into the cochlea with external transmitter and microphone) for profound loss with little or no benefit from hearing aids (see "Additional Information").
   G. Few treatable causes of SNHL, such as autoimmune inner ear disease (cortisone), syphilis (penicillin and cortisone), and perilymph fistula (repair).
   H. Screen vision to rule out problems because hearing-impaired individuals rely heavily on their vision, and impairments in these senses often are associated.
VI. **Additional Information**
   A. SNHL usually is not corrected through use of medication or surgery; thus prevention is the best approach. Preventive measures include genetic counseling, early prenatal care, immunizations, control of noise levels, and identification of ototoxic drugs.
   B. Prenatal (nonhereditary) causes of SNHL include rubella, influenza, Rh factor, syphilis, cytomegalovirus, anoxia, accumulation of toxic substances in the mother's bloodstream, and cerebral palsy, which has its own causes.
   C. Perinatal causes include anoxia, prematurity and multiple births, exposure to contagious disease such as hepatitis, exposure to high noise levels, and trauma (e.g., violent contractions during birth, use of high forceps).
   D. Postnatal causes include measles, mumps, whooping cough, influenza, syphilis, excessive fever, autoimmune inner ear disease, bacterial meningitis, scarlet fever, diphtheria, encephalitis, diabetes, ototoxic drugs, accumulation of toxic substances in the blood from kidney disease, acoustic nerve tumors, head trauma, and sound trauma.

E. Exposure to intense and frequent noise levels can cause temporary or permanent damage to the hair cells in the cochlea. The reduction in sensitivity occurs in the higher frequencies. *Noise-induced hearing loss (NIHL)* may occur over time and generally is so gradual and subtle that it is not noticed. It is one of the most common chronic conditions of childhood (Nash et al, 1997). NIHL also may be related to a single noise exposure. Firecrackers, fireworks, model airplane engines, and toy firearms have produced permanent hearing loss in children. A single gunshot generates the same deafening effect as listening to the roar of a motorcycle or loud rock music for 40 hours. Many teenagers incur temporary or permanent sensorineural impairment because of exposure to loud music. Temporary threshold shift largely disappears within 16 hours after exposure. Permanent damage may occur with extended exposure to sounds louder than 85 dB. The sound of a rock band at a distance of 30 ft is 110 dB. A power mower, the roar of a motorcycle, and the siren of an ambulance all exceed the safe limit. When the listener must strain to hear someone at an arm's length away, the surrounding noise is dangerous. Minimum safe exposure is for ½-hour segments without ear protection. Ear defenders may reduce the risk of NIHL. Exposure to loud sounds is especially traumatic for children with hearing aids because the sound is amplified.

F. Environmental, occupational, or household noise also causes stress-related problems, including fatigue, reduced sleep, increased frustration, difficulty in concentrating, and hypertension. Effects can be gradual, cumulative, and so subtle that they remain untreated with no determination of the underlying cause until permanent damage has occurred. Americans are losing their hearing at an increasingly younger age. The greatest increase of hearing loss has been in the 45- to 65-year age group, which is 20 years younger than expected. This increase in NIHL has led to a national campaign announced by the National Institutes of Health in 1999. The campaign, WISE EARS!, with a goal of reduced NIHL, is sponsored by the National Institute on Deafness and Other Communication Disorders (NIDCD) in collaboration with the National Institute for Occupational Safety and Health (NOSH) (see Web Sites).

G. *Cochlear implants,* also called *cochlear prostheses,* act as a substitute for the hair cells of the organ of Corti and directly stimulate the nerve fibers in the cochlea. The devices may be implanted as early as 12 months of age; results are better with earlier implantation. Increased listening is the first indication of success. Development of some speech usually occurs 2 to 3 years after implantation. Cochlear implants do not restore normal hearing but increase the ability to hear environmental sounds. Binaural implants are now available and improve hearing by reducing the distraction of environmental noises. Hearing-impaired adults may be disinclined to consider cochlear implants for their child because this may disconnect the child from their deaf culture. Cochlear implants are contraindicated with findings of an abnormal acoustic nerve.

H. The FDA approved a new implanted hearing device in 2000 for use in teenagers and adults with neurofibromatosis type 2 when tumors growing on the cranial nerves must be surgically removed. Surgery requires severing the nerve, resulting in total loss of hearing. The device is an auditory brainstem implant system that has restored at least some degree of hearing in all patients in whom the device was implanted correctly.

I. Genetic counseling is indicated when SNHL has been identified in one offspring.

MIXED CONDUCTIVE-SENSORINEURAL HEARING LOSS

I. **Definition**
   A. Hearing loss produced by abnormalities in the middle ear and along the neural pathways.

II. **Etiology**
   A. Recurrent OM may cause cochlear degeneration. Although otosclerosis generally is associated with a CHL, this disease may invade the inner ear and cause sensorineural impairment. A child with a diagnosed SNHL could develop a mixed loss when middle ear pathological conditions interfere with the conduction of sound waves through the middle ear.

III. **Signs, Symptoms, and History**
   A. A child will demonstrate signs and symptoms of both types of loss. (Refer to previous sections on CHL and SNHL.)

IV. **Effects on Individual**
   A. Delayed development of speech and language skills.
   B. Learning problems resulting from language deficit.
   C. Poor self-concept from reduced communication skills and poor academic achievement.
   D. Social isolation because of difficulty in hearing and poor articulation.

V. **Management/Treatment**
   A. Hearing aid.
   B. Treatment of conductive component.
   C. Preferential classroom seating as needed. Seating in the center of second row is preferred so that the child is close to the teacher but able to pick up visual cues from other students. Seat away from noise sources, such as air conditioners, open doors, windows, pencil sharpeners, computer centers, and aquariums.
   D. Select a "buddy" to alert the student when particularly important information is presented, to take notes, or to help clarify spoken language.
   E. Screen vision, since hearing-impaired individuals rely heavily on their vision; vision and hearing impairments are often associated.

CENTRAL AUDITORY PROCESSING DISORDERS

I. **Definition**
   A. Central auditory processing disorder (CAPD) is a decrease in auditory comprehension rather than a reduction in hearing acuity. A normal brainstem-evoked response may be present, but the child is

unable to recognize or understand speech. May have normal cognitive skills but is unable to process auditory information. Condition may be mild (e.g., learning disability) to more severely involved (e.g., autism).

II. Etiology

A. *Organic type* is caused by a congenital malformation of the auditory center; damage to the eighth cranial nerve by injury, disease such as meningitis, encephalitis, poisoning; or child abuse (head trauma). May be aphasic (expression), agnosia (sounds), or dysacusia (distortion). *Functional type* occurs as a result of sensory and/or experiential deprivation, autism, childhood schizophrenia, or conversion hysteria (withdrawal from hearing to prevent remembrance of a traumatic event).

III. Signs, Symptoms, and History

A. Unresponsive or inconsistent responses to caregiver.

B. May localize to sounds and may be sensitive to loud sounds, but speech is meaningless.

C. May be unable to inhibit response to loud sounds because of lack of cerebral control.

D. Problem areas affecting school and home behaviors include auditory figure-ground (distracted by background noise), auditory memory (difficulty remembering information such as lists and directions), auditory discrimination (difficulty distinguishing between similar-sounding words), auditory attention (cannot maintain focus), and auditory cohesion problems (difficulty drawing inferences, comprehending abstract information, or solving riddles).

IV. Effects on Individual

A. Development of speech and language skills is lacking or very limited.

B. Frustration caused by inability to communicate.

C. Development of self-stimulatory behaviors.

D. Difficulty following directions.

E. Unusually bothered or easily distracted by loud or sudden noises.

F. Withdrawal.

G. Tendency to confuse similar-sounding words.

V. Management/Treatment

A. Use of signing or simple communication.

B. Close attention and response to child's cues.

C. Use of communication board.

D. Reduce background noise.

E. Use of simple meaningful sentences, speaking more slowly.

F. Have student repeat directions back.

G. Taking notes and making lists, wearing a watch.

VI. Additional Information

A. Several techniques have been developed for use with children with severe CAPD or autism. One technique is auditory integration training (AIT), developed by Guy Berard. AIT uses filtered electronically, modulated music (Berard, 1993). AIT is completed in 10 hours over a 10-day period. The American Academy of Audiology published a position statement declaring these techniques to be experimental and urging more research to establish their efficacy (American Academy of Audiology, 1993).

UNILATERAL HEARING LOSS

I. Definition
   A. Hearing loss in one ear with normal hearing in the other ear. Prevalent data suggest that 16 to 19 children in 1000 have unilateral losses that are potentially educationally significant (ASHA, 1993).

II. Etiology
   A. May be conductive or sensorineural.

III. Signs, Symptoms, and History
   A. Usually have difficulty localizing sounds and voices.
   B. May have difficulty hearing faint or distant speech.
   C. Background noises impede speech detection.

IV. Effects on Individual
   A. May become fatigued because of greater effort needed to listen.
   B. May be perceived as having selective hearing or to be inattentive because of discrepancies in ability to understand speech in quiet versus noisy environment.
   C. Frustration may lead to behavior problems.
   D. On average, children with unilateral hearing loss are one full grade behind their peers academically.

V. Management/Treatment
   A. Generally given preferential seating.
   B. Hearing aid, may have a contralateral routing of signals (CROS) hearing aid.
   C. May benefit from a personal or soundfield frequency modulation (FM) system.
   D. Close monitoring is needed to avoid secondary complications, since a child may be thought to be noncompliant or inattentive, which may lead to behavior disorders.

VI. Additional Information
   A. Many children with hearing impairment may be overactive, probably because poor auditory input results in inattention followed by overcompensation or hyperactivity. They may be easily distracted from tasks because auditory input is diminished. Students with hearing loss may tend to have an external locus of control. They feel a loss of personal control and may place responsibility on parent, teacher, or hearing aids rather than accepting it for themselves.
   B. Use of a hearing aid alone does not achieve optimal listening condition because the aid amplifies both the teacher's voice and environmental noise. Classroom noise can be reduced by use of carpets, sound-absorbing tiles and drapes, and by closing doors and windows. Noise, reverberation, and distance (NRD) are factors affecting the ability to hear in a classroom. Noise masks speech, the echo in a classroom smears speech, and the distance from teacher to student affects the decibel level of the speech and limits visual cues. NRD affects consonants more than vowels because vowels are louder. Consonant sounds are low energy and do not become louder even when

the voice is raised. English is a consonant-dependent language, and speech is garbled when the consonants are lost.

C. The signal-to-noise ratio is significant; this relates to the loudness of the teacher's voice compared with the environmental noise. For students with normal hearing, the teacher's voice should be +6 dB; for those with hearing impairment, it should be +15 dB. Typical signal-to-noise ratio in a classroom is −7 to +5 dB. This can be overcome by using a personal or soundfield FM system. Classroom acoustics also are critical for students with attention deficit hyperactivity disorder (ADHD), CAPD, and those with English as a second language.

HEARING AIDS

EVALUATING HEARING AID FUNCTIONING

The following factors can affect the proper functioning of hearing aids:

I. **Insufficient Amplification**
   A. Dead batteries.
   B. Wires or tubing detached.
   C. Aid turned off; volume too low.
   D. Improper mold.
   E. Wax or other material in ear or mold.
   F. Unsuitable aid for degree of loss.

II. **Acoustic Feedback**
   A. Lower the volume of the aid.
   B. Reinsert the aid, making certain no hair is caught between ear mold and canal.
   C. Clean the ear mold/ear.

III. **Whistling Noise**
   A. Improperly worn.
   B. Improperly made.
   C. Worn out—crack in the tubing.
   D. Hearing may be worse, and child is turning volume up too high.

IV. **Discomfort from Mold**
   A. OM.
   B. Ear tumor.
   C. Improperly fitted mold.
   D. Ear skin or cartilage infection.

CAUTION: Batteries may cause severe injury or death if swallowed; batteries are difficult to remove from the esophagus. Batteries should be kept in a child-proof place and should not be changed in the presence of young children.

Box 2-4	*Hearing Aid Settings*

O = Off
T = Telecoil/telephone for telephone pickup or FM usage
M = Microphone/telecoil for hearing others and own voice
DAI = Direct audio input for connection with assistive listening devices

Table 2-6	*Classifications of Hearing Function**
Hearing Loss (dB)	**Effects/Educational Implications**
Mild (26-40)	Soft or distant speech may be difficult. At 30 dB, child can miss up to 10% of speech signals. Preferential seating indicated. Auditory learning dysfunction: mild language delay, mild speech problems, inattention may manifest. Child may experience fatigue because of listening effort needed. Auditory training, FM systems, speech therapy beneficial. Without amplification, child with 35-40 dB loss can miss at least 50% of class discussion; 25 dB HL is approximately amount heard with fingers in both ears.
Moderate (41-55)	Conversation speech understood at distance of 3-5 ft (face-to-face). Without amplification, child with 50 dB loss may miss 80%-100% of speech signal. May have limited vocabulary and articulation difficulties but should have good rhythm. Preferential seating, hearing aid, auditory training/FM system, and speech therapy indicated. Able to speak on telephone; can usually understand speech by hearing alone. Children rarely attend special schools or classes for deaf.
Moderately severe (56-70)	Others must speak loudly to be understood. Difficulty participating in classroom discussions. Usually cannot understand speech by hearing alone. Able to speak on telephone. Visual cues increase acquisition of speech and language. Speech should have good rhythm, tone, and articulation. Full-time amplification is essential. Preferential seating, speech and language therapy indicated. Requires resource specialist or special class depending on extent of language delay.
Severe (71-90)	May hear voices close to ear (about 1 ft). May discriminate environmental sounds. May distinguish vowels, but many consonants will be distorted. Language may not develop spontaneously and will be defective if hearing loss occurs before age 1 yr. May benefit from total communication approach, especially in early years. Auditory amplification necessary. Special education that focuses on speech, language, and auditory training needed. After sufficient training in special education, child may enter regular classroom but still requires speech therapy.
Profound (≥91)	Some loud noises may be audible. Vision is primary method for learning and communication. Speech and language are defective; if loss is present before 1 yr, will not develop spontaneously. Requires special education or schools for deaf. Amplification is used for auditory awareness, voice control, and spatial orientation. May be considered for cochlear implant as young as 12 mo (FDA approval granted in 2000). Vibrotactile or electrotactile hearing aids may be used to support lip-reading, increase awareness of environmental sounds, and for training of speech production and reception.

*These descriptions are meant as guidelines only. They are not intended for use as labels or to influence expectations for the development of communication. The ability to develop communication in a variety of modalities varies among individuals.

TESTING PROCEDURES

PURE TONE SCREENING

Children as young as 3 years old frequently can be conditioned for pure tone audiometric screening. Early identification of hearing and communicative problems is vital because intervention in the early years can avoid or minimize educational difficulties when the child begins academic activities.

I. **Screening Criteria**
    A. In 1997 the American Speech-Language-Hearing Association (ASHA) issued new *Guidelines for Audiologic Screening*. The guidelines are age-based, with separate criteria for 7 months through 2 years, preschool children ages 3 to 5 years, and school-age children ages 5 through 18 years.
    B. The National Association of School Nurses (NASN) has published a manual, *The Ear and Hearing: A Guide for School Nurses* (1998). In the absence of state or district guidelines, pure tone audiometric screening is recommended for students as follows:
        1. In prekindergarten, kindergarten, and grades 1, 3, and 5.
        2. In higher grades as time allows.
        3. Newly enrolled students in school without record of passing a hearing screening.
        4. Referred for or in special education (as required by PL 94-142).
        5. Failing previous screenings.
        6. Having frequent upper respiratory infections or middle ear problems.
        7. Referred by student, teacher, parent, or concerned third party.
    C. ASHA adds screening in the second grade, eliminates screening in the fifth grade, but adds screening in seventh and eleventh grades. The upper grades are added because of the increased potential for hearing loss among adolescents because of overexposure to high levels of noise and the importance of identifying hearing impairment that may affect their educational or career opportunities after graduation.

II. **Screening Procedure**
    A. NASN recommends screening at 25 dB when there is no sound proof room. ASHA guidelines recommend screening at 20 dB.
        1. Select quietest room possible.
        2. Let audiometer warm up for approximately 10 minutes.
        3. Check that earphones are plugged into correct jacks in audiometer.
        4. Put on earphones and verify that audiometer and earphones are working properly by testing all frequencies bilaterally at comfortable hearing level.
        5. Determine what form of signal will be most appropriate to indicate that tone has been heard (e.g., raising hand or fingers, saying "yes," or using signal light). Be certain individual understands that signal must be given the first time tone is heard, even if the tone is barely audible.
        6. Place earphones on each ear (red on right and blue on left) and adjust them for proper fit.

7. Set hearing threshold level (HTL) at 25 dB.
8. Starting with right ear, present tone at 2000 Hz for 1 to 2 seconds, proceed to 4000 Hz, finish at 1000 Hz.
9. Repeat same procedures for left ear.
10. Tone may be repeated, but not above 25 dB.
11. Do not establish a pattern or rhythm; vary length of tone and pauses.

III. **Failure Criteria**
   A. NASN recommends rescreening after 2 to 3 weeks if one frequency is missed in either ear. ASHA recommends rescreening at the same session if possible, after reinstructing the student and repositioning the earphones. Each state generally has its own standards and criteria.

IV. **Action**
   A. Both NASN and ASHA recommend referral for professional evaluation after failing two sweep-check screenings. Some states, school districts, and public funding agencies require pure tone threshold testing before making a referral.

PURE TONE THRESHOLD

I. **Screening Criteria**
   A. Those who have failed the pure tone screening should be tested at 250, 500, 1000, 2000, 4000, and 8000 Hz, plus 3000 and 6000 Hz at times. A modified threshold test includes testing at 1000, 2000, and 4000 Hz and is the method described here.
   B. The first six steps are pure tone screening procedure.
      1. Begin testing the right ear at 1000 Hz at 40 dB. Maintain each tone presented during testing for 1 to 2 seconds.
      2. If there is response at 40 dB, drop back in 10-dB steps until there is no longer a response, then increase in 5-dB steps until sound is audible.
      3. If there is no initial response at 40 dB, present the tone at 60 dB. If there is no response at 60 dB, stop testing at that frequency and indicate on student record "does not hear at 60 dB."
      4. If the student responds at 60 dB, drop back in 10-dB steps until there is no longer a response, then increase in 5-dB steps until sound is audible.
      5. Drop back 10 dB and ascend in 5-dB steps two more times to determine accuracy of threshold. Threshold is lowest level at which correct response is given two out of three times a tone is presented.
      6. As you obtain thresholds for each frequency, record results numerically or in graph form (audiogram) on data sheet.
      7. Impedance should be administered and results added to those obtained from pure tone audiometry.
      8. When testing children, particularly younger ones, periodically remind them that signal must be given as soon as they hear the tone.
      9. Conditioned play audiometry (CPA) is an effective method of testing 3- and 4-year-olds; CPA is described in the section "Infant, Preschool, and Special Education Screening."

II. Failure Criteria
A. NASN recommends that children be referred for threshold level of 30 dB or more for two or more sounds in one ear and threshold level of 35 dB or more for one tone in either ear. ASHA recommends rescreening at the same session if possible, after reinstructing the student and repositioning the earphones. Each state generally has its own standards and criteria.

III. Action
A. Notify parents of results and recommend evaluation by a physician, otolaryngologist, or audiologist. Give parents a form letter that includes test results and space for the physician's report and recommendations.

IV. Additional Information
A. A screening tool developed for use by teachers is the Screening Instrument for Targeting Educational Risk (SIFTER). It consists of 15 questions relating to a student's school performance when hearing problems are suspected. Areas covered are academics, attention, communication, class participation, and school behavior. Completion of the questionnaire provides information helpful to the nurse and audiologist in completing more thorough testing; helpful as a pretest and posttest when evaluating the benefit of personal or classroom amplification; also used as in-service instrument with teachers to discuss possible effects of hearing impairment on learning. Available through Educational Audiology Association at 1-800-460-7322 or at http://www.edaud.org.

IMPEDANCE/IMMITTANCE AUDIOMETRY

Impedance (immittance) is an objective, rapid, efficient, and noninvasive means of measuring the compliance/mobility of the tympanic membrane and air pressure of the middle ear. It can be used for screening large populations of children but is best used as a part of a comprehensive screening program rather than as a single measure. No special testing environment is necessary, and no response from the child is required.

In a normal ear, loud sounds cause the stapedius muscle to momentarily contract, which stiffens the ossicles and immediately lowers the membrane compliance. The muscles in both ears contract in response to a stimulus delivered in only one ear (bilateral response). This stapedial reflex generally is absent when a conductive hearing loss exists. The muscle contraction has little effect on a tympanic membrane immobilized by fluid or by fixation of the ossicle. No observable effect is present in cases of perforated membrane or discontinuity of the ossicular chain.

Impedance also determines whether the stapedial reflex is present. Some instruments also include a report of physical volume, which provides the examiner with the cavity size of the external ear canal measured in cubic centimeters. A shortened physical volume may indicate blockage or presence of a foreign object. A report of physical volume can be helpful when a child has had tubes inserted for chronic OM. When tubes are intact and functioning, the physical volume is above normal limits. If the tubes have become dislodged or are blocked by drainage or wax, the volume is normal.

I. **Screening Criteria**
    A. ASHA recommends screening all children at risk for middle ear problems, especially those younger than age 7 (ASHA, 1993).

II. **Screening Procedure**
    A. Before testing, examine external auditory canal with an otoscope for size, obstruction, inflammation, or any abnormalities. Do not test if pain, drainage, or apparent problem is present, which indicates immediate referral to a physician.
    B. Explain procedure and offer reassurance that test is not painful.
    C. Use appropriate probe tip; it should be larger than meatus because objective is to obtain airtight seal.
    D. To obtain best seal, ear canal must be straightened. In ages 12 months to 3 years, pinna must be pulled downward and backward. For children older than 3 years, pull the pinna upward and back, with the head tilted slightly away from examiner.
    E. Apply the probe firmly to canal opening.
    F. Hold probe steady until machine indicates test is completed. Remove probe.
    G. Results may be in numerical or digital display or form depending on the type of instrument used.
    H. A number of impedance machines are available on the market; each machine has its own method of operation; therefore follow manufacturer's guidelines.
    I. Record results and make appropriate referral if needed.

III. **Additional Information**
    A. To check compliance of the tympanic membrane, introduce positive pressure into the external ear canal with a probe tip. As this positive pressure (measured in millimeters of water, mm H_2O) is released, it gradually changes to negative pressure, and the membrane moves. The degree of movement is known as *middle compliance* (measured in cubic centimeters, cm^3) and is recorded by numerical digital display or on a graph. The air pressure required for the membrane to reach maximum compliance is recorded as middle ear pressure. Results of compliance and air pressure convey information regarding the state of the middle ear and function of the eustachian tube. Abnormal readings identify the possibility of middle ear disease.
    B. Often young children become very fearful of the probe, regardless of how well the examiner explains what will be heard and offers assurance of no discomfort. Sometimes the child's fear is alleviated if the testers demonstrate on themselves, a doll, or a stuffed animal. (If possible, the examiner can place the probe on the child's hand because contact with the skin will cause the same humming sound as when the probe is placed in the canal.) Rather than upsetting the child and ruining the chance of a later attempt, the examiner should offer reassurance and understanding and let the child watch while others are tested. When an entire class is to be screened, demonstration of the procedure to the group before individual testing is recommended.

C. Pure tone screening is inadequate for detecting a large percentage of children with OM because the conductive hearing loss may not be significant enough for the child to fail screening standards. Pure tone screening and impedance complement each other; inclusion of both in a hearing screening program is highly recommended.

D. The complete impedance/immittance testing battery includes tympanometry, static compliance, acoustic reflex threshold measurement, ear canal physical volume test (PVT), and behavioral observation.

INFANT, PRESCHOOL, AND SPECIAL EDUCATION SCREENING

Several developmental screening tools and methods can be used to screen an infant's or young child's hearing. Numerous states have passed newborn screening legislation that mandates auditory screening of newborns and should greatly increase the number of infants identified with hearing losses; this practice hopefully will result in early intervention. This section provides screening criteria and descriptions of several of the better-known tests, including the appropriate age group and source of further information. When a hearing loss is suspected, the physician and audiologist should perform a complete medical and audiological assessment as soon as possible.

EARLY CHILDHOOD SCREENING CRITERIA

The JCIH recommends a hearing evaluation every 6 months until 3 years of age if certain high-risk indicators are present, even when results of birth screening are negative (see Table 2-5). Monitoring should continue at appropriate intervals to detect delayed onset of sensorineural or conductive hearing loss.

I. **Otoacoustic Emission (OAE) Response**
   A. Appropriate age.
      1. Newborns; infants, and preschoolers who cannot follow instructions for behavioral procedures.
   B. Summary of test.
      1. Both transient evoked otacoustic emissions (TEOAEs) or distortion product otacoustic emissions (DPOAEs), are sensitive to hair cell dysfunction. OAE is a measurement of the inner ear (cochlear) response to a sound introduced into the external ear. This response is obtained by placing a microphone in the external ear and connecting it to a computer that provides an objective interpretation. OAE detects both sensory (cochlear or inner ear) and recurrent CHL and is measured in decibel sound pressure level (dBSPL).
      2. OAEs do not detect neural (eighth nerve) loss or auditory brainstem pathway dysfunction. Factors affecting quality of testing include probe fit, environmental noise, and internal (subject) noise. Newborns have a considerable amount of internal noise that decreases by 4-5 months of age.
   C. Additional information.
      1. Devices are now easier to use and available for use in the schools from school health supply suppliers. As the technology improves, OAEs will play an increasingly important role in screening and may eventually replace pure tone audiometry.

II. Electrophysiological Procedures
    A. Appropriate age.
        1. Birth through preschool or older children who are difficult to test or have developmental/cognitive or physical impairments.
    B. Summary of test.
        1. These procedures may be called *automated auditory brainstem response (AABR), auditory brainstem response (ABR), brainstem auditory evoked response (BAER),* or *evoked response audiometry (ERA).* The child must be relaxed or sleeping, which usually requires mild sedation. Rapid clicking sounds are presented through earphones, and brain wave patterns are recorded as measured through electrodes placed on the child's scalp. Activity of the cochlea, eighth cranial nerve, and auditory brainstem pathway are measured and can detect auditory neuropathy or neural disorders. Use of bone conduction AABR in conjunction with the traditional air conduction AABR discriminates CHL from SNHL and assesses the extent of conductive involvement.
    C. Additional information.
        1. Both OAEs and ABRs can produce false-negative results; behavioral testing is recommended in high-risk infants or when language delay is noted.

III. Visual Reinforcement Audiometry (VRA)
    A. Appropriate age.
        1. Approximately 6 to 24 months, or children unable to tolerate earphones.
    B. Summary of test.
        1. Behavioral testing, which also may be called *conditioned orientation reflex (COR)* or *condition orienting response audiometry (CORA)* is a subjective measure of hearing. The child is seated in a sound-conditioned booth on an adult's lap. Lighted mechanical toys are flashed on simultaneously with an auditory signal (speech or warble tone) to the right or left of the child's visual field. The child responds by turning toward source of sound and is rewarded by seeing the lighted action toy. In this sound field testing environment, results provide measurement of hearing for the better ear only because the child is using both ears to respond to the sounds. When the child is able to tolerate earphones, further testing should be done to obtain ear-specific information.

IV. Conditioned Play Audiometry
    A. Appropriate age.
        1. CPA can be used for pure tone screening of children 2½ to 5 years old and children with developmental delay.
    B. Summary of test.
        1. Before testing, the child is conditioned to drop blocks or other small objects into a container when a tone from the audiometer is presented. The earphones are left on the table, and the examiner plays the game with the child until the child's response is appropriate and consistent. The earphones are then securely

placed on the child, and the examiner proceeds with the pure tone screening or audiogram. Sounds may be presented through loudspeakers if the child is unable to tolerate earphones.

WEB SITES

American Academy of Audiology
 1-800-AAA-2336
 http://www.audiology.org
American Society for Deaf Children
 717-334-7922
 http://www.deafchildren.org/
American Speech-Language-Hearing Association
 1-800-498-2071
 Consumer site: http://www.asha.org
 Professional site: http://www.professional.asha.org/index.htm
National Association of the Deaf
 301-587-1788
 http://www.nad.org
National Institute on Deafness and Other Communication Disorders
National Institutes of Health
 301-496-7243
 http://www.nidcd.nih.gov
WISE EARS!
National campaign to combat noise-induced hearing loss
 1-800-241-1044
 http://www.nidcd.nih.gov/health/wise

GLOSSARY OF HEARING TERMS

Adventitious   Accidental, referring to relatively sudden loss of hearing.

Agnosia   Inability to understand significance of sounds.

Air conduction   Pathway of sounds conducted to the inner ear by the outer and middle ear.

Aphasia   Partial or complete loss of expressive and receptive language; most commonly an incomplete mixture of both receptive and expressive aphasia. Causes include stroke, head trauma, or prolonged hypoxia. May be transient.

Articulation   Vocal tract movements for production of speech. Articulate speech is distinct and connected.

Assistive listening device   Any device used to enhance ability to hear by reducing background noise, amplifying sound, and overcoming negative effects of distance. Includes amplified telephones, one-to-one communicators, and frequency modulation (FM) systems.

Atelectasis of tympanic membrane   Collapse or retraction of the tympanic membrane; may or may not be associated with otitis media.

Audiogram   Graphic representation of audiometric findings.

Audiologist   One skilled in the identification, measurement, and rehabilitation of people with hearing impairments and related disorders (e.g., vestibular dysfunction, tinnitus).

Auditory perception   Ability to identify, interpret, and attach meaning to sound.

Auditory prosthesis   Device that substitutes or enhances the ability to hear.

Auditory training   Lessons to assist a person with hearing loss to maximize residual hearing.

Augmentative devices   Technical tools to assist individuals with limited or no speech, such as text telephones, communication boards, and conversion software translating text to speech.

Auricle   See Pinna.

Bel   Unit of measure expressing the ratios of acoustical or electrical power.

Bone conduction   Sounds conducted to the inner ear through mechanical vibrations in the bones of the skull.

Cholesteatoma   Cystic mass in middle ear composed of cholesterol and epithelial cells as a result of a congenital defect or chronic otitis media. Requires surgical removal.

Cholesterol granuloma   A serious complication of acute otitis media in which a chronic collection of infection and cholesterol crystals have formed a solid mass.

Cochlea   Spiral bony structure in the inner ear that transforms sound waves into nerve impulses that are sent to the brain; it is part of the bony labyrinth.

Cochlear nerve   One of the main divisions of the eighth cranial nerve; responsible for hearing and balance; also called *auditory nerve.*

Compliance   Inverse of stiffness.

Contralateral routing of signal   Contralateral routing of signal (CROS) is a hearing aid for persons with normal or near-normal hearing in one ear and an unaidable loss in the other ear. This device allows a person to have two-sided hearing by channeling all the signal into the "good" ear.

Decibel (dB)   A decibel (dB) is the unit of measurement of intensity in acoustics and audiometrics; one tenth of a bel.

Dysacusia   Distortion of intensity or frequency of sounds.

Dysfluency   Disruption in smooth flow of speech.

Eustachian tube   Tube lined with mucous membrane that connects the nasopharynx and the middle ear cavity. Usually remains closed but opens during chewing, swallowing, and yawning.

Eustachian tube dysfunction   Tube does not open when needed to equalize pressure between the middle ear space and the atmospheric pressure. Most common cause is an inflammatory reaction of the membranous lining of the tube with nasal infections or allergies. Other reasons include enlargement of adenoids, developmental anomalies (e.g., cleft palate, cleft uvula), or immaturity of palatal muscles that often do not mature until after 12 months. May be acute or become chronic.

Frequency   Number of complete oscillations of a vibrating body per second. Physical attribute of sound measured in hertz (Hz).

Frequency modulation systems   Frequency modulation (FM) systems provide amplification of voice. They may be personal units or soundfield units for an entire classroom. The teacher wears a personal microphone for either method. Personal units require a receiver to be worn by the student or the placement of a boom box near the student. Sound field units require 2-4 loudspeakers mounted on the walls or ceiling. The soundfield system eliminates the identification of any one child as having special needs, and amplification has been shown to be advantageous for students with learning disabilities.

Hearing threshold level   Hearing threshold level (HTL) is the lowest level at which the pure tone audiometer stimulates normal hearing; hearing-level dial is calibrated in dB HTL.

Hertz   Hertz (Hz) is the number of cycles per second (cps).

Impedance   Term is interchangeable with immittance. Opposition to sound wave transmission, which is made up of frictional resistance, mass, and stiffness and influenced by frequency.

Incus   An anvil-shaped bone, one of the three ossicles in the middle ear; transmits sound from the malleus to the stapes.

Labyrinthitis   Infection or inflammation of the inner ear; affects balance and may cause temporary hearing loss.

Language   The structured, symbolic, and accepted system of interpersonal communication.

Malleus   One of the three ossicles in the middle ear, shaped like a hammer; transmits sounds from the tympanic membrane to the incus.

Mastoiditis   Infection of the mastoid process.

Meatus   Opening or passage.

Meniscus   A fluid line; when fluids are present in the middle ear, the meniscus is sometimes seen through the tympanic membrane.

Myringotomy   Surgical incision in tympanic membrane to relieve pressure by draining fluid or pus from the middle ear.

Neurofibromatosis type 1   Neurofibromatosis type 1 (NF-1) is also called *von Recklinghausen's disease;* an inherited multisystem disorder in which nonmalignant tumors grow on the skin and nerves that may include the cochlear nerve. Symptoms of NF-1 include café-au-lait spots, axillary and inguinal freckling, bone lesions, optic gliomas, and neurofibromas. Individuals with NF-1 often have learning disabilities.

Neurofibromatosis type 2   Neurofibromatosis type 2 (NF-2) is characterized by family history and bilateral nonmalignant tumors on the eighth cranial nerve. NF-2 may occur in the teenage years and cause hearing loss. Individuals with NF-1 often have learning disabilities.

Noise-induced hearing loss   Hearing loss caused by exposure to harmful sounds, either very loud impulse sound(s) or repeated exposure to sounds above 90-dB levels over an extended time.

Ossicular discontinuity   Disconnection of the ossicles, resulting in hearing loss. May be caused by retraction pockets, cholesteatomas, or a perforation of the eardrum.

Osteogenesis imperfecta   Hereditary disorder characterized by multiple fractures; also called *brittle bone disease.* Sixty percent of affected individuals have conductive hearing loss by adolescence or young adulthood.

Osteopetrosis   Inherited disorder with generalized increase in bone density. In severe forms, bones in the skull may become so dense that they cause compression of cranial nerves, resulting in deafness, blindness, and early death.

Otitis externa   Inflammation or infection of the external canal or auricle. Major causes are bacteria, allergies (nickel or chromium in earrings or chemicals in hair sprays or cosmetics), fungi, viruses, and trauma. Excessive swimming may wash out protective cerumen, remove skin lipids, and lead to secondary infection (also called *swimmer's ear*).

Otitis media   Acute otitis media (AOM) is fluid in the middle ear with signs or symptoms of ear infection (bulging eardrum, pain, perforated eardrum) and usually requires treatment with antibiotics. Otitis media with effusion (fluid) (OME) is otitis media without signs or symptoms of ear infection and does not usually require antibiotics.

Otoplasty   Plastic surgery of the outer ear.

Otorrhea   Malodorous discharge from the external ear. May be serous, sanguinous, purulent, or contain cerebrospinal fluid.

Otosclerosis   Formation of spongy bone in the middle ear, usually around the footplate of the stapes and oval window; a progressive conductive hearing loss results when it interferes with stapedial vibration.

Ototoxic drugs   Drugs such as a special class of antibiotics, aminoglycosides, that may have a harmful affect on the eighth cranial nerve; may cause deafness or severe hearing loss. Other such drugs include aspirin, furosemide, and quinine.

Perilymph fistula   A leak of the inner ear fluid into the middle ear; most commonly the result of head trauma.

Pinna   Projected part of the external ear (auricle); gathers sound waves from the environment.

Pressure-equalizing tubes   Pressure-equalizing (PE) tubes are inserted in the tympanic membrane to equalize pressure between the inner ear and the middle ear. Usually temporary and become dislodged, falling out in less than a year. Permanent tubes may be sutured into place when needed over long term.

Pure tone   Sound waves of only one frequency.

Pure tone average   Pure tone average (PTA) is the average hearing loss, in decibels, across all frequencies in an individual's better ear. Sometimes screened at only 500, 1000, and 2000 Hz.

Recruitment   Large increase in the perceived loudness of a signal after a relatively small increase in intensity above threshold; symptomatic of some sensorineural hearing losses.

Round window   Opening in the medial wall of the middle ear leading into the cochlea; covered by a secondary tympanic membrane.

Semicircular canals   Three bony, fluid-filled canals in the inner ear that make up the largest part of the vestibular system, which is associated with the sense of balance.

Stapedius reflex threshold   Lowest intensity at which a sound causes the stapedius muscle to contract.

Stapes   One of the three ossicles, resembles a tiny stirrup. Transmits vibrations from the incus to the inner ear.

Tadoma   Method of tactile speech transmission used by deaf-blind whereby a carefully positioned hand is used to sense vibrations, movement, and airflow on the face of the speaker.

Threshold   Level at which a tone is perceived as barely audible; usual clinical criteria demand the subject be aware of the sound 50% of the time presented.

Tinnitus   Sounds in the ear; described as ringing, roaring, buzzing, and so on.

Tympanocentesis   Process of inserting a needle through the tympanic membrane to aspirate fluid from the middle ear for evaluation or treatment.

Tympanogram   A graph plotting the compliance of the tympanic membrane at specific air pressures.

Tympanosclerosis   Calcium formations in the middle ear or on the tympanic membrane; caused by otitis media; results in loss of mobility of the conductive mechanism.

Vestibular apparatus   Structures in the inner ear related to balance and sense of position; includes the vestibule and the semicircular canals.

Vibrotactile hearing aid   Sensations produced by electrical stimulation of the nerves that lead from touch receptors in the skin. Surface electrodes on the skin deliver stimulation signals to convey sounds through sense of touch. Single-channel aids are worn on the wrist, multichannel on the forearm, neck, or abdomen. May also be called *electrotactile aids* (Tactaid, Audiological Engineering Corp, Somerville, MA; Minivib, Special Instrument AB, Lidingo, Sweden; TAM, Summit, London, United Kingdom).

ABBREVIATIONS OF HEARING TERMS

AABR Automated auditory brainstem response
ABR Auditory brainstem response
ALDs Assistive listening devices
AOM Acute otitis media
BAER Brainstem auditory evoked response
BOA Behavioral observation audiometry
CPA Conditioned play audiometry
DPOAE Distortion product otoacoustic emissions (two pure tone stimuli are presented at the same time)
dBSPL Decibel sound pressure level
EOAE Evoked otoacoustic emissions
ERA Evoked response audiometry
HTL Hearing threshold level
OME Otitis media with effusion
PET Pressure-equalizing tubes
PTA Pure tone average
SDT Speech detection threshold
TEOAE Transient evoked otoacoustic emissions (elicited by brief acoustic stimuli such as clicks or tone bursts)
TM Tympanic membrane
VRA Visual reinforcement audiometry

BIBLIOGRAPHY

American Speech-Language-Hearing Association: *Guidelines for audiologic screening,* 1997, Available online: http://www.professional.asha.org. Accessed September 2000.
American Speech-Language-Hearing Association: Guidelines for audiology services in the schools, *ASHA* 35(suppl 10):24-32, 1993.

American Academy of Pediatrics: Policy statement, *Pediatrics* 103(2):527-530, 1999.

Anshel J: *Smart medicine for your eyes,* New York, 1999, Avery.

Anshel J: *Visual ergonomics in the workplace,* London, 1998, Athenaeum Press.

Ashwill J, Droske S: *Nursing care of children: principles and practice,* Philadelphia, 1997, WB Saunders.

Atkinson J, Braddick O: Sensory and perceptual capacities in the neonate. In Straton P, editor: *Psychobiology of the human newborn,* Chichester, UK, 1982, Wiley.

Bacal DA, Wilson MC: Strabismus: getting it straight, *Contemp Pediatr* 17(2):49-60, 2000.

Batshaw M, editor: *Children with disabilities,* ed 4, Baltimore, 1997, Brookes.

Berard G: *Hearing equals behavior,* New Caanan, Conn, 1993, Keats.

Bowden K, Dickey S, Greenberg C: *Children and their families: the continuum of care,* Philadelphia, 1998, WB Saunders.

Burns CE et al: *Pediatric primary care: a handbook for nurse practitioners,* ed 2, Philadelphia, 2000, WB Saunders.

California Department of Education: *First look: vision evaluation and assessment for infants, toddlers, preschoolers, birth through 5 years of age,* (Pub No 1388), Sacramento, Calif, 1998, Special Education Division.

Chen D, editor: *Essential elements in early intervention: visual impairment and multiple disabilities,* New York, 1999, AFB Press.

Chen D, Friedman C, Cavello G: *Parents and visually impaired infants: identifying visual impairment in infants (PAVII),* Louisville, Ky, 1990, American Printing House for the Blind.

Evans A: Color-vision deficiency: what does it mean? *J School Nurs* 8(4):6-10, 1992.

Hall JW, Chase P: Answers to 10 common clinical questions about otoacoustic emissions today, *Hearing Journal* 46(10):29-32, 1993.

Hickok G, Bellugi U, Klima E: Sign language in the brain, *Sci Am* 284(6):58-65, 2001.

Hoyt C, Jastrzebski G, Marg E: Delayed visual maturation in infancy, *Br J Ophthalmol* 67:127-130, 1983.

Hubel D, Wiesel T: Brain mechanisms of vision, *Sci Am* 241(3):150-162, 1979.

Joint Committee on Infant Hearing: *Principles and guidelines for early hearing detection and intervention programs: year 2000 position statement from the JCIH,* McLean, Va, 2000, American Academy of Audiology. Available online: http://www.audiology.org.

Kotulak R: *Inside the brain: revolutionary discoveries of how the mind works,* Kansas City, Mo, 1996, Andrews & McMeel.

Kushner B: Amblyopia. In Nelson LB, editor: *Harley's pediatric ophthalmology,* ed 4, Philadelphia, 1998, WB Saunders.

Nash DB et al: When loud noises hurt, *Contemp Pediatr* 14(6):97-109, 1997.

National Institute on Deafness and Other Communication Disorders (NIDCD): *WISE EARS!* September 2000, Available online: http://www.nidcd.nih.gov/health/wise/index.htm. Accessed September 4, 2000.

Neff J: Visual acuity testing, *J Emerg Nurs* 17(6):431-436, 1991.

Nelson LB: *Harley's pediatric ophthalmology,* ed 4, Philadelphia, 1998, WB Saunders.

Niskar AS, Kieszak SM, Holmes A, et al: Prevalence of hearing loss among children 6 to 19 years of age: the Third National Health and Nutrition Examination Survey, *JAMA* 279(14):1071-1075, 1998.

Northern J, editor: *Position statement: auditory integration training,* May 25, 1993, American Academy of Audiology, Available online: http://www.audiology.org. Accessed September 4, 2000.

Pappas DG: *Diagnosis and treatment of hearing impairment in children,* ed 2, San Diego, 1998, Singular.

Payan-Langston D: *Manual of ocular diagnosis and therapy,* ed 3, Boston, 1991, Little, Brown.

Prevent Blindness America: *Children and eye problems,* Sept 18, 1998, Volunteer eye health and safety organization, Available online: http://www.preventblindness.org/children. Accessed Mar 12, 2000.

Roizen NJ, Diefendorf AO: Hearing loss in children, *Pediatr Clin North Am* 46(1):1-16, 1999.

Rosenthal O, Phillips R: *Coping with color-blindness,* New York, 1997, Avery.

Ruben RJ: Early identification of hearing impairment in infants and young children, *Int J Pediatr Otolaryngol* 27:207-213, 1993.

Russell KE, Coffin C, Kenna M: Cochlear implants and the deaf child: a nursing perspective, *Pediatr Nurs* 25(4):396-400, 1999.

Sato-Viacrucis K: The evolution of the Snellen E to the blackbird, *School Nurse* Spring:18-19, 1985.

Slattery WH III, Fayad JN: Cochlear implants in children with sensorineural inner ear hearing loss, *Pediatr Ann* 28(6):359-363, 1999.

Vohr BR: Screening infants for hearing impairment, *J Pediatr* 128(7):710-714, 1996.

Wiesel T, Hubel D: Single responses in striate cortex of kittens deprived of vision in one eye, *J Neurophysiol* 26:1003-1017, 1963.

Wong D: *Whaley and Wong's nursing care of infants and children,* ed 5, St Louis, 1995, Mosby.

Wright KW: *Pediatric ophthalmology for pediatricians,* Baltimore, 1999, Williams & Wilkins.

Wright K, Spiegel P: *Pediatric ophthalmology and strabismus,* St Louis, 1999, Mosby.

CHAPTER 3

Acute Conditions

The number of school-age children who come to school with an acute illness is difficult to estimate. Frequently, nurses in the school and community setting are the first called on to determine whether a health problem exists and if further assessment is required. Thus the nurse must be aware of signs and symptoms of individual illness, be able to provide the necessary initial management, and make appropriate and informative referrals for additional treatment when necessary. Initial management information in this chapter gives the nurse a plan of action. After assessing the problems, the nurse frequently must provide health care and comfort until a parent assumes responsibility or there is additional medical intervention.

Action may be necessary to protect other students and staff from exposure to communicable disease. Guidelines are provided for excluding the student who might have a contagious condition. Determining the length of time for home-stay and readmission is critical so as not to jeopardize the health of others in the classroom setting. The recommendations in this chapter are suggested when public health or school policies have not been established.

Because this manual defines school-age from birth through 21 years, certain health problems included here may not be relevant to the traditional school-age child. Early intervention with the special-needs child requires that the nurse have knowledge of health problems associated with the very young and be able to educate and support the teaching staff who work with these children and their families.

ACUTE UPPER AIRWAY OBSTRUCTION (CROUP)

I. **Definition**
  A. The term *croup* applies to relatively acute infections of the upper and lower respiratory tract that are characterized by a "barking" cough, hoarseness, and degrees of respiratory distress. The infection involves the larynx, trachea, and at times, the bronchi. Although all areas of the upper respiratory tract may be involved, croup receives its name from the primary area affected. The four forms of croup are:
    1. Croup or acute laryngotracheobronchitis.
    2. Spasmodic laryngitis.
    3. Acute infectious laryngitis.
    4. Acute epiglottitis.
II. **Etiology**
  A. Acute laryngotracheobronchitis is a viral condition, as is spasmodic laryngitis. Parainfluenza viruses cause acute infectious laryngitis. *Haemophilus influenzae* type B (HIB) generally causes acute epiglottitis,

although *Streptococcus pyogenes, Streptococcus pneumoniae,* and *Staphylococcus aureus* may be associated. However, the use of HIB vaccine has nearly eliminated HIB as a cause of epiglottitis.

B. The incidence of croup is highest in males and occurs primarily in the winter season. There is a strong family history of croup in 15% of children, and recurrence is common in the same child (Behrman, Kliegman, and Jenson, 2000).

III. **Signs, Symptoms, and History**
   A. Croup, acute laryngotracheobronchitis (6 months-5 years).
      1. Most common form of acute upper airway obstruction (AUAO).
      2. Major findings; inflammatory edema, destruction of ciliated epithelium and exudate.
      3. Upper respiratory tract infection (URI) for several days before raspy cough.
      4. Mild fever or no fever.
      5. Mildly edematous and reddened epiglottis.
      6. Difficult inspirations with prolonged and labored expirations, inspiratory rales.
      7. Bilateral diminished breath sounds.
      8. If continues, cough worsens, nasal flaring, and intercostal, substernal, and suprasternal retractions occur.
      9. Rapid respiratory failure may develop.
      10. Can last several days and occasionally many weeks.
   B. Acute spasmodic laryngitis/croup (1-3 years).
      1. Clinically similar to laryngotracheobronchitis but no findings of family infection.
      2. Allergic and psychological triggers may be involved, as well as gastroesophageal reflux.
      3. Sudden onset, generally at night.
      4. May be preceded by mild-to-moderate hoarseness and coryza.
      5. Usually no temperature elevation.
      6. Restlessness and anxiety.
      7. Dyspnea and possible cyanosis.
      8. Inspiratory stridor and possible inspiratory retractions.
      9. Increased pulse rate, respirations decreased and labored, skin cool and moist.
      10. Minimal inflammation of posterior pharynx.
      11. Symptoms' severity decreases within a few hours, and child appears healthy, with exception of slight cough and hoarseness.
      12. Episode may occur a few more nights, and recurrence not uncommon.
   C. Acute infectious laryngitis (few months-5 years).
      1. Preceded by URI with sore throat, "barking cough," and hoarseness.
      2. Slight to no temperature elevation.
      3. Condition generally mild; however, severe respiratory distress may develop with dyspnea and rapid respirations, restlessness, retractions, and inspiratory stridor.

D. Acute epiglottitis; supraglottitis (2-7 years).
1. Observed less often because of use of HIB vaccine.
2. Sudden onset.
3. Fever of 101 degrees F (38.3 degrees C) or higher.
4. Inspiratory stridor.
5. Inflamed pharynx, muffled voice.
6. Drooling, sore throat, and dysphagia.
7. Respiratory distress from airway obstruction can occur within minutes or hours.
a. Accompanied by restlessness and anxiety, cyanosis.
b. Dyspnea and respirations 20 to 30 per minute.
c. Severe obstruction.
d. Pulse rate of 160+ per minute, inspiratory rhonchi (rattling in the throat), suprasternal and substernal retractions.
e. Child may lean forward with chin extended.
8. Death can occur without adequate treatment.

IV. Initial Management
A. Afebrile children with laryngotracheobronchitis or acute spasmodic croup can be managed at home effectively and safely. Neither condition responds to antibiotics.
B. Observe closely for signs of respiratory obstruction.
C. Steam from hot running water in a closed room or cold steam from a nebulizer may provide relief from respiratory distress or acute laryngeal spasm within moments.
D. If outdoor temperature is low and less than 100% saturated with water vapor, briefly expose individual to cold air. Sudden exposure to cold air often relieves laryngeal spasm, since it causes mucosal cooling, leading to vasoconstriction and decreased edema.
E. To prevent aspiration, do not give food or fluids to a person in respiratory distress.
F. Have someone stay with or hold person to comfort and ease apprehension and observe for signs of obstruction.
G. If breathing is impeded and respiratory obstruction is evident, immediately call parent(s) and 911 for care and transfer of student to nearest medical facility or emergency room.
H. Keep student in upright position if in distress.
I. Expiratory stridor indicates severe condition.

V. Exclusion/Readmission
A. Student should remain out of school until physically well and there has been no temperature elevation for the preceding 24 hours.

VI. Additional Information
A. Treatment for mild cases:
1. Treat fever if indicated.
2. Do not give student common cold preparations because they further dry and thicken respiratory tract secretions.
3. Do not give student cough syrups, since they contain cough suppressant, which inhibits the natural tendency to clear the airway.
4. Honey and lemon juice can be given to soothe the cough.

   5. Check during night to determine if symptoms have become more severe.
   6. Use a cool mist humidifier.
   7. Encourage clear liquids.
VII. **Web Sites**
   American Academy of Family Physicians—Croup Parent Handout
   http://www.familydoctor.org/handouts/220.html
   Virtual Children's Hospital—Electric Airway: Upper Airway Problems in Children
   http://www.vh.org/Providers/Textbooks/ElectricAirway/ElectricAirway.html

BLEPHARITIS

 I. **Definition**
   A. Blepharitis is a chronic inflammation of the eyelid margins.
 II. **Etiology**
   A. This condition may be seborrheic, staphylococcal, or a combination of the two factors.
 III. **Signs, Symptoms, and History**
   A. Condition is usually bilateral and chronic or recurrent.
   B. Redness and swelling.
   C. Crusting or scaling of the eyelids.
   D. Common symptoms, burning, itching, and irritation.
   E. Staphylococcal blepharitis; ulceration of lid margin, lashes often fall out, conjunctivitis and superficial keratitis are associated.
   F. Seborrheic blepharitis; greasy scaling, infrequent ulceration, lid margins less red.
 IV. **Initial Management**
   A. Cleanse the lid margins using a moistened cotton applicator or cloth to remove scales and crusts. This is an important treatment modality, and the student can learn how to do the daily cleansing as the nurse cleans the area and teaches at the same time.
   B. For seborrheic blepharitis: examine scalp, body, and eyebrows to determine if student and parent need information regarding control of seborrhea; concurrent treatment may be needed.
   C. For staphylococcal blepharitis: apply an antistaphylococcal antibiotic to the eye margins. Refer student, as needed, to his or her health care practitioner (HCP).
 V. **Exclusion/Readmission**
   A. If student is young, exclude from school if staphylococcal infection present.
   B. Student may return to school when lesions are healed and no further crusting is present.
 VI. **Additional Information**
   A. Treatment of staphylococcal blepharitis is usually continued for a week or more after symptoms have disappeared. The student may need the antibiotic administered at school. Unless the seborrheic condition is so severe that it is limiting, the student may remain in school while under treatment.

Box 3-1	*Administering Eye Ointment*

1. Pull down the lower lid and apply a thin line of ointment along the inner margin of the lid.
2. Ointment may cause temporary blurring of vision.
3. For seborrhea, remove crusts on lids with a moist cotton applicator before applying.

VII. Web Sites
American Optometric Association
http://www.aoa.org/conditions/blepharitis.asp

CANDIDIASIS (DIAPER DERMATITIS)

I. **Definition**
   A. Candidiasis is a form of diaper rash often seen in infants and young children. It can be associated with oral candidiasis (thrush).
II. **Etiology**
   A. *Candida albicans,* a fungus, is the main cause.
III. **Signs, Symptoms, and History**
   A. *Transmission with excretions or secretions or by poor handwashing technique.*
   B. Common in infants younger than 6 months.
   C. Red, scorched appearance to skin from perianal to anterior abdominal areas.
   D. Sharp demarcation occasionally evident.
   E. Weeping lesions, vesicles, pustules, and papules may be present.
   F. Satellite lesions may occur.
   G. Presence of oral candidiasis.
   H. History of recent antibiotics.
IV. **Initial Management**
   A. Good handwashing technique.
   B. Do not use cornstarch (provides medium for bacteria growth).
   C. Do not use plastic pants.
   D. Keep area clean and dry and leave open to air whenever possible.
   E. Nystatin cream, powder, or ointment, clotrimazole 1% cream, amphotericin cream or ointment, or miconazole 2% ointment (antifungal medications) may be used.
   F. Hydrocortisone 1% may also be used during the first few days if significant inflammation is present.
   G. Combination drugs, along with topical corticosteroids, should be carefully used, since they may lead to serious local side effects.
V. **Exclusion/Readmission**
   A. No exclusion, but child must receive appropriate medical treatment.
VI. **Web Sites**
   ### Center for Disease Control
   http://www.cdc.gov/ncidod/dbmd/diseaseinfo/candidiasis_t.htm

CONJUNCTIVITIS

I. **Definition**
   A. Conjunctivitis, commonly called *pinkeye*, is a contagious inflammation of the conjunctiva, the mucous membranes that line the eyelids and extend over the sclera.
II. **Etiology**
   A. Conjunctivitis is caused by bacteria, (*H. influenzae, S. pneumoniae,* enterococci), virus (adenovirus 3, 4, and 7, herpes simplex virus [HSV], herpes zoster, enterovirus), allergy, chemical, or other irritants.
III. **Signs, Symptoms, and History**
   A. *Incubation period is usually 24 to 72 hours for bacterial conjunctivitis and 5 to 12 days for viral conjunctivitis. Duration of disease: up to 2 weeks.*
   B. *Period of communicability for bacterial conjunctivitis is any time during the course of active infections; for viral conjunctivitis, it is usually the later part of the incubation period up to 14 days after onset.*
      1. Bacterial.
         a. *Incubation period is usually 24 to 72 hours; period of communicability is any time during the course of active infection; duration is 7 to 10 days.*
         b. Sclera red or pink, and lining of eyelid inflamed, in one or both eyes.
         c. Photophobia.
         d. Moderate tearing.
         e. Minimal or no itching.
         f. Blurred vision that clears with blinking.
         g. Purulent discharge.
         h. Dried discharge on eyelids upon awakening.
         i. Swollen eyelids.
      2. Viral.
         a. *Incubation period is 5 to 12 days; period of communicability is usually the later part of the incubation period up to 14 days after onset; duration is up to 2 weeks.*
         b. Sudden onset.
         c. Minimal itching, initially only one eye involved.
         d. Refer to ophthalmologist if photophobia or herpes lesions are present.
         e. Sclera red or pink, and lining of eyelid inflamed, in one or both eyes.
         f. Profuse tearing.
         g. Preauricular node.
      3. Allergic.
         a. Conjunctiva red.
         b. Mucosa swollen; profuse tearing, first watery, later can become purulent.
         c. Severe itching, family history of seasonal allergies.
         d. Bilateral involvement common.

IV. **Initial Management**
   A. Isolate from others dependent on etiology.
   B. Cool compresses.
   C. Discuss importance of good handwashing technique.
   D. Refer to HCP.
V. **Exclusion/Readmission**
   A. For both bacterial and viral conjunctivitis, exclude student from school.
   B. Student with a bacterial infection may return to school after treatment started; student with a viral infection may return when eyes are clear.
   C. Student with allergic conjunctivitis is not excluded from school.
VI. **Additional Information**
   A. Bacterial and viral conjunctivitis are transmitted by contact with the discharge from the conjunctiva or upper respiratory tract of infected persons or by contaminated fingers, clothing, or other articles.
   B. Treatment for bacterial conjunctivitis is ophthalmic solution or ointment, Sulfacetamide 10%, chloramphenicol 1%, erythromycin 0.5%. For allergic conjunctivitis, Vasocon 0.012%, 0.02%, 0.03%, 0.1%; refer to allergist.
VII. **Web Sites**
   American Optometric Association
   http://www.aoa.org/conditions/conjunctivitis.asp

DIAPER DERMATITIS

I. **Definition**
   A. Diaper dermatitis is an inflammatory irritation of the skin that causes a breakdown of this natural barrier.
II. **Etiology**
   A. Diaper dermatitis is caused by prolonged exposure of the skin to urine and/or feces; a sensitivity to such things as disposable diapers, soaps, and detergents; inappropriate or no cleansing of the area; or skin dermatoses, which is aggravated by wearing diapers.
III. **Signs, Symptoms, and History**
   A. Change in brand of diapers.
   B. Frequency of diaper change and method of cleansing; frequency of wet or soiled diapers.
   C. Current medications (antibiotics); use of ointment in rash area.
   D. Mechanical.
      1. Acute or chronic erythematous, hyperpigmented area along edge of diaper or plastic pants.
      2. Erythematous skinfolds.
   E. Chemical.
      1. Erythematous macular or papular rash, which is shiny and peeling in diaper area.
      2. Erythema on buttocks and around anus.
      3. Dry and erythematous around head of penis.

F. Hygienic factor.
1. Any of the above symptoms.
2. Noticeably poor hygiene.

IV. **Initial Management**
A. Change diapers frequently, keeping skin dry and clean.
B. Use warm water and mild soap to wash genital area after every diaper change.
C. Use greasy ointment when skin is dry; use protective ointment for skin irritation (e.g., Desitin, A and D ointment, zinc oxide, petrolatum). Hydrocortisone 0.5% or 1% three or more times/day for a maximum of 5 days for inflammation.
D. Do not use both disposable diapers and rubber pants.
E. Cloth diapers should be washed well, double rinsed, and hung out to dry when possible.
F. Dilute urine by increasing fluids.
G. Sitz baths, expose area to air.

V. **Exclusion/Readmission**
A. Does not apply to simple diaper rash.

VI. **Additional Information**
A. Differential diagnosis includes bacterial, viral, or monilial infections; psoriasis, atopic dermatitis, scabies, seborrhea.
B. Management is difficult with children who seem predisposed to diaper dermatitis. Complete healing can take several days. However, definite improvement should be observed within 48 to 72 hours after treatment has begun.
C. Yeast and bacterial infections may be mistaken for diaper rash. If there are small bright red scaly spots or convex shapes, use antifungal cream. Large, fragile vesicles or pustules may indicate bacterial infection, and an antibiotic may be needed.

VII. **Web Sites**
Children's Hospital Boston
http://www.childrenshospital.org/cfapps/A2ZtopicDisplay.cfm?Topic=Diaper%20Dermatitis
American Osteopathic College of Dermatology
http://www.aocd.org/skin/dermatologic_diseases/diaper_dermatitis.html

DIARRHEA

I. **Definition**
A. Diarrhea is the passage of excessive fluid and electrolytes in the stool. This condition may be acute or chronic. Chronic diarrhea is an increased frequency of unformed stool lasting longer than 2 weeks.

II. **Etiology**
A. The pathogenesis of diarrhea episodes include five known causes: (1) inflammatory processes, (2) motility disorders, (3) viral and bacterial agents, (4) secretory diarrhea, and (5) osmotic diarrhea, or combinations of these. Inflammatory processes include any surgical procedure or condition that has the ability to change the anatomy and

functional integrity of the intestine, such as bacterial invasion, celiac sprue, and irritable bowel syndrome. Acute diarrhea can result from any atypical peristalsis from any source. Motility disorders may be either delayed or rapid and can be associated with infection or bacterial overgrowth.

III. **Signs, Symptoms, and History**
   A. Watery, copious bowel movement; may have foul odor or be bloody.
   B. Elevated temperature, abdominal pain, and vomiting.
   C. Dehydration, including decrease in urine output with increased concentration; sunken eyes; weight loss; and depressed fontanel in the infant.
   D. History of exposure in family, school site, or community.
   E. Recent travel to high-risk area and possible correlation with change in diet.

IV. **Initial Management**
   A. Take temperature.
   B. Observe frequency, consistency, color of stools, and presence of blood, pus, or mucus.
   C. Note any vomiting, abdominal cramping, irritability, and loss of appetite, fever, or other signs of distress.
   D. Give clear fluids in place of formula, milk, and solids as necessary.
   E. BRAT diet: bananas, rice, applesauce, and tea.
   F. Practice good general hygiene.

V. **Exclusion/Readmission**
   A. Student generally will not be dismissed for one or two loose stools unless other signs of illness exist.
   B. Student must be fever-free 24 hours before returning to school.
   C. Younger students, if diarrhea persists, must have written statement from HCP that no viral, bacteriological, or parasitic condition exists.

VI. **Web Sites**
   National Digestive Diseases Information Clearinghouse
   1-800-891-5389
   http://www.niddk.nih.gov/health/digest/pubs/diarrhea/diarrhea.htm

ECZEMA (ATOPIC DERMATITIS)

I. **Definition**
   A. Eczema is an acute or chronic cutaneous inflammatory condition characterized by pruritus, swelling, blistering, oozing, and scaling of the skin.

II. **Etiology**
   A. There is a strong family predisposition. The most predominant indicator is a family history of asthma, eczema, or hay fever. Infants with atopic dermatitis (AD) seem to develop allergic rhinitis and subsequent asthma. AD affects 2%-10% of children, and 90% of those children will manifest symptoms by age 5.
   B. The underlying problem is the skin's inability to retain adequate amounts of water; can be triggered by ingestion of or contact with a

substance to which an individual is sensitive (e.g., milk, fish, eggs, or inhalation of dust, pollen, or similar substances).

III. **Signs, Symptoms, and History**
   A. T-cell dysfunction and elevated immunoglobulin E (IgE) occur.
   B. There are three distinct stages: (1) infantile, (2) childhood, and (3) preadolescent or adolescent.
   C. Usually begins in infancy, age 2 to 3 months, or can be delayed.
   D. Chronic lesions or red macular areas on face, neck folds, scalp, hands, behind ears, antecubital and popliteal areas.
   E. Erythematous papules, vesicles, pustules, scales, crusts, or scabs, alone or in combinations; they may be dry or with watery discharge.
   F. Severe itching or burning with overall dry skin.

IV. **Initial Management**
   A. Disorder can be controlled but not cured.
   B. Teach avoidance of allergens and extreme temperatures; sweating leads to itching and irritation.
   C. Treatment:
      1. Keep fingernails short to prevent scratching and secondary infections.
      2. Keep skin moist; apply wet compresses for weeping, oozing lesions.
      3. Aveeno or oatmeal bath to soothe.
      4. Colloidal bath will soothe dry, itchy skin; use 2 cups cornstarch in a bathtub of water.
      5. Limit bathing time to 5 to 10 minutes to prevent depletion of natural skin oils; apply oil/ointment immediately to moist skin.
      6. If infrequent bathing is prescribed, use Cetaphil cleanser, a nondrying, soap-free cleanser.
      7. May prescribe antihistamines to decrease itching, such as hydroxyzine (Atarax) and diphenhydramine (Benadryl).

V. **Exclusion/Readmission**
   A. Does not apply.

VI. **Web Sites**
   American Academy of Dermatology—Eczema
   http://www.aad.org/pamphlets/eczema.html
   American Academy of Dermatology—EczemaNet
   http://www.skincarephysicians.com/eczemanet/index.htm

ERYTHEMA INFECTIOSUM (FIFTH DISEASE)

I. **Definition**
   A. Erythema infectiosum is a mild, nonfebrile erythematous skin eruption that usually occurs in children ages 2-13 but can occur in adults. Usually seen in late winter and early spring but can occur anytime. It is named *fifth disease* because it was the fifth eruptive rash characterized.

II. **Etiology**
   A. Fifth disease is caused by the human parvovirus B19, transmitted in blood and respiratory secretions from an infected individual.

III. Signs, Symptoms, and History
A. *Incubation period is less than 1 month.*
B. *Period of communicability is up to the appearance of the rash.*
C. Usually benign and self-limited disease.
D. Prodrome: Rash preceded by low-grade fever (up to 102 degrees), malaise, sore throat, and headache.
E. Secondary stage: Face has "slapped cheek" appearance, erythema, and a pallor that lasts 1 to 2 days.
F. Over the next several days, appearance of "lacy rash," a maculopapular eruption that progresses from proximal to distal surfaces of the trunk and extremities.
G. Rash may last days or weeks.
H. Rash may reappear months later in response to certain external stimuli: sunlight, temperature extremes, exercise, trauma, and emotional stress.
I. Studies demonstrate that about 20% of children are asymptomatic.

IV. Initial Management
A. No specific management.
B. Treat symptomatically, take temperature, assess rash area, isolate from other children.
C. Educate teachers and staff of childbearing age, including those working in preschools.

V. Exclusion/Readmission
A. Exclude from school with temperature and until rash has erupted. Not thought to be contagious after eruption of rash.
B. The effectiveness of immunoglobulin (IG) injection for prevention is unknown.

VI. Additional Information
A. Laboratory test used for detection is B19-specific immunoglobulin M (IgM)-antibody assay. When assay is positive, it only indicates infection within the past several months.
B. In older students and adults, arthralgias and arthritis are associated with B19 parvovirus. Affected joints in the hands may be the only symptom. Joint symptoms and rash generally occur 2-3 weeks after infection and can persist for many months afterward.
C. Fifth disease can be dangerous to the fetus of pregnant women who contract the disease. No birth anomalies have been reported by the March of Dimes to date, but there is a small risk for an infected fetus to develop anemias and heart failure, which can lead to miscarriage or stillbirth. Alert pregnant women to contact their HCP and possibility of avoiding the classroom or school situation in which there is an exposure or which exposure of fifth disease is likely.
D. This disease can also precipitate an aplastic crisis in children with sickle cell disease or those with autoimmune hemolytic anemia and α-thalassemia. For those individuals with immunodeficiencies, the infection with H19 virus can lead to severe chronic anemia.

VII. Web Sites
Dermatology Channel
http://www.dermatology.net/viral_infection/erythema_infectiosum.shtml

FEVER

I. Definition

A. Fever is an elevation of the body's normal temperature of 37 degrees C (98.6 degrees F) and ranges from 36 degrees C to 37.5 degrees C (96.8 degrees to 99.5 degrees F). If the temperature is measured axially, the norm would be 0.5 degrees C (1 degree F) *lower;* if measured rectally, the norm would be 0.5 degrees C (1 degree F) *higher* than orally.

B. *Low-grade* fever is 37.5 degrees to 38.2 degrees C (99.5 degrees to 101 degrees F) when taken orally.

C. *High-grade* fever is 38.2 degrees C (101 degrees F) when taken orally.

D. Temperature can be temporarily affected by age, physical activity, ovulation, and emotional stress.

II. Etiology

A. A fever develops in response to a disturbance in the homeostatic mechanisms of the hypothalamus, where a balance between heat production and peripheral heat loss is maintained. Pyrogens (a protein substance released by leukocytes) are produced within the body whenever inflammatory and infectious processes occur.

B. In inflammatory processes, such as those that occur in tissue damage, cell necrosis, malignancy, antigen-antibody reactions, and rejection of transplanted tissues, fever is due to the action on endogenous pyrogens, which act on the thermoregulatory center in the hypothalamus. Exogenous pyrogens occur in the body when it is invaded by bacteria, viruses, fungi, and other types of infectious organisms.

III. Signs, Symptoms, and History

A. First stage:
1. Chilling and shivering results from the body's attempt to raise the temperature.
2. This reaction produces thirst, increased respirations, and increased pulse rate of about 8-10 beats per minute for each degree of temperature increase.

B. Second stage:
1. Fever persists, fluid and electrolyte losses are more severe, and evidence of cellular dehydration exists.
2. This stage is when convulsions in infants and children and delirium in older individuals occurs.

IV. Initial Management

A. Observe for any appearance of symptoms of disease process.

B. Note any recent illnesses and/or medication.

C. Treat symptomatically until parent is able to pick up from school.

D. During a chill, cover and protect from drafts; chilling raises body temperature.

E. If no chill present, remove as much clothing as possible.

F. Apply cold compresses to the forehead.

G. Sponge with tepid water, only uncovering small areas. When skin cools, accompany sponging with rubbing to encourage circulation of blood through skin.

H. When giving sponge bath, continue for as long as necessary to lower temperature; quick splash may only stimulate heat production.
I. If possible, give clear fluids by mouth.
V. **Exclusion/Readmission**
A. Student with temperature of 37.7 degrees C (100 degrees F) or above may be dismissed from school.
B. If student appears well and fever is low-grade, consider other varying factors, recent exercise or emotional state. Retake temperature in 15 minutes.
C. Student may be readmitted to the classroom if there has been no fever in preceding 24 hours.
VI. **Additional Information**
A. Oral temperature is contraindicated when seizure disorder, irrational behavior, or mouth breathing exists; when infants/toddlers are involved; or there is disease, surgery, or structural anomaly of the oral cavity.
VII. **Web Sites**
KidsHealth for Parents: What is fever?
http://www.kidshealth.org/parent/general/sick/fever.html

FROSTBITE

I. **Definition**
A. Frostbite is an injury to the tissues and impaired circulation to the affected area, which can lead to cell destruction. Areas that are prone to freeze first are the cheeks, nose, ears, fingers, toes, and feet.
II. **Etiology**
A. Because of prolonged exposure to cold ranging from -2 degrees to -10 degrees, nerve, blood vessel, and other cells are temporarily frozen. Many factors can potentiate effects of cold and include fatigue, injury, high altitude, immobility, dependency of the extremity, general health, duration of exposure, and increased wind velocity. Frostbite can be mild to severe. Exposure to extremely cold chemicals such as liquid oxygen produces immediate frostbite.
III. **Signs, Symptoms, and History**
A. Exposure to cold.
B. Early signs are shivering, low body temperature, skin pain, tingling, and numbness.
C. Skin red initially, then pale, slightly yellow, or waxy white.
D. Tissue blanches early on, then may feel rock-hard or doughy.
E. Previous history of frostbite will have increased sensitivity in same area to cold.
F. On rewarming, extent of tissue damage can be determined accurately.
G. Frostnip or superficial frostbite:
   1. Discomfort and redness.
   2. Skin seems to be normal within a few hours.
   3. Can be cared for at home with medical follow-up.
   4. Usually no significantly damaged tissue.

H. Deep frostbite:
 1. Erythema and swelling.
 2. Cyanosis or mottling.
 3. Numbness associated with burning pain.
 4. Bullae and vesicles that appear within 24 to 48 hours; however, if necrosis of tissue occurs from inadequate circulation in involved area(s), blisters do not occur.
 5. Gangrene.

IV. **Initial Management**
 A. Take temperature to determine if hypothermic: a condition where body core temperature is at or below 35 degrees C (95 degrees F) and is life threatening.
 1. Minor is 32-36 degrees C (89.6-96.8 degrees F).
 2. Moderate is 30-32 degrees C (86-89.6 degrees F).
 3. Severe is less than 30 degrees C (86 degrees F).
 B. Remove wet clothing.
 C. Do not massage or rub area with snow.
 D. Do not rewarm area if there is possibility of refreezing.
 E. Rewarm area rapidly (do not use dry heat, such as radiator or oven). May use warm clothing, blanket, or another body surface.
 F. Protect area from further trauma.
 G. Keep other areas of body warm by covering them with blanket.
 H. Severe frostbite must be managed by emergency specialists.

V. **Exclusion/Readmission**
 A. Does not apply.

VI. **Additional Information**
 A. Education of school staff, students, and sending newsletters home to caregivers regarding prevention and initial management of frostbite are necessary tasks. Knowledge for initial management is important to include in the education; contraindications should also be included.
 B. To prevent frostbite, make sure children wear several layers of loose protective clothing, such as face masks, hats, earmuffs, mittens, and appropriate boots. Have extra socks, mittens, and hats on hand (mittens are usually warmer than gloves). During severe cold weather, check children's cheeks and hands periodically for symptoms of frostbite. If there are suspicious signs, warm the affected area with body heat (place hands in groin area or axilla).
 C. Older children and adolescents should avoid alcohol and cigarettes while they are exposed to cold. Alcohol causes peripheral vasodilation, which increases the rate of heat loss from the skin. Nicotine, by vasoconstriction, inhibits peripheral blood flow.

VII. **Web Sites**
 KidsHealth for Parents: Frostbite
 http://www.kidshealth.org/parent/firstaid_safe/emergencies/frostbite.html
 McKinley Health Center: Frostbite (handout)
 http://www.mckinley.uiuc.edu/health-info/dis-cond/misc/frostbit.html
 eMedicine: Frostbite
 http://www.emedicine.com/emerg/topic209.htm

GIARDIASIS

I. **Definition**
  A. Giardiasis is a flagellated protozoan infection of the small intestine and duodenum. It ranges from asymptomatic infection to acute or chronic diarrhea and malabsorption. This is the most commonly identified parasite in stool specimens in the United States.

II. **Etiology**
  A. The cause is the parasite *Giardia lamblia,* also called *Giardia intestinalis.*

III. **Signs, Symptoms, and History**
  A. *Incubation period is usually 1-2 weeks.*
  B. *Period of communicability can be the duration of the infection.*
  C. *Transmission is by direct person-to-person contact and contaminated food and water. Can be epidemic in day care centers and custodial institutions.*
  D. Acute infection usually lasts 1-3 weeks; can become chronic.
  E. Usually asymptomatic in both children and adults.
  F. Failure to thrive in young infants and toddlers.
  G. Limited phase of acute infection with or without anorexia and weight loss, nausea, and low-grade fever.
  H. Abdominal distention, cramps, flatulence, nausea, vomiting, and fatigue.
  I. Initially watery stools, which later become greasy (steatorrhea), malodorous, and may float. No blood or mucus in stools.
  J. May have intermittent periods of normal bowel movement and constipation.
  K. Chronic infection may cause malabsorption and debilitation.

IV. **Initial Management**
  A. Maintain good hygiene practices.
  B. Refer to primary HCP.
  C. Provide clear liquids; discontinue formula, milk, juices, and food.
  D. Dispose of feces/diapers using sanitary precautions.
  E. Use petroleum jelly on perianal area to prevent excoriation.
  F. Treatment: metronidazole (Flagyl) and furazolidone (Furoxone).

V. **Exclusion/Readmission**
  A. Exclude children and adults with acute diarrhea in day care settings.
  B. Exclude others from school if laboratory tests are positive and diarrhea is untreated.
  C. Readmit student after diarrhea has stopped or treatment has started: check school or state guidelines and Department of Health standards, since they vary among states.

VI. **Additional Information**
  A. Follow universal handwashing precautions. For objects that cannot be cleaned in a dishwasher, use disinfectant solutions such as bleach and water. Solutions are weakened by light, heat, and evaporation. Must be mixed fresh every day.

VII. **Web Sites**
  Association of State and Territorial Directors of Health Promotion and Public Health Education (ASTDHPPHE)
  http://www.astdhpphe.org/infect/giardiasis.html

| Box 3-2 | *Disinfectant Solution* |

¼ cup bleach (5.25% sodium hypochlorite) to 1 gal cool water.
  OR
1 tablespoon bleach, per 1 qt cool water.

HAND, FOOT, AND MOUTH DISEASE

I. Definition

  A. This highly contagious viral disease is characterized by pharyngitis, fever, and exanthem, particularly on the hands and feet. More common in the summer and early autumn and in children younger than 10.

II. Etiology

  A. Coxsackie virus A16 is the major cause. Enterovirus 71 is another causative factor, is more severe, and has been associated with meningitis, encephalitis, and paralytic disease.

III. Signs, Symptoms, and History

  A. *Incubation period is 4-6 days.*

  B. *Period of communicability is during the acute phase of illness but can be longer.*

  C. *Transmission is from person to person by direct contact with nose and throat discharges or the stool of infected persons.*

  D. Rash may persist 1 week or longer. Rash does not itch.

  E. Low-grade fever, 102 degrees F (39.3 degrees C).

  F. Pharyngitis; vesicular lesions on posterior pharynx and possibly gums, side of tongue, or buccal surfaces of cheeks.

  G. Lesions rupture, leaving shallow ulcers; malaise.

  H. Symmetrical maculopapular eruptions on palms and soles in addition to oral lesions. Lesions may occur on buttocks.

  I. Virus may produce vesicular lesions on hands, feet, and buttocks without oral lesions. Lesions more frequently on the dorsal surface of the hands and feet.

IV. Initial Management

  A. Good handwashing technique.

  B. Isolate student from others.

V. Exclusion/Readmission

  A. Exclude student from school during the acute phase and until fever-free for 24 hours.

VI. Web Sites

  Lucile Packard Children's Hospital: Hand Foot and Mouth Disease
  http://www.lpch.org/HealthLibrary/ParentCareTopics/SkinWidespread
  Symptoms/HandFootMouthDisease.html

HEPATITIS A

I. Definition

  A. Hepatitis A is the most common type of hepatitis in the United States. It is an inflammation of the liver that occurs sporadically or in epidemics. About 15% of people infected with hepatitis A virus (HAV) will have prolonged or relapsing symptoms over a 6- to 9-month period (see Table 4-7).

II. Etiology

A. It is caused by HAV. The highest rates of HAV are among children 5-14 years of age, with approximately one third of reported cases occurring among children under 15 years of age.

III. Signs, Symptoms, and History

A. *Incubation period is 15 to 50 days, with an average of 28 days.*

B. *Period of communicability of virus is up to 2 weeks before symptoms appear.*

C. *Transmission of HAV is by the fecal-oral route, with the virus being transmitted from person to person between household contacts or sex partners, or by contaminated food or water.*

D. There is no chronic, long-term infection, nor is there crossover to other types of hepatitis.

E. There is immunity to hepatitis A after infection.

F. The disease is generally noninfectious after 1 week of jaundice.

G. History of direct exposure.

H. History of eating contaminated shellfish or drinking contaminated water.

I. Children generally asymptomatic.

J. Onset is abrupt with adults and older children.

K. Prodromal phase: fever, anorexia, nausea and vomiting, malaise, abdominal pain, headache, enlarged or tender liver.

L. Icteric phase, 5 to 7 days after initial symptoms: sclera and skin jaundiced, urine darkened, light-colored stools.

IV. Initial Management

A. Refer those with presenting symptoms for medical care. Treatment and management of HAV infection is supportive.

B. HAV is a reportable disease in all states.

C. Use good handwashing techniques after toileting and before and after eating or preparing food.

D. Dispose of feces in a sanitary manner.

E. Determine type of health education needed by client, family contacts, school staff, and community.

F. Refer close contacts to their HCP or health department for information regarding immunoglobulin.

G. Inform school staff who may be at risk (e.g., staff providing special health services, custodians, bus transportation personnel) of any necessary cleaning or precautions.

H. Review and implement Occupational Safety and Health Administration (OSHA) regulations.

I. There are no specific measures for treatment.

V. Exclusion/Readmission

A. Exclude student from school.

B. Student may return after a minimum of 1 week after onset of jaundice.

VI. Additional Information

A. Examples of transmission include drinking water or using ice contaminated with HAV, eating raw or partially cooked shellfish harvested from waters containing raw sewage, and eating vegetables, fruits, or other uncooked contaminated foods. Diaper changing tables, when not cleaned or cared for properly, may facilitate the spread of hepatitis A. HAV can survive on an object or surface for months.

B. The Advisory Committee on Immunization Practices (ACIP) recommends routine childhood immunization against hepatitis A in those states with rates of the disease that are twice the national average or greater. Consult local or state health department for current recommendations. The vaccine dosages and schedules vary according to age and type of vaccine. Advise families to check with their HCP.

C. Hand washing is the most important measure for prevention and control. Young children are more likely to have poor handwashing habits, making education an important role of the school nurse.

D. Maintain strict OSHA protocols. Heating foods to 185 degrees F for 1 minute or washing surfaces with a 1:10 solution of household bleach to water can inactivate HAV.

E. IG injections should be given as soon as possible and no later than 2 weeks after exposure. Staff and children in day care centers or schools that care for children in diapers should receive injections if there is more than one case a month. In addition, all members of households whose diapered children attend the center/school should get injections when the disease exists among three or more families. If the infected person is directly involved in handling foods that will not be cooked or in handling cooked foods before they are eaten, other kitchen employees and possibly those served should be injected. Individuals should contact their local or state public health department for current recommendations.

VII. Web Sites

KidsHealth for Parents: Hepatitis
http://www.nlm.nih.gov/medlineplus/hepatitis.html

Non-Profit Organizations and Immunization and Hepatitis Resources
http://www.immunize.org/resources/noprofit.htm

Teenhealth: How Hepatitis Can Hurt You.
http://www.kidshealth.org/teen/infections/stds/hepatitis.html

Centers for Disease Control and Prevention (CDC) Resources
http://www.immunize.org/resources/cdc.htm

American Academy of Pediatrics
http://www.medem.com/MedLB/article_detaillb.cfm?article_ID=ZZZ9VB53R7C
&sub_cat=107

HERPANGINA

I. Definition

A. Herpangina is an acute viral infection characterized by a rapid onset.

II. Etiology

A. Herpangina is caused by the Coxsackie virus A, which is in the Enterovirus family. The infection generally occurs in summer and early fall; it is most commonly reported in children 1 to 4 years of age.

III. Signs, Symptoms, and History
   A. *Incubation period is 3 to 6 days.*
   B. *Period of communicability is during the acute phase or longer. The virus persists in stools for several weeks.*
   C. *Transmission is by direct contact with nasal and oral discharge, as well as feces from an infected person or by droplets.*
   D. Self-limiting infection and complete course lasts 4-6 days.
   E. Abrupt onset with fever of 103-105 degrees F (39.4-40.5 degrees C) lasting 1-4 days.
   F. Loss of appetite, dysphagia, and sore throat.
   G. Vomiting and abdominal pain.
   H. Older children generally complain of headache and backache.
   I. Small gray-white vesicles (1 to 2 mm in diameter) with red areolas usually on the anterior tonsillar pillars; they also appear on the tonsils, uvula, pharynx, posterior buccal surfaces, and edge of the soft palate.
   J. Vesicles quickly rupture, producing pain and shallow ulcers.

IV. Initial Management
   A. Treatment is symptomatic.
   B. Practice good handwashing technique.
   C. Isolate student from other students.
   D. Take special cleaning precautions with eating utensils, drinking fountains, and so on.

V. Exclusion/Readmission
   A. Exclude child from school until temperature-free for 24 hours and oral lesions have disappeared.

VI. Web Sites
   MedlinePlus Health Information: Herpangina
   http://www.nlm.nih.gov/medlineplus/ency/article/000969.htm
   Family Practice Notebook: Herpangina
   http://www.fpnotebook.com/ENT99.htm

HERPES ZOSTER (SHINGLES)

I. Definition
   A. Herpes zoster (HZ) is an acute viral infection characterized by inflammation of the spinal ganglia and vesicular eruptions along a sensory nerve distribution. Commonly called *shingles,* it seldom occurs in children younger than 10.

II. Etiology
   A. HZ is a latent complication of the varicella virus (chickenpox). It may be caused by reactivation of or additional exposure to the virus.

III. Signs, Symptoms, and History
   A. *Period of communicability is until lesions are crusted.*
   B. *Transmission is by direct contact with uncrusted lesions.*
   C. First symptom may be pain at the site before appearance of rash.
   D. Rash consists of maculopapular lesions that quickly vesiculate with an erythematous base. These blisters eventually crust.

E. Rash follows along distribution of lumbar and thoracic nerves and is generally unilateral, ending at body's midline. Lesions can also occur along trigeminal nerve.

F. Severe pain, itching, and paresthesia (burning or tingling sensation) common, although less frequent in children.

IV. Initial Management

A. Cool compresses or Burrow's solution.

B. Calamine lotion may help dry the lesions and decrease itching.

C. Antihistamines for itching and analgesics for pain.

D. Refer for immediate ophthalmologic evaluation if lesions occur on forehead, eyes, or nose.

E. Medications include acyclovir (Zovirax) and famciclovir (Famvir).

V. Exclusion/Readmission

A. Exclude student from school until lesions are crusted; may be 1-2 weeks. Those with altered immunity may have prolonged contagion.

B. May return to school if lesions can be covered.

VI. Additional Information

A. African-Americans have a significantly lower risk of developing HZ than Caucasians. HZ may be an early indication of human immunodeficiency virus (HIV) infection in young African-Americans.

B. A major complication is bacterial infections. Severe ophthalmic infection may cause corneal opacification or secondary bacterial infection.

C. Varicella vaccine has reduced incidence of chickenpox and HZ.

VII. Web Sites

American Academy Of Dermatology: Herpes Zoster
http://www.aad.org/pamphlets/herpesZoster.html

IMPETIGO

I. Definition

A. Impetigo is a highly contagious skin disease characterized by pustular eruptions. It is seen primarily in infants and children.

II. Etiology

A. Impetigo is caused primarily by *S. aureus;* group A beta-hemolytic streptococcus (GABHS), alone or in combination, is also associated with the infection.

III. Signs, Symptoms, and History

A. *Incubation period is 2 to 5 days.*

B. *Period of communicability lasts until the lesions are dry.*

C. *Transmission is by direct contact.*

D. Lesions are most commonly found on the face and extremities.

E. Secondary infection to insect bites, abrasions, chickenpox, scabies, burns, and any break in the skin.

F. Rapid progression from macules to vesicles to pustules.

G. Pustules rupture, producing an oozing, sticky, honey-colored crust.

H. Pruritus.

I. Exposure to others with impetigo.

IV. **Initial Management**
   A. Good handwashing technique. Scrub area with soap and water. Cover with clean dressing if possibility of exposure to others, or leave open to air.
   B. Clean toys and items the child uses.
V. **Exclusion/Readmission**
   A. Exclusion depends on student's age and ability to practice good personal hygiene.
   B. Day care students are excluded until 24 hours after treatment has been initiated.
   C. Without medical treatment, student cannot return to school until lesions are dry.
VI. **Additional Information**
   A. Medical treatment is with antibiotic of choice applied locally or systemically. Baciguent (Bacitracin) and mupirocin (Bactroban) are used topically, whereas cephalexin (Keflex), cloxacillin (Cloxapen), dicloxacillin (Dynapen), and erythromycin (E-mycin) are used systemically. Topical is used for isolated lesions, but if no improvement within 3 days, oral medication is prescribed. Oral medication is used for widespread lesions when deeper tissue is involved and/or with constitutional symptoms.
   B. Complications are rare. One complication is acute glomerulonephritis, which usually causes the urine to turn dark brown and which is often accompanied by a headache and elevated blood pressure. Other complications include osteoarthritis, septicemia, septic arthritis, and pneumonia.
VII. **Web Sites**
   KidsHealth for Parents: Impetigo
   http://www.kidshealth.org/parent/infections/bacterial_viral/impetigo.html
   University of Iowa, Department of Dermatology: Impetigo (photo)
   http://tray.dermatology.uiowa.edu/Impetigo004.htm

KAWASAKI DISEASE

I. **Definition**
   A. Kawasaki disease is an acute febrile vasculitis that affects the arterioles, venules, and capillaries, mainly in infants and children. In the United States and Japan, it is the leading cause of acquired heart disease in children. It is also known as *mucocutaneous lymph node syndrome (MCLS)*.
II. **Etiology**
   A. The cause of Kawasaki disease is not known, but it is thought to be infectious and viral. It is more prevalent in Asian children, seen more in males than females, and is rare in children over 8 years of age.
III. **Signs, Symptoms, and History**
   A. Acute phase lasts up to 14 days.
      1. Significant irritability.
      2. Fever of 101 degrees F (38.5 degrees C). Can spike to 104 degrees F or higher.

3. Reddened oral cavity.
4. Reddened conjunctiva with no discharge.
5. Edema of hands and feet with reddening of palms and soles.
6. Strawberry tongue.
7. Erythematous, nonpruritic rash.
8. Dry and red lips with fissuring (cracking).
9. Swelling of cervical lymph nodes.
10. Tachycardia and gallop rhythm.
B. Subacute phase, around tenth to twenty-fifth day.
   1. Peeling of fingers and toes.
   2. Fever subsides.
   3. Rash desquamates (shedding of skin cells).
   4. Possible arthritis and arthralgia (joint pain).
   5. Possible cardiac complications; arrhythmias, aneurysms or thrombosis, congestive heart failure, pericardial effusion, mitral valve insufficiency with resulting heart murmur. Risk of sudden death.
C. Convalescent phase, 25 to 60 days.
   1. All signs of illness have disappeared.
   2. Preceding coronary complications may also occur during this phase.
   3. Transverse grooves on fingernails and toenails.

IV. Initial Management
A. Isolate student from other children and call parent(s).
B. Refer to primary HCP.

V. Exclusion/Readmission
A. Exclude student from school as you would any student with elevated temperature.
B. Readmit student on HCP's release.
C. Consult with HCP upon student's return regarding level of activity, medications, and signs of complications.

VI. Additional Information
A. Illness is self-limited, but treatment of intravenous immunoglobulin (IVIG) and high dose of aspirin is given as soon as possible after diagnosis. This treatment helps to diminish the risk of coronary aneurysm or disease. Recovery is generally complete for those without coronary disease, and prognosis with coronary disease depends on the severity.

VII. Web Sites
Kawasaki Disease Foundation
http://www.kdfoundation.org/
Lucile Packard Children's Hospital: Kawasaki Disease
http://www.lpch.org/DiseaseHealthInfo/HealthLibrary/cardiac/kawasaki.html

LYME DISEASE (TICK-BORNE DISEASE)

I. Definition
A. Lyme disease, also called *Lyme arthritis,* is a recurrent multisystemic disease named for Old Lyme, Connecticut, where the first well-known U.S. outbreak occurred in 1975. It is transmitted by a tick and can take 24 to 48 hours to transmit the bacteria. Symptoms resemble those of

many other diseases, which makes diagnosis difficult. There is a direct detection test for confirmation of active disease. It is reported worldwide and in most U.S. states.

   B. Ticks can harbor more than one disease-causing agent and can transfer these to their human hosts. Co-infective agents include *human granulocytic ehrlichiosis (HGE), human monocytic ehrlichiosis (HME)*, and *babesiosis.*

   C. Prime time for infection is in the spring when the tick is in the nymph stage (about the size of a pinhead) and is difficult to see. In the fall, the adult stage is larger, and thus the tick is easier to detect.

II. Etiology

   A. The disease is caused by the spirochete, *Borrelia burgdorferi.* Incubation period can be 3 to 31 days. On the East Coast, the deer tick, *Ixodes scapularis,* transmits bacteria for Lyme disease, HGE, and HME, along with the parasite that causes babesiosis. On the West Coast, the Western black-legged deer tick, *Ixodes pacificus,* spreads Lyme disease and HGE bacteria. It is not known which tick species transmits the HME bacteria and the babesiosis parasite. Lyme disease is the most common tick-borne illness in the United States.

III. Signs, Symptoms, and History

   A. Prime season for Lyme disease is April through July; for HGE, prime season is November through May; currently season unknown for HME and babesiosis organisms.

   B. First stage: early localized disease.
      1. Lyme, ehrlichiosis, and babesiosis disease.
         a. Sudden appearance of a bull's eye rash is 1 in 2 Lyme disease cases and 1 in 5 ehrlichiosis cases. There is no rash with babesiosis. Rash usually circular but can be oblong and hot to the touch; appears as a bruise on dark skin and red on light skin.
         b. Flu-like symptoms: fatigue, joint pains, muscle aches, headaches, and low-grade fever.
         c. With ehrlichiosis and babesiosis: may have nausea, vomiting, diarrhea, and appetite loss, along with flu-like symptoms.
         d. With babesiosis: may have drenching sweats.
         e. Without treatment, early Lyme disease symptoms disappear within 3 to 4 weeks. Illness may return weeks or months later and manifest in late stages, with debilitation symptoms such as memory or mood disturbances and arthritis.
         f. Without treatment, ehrlichiosis symptoms disappear without long-term concerns, but some individuals develop life-threatening complications, and about 5% die.
         g. Babesiosis is usually mild, even without treatment, but can develop severe anemia, kidney failure and other life-threatening complications, and death.

   C. Second stage: early disseminated disease.
      1. Lyme disease.
         a. Infection of the eye; retinitis, conjunctivitis, uveitis.
         b. Infection of the bone; osteomyelitis, mild arthritis.

       c. Infection of the heart; pericarditis, myocarditis, with palpitations, heart pain (if inflammation of the heart muscle).
       d. Infection of the liver; hepatitis.
       e. Infection of central nervous system (CNS); meningitis, facial paralysis, drooping eyelids.
    2. Babesiosis.
       a. Malaria-like illness when red blood cells are attacked.
       b. Weakened immune systems.
  D. Third stage: late disease.
    1. Lyme disease.
       a. May take months or years to occur.
       b. Pauciarticular—involvement of less than 5 joints.
       c. Arthritis, which may be recurrent with painful swollen joints, usually the knees.
       d. Late neurological concerns of deafness, chronic encephalopathy, and keratitis.
    2. HGE.
       a. Toxic shock and death.
    3. Babesiosis.
       a. Anemia and kidney failure.

IV. Initial Management

  A. Remove tick as soon as possible, preferably with tweezers.
  B. Pull steadily outward and away from the skin; do not twist or jerk the tick.
  C. Protect fingers and hand with a tissue, paper towel, or glove.
  D. Apply alcohol or disinfectant to area after tick removal.
  E. Place tick in jar of alcohol and keep for identification.
  F. Wash hands with soap and water.
  G. Observe the site for signs of a rash for at least a month.
  H. Notify parents, and discuss further follow-up.
  I. The disease is not treated until symptoms appear. Lyme disease and ehrlichiosis infections are treated with antibiotics. Antibiotics plus medication, used for therapy with malaria, can cure babesiosis. Antibodies remain in the system, and the individual may continue to test positive.

V. Exclusion/Readmission

  A. Does not apply.

VI. Additional Information

  A. A vaccine approved by the Food and Drug Administration (FDA) has been available since 1998 and is given in a series of three injections. It is approximately 75% effective and does not protect against HGE and HME ehrlichiosis or babesiosis. Research indicates safeness in only those individuals between 15 and 70 years old. An untreatable, degenerative form of arthritis has been reported. When living in an area where ticks and animals harbor the disease or if the individual has had Lyme disease and remains vulnerable, these risks should be discussed with the individual's HCP.

| Box 3-3 | *Precautions to Avoid Tick Bites* |

1. Cover skin with clothing.
2. Wear light-colored, long-sleeved shirts and long pants.
3. Tuck pant legs into socks and button shirts.
4. Apply tick repellents containing diethyltoluamide (DEET) to your skin and clothing. Reapply every few hr and read/follow instructions, since DEET can be toxic.
5. Cover ground area with a blanket when sitting.
6. Apply medication to kill ticks on pet dogs and cats that go outside.
7. Check clothing and full-body skin for ticks on returning from a potentially tick-infected area such as a grassy or woodland area. Include head and back of body.
8. Wash clothing on return, and dry for at least 20 minutes.

VII. Web Sites
Centers for Disease Control Lyme Disease Home Page
http://www.cdc.gov/ncidod/dvbid/lyme/index.htm
Lyme Disease Network
http://www.lymenet.org/

MEASLES (RUBEOLA)

I. Definition
A. Measles is a contagious childhood disease marked by fever and skin eruption. It is a vaccine-preventable disease.

II. Etiology
A. The cause is the measles virus. One attack almost invariably confers immunity, although second occurrences have been recorded.

III. Signs, Symptoms, and History
A. *Incubation period is 10 to 12 days.*
B. *Period of communicability is for at least 7 days after the onset of the first symptoms.*
C. *Transmission is respiratory droplet and by contact with articles freshly contaminated by nose, throat, mouth, and eye secretions.*
D. Prodromal phase, 4 to 5 days.
   1. Fever, malaise, runny nose, cough, conjunctivitis.
   2. Koplik spots (small, irregular, red spots with minute grayish-white center on buccal mucosa) that usually disappear 1 or 2 days after onset of rash.
E. Rash, 3 to 4 days later.
   1. Abrupt rise in temperature as rash appears.
   2. Fine, reddish brown eruptions.
   3. Begins on face, hairline, and behind ears and gradually spreads downward.

4. Rash is more severe in earlier sites and less intense in later sites.
5. About 2 days after rash appears, symptoms begin to subside.
6. Complications include otitis media, pneumonia, laryngotracheo-bronchitis and obstructive laryngitis, encephalitis, and permanent disability or death.

IV. Initial Management

A. Treatment is symptomatic and supportive.
B. Good handwashing technique by school personnel.
C. Proper disposal of soiled tissues.
D. Isolate student from other students.
E. Review immunization records of all students for measles vaccination.
F. Notify parents and parents of any student not immunized, following school and county guidelines.
G. Notify and follow local health department regulations regarding reporting of disease.
H. Closely observe all students for possible additional cases.
I. Those with severe measles have low vitamin A levels. A one-time dose of 100,000 units of vitamin A for children 6 to 12 months of age and 200,000 units for children 1 year of age or older can be given. The dose is repeated the following day and 1 month later if ophthalmologic evidence of vitamin A deficiency exists.

V. Exclusion/Readmission

A. Immediately exclude student from school.
B. Student may return to school a minimum of 5 days after rash appears.

VI. Additional Information

A. Measles vaccine is administered as part of the measles, mumps, and rubella (MMR) series to children, starting at 12 to 15 months and again at 4 to 6 years of age or 11 to 12 years. Adults born before 1957 are thought to be immune. Adults born in 1957 or later should receive 1 to 2 doses of MMR vaccine, unless (1) they can provide proof of one dose given at 12 months of age or later, (2) they have documented proof from a physician of prior measles diagnosis, or (3) they have laboratory evidence of immunity.
B. Contraindications for MMR include immunocompromised individuals, febrile individuals, pregnant women, and recipients of recent blood products or IG, in which case the vaccine should be postponed for 3 months.
C. IG (0.25 ml/kg) may be given to a susceptible, exposed individual within 5 days for prevention of disease, but if given after 5 days, it will reduce severity of illness. HIV-infected children, regardless of vaccination status, should be given IG if measles exposure has occurred.

VII. Web Sites

McKinley Health Center: Measles (Rubeola) Self Care Instructions
http://www.mckinley.uiuc.edu/health-info/dis-cond/commdis/meas-sci.html
KidsHealth for Parents: Measles (Rubeola)
http://www.kidshealth.org/parent/infections/lung/measles.html

INFECTIOUS MONONUCLEOSIS

I. **Definition**
   A. Infectious mononucleosis, also referred to as the *kissing disease,* is an acute, self-limiting viral disease that can occur at any age but is most commonly seen in adolescents and young adults. The infection is characterized by increased mononuclear leukocytes in the blood.

II. **Etiology**
   A. Mononucleosis is usually caused by the Epstein-Barr virus (EBV) and can occur in both sporadic and epidemic forms. Infrequently, cytomegalovirus, HIV, toxoplasma gondii, and human herpesvirus type 6 cause the infection.

III. **Signs, Symptoms, and History**
   A. *Incubation period is 3 to 7 weeks.*
   B. *Period of communicability may last for months in viral excretions, making asymptomatic carriers common.*
   C. *Transmission is generally by direct, intimate contact with infected saliva and rarely by blood transfusions or bone marrow transplantation. Repeated and prolonged contact with infected oral secretions is thought to be required, making the contact unknown.*
   D. Generally mild illness and difficult to recognize in children, but overt illness in adolescents and young adults. Usually mild but can be serious with complications.
   E. Symptoms vary in type, duration, and severity.
   F. Prolonged fever with generalized lymphadenopathy and splenomegaly.
   G. Malaise, fatigue, and persistent low-grade headache.
   H. Epistaxis, severe sore throat, frequently exudative or accompanied by palatine petechiae.
   I. Discrete maculopapular skin rash may occur, particularly over trunk. Occurs more often in young children, whereas older ones have abdominal pain.
   J. Jaundice from hepatic involvement.
   K. Spleen enlargement.
   L. Can be confused with many conditions, including those characterized by neurological and cardiac symptoms.

IV. **Initial Management**
   A. Refer student with presenting symptoms to HCP for diagnostic laboratory tests, especially if abdominal pain, sore throat, making student unable to drink or eat, and difficulty breathing.
   B. Properly dispose of or disinfect all articles that may have been soiled with nose and throat discharges.
   C. Determine type of information needed for education of infected person, family, and contacts.
   D. Avoid administering live vaccines until several months after recovery.
   E. Treatment is usually symptomatic.
   F. Acute symptoms typically disappear within 2 to 4 weeks, with some students needing restricted activities for 2 to 3 months because of continued fatigue, malaise, or enlarged spleen.

V. Exclusion/Readmission
A. Exclude student from school.
B. Student may return after acute symptoms have disappeared.
C. Discuss with parent/HCP any restriction on activities and any recommendations regarding rest or reduced school day.
D. On student's readmission to school, discuss with student and staff necessity for proper disposal of articles soiled with throat and nose discharges and good handwashing. EBV can be shed in oral secretions up to 6 months after acute infection and intermittently throughout life.
E. Allow time for students to express feelings and concerns regarding illness or limitations of sports and social activities and provide a safe place to vent their anger and frustration when they return to school.
F. Student may need additional rest and regulation of activities according to tolerance.

VI. Additional Information
A. Clinical manifestations; positive heterophil agglutination test and an increase in atypical leukocytes in a peripheral blood smear generate diagnosis; spot test (monospot) and heterophil antibody test.
B. Rest and symptomatic treatment is the management approach. Oral penicillin is occasionally prescribed for a sore throat, especially GABHS. Acyclovir and corticosteroids decrease oropharyngeal shedding and viral replication but do not change the severity or duration of symptoms or clinical outcome. The level of individual tolerance and symptoms dictates regulation of activities. Severe manifestations are often treated more aggressively.

VII. Web Sites
KidsHealth for Parents: Infectious Mononucleosis
http://www.kidshealth.org/parent/infections/bacterial_viral/mononucleosis.html
Food and Drug Administration: On the Teen Scene: When Mono Takes You Out of the Action
http://www.fda.gov/fdac/features/1998/398_mono.html
Teenhealth
http://www.kidshealth.org/teen/infections/common/mononucleosis.html

MUMPS (INFECTIOUS PAROTITIS)

I. Definition
A. Mumps is an acute, contagious, febrile disease marked by inflammation of the salivary glands. It was widespread worldwide but occurs less frequently as a result of the 1967 introduction of the MMR vaccine.

II. Etiology
A. The cause of mumps is an ribonucleic acid (RNA) virus of the genus *Paramyxovirus.*

III. Signs, Symptoms, and History
A. *Incubation period is 14 to 24 days.*
B. *Period of communicability is approximately 6 days before and 9 days after salivary gland swelling has appeared.*
C. *Transmission is by direct contact, airborne droplets, saliva, and possibly by urine from an infected person.*

    D. Prodromal, first 24 hours:
        1. Fever, headache, malaise, and loss of appetite.
        2. Earache aggravated by chewing.
    E. Third day:
        1. Swelling, unilateral or bilateral, of one or more salivary glands, usually parotid, accompanied by pain and tenderness.

IV. Initial Management

    A. Treatment is symptomatic and supportive.
    B. Follow appropriate separation practice from other students.
    C. Good handwashing techniques by school personnel.
    D. Proper disposal of soiled tissues.
    E. Review immunization records of all students for mumps vaccination.
    F. Notify parents, and parents of unimmunized students, and follow school and county guidelines.
    G. Notify and follow local health department regulations regarding reporting of disease.
    H. Be aware of other students for symptoms and refer for care.

V. Exclusion/Readmission

    A. Isolate and exclude student from school.
    B. Student may return to school a maximum of 9 days after start of swelling.

VI. Additional Information

    A. Mumps vaccine is administered as part of the MMR series to children, starting at 12 to 15 months and again at 4 to 6 years of age or 11 to 12 years. See Appendix B: Immunizations.
    B. Complications of mumps disease include sensorineural deafness, epididymitis/orchitis, myocarditis, postinfectious encephalitis, arthritis, hepatitis, mastitis, and sterility (seldom in adult male). Pregnant women should contact their primary care provider, since exposure to the virus in the first trimester of pregnancy may increase the likelihood of spontaneous abortion.

VII. Web Sites

Intelihealth: Mumps
http://www.intelihealth.com/IH/ihtIH/WSIHW000/9339/10973.html

OTITIS MEDIA

I. Definition

    A. Otitis media (OM) is an inflammation of the middle ear and the most common cause of conductive hearing loss in children. It can be described as acute otitis media (AOM) with or without effusion, chronic otitis media with effusion, OM with or without cholesteatoma, and atelectasis of the tympanic membrane/middle ear/mastoid. If it lasts 6 weeks or more it is considered to be *chronic otitis media*.

II. Etiology

    A. *S. pneumoniae* or *H. influenzae* are major causes. Frequently, OM is associated with allergic rhinitis or hypertrophy of the adenoids. Secondhand smoke is a significant factor contributing to the incidence of OM.

III. **Signs, Symptoms, and History**
    A. Most commonly a result of eustachian tube dysfunction.
    B. Concurrent upper respiratory or pharyngeal infection.
    C. Pain, fever, malaise, irritability, and lethargy.
    D. Anorexia, nausea, vomiting, diarrhea, and headache occur less often.
    E. Enlarged postauricular and cervical lymph glands.
    F. Infant may become irritable, pull at ears, and roll head from side to side.
    G. Middle ear fluid may be serous (thin), mucoid (thick), purulent (pus-filled), or combination.
    H. Otoscopic exam reveals bright red bulging tympanic membrane with no visible landmarks or light reflex; indicates effusion.
    I. Impedance testing shows negative pressure and low compliance.
    J. Foul smell may result from eardrum rupture.
    K. Feeling of fullness in ear; popping sensation with swallowing.
    L. Fever or severe pain often absent with OM and may seem well.
    M. Babies who are put to bed with a feeding bottle are more likely to have increased incidence of OM.

IV. **Initial Management**
    A. Call parent(s) and discuss referral of care to HCP.
    B. Treat discomfort and fever.
    C. Monitor impedance and hearing acuity testing.
    D. Discuss hearing acuity variance with speech therapist for ongoing monitoring.
    E. If pressure-equalizing (PE) tubes are placed, use precautions for water play to avoid middle ear infections. Provide impedance testing to monitor patency of tubes.
    F. Symptoms of conductive hearing loss; see Chapter 2.

V. **Exclusion/Readmission**
    A. Does not apply.

VI. **Web Sites**
    American Speech-Language-Hearing Association: Questions and Answers about Otitis Media, Hearing and Language Development
    1-800-638-8255
    http://www.kidsource.com/ASHA/otitis.html
    National Institute on Deafness and Other Communication Disorders
    http://www.nidcd.nih.gov/health/parents/otitismedia.htm

PEDICULOSIS CAPITIS (HEAD LICE)

I. **Definition**
    A. This condition is an infestation of lice in the scalp and facial hair. Three types of human lice are head, body, and pubic. They all have similar life cycles. However, head and pubic lice spend their life cycles on the skin of the human host, whereas body lice live in clothing, coming to the skin only to feed. Head lice generally can not live longer than 24 hours without access to a human host; however, nits (eggs) may survive up to a week. The female louse lays 3-5 eggs per day, which take 7-10 days to hatch and another 7-10 days to mature and lay eggs. Lice do not jump, fly, or live on animals.

II. **Etiology**
   A. The louse *Pediculus humanus capitis* is the cause of the infestation.
III. **Signs, Symptoms, and History**
   A. Itching of scalp and/or back of neck.
   B. Presence of louse.
   C. Presence of nits on hair shaft.
      1. Observed on hair shaft close to head; difficult to remove with fingernails.
      2. Nits resemble dandruff, but dandruff can be easily removed from hair shaft, whereas lice nits cannot.
      3. Lice nits are small, grayish white, tear-shaped, and hatch in 1 week.
      4. Nits ½ inch or more from the scalp are nearly always hatched and do not indicate active infestation.
   D. Reddened areas around scalp, behind ears and neck.
IV. **Initial Management**
   A. Be aware of school/district policy and standards.
   B. Practice good handwashing techniques.
   C. Isolate child from other children without embarrassment.
   D. Examine all children in the class, as well as siblings of those identified as having head lice.
   E. Advise parent to consult HCP for prescription or purchase over-the-counter medication and follow instructions on product.
   F. All individuals living in the household should be inspected and *only treated* if infested. Encourage parent to notify relatives and other contacts of infestation.
   G. Advise family to wash all bedding, linens, combs, brushes, and headgear in hot soapy water.
   H. Objects that cannot be laundered or dry cleaned may be sealed in plastic bag for a week.
   I. Educate family about the transmittal of lice by sharing hats, combs, and so on.
   J. Allow time for student to express his or her feelings, since psychological impact is stressful.
   K. Educate public regarding prevention, transmission, detection, and treatment.
V. **Exclusion/Readmission**
   A. Exclude from school until hair has been properly treated and no nits are present.
   B. Recheck on return to school and evaluate the student in 7 to 10 days to determine if he or she has become reinfected with nits; may require second treatment for newly hatched eggs.
   C. School nursing organization policies differ on nit-free guidelines. Refer to your district or school policy, check the National Association of School Nurses (NASN) (www.nasn.org), and your state school nurse organization for specific policies and guidelines. Some chronic infestations require more stringent management, but the potential for epidemic spread is minimal and unnecessary exclusion causes children to miss school and parents to lose time from work.

Box 3-4	*Instructions for Pediculicide Products*

1. Infected household members must be treated at the same time.
2. Apply permethrin-based products, synthetic molecule, (NIX and Elimite cremes) to freshly shampooed, towel-dried hair. Hair must be partially dry for product to be effective.
3. Apply pyrethrum-based shampoos, natural product, (RID, Clear, Pronto, A-200, and various generic products) to dry hair.
4. Entire scalp and hair close to scalp should be saturated. It is usually not necessary to treat long hair to the ends, since lice rarely travel far from the scalp.
5. Application is more effective when a few drops are placed over various parts of the head, rather than putting a large amount in the middle and spreading out from there.
6. Leave all treatments in hair for time period indicated by product instructions to avoid scalp irritation. Do not cover with shower cap.
7. Begin nit comb-out process at the nape of the neck, around the ears, and work upward. Several combs are available; the National Pediculosis Association recommends the "Lice Meister" metal comb.
8. Apply second application in 7 to 10 days as recommended to kill any newly hatched lice.

VI. Web Sites
   National Pediculosis Association
   1-800-446-4672
   http://www.headlice.org
   Harvard School of Public Health: Head Lice: Information and Frequently Asked Questions
   http://www.hsph.harvard.edu/headlice.html
   Head Lice Infestation (Pediculosis) Fact Sheet
   http://www.cdc.gov/ncidod/dpd/parasites/headlice/factsht_head_lice.htm

PINWORMS (ENTEROBIASIS)

I. **Definition**
   A. Pinworms, or enterobiasis, are white threadlike parasites that live in the large intestine and are found in and about the rectal area. They are the most common helminthic infection in the United States. Infections are more frequent in preschool and younger school-age children and in crowded living conditions.
II. **Etiology**
   A. The cause is a parasitic infection with *Enterobius vermicularis*.
III. **Signs, Symptoms, and History**
   A. *Incubation period starts when eggs are inhaled or ingested. See cycle in "Additional Information."*
   B. *Period of communicability is the entire time the eggs exist in the environment.*
   C. *Transmission is either directly by the transfer of infective eggs by hand from the anus to the mouth or indirectly through articles contaminated with eggs.*

| Box 3-5 | *Instructions for Tape Test* |

1. Collect while child is asleep, or on awaking and *before* a bowel movement or a bath.
2. May need to perform task more than once to collect eggs.
3. Loop transparent tape, sticky side out, around end of a tongue depressor.
4. Press firmly against child's perianal area.
5. Place in plastic bag or glass jar.
6. Take in for microscopic examination.
7. Commercial kit available.

The eggs can survive up to 2 weeks without a human host on objects such as bed linen, underwear, food, shared toys and bath items, door knobs, and toilet seats.

  D. May be no symptoms.
  E. Perianal itching and scratching, especially at night.
  F. Vaginal and anal irritation because of scratching.
  G. Migration of worms to vagina or urethra may cause infection.
  H. Sleeplessness, irritability, restlessness, distractibility, and short attention span found in young children.
IV. **Initial Management**
  A. Call parent(s) immediately and discuss assessment using the *tape test* or a flashlight to observe the area 2-4 hours after child is asleep. See "Additional Information."
  B. Bed linens, hand towels, and clothing should be machine washed using hot water and dried using a heat setting.
  C. Notify teaching staff and provide education.
    1. Follow standard hygienic procedures.
    2. Washing hands after toileting and before eating or preparing food.
    3. Provide adequate toilet and handwashing facilities and time.
    4. Discourage habits of nail biting and scratching bare perianal area.
    5. Clean infected area(s) and routinely disinfect.
    6. Remove sources of infection by treating cases.
V. **Exclusion/Readmission**
  A. Exclude young child from school until 24 hours after treatment has been initiated.
VI. **Additional Information**
  A. After the eggs are inhaled or ingested, they hatch in the upper intestine, maturing in 2 to 8 weeks, and migrate to the cecal area. Females mate and migrate out of the anus, where they lay up to 17,000 eggs (American Academy of Pediatrics, 1997). The movement of worms on the skin and mucous membranes causes intense itching. The eggs adhere to many surfaces because of their adhesiveness and durability. While scratching or during toileting, eggs can easily be deposited on hands or under fingernails, which can create reinfestation of young children in preschool care.

B. Treatment includes mebendazole (Vermox), pyrantel pamoate (Antiminth), piperazine phosphate, and pyrvinium pamoate (Provan). Mebendazole is the drug of choice. It is safe, convenient, and effective with few side effects; however, it is not recommended for children under 2 years of age. Pyrvinium pamoate stains stool and vomitus bright red, along with skin and clothing that come into contact with the drug. Mebendazole may cause abdominal pain and diarrhea. Treatment is a one-time dose. Reinfection is common, and in certain cases, entire families require treatment.

VII. **Web Sites**

Centers for Disease Control: Pinworm Infection—Fact Sheet
http://www.cdc.gov/ncidod/dpd/parasites/pinworm/factsht_pinworm.htm
Centers for Disease Control: Pinworms in the Child Care Setting
http://www.cdc.gov/ncidod/hip/abc/facts29.htm
FamilyDoctor.org: Pinworms (handout—also available in Spanish)
http://www.familydoctor.org/handouts/139.html

POISON IVY, OAK, AND SUMAC DERMATITIS

I. **Definition**

A. Contact with dry or succulent segments of poison ivy, oak, or sumac can induce a potential serious dermatitis. Poison ivy is common in the Rockies; poison oak is generally west of the Rockies; and poison sumac is usually observed in swamp areas of the Southeast.

II. **Etiology**

A. The cause is an oil substance, urushiol, that transverses the roots, stems, leaves, and fruit of the plant. It can also result from contact with smoke, burning leaves, contaminated clothing, tools, or the fur of a cat or dog.

III. **Signs, Symptoms, and History**

A. Rash may begin within 6 hours to 6 or more days after exposure.

B. Redness, itching, and swelling.

C. Multiple blisterlike lesions that appear in linear streaks.

D. Lesions usually rupture, followed by oozing of serum and subsequent crusting.

E. Itching stops after 10 to 14 days, and healing occurs spontaneously.

IV. **Initial Management**

A. With known exposure, immediately flush with cold running water to neutralize the oil that has not bonded to skin; may leave clothes on and rinse skin and clothing.

B. Use of mild soap may be helpful, but harsh soap removes protective skin oil.

C. Hard scrubbing may further irritate skin.

D. Clothing should be carefully removed and laundered in hot water and detergent.

E. Treatment is symptomatic.

F. Blistering phase can be soothed by cool soda baths (1 cup soda per tub), Aveeno baths, calamine lotion, and Burrow's solution compresses.

G. Oral corticosteroid gel applied before blister formation may relieve or prevent inflammation. Topical corticosteroids and sedatives such as diphenhydramine (Benadryl) are used for severe reactions. Encourage student not to scratch, since this may cause secondary infections.

V. **Exclusion/Readmission**

A. Student may remain in school as long as itching does not interfere with ability to function in classroom.

VI. **Additional Information**

A. Prevention is best accomplished by teaching staff and students to recognize the plants so as to avoid them. Those who are known to be allergic can secure a protective cream for exposed skin, Stokoguard.

VII. **Web Sites**

American Academy of Dermatology
http://www.aad.org/pamphlets/PoisonIvy.html
MedlinePlus Health Information: Poison ivy-oak-sumac injury
http://www.nlm.nih.gov/medlineplus/ency/article/000027.htm

UPPER RESPIRATORY TRACT INFECTION (COMMON COLD)

I. **Definition**

A. The common cold is an acute infection of the upper respiratory tract, nose, and pharynx, usually lasting 5 to 7 days. URIs are the most common occurring childhood illness and account for the highest number of absences from school. Colds occur more frequently in the fall and winter.

II. **Etiology**

A. URIs are known to be caused by more than 200 viruses, with rhinoviruses composing more than one third of these. Respiratory syncytial virus (RSV) is seen in infants.

III. **Signs, Symptoms, and History**

A. *Incubation period is 2-5 days and can be up to 8 days.*

B. *Transmission is directly from contaminated large or small particle droplets or indirectly from contaminated secretions on hands or objects.*

C. Symptoms depend on age, living environment, and preexisting health concerns.

D. Infection rate appears to be higher in the toddler and preschool-age child. Infants younger than 3 months have a lower infection rate, and those over age 5 have URIs less frequently.

E. Disease is self-limiting and can last up to 10 days.

F. General malaise.

G. Fever appears abruptly in ages 3 months to 3 years and is associated with irritability, restlessness, and decreased activity and appetite. Older children have a low-grade temperature.

H. Nasopharyngitis, which is more severe in infants and younger children.

I. Older child exhibits dry and irritated nasal passages and pharynx, followed by chilly sensations, muscular aches and pains, sneezing, nasal discharge, and unproductive cough.

    J. Nasal inflammation can lead to obstruction and open-mouth breathing.

    K. Nasal discharge.

    L. Red and watery eyes.

IV. **Initial Management**

    A. Management is symptomatic.

    B. Emphasize good general hygienic measures (e.g., use of individual eating/drinking utensils, proper disposal of tissues, washing hands).

    C. Notify parent(s).

    D. Determine temperature; *antipyretics* are used for mild fever and any discomfort.

    E. Note consistency and color of nasal discharge. *Decongestants* may be prescribed for infants 6 months and older to decrease swollen nasal openings. Nasal congestion may make sleeping and feeding laborious.

    F. If cough is present, note frequency and whether or not productive. When cough is dry and hacking, *cough suppressants* containing dextromethorphan may be prescribed. Suppressants that contain alcohol should not be administered to young children.

    G. Antihistamines may be used, but they cause drowsiness or have the opposite effect of stimulation. They may only have small benefits as some of the other symptomatic drugs, with the exception of ibuprofen and acetaminophen.

    H. Aspirin should not be given because of the association with Reye's syndrome.

V. **Exclusion/Readmission**

    A. It is difficult to exclude from school every child who has a simple cold, and decisions regarding dismissal depend on individual circumstances (e.g., student's age, personal hygiene, classroom setting, developmental level). Student may be dismissed from school for any of following reasons:

        1. Purulent or discolored nasal discharge.

        2. Temperature of 100 degrees F or above.

        3. Student too ill or uncomfortable to adequately function in classroom setting.

        4. Student can return to school when temperature-free for 24 hours, nasal drainage is clear, and ceases to be threat to well-being of others.

VI. **Web Sites**

    KidsHealth for Parents: Common Cold

    http://www.kidshealth.org/parent/infections/common/cold.html

RINGWORM OF THE BODY (TINEA CORPORIS)

I. **Definition**

    A. Ringworm of the body is a shallow fungal infection of the skin, hair, and nails. Ringworm is generally but not always ring-shaped.

II. **Etiology**

    A. Ringworm is caused by *Trichophyton tonsurans, Microsporum canis dermatophytes,* and *Epidermophyton fungi.*

III. **Signs, Symptoms, and History**
    A. Rash begins as small, red, colorless, or depigmented circle that progressively becomes larger.
    B. Circular border is elevated and perhaps scaly and dry or moist and crusted.
    C. Center of circle starts to heal as area becomes larger.
    D. Mild pruritus, pain, and scaling.
    E. Close contact with infected animals (dog, cat, pet mice) or human beings.
    F. Usually seen on arms, face, and neck but may occur elsewhere on body.
    G. Most common cause of alopecia.

IV. **Initial Management**
    A. Cover area; younger student excluded from school; older student may return to class.
    B. Use good handwashing techniques.
    C. Clean toys or items contaminated by infected younger student.
    D. Tinea capitis (ringworm of the scalp) must be treated by oral administration of griseofulvin.

V. **Exclusion/Readmission**
    A. Depends on the age and developmental level of student. If younger student or disabled and lesion cannot be covered, exclude student from school until treatment has started.
    B. After treatment, recheck in 1-2 weeks for improvement; if no improvement, refer student back to primary care practitioner.

VI. **Web Sites**
    American Academy of Family Physicians. Tinea Infections: Athlete's Foot, Jock Itch, and Ringworm (handout)
    http://www.familydoctor.org/handouts/316.html
    MedlinePlus Health Information: Tinea Corporis
    http://www.nlm.nih.gov/medlineplus/ency/article/000877.htm
    MedlinePlus Health Information: Ringworm (photos)
    http://www.nlm.nih.gov/medlineplus/ency/article/001439.htm

ROSEOLA (EXANTHEM SUBITUM)

I. **Definition**
    A. Roseola is an acute illness of children younger than 4; it commonly occurs around 1 year of age. The incidence is highest in the spring.

II. **Etiology**
    A. The cause of roseola is human herpesvirus type 6 (HHV-6).

III. **Signs, Symptoms, and History**
    A. *Incubation period is approximately 5 to 15 days.*
    B. *Period of communicability is unclear.*
    C. *Transmission is unknown.*
    D. Illness is self-limiting.
    E. Sudden fever as high as 104 degrees to 106 degrees F (40-41.1 degrees C) lasting 3 to 5 days; temperature drops with appearance of rash.

F. Discrete rose-pink maculopapular rash, initially on trunk, then spreading to face, neck, and extremities. Fades on pressure, nonpruritic, and lasts from 1 to 2 days.

G. Cervical/postauricular lymphadenopathy.

H. Reddened pharynx, coryza, cough.

I. Complications are rare but include encephalitis, recurrent febrile seizures, and mononucleosis-like illness.

IV. **Initial Management**

A. Treatment is supportive and symptomatic.

B. Isolate child from other children.

C. Treat fever (refer to fever discussion).

D. If prone to febrile seizure, discuss precaution with parent(s).

V. **Exclusion/Readmission**

A. Exclude student from school.

B. Student may return to school when fever and rash have gone.

VI. **Web Sites**

eMedicine: Pediatrics, Roseola Infantum
http://www.emedicine.com/emerg/topic400.htm
Virtual Children's Hospital: Roseola
http://www.vh.org/Patients/IHB/Peds/CQQA/roseola.htm

RUBELLA (GERMAN MEASLES)

I. **Definition**

A. Rubella is a mild infectious childhood disease that was widespread but is now infrequent because of the availability of a vaccine. The greatest danger of rubella is its effect on a fetus.

II. **Etiology**

A. The cause is an RNA virus of the genus *Rubivirus*.

III. **Signs, Symptoms, and History**

A. *Incubation period is 14 to 21 days.*

B. *Period of communicability is from 7 days before rash appears to at least 5 days after the rash appears. Immunization prevents the disease.*

C. *Transmission is by direct contact with nasopharyngeal secretions, feces, or urine from infected individual.*

D. Prodromal stage is first 1 to 5 days and then subsides 1 day after rash has appeared.

E. Low-grade fever, headache, malaise, anorexia, mild conjunctivitis, nasal discharge, cough, pharyngitis, and swelling of lymph nodes behind ears.

F. Rash, distinct faint pink; appears first on face and rapidly spreads downward. Disappears in same order as began; usually gone by third day. Sometimes resembles measles or scarlet fever.

IV. **Initial Management**

A. Treatment is supportive and symptomatic.

B. Follow appropriate isolation practice from other students.

C. Good handwashing techniques and hygienic procedures by school personnel.

D. Proper disposal of soiled tissues.

E. Review immunization records of all students for rubella.

F. Notify parents and parents of any student not immunized, following school and county health guidelines.

G. Notify and follow local health department regulations regarding reporting of disease.

H. Be aware of other students, staff, or family members for symptoms and refer for care as needed.

I. Complications are rare but include arthritis, encephalitis, and purpura.

J. Refer any pregnant woman exposed to rubella to her HCP. In early pregnancy rubella may cause congenital rubella syndrome, which is a serious multisystem disease resulting in heart damage, blindness, deafness, mental retardation, or miscarriage and stillbirth.

V. Exclusion/Readmission

A. Immediately isolate and exclude student from school.

B. In preschools and day care centers, any child under 12 months without vaccination against rubella should be excluded until immunized or until 3 weeks after the onset of rash in the last case.

C. Student may return to school minimum of 6 days after rash has appeared.

VI. Web Sites

KidsHealth for Parents: Rubella (German Measles)

http://www.kidshealth.org/parent/infections/skin/german_measles.html

SCABIES

I. Definition

A. Scabies is a highly pruritic, communicable infection of the skin.

II. Etiology

A. Scabies is caused by the itch mite *Sarcoptes scabiei.* The female pregnant mite burrows beneath the stratum corneum layer of the epidermis and deposits her eggs and fecal material. These burrows are minute, linear, grayish-brown, threadlike lesions that are a distinctive sign; the mite may be seen at the end of the lesion, appearing as a black dot.

III. Signs, Symptoms, and History

A. *Incubation period is 4-6 weeks for new infestation. In a person who has had scabies previously, symptoms appear within a few days.*

B. *Period of communicability is while mite is alive. The mite cannot live over 48 to 72 hours away from a host.*

C. *Transmission is by direct contact or indirect contact of infected garments or linens.*

D. Intense itching, more severe at night.

E. Raised grayish-white, linear burrows, papules, or vesicles.

F. Child under 2 years, largest eruption usually found on feet and ankles.

G. Child over 2 years, largest eruption usually found on hands and wrist.

H. Skin eruptions are commonly found in the webbing of the fingers; the skinfolds of the wrist, elbow, or knee; the penis; the breast or shoulder blades; the axillary folds; and the abdomen, buttocks, and groin.

Box 3-6	*Instructions for Permethrin 5%*

1. Infected household members must be treated at the same time.
2. Treatment is most easily applied at bedtime.
3. Bath or shower and dry skin completely.
4. Trim nails and with brush, apply product under fingernails.
5. Apply lotion from neck down to the soles of the feet, massage into all surfaces, including skinfolds.
6. If lotion gets into eyes, immediately flush with water.
7. Leave on overnight, 8 to 14 hours, following pharmaceutical instructions.
8. Remove during a warm bath, shower, and shampooing of hair.
9. Stinging or mild stinging may occur, may be normal for some individuals.
10. Change and wash or dry clean all clothing, linens, and towels used. Dry in hot dryer.

    I. Pustules present, with secondary infection from scratching.

    J. Exposure to scabies at home or school.

IV. **Initial Management**

    A. Isolation depends on the age and development level of the student and the location of the lesions.

    B. Good handwashing technique.

    C. Instruct parent(s) that all family members should be treated. Also, the need to wash all bed linens, towels, underwear, and so forth, in hot water (140 degrees F).

    D. Treatment with permethrin 5% (Elimite) is safe and requires one application. Instructions of medication must be followed.

V. **Exclusion/Readmission**

    A. Exclude student from school until 24 hours after treatment has been completed.

VI. **Web Sites**

    Center For Disease Control Division of Parasitic Diseases: Scabies
    http://www.cdc.gov/ncidod/dpd/parasites/scabies/factsht_scabies.htm
    McKinley Health Center: Scabies (handout)
    http://www.mckinley.uiuc.edu/health-info/dis-cond/commdis/scabies.html

SCARLET FEVER

    I. **Definition**

    A. Scarlet fever is an acute, systemic, contagious childhood disease, usually occurring in spring or late winter. It is also called *scarlatina* (a small scarlet rash).

    II. **Etiology**

    A. The cause is GABHS, generally following streptococcal pharyngitis.

    III. **Signs, Symptoms, and History**

    A. *Incubation period ranges from 1 to 7 days.*

    B. *Period of communicability is during incubation period, and active phase of illness is approximately 10 days but may persist for months.*

C. *Transmission is by direct contact with an infected person, by droplet spread, or by indirect contact with contaminated articles and ingestion of contaminated food (e.g., milk, milk products, deviled eggs).*

D. Complications are otitis media, rheumatic fever, glomerulonephritis, peritonsillar abscess, sinusitis and carditis, and polyarthritis.

E. Prodromal lasts 1 to 2 days.
   1. Abrupt fever from 102 degrees to 104 degrees F (39-40 degrees C); increased pulse, which is out of proportion to fever, headache, pharyngitis, chills, and malaise.
   2. Abdominal pain may occur.

F. Exanthem, skin
   1. Rash appears 12 to 48 hours after onset of pharyngitis; red, punctiform lesions (pinpoint) with fine papules on trunk and extremities.
   2. Increased redness in Pastia's lines (lines in inguinal, antecubital, or other skinfolds), which do not blanch upon pressure; skin feels rough or like sandpaper; rash persists for about 1 week. Desquamation occurs on fingers and toes, occasionally on palms of hands, and soles of feet. May be complete by 3 weeks or longer.

G. Exanthem, in mouth
   1. Red pharynx and uvula, tonsils enlarged, red, edematous and covered with gray-white exudate.
   2. Tongue is swollen, red, and has a white coating from which red papillae project for 1 to 2 days (white strawberry tongue); white sloughs off, displaying prominent papillae and palate, which persist with erythematous punctuate lesions (red strawberry tongue) by 4 to 5 days.

IV. **Initial Management**
   A. Isolate child from other students.
   B. Good handwashing technique.
   C. Supportive measures.
   D. Call parent to have evaluation by HCP and to report diagnosis so other children can be observed.
   E. Treatment of choice is penicillin, erythromycin for sensitive children; fever usually subsides 24 hours after initiation of therapy.

V. **Exclusion/Readmission**
   A. Exclude student from school.
   B. Student may return to school 24 hours after antibiotic therapy has been initiated and has been fever-free for 24 hours.

VI. **Web Sites**
   KidsHealth for Parents: Scarlet Fever
   http://www.kidshealth.org/parent/infections/bacterial_viral/scarlet_fever.html

SHIGELLOSIS (ACUTE DIARRHEA)

I. **Definition**
   A. Shigellosis is a dysentery-like acute diarrhea involving the large and distal small colon. It can be a serious disease, particularly in children younger than 2. It can be epidemic in day care centers and institutions.

II. Etiology
    A. Shigellosis is caused by *Shigella dysenteriae;* there are 4 subgenera of bacilli. The pathogen stimulates loss of fluids and electrolytes. Peak incidence is in late summer.

III. Signs, Symptoms, and History
    A. *Incubation period is 1-7 days.*
    B. *Period of communicability is during acute infection and until bacteria are no longer present in feces, 1-4 weeks.*
    C. *Transmission is directly or indirectly by an infected individual.*
    D. Onset is variable but generally abrupt.
    E. Fever up to 104 degrees F (40 degrees C), nausea and vomiting and sometimes toxemia.
    F. Watery diarrhea with mucus and pus 12-48 hours after onset.
    G. Convulsions associated with fever in young children.
    H. Stools preceded by abdominal cramps, tenesmus, and straining.
    I. Headache, nuchal rigidity, delirium.
    J. Severe dehydration and collapse is a complication.
    K. Usually self-limiting, lasting several days to weeks, average time 4-10 days.

IV. Initial Management
    A. Good handwashing techniques (e.g., after diapering, toileting, and fecal accidents).
    B. Call parent(s) and advise going to HCP.
    C. Discontinue formula, milk, and solids.
    D. Provide clear liquids.
    E. Treat fever.
    F. Treatment is with antibiotics.
    G. Educate school staff and parents about outbreaks caused by contaminated water, which can occur in youth activity groups, such as sports teams, or on field or overnight trips.

V. Exclusion/Readmission
    A. Depends on age of child and physical involvement.
    B. Exclude from school until diarrhea has stopped and local health department recommendations have been met for any young child or adult.

VI. Web Sites
Center for Disease Control: Shigellosis
http://www.cdc.gov/ncidod/dbmd/diseaseinfo/shigellosis_g.htm

BACTERIAL SKIN INFECTION

I. Definition
    A. Bacterial skin lesions are abscesses, carbuncles, cellulitis, folliculitis, furuncles, impetigo, and pyoderma. These lesions are generally localized and discrete. They occur more frequently in the younger child, decreasing with increased age.

II. Etiology

A. Bacterial skin infections are caused by various strains of staphylococcus and streptococcus pathogens. This bacterium is normal flora of the skin and becomes pathogenic, depending on the individual's skin integrity, the barrier, the individual's immune and cellular defenses, and the invasiveness and toxigenicity of the particular organism.

III. Signs, Symptoms, and History

A. Those with immunodeficiency disorders, debilitating conditions, on immunosuppressive therapy, or disabled individuals with poor hygiene habits and behaviors are at an increased risk.

B. Primary finding is lesion or lesions that contain pus.

C. Carbuncles (multiple or cluster of boils).
  1. Develop more slowly than single furuncle.
  2. Most common in males and on nape of neck.
  3. Fever and prostration may occur.
  4. Systemic effect, when severe, is malaise.
  5. Treatment: cleansing and topical or systemic antibiotics depending on severity.

D. Folliculitis (infection of hair follicle).
  1. Pinhead-sized lesions or larger pustules surrounded by redness.
  2. Usually on scalp or extremities.
  3. Generally number of pustules are present in same area.
  4. Can be mildly pruritic.
  5. Systemic effect, when severe, is malaise.
  6. Treatment: cleansing and topical or systemic antibiotics depending on severity.

E. Furuncles (boils).
  1. Lesion is larger than a pimple.
  2. Redness, elevation, and tenderness.
  3. Initial nodule becomes a pustule with central necrosis.
  4. Sanguineous purulent discharge.
  5. Occur frequently on neck, face, buttocks, breasts, and axillae.
  6. Systemic effect, when severe, is malaise.
  7. Treatment: cleansing and topical or systemic antibiotics depending on severity.

F. Cellulitis.
  1. Inflammation of skin and subcutaneous tissues, swelling, extreme redness.
  2. Lymphangitis "streaking" usually observed.
  3. May progress to abscess.
  4. Regional lymph nodes often involved.
  5. Systemic effects include fever, malaise.
  6. Treatment: oral or parenteral antibiotics; moist, hot compresses; immobilization of affected area; and rest.

G. Impetigo (see "Impetigo").

H. Pyoderma *(Staphylococcus, Streptococcus)*.
  1. Infection extends into dermis.
  2. Tissue reaction more severe.

     3. Systemic effects include fever, lymphangitis.
     4. Contagious and autoinoculable.
     5. Treatment; antibacterial soap bathing as prescribed, wet compresses, soap and water bathing.
     6. Scarring may or may not occur.
  I. Scalded skin syndrome *(S. aureus).*
     1. Macular erythema, with a "sandpaper" texture of involved skin.
     2. Epidermis becomes wrinkled, and large blisters appear.
     3. Superficial exfoliation of the skin.
     4. May be misidentified as child abuse or neglect.
     5. Treatment: systemic and topical antibiotics; gentle cleaning with saline, Burrow's solution, or silver nitrate compresses (0.25%); adequate fluid intake.

IV. Initial Management
  A. Careful handwashing before and after contact with student.
  B. Isolate from others, depending on child's age and hygiene habits, call parent(s).
  C. Teach child and all other students the importance of handwashing and care of infectious skin lesions.

V. Exclusion/Readmission
  A. Exclusion depends on extent of condition, student's age, level of understanding, and need for medical intervention.

VI. Web Sites
American Academy of Family Physicians: Skin and Wound Infections: An Overview
  http://www.aafp.org/afp/980515ap/odell.html
Merck Manual of Diagnosis and Therapy: Bacterial Infections of the Skin
  http://www.merck.com/pubs/mmanual/section10/chapter112/112a.htm

STREPTOCOCCAL PHARYNGITIS (STREP THROAT)

I. Definition
  A. Streptococcal sore throat is an inflammation of the upper airway. The infection is not serious but the complications are (e.g., acute rheumatic fever [ARF], acute glomerulonephritis).

II. Etiology
  A. The cause is GABHS.

III. Signs, Symptoms, and History
  A. *Transmission is person-to-person by contact with infectious respiratory secretions.*
  B. High percentages of acute pharyngitis are viral, making a throat culture necessary.
  C. Acute onset of pharyngitis.
  D. Headache, fever, nausea, and abdominal pain.
  E. Pharynx and tonsils may be inflamed and covered with exudate.
  F. Petechiae may be present against background of diffuse redness.
  G. Tender anterior cervical lymph nodes.
  H. Pain is mild to severe and makes swallowing difficult.

I. Clinical symptoms subside in 3-5 days unless complications occur; complications include acute glomerulonephritis, which can occur in about 10 days, and rheumatic fever in about 19 days; Sydenham's chorea may occur several months later, as well as rheumatic heart disease.

IV. **Initial Management**
A. Isolate individual from others and call parent(s).
B. Good handwashing technique.
C. Control fever elevation with cooling measures (see "Fever").
D. Advise parents to seek throat culture to rule out GABHS. Office/clinic setting test kits are available for identification, but if test results are negative, a confirmatory throat culture is recommended (American Academy of Pediatrics, 1997).
E. Treatment is oral antibiotics for approximately 10 days.
F. Advise parents to complete prescribed length of medication to eliminate organism that may lead to rheumatic fever symptoms.
G. Remind student/parent when there is a positive throat culture for GABHS to discard toothbrush and replace after 24 hours of antibiotic treatment.
H. Share information with other parent(s) and staff, since GABHS can be epidemic in day care and school sites.

V. **Exclusion/Readmission**
A. Call parent(s) and dismiss student from school.
B. Readmit student after 48 hours of antibiotic treatment, if no fever for preceding 24 hours and when no symptoms are present that interfere with school.

VI. **Web Sites**
FamilyDoctor.org: Strep Throat
http://www.familydoctor.org/handouts/670.html
Virtual Children's Hospital: Streptococcal Pharyngitis (Strep Throat, Strep Tonsillitis)
http://www.vh.org/Providers/ClinRef/FPHandbook/Chapter20/08-20.html

STY (HORDEOLUM)

I. **Definition**
A. A sty is a localized inflammation of the sebaceous gland near the eyelashes and is generally on the lower eyelid. Also spelled stye.

II. **Etiology**
A. The most common cause is *S. aureus.*

III. **Signs, Symptoms, and History**
A. Localized edema and redness.
B. Tenderness or pain.
C. Often comes to a head and resembles a pimple in 2 to 3 days.
D. Can be an *internal sty,* in which the abscess is large and may be observed through the skin or conjunctival surface, or an *external sty,* which is smaller, superficial, observed at the lid margin, and involves the gland.
E. Usually unilateral.
F. Visual acuity not affected.

IV. Initial Management
  A. Ask student or call parent(s) and inquire if aware of the problem and if treatment has been initiated.
  B. Good handwashing technique by school staff to prevent spread of organism.
  C. Instruct student not to rub or touch eyes because doing so may spread infection. Do not attempt to squeeze sty.
  D. Frequent warm compresses applied 2 to 3 times a day to bring sty to a head.
  E. If spontaneous rupture does not occur and sty is large and edematous, may need surgical incision and drainage.
  F. Topical antibiotics can be prescribed.
  G. If no result from medication, return to primary care practitioner for systemic antibiotic.
  H. When untreated, cellulitis of the lid or orbit may develop, requiring systemic antibiotics.
 V. Exclusion/Readmission
  A. Depends on student's age, level of functioning, and personal habits.
  B. Excluded student may return after treatment has been initiated.
VI. Web Sites
  Intelihealth: Sty (Hordeolum)
  http://www.intelihealth.com/IH/ihtIH/WSIHW000/9339/10151.html
  McKinley Health Center: Sty (Hordeolum) (handout)
  http://www.mckinley.uiuc.edu/health-info/dis-cond/misc/sty.html

TAPEWORM

A tapeworm is composed of a small head (scolex) and up to 4000 proglottids (segments). It has a characteristic ribbonlike shape and can be up to 30 ft long. Although infestation is not particularly common in the United States, it is frequent in other parts of the world. Because of the large number of visitors and immigrants entering the United States daily, health personnel are seeing an increased number of infected persons. The types of tapeworm are beef, pork, fish, and dwarf.

BEEF, PORK, FISH, AND DWARF TAPEWORMS

  I. Definition
  A. A parasitic infestation of the intestinal tract.
 II. Initial Management
  A. Refer suspected cases to HCP for diagnosis and treatment.
  B. Good handwashing technique.
III. Exclusion/Readmission
  A. Exclude student from school until treatment can be verified.
IV. Web Sites
  Center for Disease Control: Dipylidium Infection
  http://www.cdc.gov/ncidod/dpd/parasites/dipylidium/factsht_dipylidium.htm
  Food Safety Inspection Service
  http://www.fsis.usda.gov/OA/pubs/parasite.htm

Table 3-1 *Etiology, Symptoms, Treatment, and Prevention of Tapeworm Infestation*

Tapeworm	Etiology	Signs, Symptoms, History	Treatment	Prevention
Beef				
Adult worm is 15-30 ft long	*Cestode Taenia saginata* Transmission only by raw or poorly cooked infected beef	Usually asymptomatic; epigastric pain, diarrhea, weight loss Active proglottid may be felt crawling in anus, visible in stool	Praziquantel (Biltricide), 20 mg/kg per day in 4 divided doses for 1 day Niclosamide (Yomesan, Niclocide) also effective	Thoroughly cook beef Freezing below temperature of −5 degrees C (23 degrees F) for more than 4 days Adequate toilet facilities and meat inspection help to control
Pork				
Adult worm is 8-10 ft long	*Cestode Taenia solium* Transmitted directly through ingestion of egg-infested food or water, directly from contaminated feces to oral cavity	Usually asymptomatic; heavy larval infestations may cause muscle pains, weakness, fever If CNS involved, meningoencephalitis or seizures Eggs around anus or in stool	Same as beef	Thoroughly cook pork Same as beef prevention

Continued

Table 3-1 *Etiology, Symptoms, Treatment, and Prevention of Tapeworm Infestation—cont'd*

Tapeworm	Etiology	Signs, Symptoms, History	Treatment	Prevention
Fish				
Adult worm is 15-30 ft long	Cestode *Diphyllobothrium latum* Transmitted directly through ingestion of egg-infested fish or water; directly from contaminated feces to oral cavity	Usually asymptomatic; mild GI symptoms Eggs or segments of the worm in stool	Praziquantel (Biltricide) or niclosamide (Niclocide) are drugs of choice	Thoroughly cook all fresh fish or freeze at −18 degrees C (0 degrees F) for 24 hr All fish and shellfish for raw or semiraw consumption should be blast frozen to −35 degrees C or −31 degrees F or below for 15 hr
Dwarf				
Children more susceptible	Cestode *Hymenolepis nana* Transmitted directly through ingestion of egg-infested food or water; directly from contaminated feces to oral cavity; ingestion of larvae-carrying insects	May be asymptomatic; diarrhea, abdominal discomfort, dizziness, lethargy in children Eggs in stool	Same as beef	Elimination of rodents from home environment Protect food and water from contamination Education regarding hygienic practices and personal hygiene

TESTICULAR TORSION

I. **Definition**
   A. Testicular (spermatic cord) torsion (TT) is an acute loss of blood supply to the testis causing ensuing ischemic injury and possible tissue death of the testicle.

II. **Etiology**
   A. May follow trauma but most often occurs without known cause. Peak incidence is 12 to 18 years of age, but may occur at any age. Left testicle more likely to be involved because of longer spermatic cord.

III. **Signs, Symptoms, and History**
   A. Sudden onset of abdominal or testicular pain, which is excruciating and unremitting.
   B. Frequently occurs during sleep.
   C. Scrotum may be edematous, reddened, and warm to touch.
   D. Often bilateral.
   E. Minimal elevation of the testis increases the pain.
   F. Earlier episodes of transitory pain reported in about one half of the cases.
   G. Absence of blood flow to the testis for 4 to 6 hours may cause loss of spermatogenesis.

IV. **Initial Management**
   A. This is an emergency.
   B. Contact parent regarding prompt evaluation by physician.
   C. Treatment must begin within 6 to 12 hours from onset of pain.
   D. May be reduced manually if pain less than 4 to 6 hours, but usually requires surgical exploration and detorsion to prevent reoccurrence and to preserve fertility.
   E. Infection, tumor, trauma, hydrocele, kidney stone, or hernia needs to be ruled out.
   F. Complications of untreated TT include testicular atrophy, abscess, and loss of testis or decreased fertility.

V. **Exclusion/Readmission**
   A. Does not apply.

VI. **Web Sites**
   The Medical Center of Central Georgia: Testicular Torsion
   http://www.mccg.org/childrenshealth/urology/testor.asp

URINARY TRACT INFECTION

I. **Definition**
   A. Urinary tract infection (UTI) is a clinical condition that involves primarily the growth of bacteria within the urinary tract that is normally sterile. May involve the *lower urinary tract:* urethra and bladder, and/or the *upper urinary tract:* ureters, renal pelvis, renal calyces, and renal parenchyma. There are three classifications of UTI: (1) asymptomatic bacteriuria, (2) cystitis, and (3) pyelonephritis.
   B. Peak incidence, not including structural anomalies, occurs in children between 2 and 6 years of age. At age 1 year and older, the incidence is

higher in males; occurs more frequently in uncircumcised boys. Beyond age 2, it is more common in females (Behrman, Kliegman, and Jenson, 2000).

II. Etiology

A. The most common cause of UTI is bacteria. The most prominent bacterial organism is *Escherichia coli*, followed by *Klebsiella, Proteus,* and then *Pseudomonas, S. aureus, Haemophilus,* and coagulase-negative *Staphylococcus*. Viral infections, especially adenovirus, are a cause for cystitis.

B. Increased incidence of bacteriuria in the female is due in part to the short urethra, about ¾ in (2 cm), in young females and 1½ in (4 cm) in mature women. The length of the male urethra, 8 in (20 cm) accounts for inhibition of entry and growth of pathogens. In the uncircumcised male, bacterial pathogens ascend the urethra from the flora beneath the prepuce.

III. Signs, Symptoms, and History

A. Manifestations depend on age.

B. Unrecognized symptoms referred to as *asymptomatic bacteriuria,* occur most frequently in girls. Have day or nighttime incontinence or perineal discomfort and a positive urine culture, usually benign infection, unless pregnant, when if not treated can result in symptoms.

C. *Cystitis* is an inflammation of the bladder and ureters; there is no fever or renal injury.

D. *Pyelonephritis* is an infection involving the upper urinary tract and renal parenchyma.

E. In newborns and those under age 2:
1. Poor feeding; failure to thrive; vomiting, diarrhea, and abdominal distention; and jaundice.
2. Fever or hypothermia, sepsis.
3. Altered voiding pattern, strong-smelling urine, irritability and squirming, persistent diaper rash.

F. In preschool and those over age 2:
1. Fever.
2. Increased frequency of urination, dysuria, or urgency.
3. Lower abdominal pain or costovertebral tenderness.
4. Pyelonephritis indications: high fever with chills, severe abdominal or flank pain, malaise, vomiting, diarrhea, jaundice in the neonate.

G. In adolescents (classic signs):
1. Lower tract infection: fever often absent, frequency and urgency, dysuria (pain and burning), enuresis.
2. Upper tract infection: fever and chills, flank pain, lower tract symptoms occur a few days later, lower abdominal pain, costovertebral tenderness.
3. May develop UTI after first time intercourse.

IV. Initial Management

A. Discuss clinical manifestations and need for diagnostic evaluation with parent(s) and stress need for follow-up.

Box 3-7	***Preventive Education for Urinary Tract Infections***

1. Discuss diet high in animal protein to avoid alkaline urine.
2. Encourage generous fluid intake.
3. Good perianal hygiene, wipe from front to back.
4. Teach avoidance of holding urine.
5. Avoid wearing tight panties.
6. Use cotton underwear instead of synthetic underwear.
7. Avoid use of bubble baths if susceptible to UTIs.
8. Educate sexually active teenagers to void after intercourse.
9. Treat vaginitis or pinworm infestation to avoid irritation/scratching.

    B. Treat the fever, follow school guidelines/procedures.

    C. If enuretic, assure student it is only symptom of the infection.

    D. For infants and toddlers, check diaper every ½ hour to determine signs of discomfort, straining, intermittent starting or stopping, dripping of small amounts, frequency, and odor.

    E. Educate about prevention and treatment of infection with child and parent.

    F. Treatment:

        1. Midstream urine culture for identification.

        2. Mild symptoms: treatment is delayed until culture results available, nitrofurantoin, amoxicillin.

        3. Severe symptoms: culture is obtained and treatment begins immediately, therapy with trimethoprim-sulfamethoxazole suggested, but the previous treatment is also used.

        4. Acute febrile infections suggesting pyelonephritis is treated with broad-spectrum antibiotic for 14 days.

        5. Hospitalization for acute symptoms of pyelonephritis with parenteral antibiotics.

        6. Single antibiotic dose or 3-day treatment for adolescent girls can be considered for uncomplicated UTI.

        7. When younger than 5, complicated UTI, radiological evaluation of kidneys and bladder is done to rule out renal scarring.

V. Exclusion/Readmission

    A. Does not apply.

VI. Web Sites

    The National Kidney and Urologic Diseases Information Clearinghouse: Urinary Tract Infections

    http://www.niddk.nih.gov/health/urolog/pubs/utichild/utichild.htm

VARICELLA-ZOSTER VIRUS (CHICKENPOX)

I. Definition

    A. Chickenpox is a highly contagious, self-limiting disease marked by an eruption on the skin and mucous membranes. The initial infection results in a lifelong dormant infection of the sensory ganglion nerve cells. Reactivation of this latency condition is the cause of HZ or shingles.

II. Etiology

    A. Varicella-zoster virus (VZV) is a human herpesvirus. It is the cause of primary, latent, and recurrent infections. Epidemics are most frequent in winter and spring.

III. Signs, Symptoms, and History

    A. *Incubation period is 10-21 days.*

    B. *Period of communicability is from 1 day before the rash to 5 to 6 days after the onset of the rash.*

    C. *Transmission is by secretions from the respiratory tract of infected persons and to a lesser degree, discharge from skin lesions and scabs until dry.*

    D. Generally mild illness in childhood.

    E. In adolescents and immunocompromised children there can be increased morbidity and mortality.

    F. Predisposes individual to GABHS and *S. aureus* infections.

    G. Prodromal (initial stage):

        1. Slight fever.

        2. Malaise.

        3. Anorexia.

        4. Headache.

        5. Mild abdominal pain.

    H. Rash

        1. First appears on back and chest, spreading outward to face and extremities; but sparse on distal limbs. May be limited to a few lesions.

        2. Continues to make its appearance for 3 to 7 days.

        3. Begins as a flat red macule that rapidly progresses to lesions resembling insect bites, itchy.

        4. These lesions develop into blisters with an amber fluid.

        5. Blisterlike eruptions are in crops; after they rupture, crusts form.

        6. All stages present in varying degrees at one time: macules, papules, vesicles, and scabs.

IV. Initial Management

    A. Isolate student from other students.

    B. Maintain good handwashing technique.

    C. Keep infected student isolated from immunosuppressed individuals and those with eczema, malignancies, and human immunodeficiency syndrome/acquired immunodeficiency syndrome (HIV/AIDS), since they are at high risk for greater complications.

    D. Disease can be prevented by immunization with a live-attenuated VZV vaccine. Required now for children in some states.

    E. If high-risk students are exposed, varicella zoster immunoglobulin (VZIG) given within 72 hours may alter the course of the disease.

V. Exclusion/Readmission

    A. Exclude student from school.

    B. Student may return to school minimum of 7 days after onset of rash; all vesicles (blisters) must have crusted.

VI. **Additional Information**
   A. Gestational chickenpox can cause a severe reaction in a pregnant woman and a rare but identifiable syndrome in the fetus. The infection can be life threatening to the fetus.
VII. **Web Sites**
   Centers for Disease Control: Chickenpox (Varicella)
      http://www.cdc.gov/nip/diseases/varicella/
   National Foundation for Infectious Diseases
      http://www.nfid.org
   National Immunization Program
      http://www.cdc.gov/nip
   Parents of Kids with Infectious Diseases
      http://www.pkids.org

BIBLIOGRAPHY

American Academy of Pediatrics, Committee on Infectious Diseases: Peter G, editor: *Red book: report of the committee on infectious diseases,* ed 24, Elk Grove Village, Ill, 1997, The Academy.

Anderson K, editor: *Mosby's medical, nursing, and allied health dictionary,* ed 5, St Louis, 1998, Mosby.

Behrman RE, Kliegman RM, Jenson HB: *Nelson textbook of pediatrics,* ed 16, Philadelphia, 2000, WB Saunders.

Benenson A, editor: *Control of communicable diseases manual,* ed 17, Washington, DC, 2000, American Public Health Association.

Bowden VR, Dickey SB, Greenberg CS: *Children and their families: the continuum of care,* Philadelphia, 1998, WB Saunders.

Burns CE et al: *Pediatric primary care: a handbook for nurse practitioners,* ed 2, Philadelphia, 2000, WB Saunders.

Centers for Disease Control and Prevention: *Epidemiology and prevention of vaccine-preventable diseases,* ("Pink Book"), ed 6, Waldorf, Md, 2000, Public Health Foundation.

Centers for Disease Control and Prevention: *Giardiasis,* September 13, 2000, Available online: http://www.cdc.gov/ncidod/dpd/parasites/giardiasis/default.htm. Accessed on August 8, 2001.

Centers for Disease Control and Prevention: Prevention of hepatitis A through active or passive immunization: recommendations of the Advisory Committee on Immunization Practices (ACIP), *MMWR Morb Mortal Wkly Rep* 48(RR-12):1-37, 1999.

Centers for Disease Control and Prevention: *Preventing emerging infectious diseases: a strategy for the 21st century,* Atlanta, Ga, 1998, The Centers, Available online: http://www.cdc.gov/ncidod.

Dychkowski L: Understanding the common viral infection among school-age children, *School Nurse News* 15(5):2-4, 1998.

Finberg L: *Saunders manual of pediatric practice,* Philadelphia, 1998, WB Saunders.

Giardina RG, Psota CE: Universal precautions and infection control in a school setting. In Porter S, Haynie M, Bierle T, et al, editors: *Children and youth assisted by medical technology in educational settings: guidelines for care,* Baltimore, 1997, Paul H Brookes.

Gildea J: *Human parvovirus B19: flushed in face though healthy (fifth disease and more),* *Pediatr Nurs* 24(4):325-329, 1998.

Hodgson BB, Kizior RJ: *Saunders nursing drug handbook 2001,* Philadelphia, 2001, WB Saunders.

Jackson PL, Vessey JA: *Primary care of the child with a chronic condition,* ed 3, St Louis, 2000, Mosby.

Jacobs R, Margolis H, Coleman P: The cost-effectiveness of adolescent hepatitis: a vaccination in states with the highest disease rates, *Arch Pediatr Adolesc Med* 154:763-770, 2000.

O'Toole M, editor: *Miller-Keane encyclopedia and dictionary of medicine, nursing, and allied health,* ed 6, Philadelphia, 1997, WB Saunders.

Pollack RJ: *Head lice information,* August 7, 2000, Department of Immunology and Infectious Disease (DIID), Laboratory of Public Health Entomology, Harvard School of Public Health, Available online: http://www.hsph.harvard.edu/headlice.html. Accessed on Sep 22, 2001.

Rakel R: *Saunders manual of medical practice,* Philadelphia, 1996, WB Saunders.

Shor E: *Caring for your school-age child,* Elk Grove Village, Ill, 1995, American Academy of Pediatrics.

Shovein M, Damazo R, Hyams I: Hepatitis A: how benign is it? *Am J Nurs* 100(3):43-47, 2000.

Siberry G, Iannone R, editors: *The Harriet Lane handbook,* ed 15, St Louis, 2000, Mosby.

Wong DL et al: *Nursing care of infants and children,* ed 6, St Louis, 1999, Mosby.

CHAPTER 4

Chronic Conditions

*T*he school-age population with chronic illness is increasing and will continue to increase as medical technology saves and extends the lives of affected students daily. The physical, emotional, intellectual, and social impact of chronic illness on children is immense, and nurses and educators contribute greatly to the goal of enabling each individual to achieve maximum potential in all areas of functioning.

This chapter provides comprehensive, concise information on 28 chronic conditions found in the school-age child that require nursing assessment and management. Each chronic condition uses the same format for usability and cohesiveness in reading and use by the nurse. The complexity of the chronic condition and the need for the school nurse to be aware of current, necessary knowledge dictate the information found in this chapter.

As the nurse reads the individual chronic conditions in this chapter, a picture of the great number of health concerns and emergencies each condition could produce will emerge. There is no question as to the importance of nursing care to the physical well-being and safety of each student with a chronic illness. The school nurse is in a position to facilitate a networking and learning environment between school staff and community health care providers (HCPs), which will bridge the gap of understanding the unique school health care and support provided during the school day to students and their families.

Individualized health care plans (IHCPs) and individualized emergency care plans (IECPs) are now a part of the student's school records. Subsections included with each condition will assist in developing these plans.

The "Effects on Individual" section provides some insight into the stress and uncertainty that may accompany each condition. Recognition of the psychological effects of long-term illness on both child and family will better equip the nurse to help students and their families cope and adjust to the many difficulties of living with a chronic illness. The nurse can have a positive influence on attitudes among staff and families by emphasizing the child's strengths rather than focusing on deficits.

AMBIGUOUS GENITALIA

I. Definition
   A. Normal sexual differentiation occurs in utero with external and internal genitalia consistent with the sex chromosome of either 46 XX (female) or XY (male). Embryos have the potential to develop as either males or females with differentiation into testes or ovaries during the seventh or eighth week of gestation. Errors in the embryonic sex determination and differentiation result in diverse degrees of intermediate sex, a condition known as *hermaphroditism* or *intersexuality.*

The condition where the chromosomal sex is different from the phenotype sex is often referred to as *intersex.*
B. *Hermaphroditism* suggests a discrepancy between the morphology of the gonads, ovaries/testes, and the appearance of the external genitalia.
C. *True hermaphroditism* presents itself with both ovarian and testicular tissue as separate organs or combined in the same organ (ovotestis), an extremely rare condition in which 80% have a 46 XX chromosome constitution (Behrman, Kliegman, and Jenson, 2000). *Female pseudohermaphrodites* have ovaries, and *male pseudohermaphrodites* have testes; both have ambiguous genitalia.
D. *Intersexual* conditions are classified by the histological appearance of the gonads but are sometimes referred to as a situation where the chromosomal and phenotype sex are different.
II. **Etiology**
A. May be caused by atypical differentiation of primitive gonads, and differentiation and development of internal duct systems and external genitalia. Alteration in these processes may result in a defect of embryogenesis, abnormalities of chromosomal complement, and biochemical abnormalities (androgen insensitivity, defective sex hormonal synthesis in a male, placental transfer of masculinizing agents in a female, or congenital adrenal hyperplasia [CAH], also called *adrenogenital syndrome*). CAH is the most common cause of ambiguous genitalia.
B. *Female pseudohermaphroditism* usually occurs when the female fetus is exposed to excessive androgens, and in the male pseudohermaphroditism usually occurs from androgen insensitivity. True hermaphroditism is not completely understood. See "Additional Information" for other ambiguous sexual conditions.
III. **Characteristics**
A. *True hermaphroditism.*
1. Has both an ovary and a testis or an ovotestis, which are usually nonfunctional.
2. Often raised as a female (Behrman, Kliegman, and Jenson, 2000).
B. Other.
1. The phenotype may be female or male; however, the external genitalia are ambiguous.
2. Gender assignment may not be the same as genetic or gonadal sex.
IV. **Health Concerns/Emergencies**
A. An electrolyte imbalance such as CAH can be life threatening if unidentified and/or untreated at birth.
B. Gender assignment of sex, when doubt exists, is a social emergency for the newborn and family and continues throughout life.
C. Need hormones or assistive medications during particular times of life.
D. May have lifelong emotional difficulties.
E. Need for long-term management.

V. Effects on Individual

A. Will need to process and make decisions about sexual identity, a developmental process that lasts through childhood, adolescence, and into adulthood.

B. Emotional/psychological.
 1. Have feelings of guilt and shame, as may parents.
 2. May not have been told or know their gender assignment.
 3. Cannot understand development of sexual body parts so may have feelings of inadequacy, shame, or inferiority.
 4. May not identify or feel like the gender selection that has been made.

C. Social/interrelations.
 1. Not accepted by one or both parents.
 2. Has to learn to face criticism, comments, and judgments because of sexual differences.
 3. May lack or not identify with parent role model.

VI. Management/Treatment

A. Listen to and support student.

B. Be supportive, understanding, honest, and encouraging with parents.

C. Teach staff and others teaching or working with student about condition in honest and supportive ways.

D. Be aware of medication and any side effects.

E. Monitor anthropometry.

F. Be alert for mental health issues and need for consulting services.

G. At birth: Four conditions that produce ambiguous genitalia requiring prompt and accurate assessment are: (1) female pseudohermaphroditism, (2) male pseudohermaphroditism, (3) true hermaphroditism, and (4) mixed gonadal dysgenesis.
 1. It is imperative that sexual identification be determined immediately and accurately because of associated physical conditions and need for family therapy.
 2. Gender determination may take days or weeks; tests may include history, physical examination, chromosomal analysis, endoscopy, and ultrasonography, radiographic contrast tests, biochemical tests, and laparotomy or gonad biopsy.
 3. Consideration of gender determination should include both anatomical findings and genetic sex determinations.

H. Treatment is centered on the cause and the degree.
 1. *Hermaphroditism* and mixed gonadal dysgenesis: choosing an appropriate gender, maximizing potential for adult sexual function, decreasing psychosocial difficulties. After gender decision, surgical intervention is usually done, and hormonal replacements are given at puberty.
 2. Defective testosterone biosynthesis of male infant: testosterone injections in adolescence and adulthood to initiate puberty and sustain adult masculinization.
 3. Controversy exists regarding treatment and surgery before the child's participation in the decision.

VII. Additional Information

    A. The Intersex Society of North America, established in the 1950s, supports a paradigm for the management of intersexual children. Their purpose is threefold:

        1. Provide qualified professional mental health care for the child and family.

        2. Empower intersexual individuals to understand their health and to choose or refuse any medical intervention.

        3. Avoid harmful or unnecessary surgery.

    B. *Female pseudohermaphroditism:* These individuals have chromatin-positive nuclei and a 46 XX chromosome constitution. This anomaly occurs when the female fetus is exposed to excessive androgens that affect the external genitalia, resulting in clitoral enlargement and labial fusion. Ovarian abnormalities do not exist, but the most common cause of this condition is increased production of androgens, which produces masculinization of the external genitalia. This varies from enlargement of the clitoris to almost masculine genitalia.

        1. The most common cause of this condition is CAH. Androgenic agents administered during pregnancy may cause similar anomalies to the external genitalia. This condition may also result from benign adrenal adenoma, ovarian tumors, and the treatment for threatened abortions.

        2. Untreated CAH results in early sexual maturation with development of facial, axillary, and pubic hair, acne, early sexual maturation, deepening of voice, and noticeable increase in musculature toward an adult male physique. The females do not develop breasts and are amenorrheic and infertile. The male testes remain small, and spermatogenesis does not occur.

    C. *Male pseudohermaphroditism:* These individuals have chromatin negative nuclei and a 46 XY chromosome constitution. External and internal genitalia vary according to degree of development of the external genitalia and internal female organs. These anomalies are caused by defects in testicular differentiation, inadequate production of testicular hormones, and/or defects in androgen action.

    D. *Androgen insensitivity syndrome* (testicular feminization): This syndrome follows X-linked recessive inheritance. Individuals with this condition, 1 in 20,000, appear as normal females despite the presence of testes and a 46 XY chromosome state. External genitalia are female, the vagina generally ends blindly, and the uterus and uterine tubes are absent or rudimentary. Normal development of breasts and female characteristics occur during puberty; however, pubic hair is scant or absent, and menstruation does not take place. Psychosexual orientation is usually completely female, and medically, socially, and legally, they are females.

        1. Testes are generally in the abdomen or inguinal canals but can descend into the labia majora. These individuals are not considered ambiguous because of normal external genitalia even though embryologically, these females represent an extreme

form of male pseudohermaphroditism. Testes are removed on discovery, since approximately one third develop malignant tumors by age 50 (Behrman, Kliegman, and Jenson, 2000).

E. *Mixed gonadal dysgenesis:* This condition is very rare, and individuals have chromatin-negative nuclei: a testis on one side and an undifferentiated gonad on the other. Internal genitalia are female, but male derivatives can be present. External genitalia range from normal female through intermediate to normal male states. Neither breast development nor menstruation occurs during puberty. Differing degrees of virilization are common.

F. *Hypospadias:* Hypospadias occurs in one of every 300 male infants. With this condition, the external urethral orifice is on the ventral surface of the glans of the penis or on the ventral surface of the body (shaft) of the penis. The penis is generally underdeveloped and curved ventrally, known as *chordee.* There are four types of hypospadias, but glandular and penile types make up 80% of cases.

1. This condition is the result of inadequate production of androgens by the fetal testes and/or inadequate receptor sites for the hormones. In perineal hypospadias, the labioscrotal folds fail to fuse, and the external urethral orifice is found between the unfused halves of the scrotum. Because in this severe type of hypospadias the external genitalia are ambiguous, those individuals with perineal hypospadias and cryptorchidism (undescended testes) are occasionally diagnosed as male pseudohermaphrodites.

G. *Epispadias:* This condition occurs in about one of every 30,000 male infants. The urethra opening is on the dorsal surface of the penis.

H. *Agenesis of the penis:* This is a rare condition in which the urethra usually opens into the perineum near the anus. This is the result of failure of the genital tubercle to develop.

I. *Bifid penis* and *double penis:* These anomalies are very rare. Bifid penis occurs when two genital tubercles develop. It is often associated with exstrophy of the bladder, urinary tract abnormalities, or imperforate anus.

J. *Micropenis:* The penis is almost hidden, since it is so small. This abnormality results from a hormonal deficiency of the fetal testes and is often associated with hypopituitarism. A number of uterine and vaginal anomalies result from arrests of development of the uterovaginal primordium during the eighth week of gestation.

K. *Double uterus:* This results from failure of fusion of the inferior parts and can be associated with a double or a single vagina. Occasionally the uterus appears normal externally but is divided internally by a thin septum. When only the superior portion of the body of the uterus is involved, the condition is called *bicornuate uterus.* When one duct has retarded growth and it does not fuse with the other one, a bicornuate uterus with a rudimentary horn develops.

L. *Absence of vagina and uterus:* This condition occurs one in every 4000 female births. It results from failure of the sinovaginal bulbs to develop and from the vaginal plate. If the vagina is absent, then the uterus is generally absent, since the developing uterus induces the formation of the vaginal plate.

M. *Vaginal atresia blockage:* This vaginal condition occurs as a result of failure of canalization of the vaginal plate. Failure of the inferior end to perforate results in an anomaly known as *imperforate hymen.*

VIII. Web Sites
eMedicine
http://author.emedicine.com/PED/topic1492.htm

IRON DEFICIENCY ANEMIA

I. Definition
A. In iron deficiency anemia, the blood is deficient in erythrocytes (red blood cells [RBCs]) and hemoglobin (oxygen-carrying pigment in RBCs). This is the most common type of nutritional anemia in all age groups.

II. Etiology
A. Factors causing anemia are:
 1. Inadequate iron stores at birth from prematurity, low birth weight, severe maternal iron deficiency, and fetal or maternal blood loss.
 2. Insufficient daily iron intake during rapid growth rate of children 3 months to 6 years old, during adolescent years combined with poor eating habits, and during adolescent pregnancy.
 3. Excessive milk intake (milk is extremely low in iron) delays or reduces the addition of solid food to the infant's diet; may also cause infant to be chubby although nutritionally deficient.
 4. Iron loss from acute or chronic hemorrhage or parasitic infection.
 5. Impaired absorption of iron from chronic diarrhea and/or gastrointestinal (GI) disturbances.
 6. Blood loss rather than poor nutrition in children older than 2 (severe form).
 7. Inability to form hemoglobin because of lack of vitamin B_{12} and folic acid deficiency.

III. Characteristics
A. Obscure and insidious symptoms; severity directly related to length of nutritional deficiency.
B. Condition characterized by microcytes (small) and hypochromic (pale) erythrocytes.
C. Fatigue and shortness of breath occur from reduced hemoglobin levels, which decrease oxygenation of tissues.
D. Early symptoms are:
 1. Pale skin and mucous membranes.
 2. Decreased activity and apathy.
 3. Prone to infections.
 4. May be asymptomatic and not diagnosed until routine physical examination.

E. Late symptoms are:
1. Easy fatigue, irritability, and anorexia.
2. Headaches, dizziness.
3. Slow nail growth.
4. Poor muscle tone.
5. Soft systolic precordial murmur.
6. Enlarged spleen.
7. Pica, usually ice.
8. Psychological disturbances (e.g., hyperactivity, decreased attention span).

IV. **Health Concerns/Emergencies**
A. Iron preparations may cause GI upset, nausea, anorexia, diarrhea, and constipation.
B. Liquid iron temporarily stains teeth; straw or medicine dropper placed at back of throat may be used for administration. Brushing teeth after dosage may lessen discoloration.
C. Black or dark green stools when iron preparation is given; absence of discolored stools may indicate medication is not being administered or poor compliance.
D. Individuals with iron deficiency absorb lead more easily and are at higher risk for lead poisoning.

V. **Effects on Individual**
A. May have difficulty in academic performance because of low energy level, frequent headaches, and dizziness.
B. Difficulty with sports participation because of poor muscle development and easy fatigue.
C. Frequently absent from school because of recurrent infections.
D. Fatigue may limit student's participation play/social activities.
E. Cognitive and psychomotor development may be affected.

VI. **Management/Treatment**
A. Avoid giving medication with meals; juices with vitamin C enhance absorption. Coffee, tea, bran foods, milk, and antacids impede absorption of iron. If iron causes vomiting and diarrhea, give with meals.
B. Avoid giving solid food at or near breast feedings because it interferes with bioavailability of the small amount of iron in human milk.
C. Achieve normal hemoglobin level by replenishing depleted iron stores.
D. Diagnosis of underlying conditions (e.g., bleeding ulcer).
E. Assist family in meal planning; provide list of foods high in iron; educate family regarding disease, medication, and dietary compliance.

VII. **Additional Information**
A. Iron medication is highly toxic, and must be kept out of the reach of children. If it is in the classroom, keep it locked in a drawer or cabinet. Usual dosage is 3-5 mg of elemental iron per kg per day. Commonly prescribed ferrous iron is more readily absorbed than ferric iron.

B. In cultures where tea is a common beverage, advise giving iron with another beverage, since tea forms an insoluble complex with iron. Some herbal tea may have a negative effect on the absorption of iron.

C. There are various nutritional recommendations; give infants iron-fortified formula. Give foods containing iron. The best sources are meat, fish, poultry, any organ meat; soybeans; dried legumes; dry enriched cereals; and whole grain breads. Other sources are egg yolks; dark green leafy vegetables; dried fruits, apricots, peaches, prunes, and raisins; nuts and peanut butter; and molasses.

D. Vitamin C helps the body absorb iron. A deficiency of vitamins B_6, B_{12}, and E can contribute to anemia. Preparing foods in iron skillets increases foods' iron content.

SICKLE CELL ANEMIA

I. **Definition**
   A. Sickle cell disease (SCD) is the term used to describe a number of diseases called *hemoglobinopathies,* of which sickle cell anemia is the most common. It is a severe, chronic, incurable, anemia characterized by sickle-shaped red blood cells, and it results in acute and chronic organ damage. RBCs with sickle-cell hemoglobin (Hb S) change and become crescent-shaped with the following conditions: low oxygen tension, dehydration, and acidosis.

II. **Etiology**
   A. Sickle cell anemia is inherited by an autosomal recessive pattern. The abnormality occurs in the globin portion of the hemoglobin. The hemoglobins (Hb) are identified by letters. Hb A denotes *normal adult hemoglobin,* Hb AS refers to *heterozygous sickle cell trait* (carrier state of one normal hemoglobin gene and one sickle hemoglobin gene), and Hb SS designates *homozygous sickle cell anemia.* Those with SCD have parents who both have the trait. It is one of the most common genetic disorders affecting persons of African descent. The gene is also found in ethnic groups from sections of Turkey, the Middle East, India, the Mediterranean area, and the Caribbean. Those with Hb AS demonstrate a mutation with the ability to resist malarial parasites.

   B. In the United States, 1 in 12 African-Americans are carriers of the sickle cell trait, and 1 in 600 manifest the disease. Sickle cell anemia affects 1 out of 375 African-American infants.

III. **Characteristics**
   A. Disease most commonly recognized after infant reaches 2 to 4 months of age, which parallels replacement of the fetal hemoglobin with Hb S.

   B. Around 5 or 6 months of age, other clinical manifestations may be observed.

   C. Dactylitis occurs; it is characterized by painful, nonpitting edema of hands and feet and is often accompanied by a fever as high as 103 degrees F (39.4 degrees C); it most frequently occurs from 6 months to 4 years of age.

D. Enlarged spleen in early childhood because of its function in removing sickle cells from the circulation; functional activity is generally lost during first few years of life.

E. From approximately 6 to 8 years, spleen decreases in size from repeated infarcts and is replaced by fibrous mass.

F. Splenic sequestration crisis (sudden pooling of blood in spleen) generally occurs between 4 months and 3 years of age.

G. Bacterial infections from functional asplenia are a major cause of death in all age groups. Infective organisms: *Haemophilus influenzae, Streptococcus pneumoniae,* and *Neisseria meningitis.*

H. Aplastic anemia crisis, which is caused by a decrease in RBC production secondary to an infection.

I. Painful vasoocclusive crisis; sickle cells obstruct blood vessels, which causes occlusion, ischemia, and possible necrosis; potentially, every organ in body affected; in older child, there is pain and tenderness in bones, back, and joints of extremities from infarctions.

J. Central nervous system (CNS) infarction or stroke may appear at any age and can cause paralysis or death.

K. In middle childhood, a zinc deficiency may contribute to underweight and delayed puberty.

L. Older children may have cardiomegaly, symptomatic gallstone formation, and damage of the liver, pancreas, and heart from the increased iron absorption.

M. Skeletal problems, including osteoporosis, skeletal deformities, and osteomyelitis.

N. Other possible clinical manifestations are growth retardation, underweight, delayed sexual maturation, frontal protuberance, retinopathy, sensorineural hearing loss, priapism (abnormal, constant, painful penile erection) and urinary retention, leg ulcers, and renal complications.

IV. **Health Concerns/Emergencies**

A. Young children with fever, nonproductive cough, pain, or respiratory distress may have acute chest syndrome (ACS), a life-threatening pulmonary complication. ACS is the second most common condition requiring hospitalization.

B. Aphasia, seizures, visual disturbances, headache, or any other neurologic symptoms may indicate cerebral insult.

C. Hematuria, enuresis, and dilute urine indicate kidney ischemia.

D. Spleen sequestration often follows an acute febrile illness, requires immediate hospitalization because it is one of the most life-threatening complications, and is responsible for the highest incidence of death in the young child; symptoms of fever, headache, and nausea may be present.

E. Eleven percent of children have strokes that can lead to lifelong disabilities. The highest risk is between 2 and 5 years of age.

F. Routine blood transfusions seem to decrease the risk for a stroke, based on research, which uses brain ultrasound data. Transfusions pose another risk by increasing amounts of iron in the body, which damage the heart and other vital organs unless steps are taken to reduce iron levels.

V. Effects on Individual

A. The toddler may interpret pain as punishment.

B. Misses school frequently, and grades, along with motivation, may drop. Pain may interfere with concentration.

C. Child may not want to spend the night at a friend's house because bed-wetting is common in some children with sickle cell anemia. Using Depends or similar diapering product may be a solution if done in privacy.

D. May be teased because of short stature.

E. Tires easily.

F. Teenager often matures later than peers, making physical appearance a concern.

G. Disfigurement, jaundice, surgical scars, and dental deformities may cause embarrassment.

H. With good treatment and supportive counseling, individual can lead a full and productive life.

VI. Management/Treatment

A. Treatment is symptomatic and supportive, since there is no cure.

B. Febrile infants with SCD should be seen immediately because of risk of bacterial and subsequent secondary infection.

C. Daily antibiotic (penicillin) treatment beginning at 2 months and continuing to age 5 or 6 can reduce serious infections by about 85%.

D. Review for or vaccinate with *H. influenzae* type B (HIB) vaccine at age 2 months to protect against life-threatening bacterial infections.

E. Encourage fluid intake because of need to maintain hemodilution; dehydration increases the sickling process.

F. Discuss extreme necessity of wearing medical alert identification.

G. Routine visual screening up to age 10 and annual retinal examination for sickle retinopathy thereafter. Referral to ophthalmologist if any eye trauma sustained.

H. Routine audiological assessments, since individual is at high risk for sensorineural hearing loss in the high-frequency range, which is caused by reduced circulation in the inner ear (vasoocclusive episodes).

I. Scoliosis screening should be done according to individual's delayed maturational level.

J. Educate teachers and other school staff regarding basic concerns during school day, field trips, sports, and other physical activities; have water available for hydration; avoid temperature extremes, stress, overexertion, and fatigue.

K. Be aware of symptoms that require urgent medical care: fever, shortness of breath, chest pain, progressive fatigue, atypical headache, abrupt visual changes, sudden loss of sensation or weakness, unrelieved pain, priapism, and abdominal distention.

L. Do not use ice on any injury because it can cause localized sickling. It is an extreme temperature change.

M. Discourage adolescent smoking, since it increases vasoconstriction.

VII. **Additional Information**
   A. Prenatal diagnosis for known carriers of hemoglobinopathies is available by chorionic villi sampling (CVS) during the first trimester. An amniocentesis can be done in the second trimester. A simple hemoglobin electrophoresis test can determine if one is a carrier of the sickle cell trait.
   B. If both parents possess the trait, there is a 25% chance that a child will have Hb S. There is also a 25% chance that the child will have neither the trait nor the disease, and there is a 50% chance that the child will have the trait like both the parents but not the disease.
   C. The drug hydroxyurea reduces the number of pain crises in about 50% of severely affected adults. The Food and Drug Administration (FDA) approves it for patients over 18 years of age. Nitric oxide gas is being explored to help prevent RBCs from sickling. Bone marrow transplant has been successful in a few children, whereas about 5% to 8% with severe hemoglobin disorders die. Gene therapy approaches are now currently being researched.
   D. Vasoocclusive episodes are caused by sickling that is precipitated by a variety of factors (e.g., weather changes, stress, menstruation in the female). A physiological process causes the accompanying pain and is associated with a psychosocial component based on the individual's tolerance and reaction to pain and family beliefs and interpretations.

VIII. **Web Sites**
   American Sickle Cell Anemia Association
   http://www.ascaa.org

JUVENILE ARTHRITIS

   I. **Definition**
   A. Juvenile arthritis (JA) is an inflammatory disease of children. There are three main forms of the disease: (1) *monoarticular* (involving one joint) or *pauciarticular* (involving four or fewer joints), (2) *polyarticular* (involving five or more joints), and (3) *Still's disease* (systemic onset). JA diagnosis is given when onset is before age 16, and duration lasts longer than 6 weeks without other known cause. The term *juvenile arthritis* is becoming popular to distinguish more clearly between JA and adult rheumatoid arthritis; previously called *juvenile rheumatoid arthritis.*

   II. **Etiology**
   A. The cause of JA is unknown; present theories include infections, autoimmunity, and genetic predisposition. Approximately 3 in 1000 children have some form of arthritis (Arthritis Foundation, 2001).

   III. **Characteristics**
   A. General characteristics:
      1. Two peak ages of onset: 2 to 5 years and 9 to 12 years.
      2. More prevalent in females than in males.
      3. Probable duration of disease, degree of disability, and eventual functional ability are based on onset, type, extent of joint

involvement, and extent of systemic involvement. Long-term prognosis is good; about 75% enter long remissions without significant impairment.

4. Early in disease process may exhibit irritability, fatigue, poor appetite, poor weight gain and growth delay, early morning joint stiffness, and walking with knees flexed to protect inflamed joints and avoid pain.

5. Most common handicapping complications are hip disease or loss of vision because of iridocyclitis (inflammation of iris and ciliary body).

B. Three types of JA:

1. *Monoarticular and pauciarticular arthritis:*
   a. Involves approximately 50% of children with JA.
   b. Mildest form and best prognosis regarding long-term joint disability.
   c. Involves four or fewer joints.
   d. May be accompanied by mild rash, low-grade fever, and other systemic involvement.
   e. Commonly seen in ankle, wrist, hip, cervical spine, and proximal interphalangeal joints, but knee joint is most commonly involved.
   f. May not complain of pain; however, can be listless and have difficulty getting up in the morning.
   g. Chronic iridocyclitis is common serious systemic complication that may precede arthritis by several years and is usually asymptomatic. Also called *uveitis* and *iritis.*

2. *Polyarticular arthritis:*
   a. Occurs in approximately 30% of children with JA.
   b. Similar to adult variety.
   c. Seen at any age but more common in older children, particularly adolescents.
   d. Low-grade fever, listlessness, and anorexia.
   e. Multiple joint involvement and most likely form to cause deformity.
   f. Joint symptoms may occur abruptly, with several joints swollen and painful.
   g. Involvement of joints usually symmetrical.
   h. High incidence of involvement of temporomandibular joint (causing a receding chin), hip, wrist carpal bones, and cervical spine.
   i. Finger and toe joints become inflamed and swollen and develop spindlelike shape.
   j. Ankylosis, immobility, and fixation of joints.
   k. Can cause growth retardation.
   l. Likely to persist into adulthood.

3. Acute systemic onset:
   a. Occurs in about 20% of children with JA.
   b. Onset usually before age 5.

      c. Temperature spikes once or twice daily and subsides without treatment.

      d. Salmon-colored macular rash frequently comes and goes with fever or may be brought on by hot shower or trauma. Appears over trunk or extremities and is nonpruritic.

      e. Joint symptoms generally do not appear for several weeks or months and at first are only subjective; warmth, swelling, and tenderness may be observed later.

      f. Other symptoms are:

        (1) Splenomegaly and hepatic enlargement.

        (2) Lymphadenopathy.

        (3) Pericarditis and pleuritis.

        (4) Elevated white blood count common.

IV. Health Concerns/Emergencies

    A. School staff should be aware that student with JA may have pain or discomfort.

    B. Work with staff to accommodate student's inability to be punctual because of morning stiffness and pain, allow rest time at school, and have extra sets of text books available, since heavy loads can increase pain. May need shortened day to decrease fatigue.

    C. Promote independence in activities of daily living (ADL) whenever possible and make available adaptive devices (e.g., railing in bathrooms, elevated commodes).

    D. Monitor weight; decreased physical activity may lead to excessive weight gain, causing increased strain on inflamed joints of lower extremities and may be secondary to decreased physical activity; weight loss can indicate arthritis of temporomandibular joint (TMJ), which causes pain while chewing, malnutrition, poor disease management, and anorexia.

    E. Discuss interactions of oral contraceptives with medications, effects of arthritis medications on fetal development, and delayed sexual maturation.

    F. Encourage good oral hygiene.

V. Effects on Individual

    A. Pain and physical limitations may interfere with daily activities and self-care and contribute to weight gain.

    B. Academic performance can suffer from frequent absences from school or inability to concentrate because of discomfort.

    C. There may be social isolation from inability to participate in many activities with peers or failure of peers to accept the child who is "different."

    D. May be irritable and demanding and feel angry and resentful.

    E. May be embarrassed because of deformities.

    F. May be anxious and concerned regarding the future and career options.

    G. May constantly depend on others if limitations prevent the child from doing even simple tasks, such as turning on a faucet, opening a door, or cutting own meat.

H. Difficulty in maneuvering steps can make the use of public transportation difficult.

I. Susceptible to increased dental caries secondary to painful TMJ and poor oral hygiene because of limited use of upper extremities.

VI. **Management/Treatment**

A. May require visual examinations 4-5 times a year because of complications such as iridocyclitis, also called *uveitis* or *iritis*. Sometimes asymptomatic, but can be detected by a special slit-lamp examination.

B. Three major management goals:
1. Prevent deformities.
2. Preserve joint function.
3. Relieve symptoms without iatrogenic complications.

C. Consult with physical therapist regarding classroom activities, exercises, and positioning that might help preserve function and prevent deformities.

D. Occupational therapists provide information and design therapy for fine motor movements, ADLs, and when TMJ is involved.

E. Periods of rest may be necessary to avoid excessive fatigue.

F. Splints, braces, and casts are used to immobilize the joints in a neutral position and prevent contractures. Passive, active, and resistive exercises are a daily routine to maintain range of motion and muscle strength. Swimming is an excellent activity.

G. Unconventional therapies introduced by family may interfere with prescribed medical treatment, such as dietary regimens and supplements.

H. Use of surgery is limited but may be performed to relieve pain, correct deformities, or restore range of motion (e.g., soft tissue releases, tendon lengthening, total/knee replacements).

I. Medication:
1. Make provisions for prescribed medication to be administered while student is at school when necessary.
2. The primary drugs for alleviating pain and inhibiting inflammation are nonsteroidal antiinflammatory drugs (NSAIDs), which include naproxen (Naprosyn), tolmetin (Tolectin), indomethacin (Indocin), and ibuprofen (Advil or Motrin). May take up to 8 to 12 weeks to observe improvement. Most common side effect for this group of medications is GI irritation, which may be avoided if taken with food.Other side effects that may interfere with school studies include dizziness, headache, and drowsiness.
3. Second-line drugs include slower acting antirheumatic drugs (SAARDs), which include gold (Solganal), d-penicillamine, and hydroxychloroquine. These are added to the schedule when NSAIDs are not effective. Gold compounds are given intramuscularly; the oral preparation is not approved for children.
4. Corticosteroids are very strong antiinflammatory drugs used when life-threatening events occur (e.g., pericarditis) or when systemic disease does not respond to NSAIDs and iridocyclitis.

5. Cytotoxic drugs are prescribed for severe debilitating disease and those not responding to NSAIDs or SAARDs. These are antineoplastics or immunosuppressants, such as cyclophosphamide (Cytoxan) and azathioprine (Imuran).
6. Regularly monitor blood levels to maintain optimal level and prevent toxicity.
7. Salicylates are seldom used, since frequent, large doses may adversely affect child, causing bleeding, acute gastritis, hyperventilation (from acidosis), drowsiness, tinnitus, and Reye's syndrome.

VII. **Additional Information**
   A. JA may last as little as several months to a year or go away indefinitely. Most children have exacerbations and remissions for many years, but the exacerbations tend to diminish over time.
   B. Remission is defined as being symptom-free for 6 months after stopping medication. Inflammation has a unique effect on the growing child. Severe arthritis can slow growth (e.g., knee inflammation can

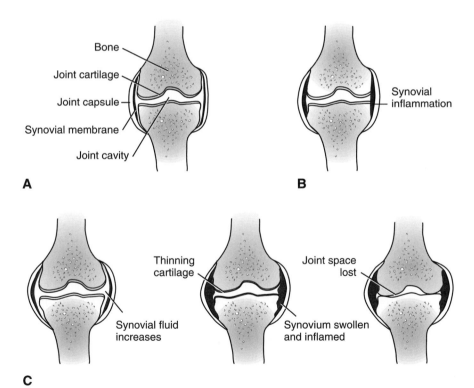

FIGURE 4-1 Juvenile arthritic process. **A,** Normal synovial joint. **B,** Early-stage synovitis. **C,** Chronic synovitis leading to joint destruction.

produce faster growth than the uninflamed knee). May resume normal growth patterns when arthritis is in remission. If the premature epiphyseal fusion has not occurred, the normal height curve will resume within 2 to 3 years.

C. The arthritic process begins with inflammation of the synovial membrane (synovitis) and joint capsule, which increases fluid in the joint, making it feel swollen and boggy (joint effusion). Chronic synovitis may lead to erosion of joint structure and loss of joint space. Over time immobilization of the joints (ankylosis), bone deformity, and subluxation (partial dislocation) occur. These inflammation processes can extend to other systems, causing pericarditis, pneumonia, uveitis, or organomegaly.

VIII. **Web Sites**

Arthritis Foundation
http://www.arthritis.org
American College of Rheumatology
http://www.rheumatology.org/patients/factsheets.html

ASTHMA

I. **Definition**

A. Asthma is a chronic inflammatory disorder of the airways characterized by airflow obstruction, which is usually reversible either spontaneously or by treatment, and bronchial hyperresponsiveness to a variety of stimuli.

II. **Etiology**

A. The inherited tendency to develop an immunoglobulin E (IgE)-mediated response to allergens, known as *atopy,* is the strongest predisposing factor for developing asthma. The allergic triggers are generally those carried in the air, such as plant pollens, molds, animal dander, house-dust mites, and secondhand smoke. In some instances, no allergic process can be detected. Asthma is a complex disorder in which biochemical, immunological, infectious, endocrine, and psychological factors are involved to varying degrees in different persons.

B. In the United States, asthma is the most prevalent cause of chronic illness, school absences in children, and a leading cause of pediatric hospital admissions (Nimmagadda and Evans, 1999). It has more than doubled in children over the past 15 years (Asthma Allergy Foundation, 2001). At a ratio of 2:1, it is more common in the male until adolescence. After age 14, the ratio reverses, with prevalence higher in females. Asthma is more common in African-Americans and Hispanics. Asthma is not usually outgrown. Adolescents or young adults may experience relief, but symptoms usually return later.

III. **Characteristics**

A. Diagnosis generally occurs between 3 and 8 years, but 50%-80% of children with asthma develop symptoms before age 5, and many have symptoms during the first year of life (NHLBI, 1997).

B. Diagnosis is based on individual's health history; family history of asthma, allergy, rhinitis or sinusitis; spirometry; and challenge tests (e.g., histamine, methacholine, cold air, response to appropriate therapy).

C. Diagnostic symptoms include:
   1. Cough, more common at night.
   2. Wheeze with prolonged expiratory phase.
   3. Cough with exercise, laughing, or crying—wheezing may not be present.
   4. Shortness of breath.
   5. Chest tightness.
   6. Symptoms worsen with precipitating factors.

D. Precipitating factors:
   1. Plant pollens, molds, dust mites, cockroaches, animal dander or secretory products, air pollutants, including secondhand smoke.
   2. Viral respiratory infections, weather changes (e.g., excessively cold, wet, or humid conditions).
   3. Physical exercise or strong emotional expressions (e.g., fear, frustration, laughing or crying hard).
   4. Medications (e.g., aspirin, NSAIDs, β-blockers, including eye drops); sensitivity increases with age and severity of asthma; aspirin is in many over-the-counter (OTC) medications, including Pepto-Bismol; these drugs may precipitate a severe or fatal exacerbation.
   5. Foods, additives, and preservatives.
   6. Endocrine changes (e.g., menses, pregnancy, thyroid disorders).

E. Prodromal (up to 6 hours) signs include anxiety, itching on neck or chest, headache, tightness in chest, rhinorrhea, loss of appetite, and fatigue.

F. Irritability, restlessness, increased anxiety, and cool clammy skin.

G. Exacerbations are caused by edema or inflammation in the bronchial wall and constriction of the small and large airways in the lungs, which results from bronchial smooth muscle spasms and excessive production of mucus.

H. Children younger than age 5 experience greater hyperresponsiveness than do older children, perhaps because of smaller airways.

I. Often associated with gastroesophageal reflux (GER).

J. About 80% of individuals with asthma have allergies in form of rhinitis or topic dermatitis (NHLBI, 1997).

K. Although the terms *minimal intermittent* and *minimal persistent* asthma are treated with a bronchodilator, a child who usually meets the criteria for "minimal" may have exacerbations during a cold that increases his or her requirement for bronchodilators (rescue medication). The illness may actually require a daily medication because of the possibility of cellular damage and ongoing repair process associated with chronic inflammation leading to permanent airway damage (restructuring), which is not responsive to treatment. Therefore early intervention is important, and use of inhaled corticosteroids is frequently the recommended treatment.

Box 4-1	*Categories of Asthma for 5 Years of Age and Older*

Individuals at any level can experience mild, moderate, or severe exacerbations.

Mild Intermittent Asthma

1. Symptoms no more than twice a week.
2. Responds to bronchodilator treatment.
3. Does not require daily medication for control.
4. Exacerbations brief (from a few hours to a few days); may vary in intensity.
5. Asymptomatic and normal peak expiratory flow rate (PEFR) between exacerbations.
6. Little interruption of school attendance.
7. Nighttime symptoms no more than twice a month.
8. PEFR no less than 80% of predicted value; PEFR less than 20% variability.

Mild Persistent Asthma

1. Symptoms more than twice a week but less than once a day.
2. Exacerbations may affect level of activity.
3. Nighttime symptoms more than twice a month but less than once a week.

4. PEFR no less than 80% of predicted value; PEFR variability 20%-30%.

Moderate Persistent Asthma

1. Daily symptoms.
2. Daily treatment with inhaled short-acting β_2-agonist.
3. School attendance and exercise tolerance affected.
4. Exacerbations at least twice a week and may last for days.
5. Nighttime symptoms more than once a week.
6. Coughing and wheezing disrupt normal activities and make it difficult to sleep.
7. PEFR 60%-80% predicted; PEFR variability greater than 30%.

Severe Persistent Asthma

1. Continual symptoms.
2. Frequent exacerbations.
3. Limited physical activity.
4. Frequent nighttime symptoms, disrupting sleep.
5. Occasional hospitalization may be needed to bring symptoms under control.
6. PEFR 60% predicted or less; PEFR variability greater than 30%.

Modified from the National Asthma Education and Prevention Program: *Expert panel report 2: guidelines for the diagnosis and management of asthma,* NIH Pub No 97-4051, Bethesda, Md, 1997, National Heart, Lung, and Blood Institute (NHLBI).

IV. **Health Concerns/Emergencies**
   A. Status asthmaticus can lead to respiratory failure and death.
   B. Acute severe prolonged asthmatic attack may result in reduced oxygenation.
   C. Silent chest may indicate severe spasm or obstruction with no movement of air (therefore no breath sounds) and requires immediate emergency treatment.
   D. Emergency symptoms:
      1. Difficulty walking or talking (e.g., unable to speak in complete sentences, using phrases or single words).
      2. Hunched over (tripod position to allow expansion of diaphragm), struggling to breathe.
      3. Sternal or intercostal retractions.

4. Perioral/nail bed cyanosis; very serious sign that indicates impending respiratory arrest.
5. Treat according to individual's emergency plan (rescue plan).

V. Effects on Individual

A. The longer the asthma attack, the greater the anxiety.
B. May feel isolated, and academic studies may suffer because of school absenteeism.
C. May be self-conscious about need for medication or monitoring and avoid going to health office for assessment or treatment.
D. May use asthma as an excuse to avoid activities.
E. May experience delay in puberty and growth because of corticosteroid use; maximal height usually possible through appropriate disease management.
F. May be negatively affected by the impact this chronic illness has on family routines, economic resources, activities, and dynamics.
G. Increasing control of the treatment plan and self-management by the student, especially in adolescence, improves compliance, diminishes exacerbations, and promotes self-empowerment.

VI. Management/Treatment

A. Individualized health care plan (IHCP).
   1. Develop in consultation with parent(s) and HCP; student should have written plan for home care as well.
      a. Prescriptions for daily, rescue, and prn medications.
      b. Peak expiratory flow rate (PEFR) monitoring instructions.
      c. Emergency contacts and plan.
      d. Guidelines for activities.
      e. Factors that increase asthma symptoms.

NOTE: Responsible student should be allowed to carry own medication and use as needed when determined by parent, school nurse, and HCP. Be knowledgeable about nursing, state, and school policy and guidelines. Refer to National Association of School Nurses' (NASN) position.

B. Prevention of exercise-induced bronchospasm (EIB).
   1. Do breathing exercises and physical training to strengthen respiratory muscles, improve breathing patterns, prevent overinflation, improve cough for clearing the airway, and provide physical and mental relaxation.
   2. Take preventive medication before exercise, as prescribed.
   3. Use combination of 2 to 3 drugs if single dose is ineffective.
   4. Do warm-up exercises.
   5. Use a scarf, muffler, or cold-weather mask to warm and humidify air as needed.
   6. Pace exercise.
   7. Maintain adequate hydration by taking in adequate fluids.

C. Monitoring.
   1. Use a daily check-off list of factors: respiratory status, medications used, PEFR, adherence to treatment plan, inhaler technique, amount of prn medications needed, side effects of medications, and sleep disturbances; provide verification of effective protocol or need for change; monitor growth, especially when

Text continued on p. 182

Table 4-1   *Key Points Regarding Management Medications*

Medication Category	Indications/Actions Per Drug Category	Possible Side Effects Per Drug Category	Comments Per Drug Category
Corticosteroids (Inhaled)			
Beclomethasone dipropionate (Beclovent, Vanceril, Beconase, Vancenase) Budesonide (Pulmicort, Rhinocort) Flunisolide (AeroBid, Nasalide, Nasarel) Fluticasone (Flovent) Triamcinolone acetonide (Aristocort, Azmacort, Kenalog, Nasacort AQ) Dosing varies by product and delivery device; usually given bid	**Indications:** Long-term prevention of symptoms; suppression, control, reversal of inflammation Decrease need for oral corticosteroid **Actions:** Antiinflammatory, reduce airway hyperresponsiveness Inhibit late-phase allergic reaction Improve PEFR Prevent exacerbations May prevent airway remodeling	Cough, dysphonia, oral thrush In high doses, systemic effects may occur (e.g., osteoporosis, growth suppression, adrenal suppression, skin thinning, easy bruising) Compare risks of uncontrolled asthma against adverse effects of drugs; potential but small risk of adverse events is well balanced by their efficacy	Spacer/holding chamber devices and mouth washing after inhalation decrease oral side effects and systemic absorption Preparations are not entirely equivalent on puff or µg basis; new delivery systems may be even more efficient Inhaled corticosteroids are most potent antiinflammatory drugs presently available Dexamethasone not included because it is highly absorbed and has long-term suppressive side effects

Corticosteroids (Systemic)

Methylprednisolone (Medrol)

Prednisolone (Delta-Cortef, Prelone, Pediapred)

Prednisone (Orasone, Deltasone, Meticorten)

Alternate-day A.M. dosing produces least toxicity when needed for long-term therapy. If daily dosing is needed, 3 P.M. is more efficacious than A.M. dose

Indications: Short term "burst" (3-10 days) for prompt control

To gain prompt control of inadequately controlled, persistent asthma

Long-term use in severe persistent asthma to suppress, control, and reverse inflammation

Actions: Antiinflammatory, reduce airway hyperresponsiveness

Inhibit late-phase allergic reaction

Improve PEFR

Prevent exacerbations

May prevent airway remodeling

Short-term use: increased appetite, fluid retention, weight gain, mood swings, hypertension, peptic ulcer, delayed wound healing, acne

Long-term use: osteoporosis, growth suppression, Cushing's syndrome, cataracts, hypothalamic–pituitary–adrenal suppression, hypertension, diabetes, muscle wasting, rarely impaired immune function

Give at lowest effective dose

Consideration should be given to conditions that could be exacerbated by systemic corticosteroids (e.g., herpes virus infections, varicella, tuberculosis)

Cromolyn sodium (Crolom, Intal, Gastrocrom, Nasalcrom, Opticrom)

Nedocromil (Tilade)

Usual dosing is qid; nedocromil has been effective on bid schedule

Indications: Long-term prevention of symptoms; may modify inflammation

Use before exercise or exposure to known allergen

Actions: Antiinflammatory; inhibit early and late-phase reaction to allergens; inhibits acute response to exercise, cold dry air, and sulfur dioxide

May have coughing with DPIs; using MDI or nebulizer may prevent cough

Occasionally unpleasant taste

Therapeutic response to cromolyn and nedocromil often occurs within 2 wk, but 4-6 wk period may be needed to measure maximum benefits

MDI cromolyn (1 mg/puff) may be inadequate, may need nebulizer delivery (20 mg/amp)

Clinical response is less predictable than response to inhaled corticosteroids

Safety is primary advantage

Continued

bid, Twice a day; *DPI*, dry powder inhalation; *MDI*, metered dose inhaler; *qid*, four times a day.

Table 4-1 *Key Points Regarding Management Medications—cont'd*

Medication Category	Indications/Actions Per Drug Category	Possible Side Effects Per Drug Category	Comments Per Drug Category
Long-Acting β₂-Agonists Inhaled: salmeterol (Serevent) Oral: albuterol, sustained release tablets Usual dosing: bid 12 hr apart	**Indications:** Long-term prevention of symptoms, especially nocturnal; used as adjunct to antiinflammatory therapy Prevention of EIB: use 30-60 min before exercise Not to be used to treat acute symptoms or exacerbations **Actions:** Bronchodilation, relaxes smooth muscles; effects last at least 12 hr	Tachycardia, skeletal muscle tremor, hypokalemia May have diminished bronchoprotective effect within wk of chronic therapy; clinical studies have not demonstrated development of tolerance	Correct use is essential Should not be used in place of antiinflammatory therapy Remind not to stop antiinflammatory therapy even though symptoms may improve significantly Not for acute symptoms or exacerbations Avoid excessive use of caffeine: colas, chocolate, coffee, tea Keep canister at room temperature; cold decreases potency Inhaled long-acting β₂-agonists preferred; are longer acting and have fewer side effects

	Indications/Actions	Side Effects	Considerations
Methylxanthines			
Theophylline sustained-release tablets and capsules (Slo-Bib, Theo-Dur, Theolair, Uniphyl) Usual dosing is 2-4 times/day at 6-12 hr intervals	**Indications:** Long-term control and prevention of symptoms, especially at night Used when not responding to inhaled medications **Actions:** Bronchodilation, smooth muscle relaxation	Effects at therapeutic dose include insomnia, increase of hyperactivity in some children, gastric upset, aggravation of ulcer or reflux Dose-related acute toxicities include tachycardia, dysrhythmias, nausea and vomiting, irritability, seizures, CNS stimulation, headaches, hematemesis, hyperglycemia, hypokalemia	Routine serum concentration monitoring essential because of significant toxicities, narrow therapeutic range, and individual differences in metabolic clearance Maintain serum concentration between 5 and 15 µg/mL Not generally recommended for exacerbations
Leukotriene Modifiers			
Zafirlukast tablets (Accolate) Usual dosing: 1 tablet bid	**Indications:** Long-term control and prevention of symptoms in mild persistent asthma for age 12 and above **Actions:** Binds to leukotriene receptors thus inhibits bronchoconstriction, reduces airway edema and smooth muscle constriction	Headache, nausea, diarrhea Increased risk of URI when used with inhaled corticosteroids	Take at least 1 hr before or 2 hr after meals Do not crush or break tablets Co-administration with warfarin increases PT; monitor PT
Zileuton tablets (Zyflo Filmtab) Usual dosing: 1 tablet qid Montelukast (Singulair) Usual dosing: 1 tablet in evening	**Indications:** Same as above **Actions:** Inhibits the enzyme responsible for producing inflammatory leukotriene products, which induce bronchoconstrictor response, enhance vascular permeability, and stimulate mucus secretion	Elevation of liver enzymes; limited reports of reversible hepatitis and hyperbilirubinemia	Inhibits metabolism of terfenadine, warfarin, and theophylline Monitor doses of these drugs

bid, Twice a day; *PT,* prothrombin time; *qid,* four times a day; *URI,* upper respiratory infection.

Table 4-2   *Key Points for Rescue Medications*

Medication Category	Indications/Actions Per Drug Category	Possible Side Effects Per Drug Category	Comments Per Drug Category
Short-Acting Inhaled B₂-Agonists			
Albuterol (Proventil, Ventolin, Airet) Bitolterol (Tornalate) Pirbuterol (Maxair) Terbutaline (Brethaire) Levalbuterol (Xopenex) Usual dosing for EIB: 1-2 puffs before exercise; for symptoms: 2 puffs tid or qid as needed	**Indications:** Acts within 30 min, relief of acute symptoms Preventive treatment for EIB **Actions:** *Bronchodilation:* Relax bronchial smooth muscle, increase vital capacity, decrease airway resistance Increasing use or lack of expected effect indicates inadequate asthma control Use of more than 1 canister/mo may indicate overreliance on this drug	Tachycardia, tremors, hypokalemia, headache, hyperglycemia, nausea, nervousness, weakness, insomnia, increased BP Inhaled route generally causes few systemic adverse effects More than 2 canisters/mo poses risk of adverse side effects	Drugs of choice for acute bronchospasm; faster and more effective than systemic route Regularly scheduled daily use not recommended; does not provide better control than prn Isoproterenol (Isuprel), metaproterenol (Alupent), isoetharine (Bronkosol), and epinephrine (Adrenalin) are not recommended
Anticholinergics			
Ipratropium bromide (Atrovent) Usual dosing: MDI 1-2 puffs qid; nebulizer 1-unit dose qid	**Indications:** Relief of acute bronchospasm (see Comments) **Actions:** *Bronchodilation:* competitive inhibition of muscarinic cholinergic receptors; may decrease mucus gland secretion	Dry mouth and decreased respiratory secretions, increased wheezing in some individuals, blurred vision if sprayed in eyes Does not have atropine's side effects	Reverses only cholinergically mediated bronchospasm; does *not* block EIB; does *not* modify reaction to antigen May provide additive effect to β₂-agonist but has slower onset of action Alternative for those with intolerance for β₂-agonists

BP, Blood pressure; *MDI,* metered dose inhaler; *prn,* as required; *qid,* four times a day; *tid,* three times a day.

Table 4-3   Peak Flow Interpretation System

Zone	Peak Expiratory Flow Rate: Personal Best or Predicted for Age	Action/Recommendation
Green—All clear	80% or better More than ____L/min	Full activity; may use preventive medication before exercise/exposure to allergens; routine management plan
Yellow—Caution needed	50%-80% Between ____L/min and ____L/min	May be having acute exacerbation, asthma not well controlled; follow plan supplied by PCP and call if student does not improve
Red—Medical alert	50% or less Less than ____L/min	Implement rescue plan immediately and call PCP if PEFR does not move to yellow or green zone after rescue medication; prepare for transport as needed

PCP, Primary care provider.

Box 4-2   Sample Questions* for the Diagnosis and Initial Assessment of Asthma

A "yes" answer to any question suggests that an asthma condition is likely.

In the past 12 months . . .

1. Have you had a sudden severe episode or recurrent episodes of coughing, wheezing (high-pitched whistling sounds when breathing out), or shortness of breath?
2. Have you had colds that "go to the chest" or take more than 10 days to get over?
3. Have you had coughing, wheezing, or shortness of breath during a particular season or time of the year?
4. Have you had coughing, wheezing, or shortness of breath in certain places or when exposed to certain things (e.g., animals, tobacco smoke, perfumes)?
5. Have you used any medications that help you breathe better? How often?
6. Are your symptoms relieved when the medications are used?

In the past 4 weeks, have you had coughing, wheezing, or shortness of breath . . .

1. At night that has awakened you?
2. In the early morning?
3. After running, moderate exercise, or other physical activity?

From the National Asthma Education and Prevention Program: *Expert panel report 2: guidelines for the diagnosis and management of asthma,* NIH Pub No 97-4051, Bethesda, Md, 1997, National Heart, Lung, and Blood Institute (NHLBI).
*These are suggested questions for student interview.

on long-term steroids; usually experience catch-up growth, avoid obesity.
2. Screen for glaucoma or cataracts when on daily high-dose systemic corticosteroids; otherwise, routine vision screening is acceptable.
D. General.
1. Controlled breathing, including pursed lips with expiration, may calm a student in respiratory distress but does not improve lung function.
2. Annual influenza vaccine recommended; pneumococcal vaccine no longer a routine recommendation (NHLBI, 1997).
3. Avoid cough suppressants, which mask symptoms.
4. Consider allergen immunotherapy when individual is sensitive, unable to avoid allergens, medications are not controlling symptoms, and reactions are noted most of the year.
E. Training: Educate teachers, coaches, bus drivers, and other school staff regarding:
1. Basic facts about asthma.
2. Signs and symptoms of respiratory distress.
3. Treatment of acute asthmatic episode and correct use of devices (e.g., metered dose and dry powder inhalers, nebulizers, space holding chambers).
4. Medications for use before exercise or exposure to known irritants.
5. Ways to minimize exposure to triggers and techniques to prevent EIB (e.g., warm-up period).
6. Individual's treatment plan with all phone numbers.
7. When to call parent(s), HCP, and/or 911.
VII. **Additional Information**
A. Pregnancy poses risks for the asthmatic, and good control is needed to avoid perinatal mortality, premature delivery, and low birth weight. Most of the medications used for asthma pose little risk to the fetus, but decongestants and antibiotics create possible risks to the fetus. Contraceptives may interact with asthma medications. Theophylline can cause the risk of toxicity because of decreased clearance when administered with contraceptives.
B. Physical activity is generally not limited; there are Olympic winners that are asthmatics, including 40 gold medal winners. EIB is associated with hyperventilation of cold, dry air. Thus ice-skating and cross country skiing are difficult, but swimming is an excellent exercise, since it builds up lung capacity without compromising the airway. EIB is caused by pulmonary loss of water and heat when hyperventilation occurs in air that is drier and cooler than the air in the lungs. EIB may be the only symptom of asthma an individual has, and he or she should be evaluated to make certain he or she is under the best control possible. Symptoms of EIB usually occur during or minutes after vigorous exercise, are generally at their worst 5-10 minutes after stopping exercise, and should resolve within a half hour.
C. School environment can aggravate or trigger asthmatic symptoms because of poor air quality, unregulated temperature, pesticides used

for pest control, animals in the classroom, and excessive humidity (e.g., mold). Environment can be evaluated and improved with tools such as the IAQ Tools for Schools Kit, which is available free through the Environmental Protection Agency (EPA), 1-800-438-4318.

D. PEFR.
  1. Peak flow monitoring provides:
     a. Means of determining effectiveness of treatment plan.
     b. Early detection of progression in the disease so changes can be instituted.
     c. Means of identifying triggers.
     d. Method of determining need for emergency care (NHLBI, 1997).
  2. PEFR personal best is the highest PEFR obtained over a 2-3 week period when asthma is in good control. Baseline should be taken 2-4 times a day: on awakening, between noon and 2 P.M., and before and after taking a short acting β_2-agonist, if prescribed. This becomes the reference point for individualized care. Charts for PEFR are available based on height and age; however, estimated normal lung function varies among racial and ethnic groups. Results cannot be applied to all populations, and the individual's personal best PEFR value is the preferred method to use for monitoring of asthma (NHLBI, 1997). The same brand of peak flow monitor should be used consistently, since various brands can give widely differing values. PEFR measurements depend on the effort and procedure used. Encouragement and frequent review of correct technique is important.
  3. Ongoing PEFR is usually taken in the morning soon after waking, before treatments, 5-15 minutes after inhaled treatments, and with increased respiratory symptoms.

NOTE: Individualized plan indicating rates and actions should be written by the HCP.

VIII. Web Sites

National Asthma Education and Prevention Program
301-592-8573
http://www.nhlbi.nih.gov/about/naepp
National Heart, Lung, and Blood Institute Information Center
http://www.nhlbi.nih.gov
American Academy of Allergy, Asthma, and Immunology
1-800-822-2762
http://www.aaaai.org
The American Lung Association
1-800-586-4872
http://www.lungusa.org
Asthma and Allergy Foundation of America
1-800-727-8462
http://www.aafa.org
U.S. Environmental Protection Agency (EPA)
Indoor Air Quality Information Clearinghouse
1-800-438-4318
http://www.epa.gov/iaq/

CEREBRAL PALSY

I. Definition
   A. Cerebral palsy (CP) is the term used to designate a number of non-progressive disorders of the CNS; it is primarily characterized by impaired muscular control and both aberrant movement and posture. The four classifications are spastic, dyskinetic, ataxic, and mixed (Minear, 1956).

II. Etiology
   A. CP can be attributed to prenatal, perinatal, and postnatal factors.
      1. *Prenatal* factors include malfunctioning placenta, intrauterine infection, teratogens, Rh incompatibility, maternal metabolic disorder, brain malformations, and genetic disorders (rare). CP occurs most commonly in the prenatal period, 44% (Eicher and Batshaw, 1993).
      2. *Perinatal* factors include premature birth, birth trauma, anoxia, low birth weight, metabolic or electrolyte disturbance, and hyperbilirubinemia.
      3. *Postnatal* factors include trauma to the head, infections of the brain (such as meningitis and toxins), cerebral hemorrhage or embolus, anoxia, and tumors of the brain. In 24% the cause appears to be unknown (Eicher and Batshaw, 1993).
   B. The neuromuscular dysfunction is directly associated to the area of the brain injured and to the stage of development when injured.

III. Characteristics
   A. Spastic CP:
      1. Most common type, 70% to 80%.
      2. Limb muscle contracts strongly with stretching or sudden attempted movement.
      3. Disorder of the adductor muscles or hip, legs crossed, scissoring.
      4. Fixed contractures common.
      5. Muscle may continue to contract and relax repetitively (clonus).
      6. In involved limbs, deep tendon reflexes are increased (e.g., ankle and knee jerk).
      7. With growth, spastic muscle becomes shorter, and pelvis, spine, and limb deformities are common.
      8. Poor control of posture and balance.
      9. Abnormal postures at rest or with change of position.
      10. Risk for hip subluxation and dislocation.
      11. Impaired fine and gross motor skills.
      12. Spastic CP is classified by limb involvement:
         a. Monoplegia—one limb involved.
         b. Hemiplegia—upper and lower limbs of one side only, 25% develop homonymous hemianopsia—sees straight ahead but not to the affected side; most common type of spastic CP.
         c. Paraplegia—lower limbs affected.
         d. Diplegia—both upper and lower limbs involved; however, lower limbs are more severely affected.

| Table 4-4 | *Educational Issues Resulting from Brain Insult* |

Class	Type	Brain Involvement	Educational Issues
Spastic	Diplegia, quadriplegia, hemiplegia	Motor cortex and pyramidal tract	Cognitive: 70% are within normal IQ range. Retardation varies from mild with learning disabilities to profound.
Dyskinesis	Athetoid, dystonic	Basal ganglia or extrapyramidal tracts	Motor skills: Both fine and gross affected, which interferes with handwriting, drawing, computer, and cutting skills, almost all
Ataxic	Range of tone and coordination; ataxic-hypotonic-atonic	Cerebellum	classroom skills. Often nonambulatory or walks with unsteady gait. Speech and language: Weak, if any perioral tone, which affects articulation. Often nonverbal. May
Mixed	Combinations of spastic and dyskinesia	Various areas in brain	benefit from augmentative communication device. Sensory integration: Impaired or limited vision, hearing, and tactile methods of learning. Dysfunctional figure ground differentiation, eye-hand coordination. Visual motor and perceptual problems. Behavioral and affective: ADHD, hyperactive, impulsivity, non-compliant and moody at times, cries

  e. Triplegia—usually one upper limb and both lower limbs affected.

  f. Quadriplegia—all four limbs involved and musculature around trunk, mouth, tongue, and pharynx may be involved, affecting speech, chewing, and swallowing; emotions more labile, inappropriate laughing/crying.

  g. Double hemiplegia—both sides of body involved, but upper extremities more involved than lower.

B. Dyskinetic (athetoid) CP:

  1. Involuntary movements are aggravated by stress.

  2. Two subtypes: athetoid and dystonic.

    a. Athetoid movements are common (slow writhing movements or chorea movements [jerky and rapid]) of extremities, neck, trunk, facial muscles, and tongue.

    b. Dystonic—slow twisting movements of trunk and extremities, resulting in an abnormal position.

3. Voluntary movements contorted.
4. Movements and rigidity disappear during sleep.
5. All extremities generally involved.
6. Drooling and dysarthria, poor speech articulation.
7. Muscles not spastic.
8. Deformities rare.
9. Impaired swallowing.
10. Motor manifestations exacerbated by emotional stress.
11. Frequently has high-frequency hearing loss or deafness.

C. Ataxic CP:
1. Walks with wide-based gait, weaving of trunk, and arms out.
2. Unable to turn rapidly, falls frequently.
3. Unable to perform rapid coordinated movements well.
4. Hypotonia during infancy and decreased tendon reflexes.
5. Tone ranges from ataxic to hypotonic to atonic.

D. Mixed cerebral palsy:
1. Combination of athetosis and spasticity.
2. Generally quadriplegic.

E. Other associated characteristics:
1. Mental retardation.
2. Seizures, particularly in spastic type.
3. Attention deficit disorder.
4. Vision and hearing impairments.
5. Tactile perception impaired.
6. Speech and language deficits.
7. Visual-motor and perceptual problems.

IV. **Health Concerns/Emergencies**
A. High-risk for injury, possibility of falls because of gross motor impairment, spasticity, and seizures.
B. At risk for status epilepticus or uncontrolled seizures.
C. Choking, aspiration, or feeding problems because of uncoordinated chewing, sucking, and swallowing.
D. Susceptible to latex allergies.

V. **Effects on Individual**
A. Depend on age, extent of involvement, and degree of mental disability.
B. Simple daily tasks (e.g., self-feeding, dressing, toileting, turning on television, answering telephone) can be monumental or impossible.
C. Student may have normal intelligence but be unable to communicate thoughts and needs verbally.
D. Those who can verbalize may encounter impatience or ridicule because of slow and inarticulate speech.
E. Delayed social development.
F. May have to face numerous surgeries to correct contractures and to provide mobility.
G. Often must depend on peers for assistance at school, thereby leaving self open to thoughtlessness or rejection.

H. Social and recreational outlets and career opportunities may be limited, but application of new technology is expanding choices in many areas.

I. Low feelings of self-worth as becomes more aware of being different from peers and siblings and the numerous problems family faces in daily management.

J. Behavior problems frequently develop because of rejection by others.

K. Constant stress from meeting with the numerous professionals involved in therapy: orthopedist, physical therapist, occupational therapist, speech therapist, neurologist, psychologist or psychiatrist, and so on.

VI. **Management/Treatment**

A. Hearing loss, vision impairment usually refractive errors (e.g., farsightedness), and strabismus must be ruled out and referred for correction if indicated.

B. Monitor medication and possible side effects:

1. Some persons with athetosis have benefited from diazepam (Valium) to control tension and excessive movement.

2. Dantrolene (Dantrium) reduces spasticity in the muscle; it may affect liver function. Botulinum toxin-A (Botox) injections and baclofen (Lioresal) also used to reduce spasticity. Baclofen given as a continuous infusion may help with ambulation.

3. Barbiturates (e.g., phenobarbital), which generally sedate, may excite individuals with brain damage. The stimulant dextroamphetamine is sometimes used to calm individuals with brain damage.

4. Anticonvulsants are administered to those with seizure involvement.

C. Caries, malocclusion, and bruxism (grinding of teeth) are common; refer for dental care when necessary.

D. Eating and feeding difficulties are prevalent because of poor perioral muscle tone and coordination. This problem, along with high caloric expenditure from spasticity and tremors, creates a calorie deficit. Evaluate, including monitoring anthropometry, and provide lists and techniques to caregiver(s) for increasing calories in diet at home and school. Some students benefit from special eating utensils; severe, unresolved problems may require gastrostomy tube placement.

E. Urinary retention and bladder control difficulties are common, as well as the inability to sense urination urge or bladder fullness. A number of medications are available.

F. High risk for pulmonary infections secondary to abnormal muscle tone, inactivity, contractures, and scoliosis. Infections last longer because of ineffective cough and ability to blow one's nose.

G. At increased risk for latex allergies. It is prudent to minimize contact with latex products.

H. Prevent breakdown of skin by encouraging staff to frequently change position of severely disabled and periodically check braces and other appliances for possible rubbing/pressure points and necrosis.

I. Awareness of safety needs:
   1. Helmet to prevent head injury.
   2. Wheelchair in good working order.
   3. Proper support when sitting balance is inadequate.
   4. Rails and other means of support should be available, particularly in toilet facilities.
   5. Evaluate usability and safety of school routine and pathways via wheelchair.
   6. Emergency evacuation plans should be in place.

J. Know physical and occupational therapy goals to determine nursing role.

K. It may be necessary to coordinate care provided by a number of professionals and community agencies while working with the parent(s). Assist parents when appropriate for respite services, meeting other parents with the same needs, finding support groups; include siblings.

L. Develop IHCP or IECP as needed. Prepare nurse assessment report for individualized education program (IEP) and participate in IEP meeting as appropriate. Nurse may be case manager for severely involved students.

VII. Additional Information

A. Common terminology associated with bracing (orthotics): ankle-foot orthosis (AFO). The metal AFO has an adjustable ankle joint; the plastic AFO keeps the foot in a fixed position. Knee-ankle-foot orthosis (KAFO) is also made of metal and plastic. The metal brace can be adjusted and lengthened for growth more easily than the plastic one. Hip-knee-ankle-foot orthosis (HKAFO) is a pelvic band that fits around the waist and is attached to a long leg brace.

VIII. Web Sites

American Academy for Cerebral Palsy and Developmental Medicine
847-698-1635
http://www.aacpdm.org
National Easter Seals Society
1-800-221-6827
http://www.easter-seals.org/
United Cerebral Palsy Association
1-800-872-5827
http://www.ucpa.org

CLEFT LIP AND/OR PALATE

I. Definition

A. A cleft of the lip results from an incomplete fusion of the medial nasal and maxillary processes. A cleft of the palate occurs because of failure of the palatal shelves to fuse. These anomalies occur during the fifth to twelfth weeks of gestation. The malformation may involve only the lip, the palate, or both the lip and palate. The severity of the defect depends on the timing of the insult on fetal development; the lip and palate develop and fuse at different times during fetal life.

B. In an incomplete unilateral cleft of the lip, only the vermilion border on either side of the lip is involved. In a complete unilateral cleft, either side of the lip is involved and extends into the nasal septum. In complete bilateral clefts, both sides of the lips are involved.

C. A unilateral complete cleft of the lip and palate extends through either side of the premaxilla alveolar arch and the lips. No fusion occurs in the premaxilla and maxilla or the bones of the hard palate and nasal septum. A bilateral complete cleft of the lip and palate extends through both sides of the premaxilla, alveolar arch, and the lips. Neither side of the premaxilla, maxilla, or palatal bones fuses together. Clefts of the palate only involve either a cleft of the soft palate or clefts of both the hard and soft palate.

II. Etiology

A. When numerous factors cause clefts, the term *multifactorial inheritance* is used to indicate a combination of chromosomal, genetic, teratogenic, and environmental factors. Over 300 syndromes exist that include clefts as a characteristic. Some syndromes are identified as chromosomal abnormalities; mutant genes or teratogens (drugs/alcohol). Environmental factors often associated with clefts are maternal vitamin deficiencies (e.g., folic acid), maternal smoking, and x-ray exposure during the first trimester of pregnancy. Each year, one out of every 700 infants is born with a cleft lip and/or palate. It is the fourth most common birth defect in the United States and appears more frequently in Asians and certain Native American tribes. It occurs less frequently in the African-American population and affects males more often than females.

III. Characteristics

A. Usually observed at birth:
   1. Notch in vermilion border of lip.
   2. Bilateral or unilateral complete separation of lip.
   3. Bilateral or unilateral opening in the roof of the mouth.
   4. Bifid uvula is associated with a submucous cleft.

B. Submucous clefts of palate are not usually observed at birth but become apparent when feeding or speech problems occur (e.g., nasal sounding).

C. Normal developmental patterns of feeding, speech, and language are disrupted.

IV. Health Concerns/Emergencies

A. Presence or severity of medical problem depends on degree of involvement.

B. Feeding difficulties with the newborn/infant is immediate problem and cause an inefficient suck, prolonged feeding time, poor weight gain/weight loss.

C. Recurrent otitis media and eustachian tube infections are common.

D. Braces and dental prosthetics increase probability of tooth decay and gum disease; regular visits to a pedodontist are necessary.

E. Displacement of maxillary arches and malposition of teeth require intervention with orthodontia.

F. Feeding problems may cause nutritional deficiencies.

G. Frequently, congenital anomalies that require additional care and medical intervention are present.

V. **Effects on Individual**

A. Child becomes frustrated because others cannot understand child's speech.

B. Facial disfigurement may cause difficulty with parent relationships and, later in life, peer groups.

C. May develop hearing loss, causing more delays in speech and language.

D. Low self-esteem because of obvious deformity.

E. Fears and trauma related to surgery and possible separation from parents.

VI. **Management/Treatment**

A. Initial concern for infant is provision of adequate nutrition and prevention of aspiration and infection:

　1. Feed in upright position.

　2. Cleft palate nipples and plastic palatal coverings are available.

　3. Use specialized nipple as needed, staying with one nipple for at least 24 hours.

　4. If unable to use nipple, infant may be gavage-fed or use medicine dropper.

B. Follow-up of periodic and complete hearing evaluations.

C. Coordinate school health with parent and cleft lip/palate clinical team.

D. Orthodontic repairs occur in stages until about age 18.

VII. **Additional Information**

A. Cleft lip surgical closure is generally done when child is 2-3 months old. Before surgery, infant should weigh minimum of 10 lbs and be free of respiratory, oral, or systemic infections. Z-plasty is the common surgery performed and minimizes notching of the lip caused by retraction of scar tissue. The surgery should enhance child's appearance and enable intake of food in a normal manner. Additional repair or revision may be needed, depending on severity of cleft lip. If the nose is involved and rhinoplasty is necessary, corrective surgery is generally delayed until adolescence, when growth has stopped.

B. Cleft palate surgical repair timing varies and should be individualized. Time of repair depends on size, shape, and degree of child's cleft palate and in healthy child can be done before 1 year of age. Surgery should unite segmented cleft, provide pleasant and intelligible speech, and prevent injury to growing maxilla. Improved techniques are lowering the age of repair to as early as 1 month. Prosthetic devices may be necessary when cleft palate interferes with dentition.

C. After palatal surgery, the nurse should frequently examine the oral cavity and report fistulas or tissue collapse to the surgeon. When not a health hazard, enlarged tonsils and adenoids create extra tissue mass that may aid in velopharyngeal function.

D. Secondary complications of cleft lip and palate include speech and language, hearing, and dental concerns. Speech and language delays occur in more than half of the affected children. Both receptive and expressive language are affected. Absent teeth may cause an interdental lisp. There may be voice problems.

E. Hearing is affected by the eustachian tube dysfunction. Cleft palate exposes the eustachian tube to food and liquids, causing a predisposition to inflammation. Upper respiratory disease also increases the incidence of middle ear and eustachian tube infections. This results in middle ear pathology, which may cause a bilateral conductive hearing loss. Dental involvement may necessitate the need for regular dental visits, preferably with a pedodontist; orthodontics; prosthodontics.

F. A child with cleft lip or palate should be evaluated by a dysmorphologist for any associated syndromes and to provide genetic consulting for the parents. The interdisciplinary management team involves at least seven people, and many more specialists are involved in the correction of the birth defect. The *pediatrician* prescribes routine health care. The *otolaryngologist* follows up middle ear pathology and eustachian tube dysfunction. The *audiologist* diagnoses hearing impairment. The *orthodontist* handles dental occlusion prevention/correction. The *prosthodontist*

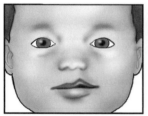
Unilateral incomplete
cleft lip

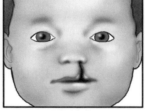
Unilateral complete
cleft lip

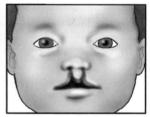
Bilateral complete
cleft lip

Soft palate
involvement only

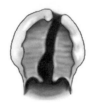
Unilateral complete
cleft palate

Bilateral complete
cleft palate

FIGURE 4-2 Cleft lip and palate.

constructs an appliance for absent teeth and/or the opening between the oral and nasal cavities. The *speech and language pathologist* oversees and remediates speech and language development. The *surgeon* repairs the cleft.

VIII. **Web Sites**
Wide Smiles
Cleft Palate and Lip Resource
209-942-2812
http://www.widesmiles.org

CYSTIC FIBROSIS

I. **Definition**
 A. Cystic fibrosis (CF) is an autosomal recessive disorder that affects multiple systems. Viscous mucus obstructs all, or nearly all, ducts of the exocrine glands. This obstruction is responsible for the clinical manifestations.

II. **Etiology**
 A. The condition is genetically transmitted, and both parents must be carriers of the gene. The CF gene is found on the long arm of chromosome 7 and is associated with production of the cystic fibrosis transmembrane conductance regulator (CFTR) protein. This defect results in abnormal electrolyte and fluid transport across cell membranes. The incidence is 1 in 3000 Caucasians in the United States, with progressively lower incidences in Hispanics, Native Americans, African-Americans, and Asians. The recessive gene is carried in 1 out of 28 Caucasians.

III. **Characteristics**
 A. Pulmonary involvement.
  1. Dry or productive cough, which may be paroxysmal.
  2. Hemoptysis not uncommon over age 10.
  3. Rapid, wheezing respirations.
  4. Shortness of breath (SOB) with increased activity, progressing to chronic SOB.
  5. Chronic sinusitis, nasal polyps.
  6. Repeated episodes of bronchopneumonia, bronchitis, bronchiectasis.
  7. Cyanosis.
  8. Clubbing of fingers and toes.
  9. Barrel chest.
 B. Gastrointestinal system.
  1. Malabsorption.
  2. Gastroesophageal reflux (GER).
  3. Meconium ileus (intestinal obstruction caused by failure to pass meconium) occurs in 7% to 10% who have the disease.
  4. Distal intestinal obstruction syndrome (DIOS) is partial or complete obstruction that may occur at any age but is more common in adolescence and young adulthood.

     5. Fibrosing colonopathy, prestricture state, or true stricture of the colon associated with excessive doses of pancreatic enzymes; greater than 6000 lipase units/kg per meal in children under age 12.

     6. Pancreatic involvement, which prohibits production of digestive enzymes and may lead to diabetes.

     7. Pancreatic insufficiency, as manifested in slow growth; failure to thrive; decreased muscle mass; voracious appetite but poor weight gain; protuberant abdomen; and frequent loose, foul-smelling, oily, floating stools.

     8. Prolapse of rectum is common in infancy and childhood.

     9. Anemia secondary to vitamin E and/or iron deficiency.

   10. Frequent bruising as a result of vitamin K deficiency.

  C. Hepatobiliary system.

     1. Prolonged neonatal jaundice.

     2. Biliary cirrhosis.

     3. Portal hypertension.

     4. Cholelithiasis.

  D. Reproductive system.

     1. Delayed puberty.

     2. Sterility in 98% of males from maldevelopment or obstruction of epididymis vas deferens and seminal vesicles.

     3. Females may be less fertile than normal because of abnormal cervical mucus.

     4. Inguinal hernia, hydrocele, and undescended testes more common.

  E. Integumentary abnormalities.

     1. Elevated concentrations of sodium and chloride in the sweat.

     2. Abnormal salt loss and dehydration secondary to electrolyte imbalance.

     3. Hyponatremic metabolic alkalosis.

     4. Heat stroke.

IV. Health Concerns/Emergencies

  A. Constipation and pain may indicate bowel obstruction.

  B. Prolapse of rectum can occur secondary to bowel obstruction.

  C. Anemia from impaired absorption of fats, which causes deficiency of fat-soluble vitamins A, D, K, and E.

  D. Pulmonary obstruction or infection:

     1. Fatigue.

     2. Irritability.

     3. Decreased appetite and exercise tolerance.

     4. Increased cough (especially at night) or sputum production.

     5. Rales, wheezes, or increased respirations.

     6. Inability to gain weight; weight loss.

     7. Intermittent low-grade fever.

  E. Excessive dosage of enzyme preparations may cause:

     1. Constipation.

     2. Frequent loose green stools.

     3. Abdominal pain.

    F. Enzymes should not remain on lips or skin because they can break down tissue.

    G. Salt loss caused by weather, vomiting, fever, or heavy exercise; symptoms:
        1. Weakness.
        2. Lethargy.
        3. Irritability.

V. Effects on Individual

    A. Demands long-term medical management.

    B. Hospitalizations may be dreaded or feared.

    C. Dependency on parents for care.

    D. Modifications of future plans may cause depression.

    E. Individual may feel different and excluded from peers because of physical limitations, medical complications, and frequent hospitalizations.

    F. Individual may experience guilt feelings because of the disruption the illness has caused the family.

    G. Puberty delayed in most young people with CF.

    H. Activities have to be built around treatment, diet, and medications.

    I. Child is subject to ridicule from peers because of retarded growth or delayed puberty.

VI. Management/Treatment

    A. Monitor height and weight.

    B. Coordinate school health management with clinical management team.

    C. Be aware of prescribed medications and side effects.

    D. Discuss using school bell sound as a reminder to do deep breathing and coughing.

    E. Encourage fluids to keep lung secretions thin.

    F. Do not restrict salt, especially during hot weather.

    G. Salt tablets may be necessary to prevent salt loss for active child.

    H. Perform chest physiotherapy (CPT) before meals when prescribed.

    I. Recognize signs of respiratory distress, and intervene before respiratory failure develops.

    J. Give enzymes at beginning of each meal and snack to facilitate absorption of fats and proteins.

    K. High-protein, high-calorie, and high-carbohydrate diet; high-fat foods not tolerated.

    L. Minimize exposure to those who have respiratory tract infections.

    M. Encourage participation in activities of interest because activity increases movement of mucus from airways.

    N. Encourage use of horn blowing instrument in the school band.

    O. Encourage peer counseling with another student who has a chronic illness.

VII. Additional Information

    A. Suspect CF in any infant who fails to thrive even with adequate intake of food. The sweat chloride test remains the best diagnostic measure. Prenatal testing is available and has a 90% sensitivity for detecting the CF gene. Multiple medications are used; antibiotics (some aerosolized) for pulmonary disease exacerbations; corticosteroids for airway inflammation and severe bronchospasm; mucous thinning drugs; enzymes for pancreatic insufficiency.

B. There are devices on the market to help maintain a patent airway. The Vest airway clearance system (Advanced Respiratory, St Paul, Minnesota) helps loosen mucus by high-frequency chest wall oscillation. The Flutter mucus clearance mechanism (Scandipharm, Inc., Birmingham, Alabama) helps to remove mucus in 5 to 15 minutes by blowing into the hand-held device. Advanced lung disease may be treated with lung or heart/lung transplant. New treatments now in clinical trials include gene therapy and CFTR protein repair. Life expectancy is into the 30s and 40s.

VIII. Web Sites

Cystic Fibrosis Foundation
1-800-344-4823
http://www.cff.org

CYTOMEGALOVIRUS

I. Definition

A. Cytomegalovirus (CMV) is a common viral infection that is found throughout the world but seldom causes clinical illness in healthy children or adults. CMV is of particular significance to pregnant women, however. It is the most common of the intrauterine infections and can result in severe mental retardation, neurological damage, and death to the fetus or newborn.

II. Etiology

A. CMV is a member of the herpesvirus group Herpesviridae. CMV is congenital or acquired and is transmitted by exposure to infected body fluids and sexual contact. A newborn without evidence of CMV can acquire it from breast milk. The exact mechanism of CMV transmission and the incubation period is unknown. It affects between 50% and 85% of adults by 40 years of age in the United States (CDC, 2001).

III. Characteristics

A. Congenitally acquired, asymptomatic CMV:

1. Of congenitally infected infants, 90% are asymptomatic (CDC, 2001) at birth *(silent infections)*. Asymptomatic infections are still a major cause of deafness, retardation, and blindness, and occasionally late manifestations appear in early childhood.

a. Progressive auditory damage (deafness).
b. Learning disabilities.
c. Neuromuscular disturbances.

2. These children excrete virus through their urine, saliva, or other bodily excretions or secretions.

B. Congenitally acquired, symptomatic CMV:

1. Also called *cytomegalovirus inclusion disease (CID)*.
2. Degree of involvement is thought to be related to gestational age of fetus at time of maternal infection.

    3. Newborns with CID exhibit some of the following abnormalities:
       a. Low birth weight.
       b. Hepatosplenomegaly.
       c. Thrombocytopenia purpura.
       d. Jaundice.
C. Those acquiring virus in childhood or as adults.
    1. Usually asymptomatic.
    2. Mononucleosis-like symptoms can occur in immunocompromised children and adults:
       a. Fever.
       b. Lymphadenopathy.
       c. Splenomegaly.
       d. Hepatitis.
    3. Reactivation; reinfection may also produce same mononucleosis-like symptoms in susceptible persons.
    4. Both asymptomatic people and those with symptoms excrete CMV through their urine, saliva, and other bodily secretions or excretions.
       a. Infected children may have prolonged periods of intermittent excretion of CMV.
       b. Infected adults may also intermittently shed virus, but is probable negligible source of transmission.
D. Immunosuppressed or immunodeficient individuals (e.g., patients with leukemia or human immunodeficiency virus [HIV], those on steroids) exposed to CMV:
    1. Susceptible to:
       a. Disseminated infection.
       b. Pneumonia.
       c. Retinitis.
       d. Hepatitis.
    2. Suffer serious morbidity and mortality.
    3. Excrete virus through their urine, saliva, and other bodily secretions or excretions:
       a. Microcephaly.
       b. Petechia.
       c. Obstructive hydrocephaly.
       d. Chorioretinitis.
       e. Cataracts.
       f. Heart disease.
       g. Encephalitis.
       h. Intracranial calcifications.
       i. Anemia.
       j. Motor disabilities.
    4. Later manifestations include:
       a. Progressive hearing loss.
       b. Visual impairment.
       c. Mental or motor retardation.
    5. Death may occur in utero; neonatal death rate is high in severely infected infants.

6. Severely involved children excrete virus through their urine, saliva, and other bodily excretions or secretions from 4-8 years of age.

NOTE: Only a very small percentage of children born with congenital CMV suffer devastating effects of classic CID.

E. Connatal (CMV acquired during or shortly after birth):
1. Almost always asymptomatic.
2. Very small percentage of children who do exhibit symptoms may have any of the following conditions:
a. Failure to thrive.
b. Hepatosplenomegaly.
c. Chronic gastroenteritis.
d. Hemolytic anemia.
e. Hepatitis.
f. Newborns will not excrete virus through their urine, saliva, and other bodily secretions or excretions until incubation period has passed.

IV. **Health Concerns/Emergencies**
A. Vary according to extent of involvement.
B. Of known congenitally infected infants who are asymptomatic at birth, 5%-20% will exhibit late manifestations of infection; these children need to be monitored for:
1. Auditory damage.
2. Neuromuscular disturbance.
3. Poor intellectual performance.
4. Learning disabilities.
C. Immunocompromised individuals are more susceptible to severe clinical manifestations and should be protected from exposure to CMV; this is a reminder that universal precautions should be practiced in all situations.

V. **Effects on Individual**
A. Congenital asymptomatic infants, who later exhibit lower intelligence quotient (IQ) levels, motor deficits, learning disabilities, and deafness, will require close clinical assessments and follow-up for special education services.
B. CID infants may die shortly after birth or be profoundly damaged, requiring lifelong care.
C. Children with mental retardation will require special education services.
D. Uninformed teaching staff and other professionals working with known infants and children may be frightened of the condition and its effects. This emotion can influence their relationship with the children and deter from their welfare and development.

VI. **Management/Treatment**
A. Varies according to extent of involvement.
B. Treatment for the student is symptomatic.
C. Severely involved students will have IEP, which includes all necessary nursing services, identifies involved personnel, and outlines procedures performed at school.

D. Educate and practice universal precautions and follow individual district/county or school site policy manual.

E. Females should receive information about the important epidemiology, transmission, and hygienic procedures concerning CMV.

F. Pregnant women should be counseled concerning the risk of acquiring CMV infection and the disease's possible effects on the fetus; women may want to be tested for CMV antibodies; refer to HCP.

G. Opportunity to be transferred to another position requiring less contact with infants and very young children should be considered.

VII. Additional Information

A. CMV is transmitted transplacentally (intrauterine); connately (during or shortly after birth); through the breast milk of an infected mother; by close or intimate contact with individuals excreting CMV through their urine, saliva, and other bodily secretions or excretions; through blood transfusions; or through transplanted organs.

B. Regarding the period of communicability:

1. Infants excrete the virus through their urine (viruria) often up to 4 years and, in the more severely involved, up to 8 years after birth. Excretion is generally intermittent.

2. Infected adults seem to excrete the virus for shorter periods of time and intermittently.

3. At present, it has not been determined how many negative urine specimens should be tested to be reasonably confident that the infant is no longer excreting CMV.

4. Infection rates vary with socioeconomic levels of the population and are higher in developing countries.

C. Prevention of CMV involves using universal precautions. Treatment is symptomatic. Drug therapy for infants is being evaluated, and vaccines are in the research and developmental stage. Evidence indicates that maternal antibody does reduce the severity of infection but does not protect the fetus from infection. Diagnosis of a maternal primary infection during pregnancy is difficult; blood tests can be performed, but isolation of CMV from the genital tract does not indicate if the infection is primary. It is currently impossible to determine if the fetus has been affected when maternal primary CMV has been documented. The National Center for Infectious Diseases does not presently recommend routine serologic testing for CMV antibodies but testing by case-by-case evaluation.

D. Recommendations concerning infants and children include:

1. Not excluding normal infants from nursing when the mother is a known excretor of CMV.

2. Because CMV can be transmitted by breast milk, the risks and benefits for its use need to be evaluated before it is given to immunosuppressed or premature infants.

3. Universal precautions should be practiced, and appropriate procedures for contaminated secretions should be exercised. For those women working with infants and high-risk children and those working in hospitals and other institutions, there is con-

cern regarding acquiring CMV. Hospital nurses appear to run a lower risk of contracting primary CMV infection from hospitalized infants and children than do community home workers, perhaps because of the short contact and the controlled environment. Research is lacking regarding the risk of community workers in contact with the disease (e.g., school nurses, teachers, and others who work directly with children with CMV). Applying universal precautions in schools should provide needed protection.

E. In immunosuppressed or immunodeficient individuals, CMV infections are a major cause of morbidity and mortality. Risk factors and the type of infection that predispose these individuals to CMV infections are not as well defined as those for the previous groups. Immunodeficient individuals include HIV and cancer patients, organ transplant recipients, hemodialysis patients, and those receiving systemic corticosteroids and immunosuppressive drugs. Posttransfusion CMV infection occurs and can be especially threatening to immunocompromised patients, infants, those receiving immunosuppressive therapy, and pregnant women.

VIII. **Web Sites**

CDC National Center for Infectious Diseases, CMV
http://www.cdc.gov/ncidod/diseases/cmv.htm
The Body: CMV
http://www.thebody.com/treat/cmv.html

DIABETES MELLITUS: TYPE 1 AND TYPE 2

DIABETES MELLITUS: TYPE 1

I. **Definition**

A. Diabetes mellitus, type 1 and type 2, are metabolic diseases caused by a deficiency in the production or in the action of the hormone insulin. Insulin converts sugar, starches, and other food into energy and is usually produced by specialized cells in the islets of Langerhans in the pancreas. There are different types of diabetes, each with its own etiology, clinical course, and treatment management. Type 1 diabetes was previously known as *insulin-dependent diabetes mellitus.* Type 2 diabetes was previously referred to as *non-insulin-dependent diabetes mellitus* and is covered later in this section.

II. **Etiology**

A. In type 1 diabetes, the body produces insufficient insulin, or the insulin produced is ineffective, resulting from a predetermined genetic susceptibility or from environmental factors that influence an autoimmune response. Particular viruses and toxins, as well as a seasonal influence, have been linked as causative factors. Changes in the body induced by obesity, pregnancy, illicit drugs, or the use of certain medications may also trigger the onset of different diabetic types.

B. Diabetes is the most common metabolic disease of childhood and adolescence; the prevalence is 1.9:1000 in school-age children and

1:360 in children at age 16 years (Behrman, Kliegman, and Jenson, 2000). Peak incidence is about 10 to 12 years of age in girls and 12 to 14 years in boys (ADA, 1996).

III. *Brain Findings*

    A. Studies on animals have demonstrated that neurons die as a result of hyperglycemia. Insulin-like growth factor 1 (IGF-1) and some antioxidant agents were found to prevent this cell death or dysfunction. Other animal studies demonstrated that uncontrolled periods of hyperglycemia damage the hippocampus, which is important for memory function. Controlling blood sugar levels with an islet cell transplant was found to protect against such damage.

IV. **Characteristics**

    A. Usually seen in children but can occur at any age.

    B. Symptoms generally manifest around preschool or school age; however, it has been diagnosed in infants as young as 6 months.

    C. Rapid onset.

    D. Presenting symptoms:

        1. Polyphagia (excessive eating).

        2. Polydipsia (excessive drinking).

        3. Polyuria (excessive urination).

        4. Weakness or fatigue.

        5. Irritability.

        6. Nausea and vomiting.

        7. Weight loss.

    E. Other manifestations:

        1. Dry skin.

        2. Skin infections that heal slowly.

        3. Blurred vision.

        4. Constipation from dehydration.

        5. Children most likely underweight and adolescents overweight.

        6. Monilial vaginitis in adolescent girls.

        7. Enuresis in previously toilet-trained child.

        8. Lethargy.

        9. Fruity breath odor.

        10. Abdominal pain.

    F. More frequently diagnosed in winter than summer.

V. **Health Concerns/Emergencies**

    A. Chronic complications:

        1. Vascular and nervous system damage.

        2. Neuropathy.

        3. Retinopathy and cataracts.

        4. Renal disease.

        5. Cardiovascular disease.

        6. Short stature and underweight.

NOTE: Must check Nurse Practice Act, state, and district policies for administration of treatment and medication before storing and giving. Also see Chapter 11 for additional emergency discussion.

Box 4-3	*Diabetic Coma: Hyperglycemia (Excess Blood Glucose) Ketoacidosis*

1. Less common than insulin reaction.
2. Slow onset.
3. Precipitating events:
   a. Undiagnosed diabetes.
   b. Too little or no insulin.
   c. Infection, illness, or injury.
   d. Emotional stress.
   e. Nonadherence to diet.
4. Symptoms:
   a. Gradual drowsiness.
   b. Increased thirst and urination.
   c. Flushed skin.
   d. Nausea, vomiting.
   e. Anorexia.
   f. Weakness, abdominal pains, generalized aches.
   g. Fruity or wine breath.
   h. Rapid pulse.
   i. Hyperventilation or tachypnea.
   j. If untreated, eventual stupor or unconsciousness.

Action:

If uncertain whether individual is hyperglycemic or hypoglycemic, the following will not do harm if person is hyperglycemic but will alleviate hypoglycemia:

1. Give conscious person sugar-containing drink; if no response, activate emergency medical services (EMS), call parent(s).
2. If unconscious, administer glucagon as prescribed; activate EMS, call parent(s).
3. To differentiate between the two, the nurse or designatee should check blood sugar level.

VI. Effects on Individual
  A. Poor self-image as a result of "being different."
  B. Parental relationships may be strained from having parent who does too much or little.
  C. May feel insulin injections are form of punishment.
  D. Altered mood and mental alertness.
  E. Unable to participate in certain sports, which may be due primarily to parental concerns.
  F. Can be healthier than peers when following recommended diet, maintaining health status, following medical regimen, and being alert to illness and fatigue.
  G. Unable to enlist in armed forces.
  H. Very little or no limitations on career or lifestyle when practices proper self care.
  I. Must check feet every day and be vigilant in looking for signs of bruising, infection, or other trauma to prevent secondary complications.
VII. Management/Treatment
  A. School nurse responsibilities:
    1. Develop IHCP for care of student.
    2. Provide appropriate diabetic care and supervise health paraprofessional or designated trained adult.
    3. Have trained back-up personnel available at all times.

Box 4-4 *Insulin Reaction: Hypoglycemia (Low Blood Sugar)*

1. Rapid onset.
2. Usually occurs before meal time and at peak effective time of insulin.
3. Precipitating events:
   a. Too much insulin.
   b. Delayed or missed meal.
   c. Excessive exercise without adequate food.

5. Blood glucose severely lowered.
6. Sweating.
7. Extreme nervousness, tremors.
8. Headache, abdominal pains.
9. Nausea and vomiting.
10. Blood pressure lowered.
11. Pulse rate increased.

Mild Reaction

1. Behavioral problems, temper tantrums, irritable, "not themselves."
2. Hunger.
3. Increased pulse and respiratory rate.
4. Hyperactivity.
5. Weakness.
6. Pallor.
7. In children, first sign may be behavioral problems.

Action

1. Provide immediate source of food, milk, fruit juice, glucose tablets, gel, or icing (milk is good because it provides lactose, protein, and fat); can follow with starch/carbohydrate snack.
2. Do not use diet drinks and do not give insulin.

Moderate Reaction

1. Cerebral function affected.
2. Confusion and disorientation.
3. Poor coordination.
4. Increased irritability.

Action

1. Check blood sugar, if indicated provide 10 to 15 g simple carbohydrates, 3 tsp sugar in water, orange juice (3 to 6 oz), apple juice, or grape juice, or treat as prescribed (e.g., glucose tablets, gel, or icing).
2. Repeat in 10 to 15 min if no response.
3. Follow with larger carbohydrate protein snack, or if meal time, allow to eat lunch.
4. Provide rest.
5. Do not give insulin.

Severe Reaction

1. Tachycardia.
2. Loss of consciousness.
3. Seizure activity.
4. Deep coma.
5. Decreased reflexes.

Action

1. Administer glucagon as prescribed, intramuscularly or subcutaneously.
2. Activate emergency medical services (EMS), notify parent(s).

4. Identify location of testing and insulin administration; arrange for safe disposal of syringes.
5. Make classroom adaptations to avoid penalizing student requiring diabetic care.
6. Check availability of glucose supply and snack foods.
7. Educate teachers and staff regarding disease and emergency procedures; include computer, music, and physical education (PE) teachers, coaches, playground supervisors, bus drivers, and cafeteria workers.
8. Advise parent(s) regarding field trips; make arrangements as needed.

9. Be aware of individual state nurse practice acts and state/district educational mandates, since they vary regarding who can be taught and who can administer glucose/insulin injections.

10. Post emergency procedures where necessary for easy access and visibility.

B. Encourage need for medical identification alert.

C. Monitor anthropometry (height and weight). Any rapid changes in weight gain or loss may be in reaction to medications and poor control.

D. Annual eye examination, with funduscopic examination (red reflex); assess teeth integrity and for skin lesions.

E. Meals and snacks should be eaten within 1 hour of scheduled time; avoid excessive protein, monitor carbohydrate intake, consistent day-to-day eating of food.

F. Drug interactions; many OTC medications contain glucose, alcohol, or glucose neurogenic substances.

G. Encourage exercise, which improves glucose utilization, and give frequent praise to overcome negative feelings and inadequacies that arise regarding reporting of and treatment for negative glucose results.

H. Sports are encouraged; however, be aware that hypoglycemic reactions can occur up to 12 hours after the event.

I. Either hypoglycemia or hyperglycemia can affect learning; be alert to classroom learning or behavioral difficulties.

J. Inappropriate behavior can be misinterpreted as acting out (e.g., belligerent, defiant) but may be due to hypoglycemia, and blood level testing should be monitored before disciplinary action or discussion.

K. Adolescent-specific issues:
1. Monitor closely, since prone to candidiasis.
2. Susceptible to hyperglycemia during menstruation.
3. Eating disorders such as bulimia and anorexia nervosa can complicate diabetic management; adolescent may manipulate or withhold insulin to control body size.
4. Pregnancy creates risks 5 times greater than to adolescent without diabetes; use low-dose estrogen contraceptive because of complications with high doses of estrogen.

L. Alcohol and drug use: Alcohol consumption inhibits the release of glycogen from the liver, causing hypoglycemia; the diabetic may be confused regarding the effects of alcohol and may self-treat with additional insulin rather than a sugary or food snack. Confusion can also occur regarding a hypoglycemic state and intoxication while in a party environment. Cigarettes and stimulants can accelerate the complications of diabetes.

M. Insulin administration technology:
1. *Insulin pens:* A cartridge of insulin is fitted into a penlike device. A special needle tip fits onto the end of the pen, and the dosage is dialed before giving. When the end of the pen is cocked and pressed, insulin is delivered. The needle is changed at every use. Cartridges hold 150 and 300 units. There are a variety of insulin

pens available. Some are completely disposable, whereas others have single dose or multidose cartridges. The insulin cartridges may or may not need refrigeration; check manufacturer's recommendations. Administration of insulin is faster, and needles are sharper, since they do not have to be inserted into a vial, and children can become independent at an earlier age.

2. *Insulin pumps:* These provide a continuous subcutaneous infusion of insulin into the site and are a bit larger than a credit card. Age for beginning use is about 10 years but is dependent on developmental level, motivation, and supportive network. The pump is computer programmed to delivery insulin from a syringe to a catheter to a needle placed in the subcutaneous tissues in the abdomen or thigh. The pump is worn on the belt or in a shoulder holster; the needle and catheter should be changed every 48 hours. After eating, a bolus can be given to cover food consumed. Can accurately delivery insulin in 0.1 unit increments. Advantages: consistent blood glucose level, reduces number of injections, improved control, convenient—can sleep late without worrying about early morning hyperglycemia, and flexibility. Disadvantages: if disconnected, individual can go into diabetic ketoacidosis (DKA), so need back-up insulin pen at school, bathing, sports, and intimate moments.

VIII. **Additional Information**

A. An expert committee to define and classify diabetes mellitus was formed under the sponsorship of the American Diabetes Association. Their published report (2000) removed the terms *insulin-dependent diabetes mellitus* and *non-insulin-dependent diabetes mellitus*. The rationale for the committee decision was to alleviate confusion with the terminology and move toward etiological classification.

B. Insulin effects vary with each preparation, and can change from person to person, by injection sites, activities, and physical/emotional well-being or within the same individual from day to day. Absorption is faster and most reliable in the abdomen, followed by the arms and legs.

C. Injection sites include upper arms, thighs, buttocks, and abdomen. Sites are rotated to various areas of the body, with approximately four to five injections given in each area. Each injection is spaced about 1 in (2.5 cm) from the previous injection.

Table 4-5 *Types of Insulin*

Insulin	Appearance	Onset	Peak	Duration
Superfast (Lispro)	Clear	5-15 min	30-90 min	3-4 hr
Fast (regular)	Clear	30-60 min	2-4 hr	3-6 hr
Intermediate (NPH or Lente)	Cloudy	1-4 hr	6-12 hr	18-24 hr
Slow (Ultralente)	Cloudy	4-8 hr	10-20 hr	16-36 hr

NPH, Neutral protamine Hagedorn (insulin).

D. *Lipodystrophy* is a complication of insulin administration. It is a localized manifestation of disordered fat metabolism and takes the form of hypertrophy or atrophy. *Hypertrophy* is a mass of fibrous scar tissue; it can cause malabsorption of insulin. *Atrophy* appears as dimpling and pitting of the skin and underlying tissue. Lipodystrophy is prevented by systematically rotating insulin injection sites, administering insulin at room temperature, and pinching up the skin before injection to ensure that the insulin goes between the fat and muscle tissue.

E. Future trends for insulin management:

1. *Intranasal insulin* is another new treatment. It is combined with bile salts and given by aerosol pump. Insulin crosses the nasal mucosa into the bloodstream, quickly increasing serum levels. It does not replace injections because of short action, but current suggested use is as a supplement at mealtime. Advantages: easy to administer; fast absorption rates. Disadvantages: some irritation of nasal mucosa; difficult to know precise dosage administration. Currently not approved by the FDA.

2. *Inhaled insulin* technology converts large or small molecules into fine-particle aerosol and delivers the insulin deep into the lungs, where it is rapidly absorbed. It is used before mealtimes, and peak values are attained within 5 to 60 minutes. Advantages: rapid delivery and peak value without injection. Disadvantage: partial loss of drug in the device, in the environment or in the oral cavity. Neither inhaled nor intranasal administration will entirely eliminate the need for injectable insulin.

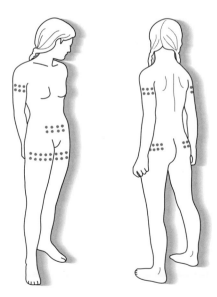

FIGURE 4-3 Rotation sites for insulin injection.

| **Box 4-5** | *Current Diabetic Research Focus* |

- Islet cell or pancreatic transplantation
- Cell therapy and beta cell development
- Laser technology
- Implanted monitors (smart pumps)
- Genetic research

3. *Glucose sensor:* Noninvasive blood glucose monitoring systems will soon be available. One appears to be and is worn like a watch. A transdermal pad is next to the skin on the wrist, which induces sweating, displaying the blood glucose level on the face of the watch. This provides continuous readings of blood glucose levels, up to 36 readings in a 12-hour period. When alarm is set, it will notify if outside of the acceptable range. Another uses a laser device to create holes in the dead outer layer of the skin, where a patch monitors the glucose concentration. A meter displays these results. Several other devices are being researched, all of which determine glucose level by measuring the concentration in the interstitial fluid (ISF) (clear fluid under the skin).

DIABETES MELLITUS: TYPE 2

I. Definition and Etiology
   A. Previously referred to as *non-insulin-dependent diabetes mellitus,* type 2 diabetes is most often found in adults. This disorder is increasing in the adolescent population. Type 2 diabetes includes those with insulin resistance, a pancreatic disease resulting in decreased insulin secretion; hormonal changes; genetic anomalies; impaired glucose tolerance; gestational diabetes mellitus; or adverse effects of drugs. Other contributing factors are heredity, obesity, sedentary lifestyles, high-fat, low-fiber diets, hypertension, and aging. Of the diagnosed diabetics, 85% to 90% are type 2.
   B. Contributing to increase in children and adolescents is being overweight, inactive or having a family history of diabetes. It is more common in African-Americans, Latinos, and Native Americans. Symptoms include being overweight (obese) with no or little weight loss, mild or no polyuria, polydipsia, manifest glycosuria without ketonuria, and acanthosis nigricans. Nurses can counsel staff, high-risk students, and others regarding development of type 2 diabetes and prevention strategies.
   C. Can often be controlled or prevented by managing weight, blood pressure, and blood lipid levels through exercise and diet, but may require oral medication if not successful. Medications for children have not been approved by the FDA; however, metformin (Glucophage) is often used, which improves insulin secretion.

II. Web Sites
   American Diabetes Association
   1-800-ADA-DISC
   http://www.diabetes.org

National Centers for Disease Control Diabetes Home Page
http://www.cdc.gov/health/diabetes.htm
Juvenile Diabetes Foundation
212-689-7868
http://www.jdfcure.org
National Diabetes Education Program
Joint Program of National Centers for Disease Control and Prevention and
National Institutes of Health
http://www.ndep.nih.gov
National Institute of Diabetes & Digestive Disorders & Kidney Diseases
http://www.niddk.nih.gov

DOWN SYNDROME

I. Definition

A. Down syndrome is a genetic disorder in which proper cell division does not occur. It is the most common chromosomal abnormality and is sometimes erroneously called *mongolism*.

II. Etiology

A. Normally an individual has 46 chromosomes in each body cell, 23 from each parent. The 46 chromosomes are in pairs of 23 and are numbered 1 to 23. An individual with Down syndrome almost always has 47 chromosomes in each cell, 23 from one parent and 24 from the other parent; the extra genetic material is responsible for the syndrome's characteristics. There are three types of Down syndrome: trisomy 21 (nondisjunction), mosaic, and translocation.

B. Down syndrome affects approximately 1 in 800 live births in the United States. The chances for an error in chromosome division increases with maternal age; at age 30 the incidence is 1:1000; age 40 is 1:100; age 45 is 42:1000. However, the majority of infants are born to women under age 35. This may be explained by prenatal detection being more common for women over 35.

C. Approximately 95% of children with Down syndrome are *trisomy 21,* which is caused by failure of the cells to divide properly during meiosis. There is an extra chromosome with the twenty-first pair of the numbered chromosomes, making three in that group. This type is more common in males and is not inherited.

D. In *mosaic Down syndrome* there is a combination; some cells have the normal number of chromosomes, and others cells are trisomy. The error in cell division occurs spontaneously after normal division has begun. This type is nonhereditary.

E. *Translocation Down syndrome* is caused by a defect in chromosomal structure rather than an error in cell division. The twenty-first chromosome attaches to another chromosome, generally the fourteenth. This form of Down syndrome may be inherited from a parent carrier. It occurs more frequently in children of younger parents and occurs more often in females.

III. Characteristics

A. No individual with Down syndrome has all the physical characteristics or same degree of mental retardation, which may range from low-average intelligence to severe mental retardation.

B. Trisomy 21 and translocation Down syndrome present the same physical characteristics.

C. Individuals with mosaic Down syndrome may have less noticeable physical features and higher intelligence than the other two types because they have a number of normal cells.

D. Physical characteristics:

1. Head.
   a. Head is generally small and round, with flattened occiput.
   b. Brachycephaly.
   c. Separated sagittal suture, enlarged anterior fontanel.
   d. Sparse hair.
   e. Undersized maxilla.
   f. Hypoplasia of midfacial bones, small, flattened nose.
   g. Short palate and narrowed nasopharynx.
   h. Susceptible to obstructive sleep apnea.
   i. Chronic rhinitis.
   j. Tongue protrudes, although it is normal in size.
   k. Teeth erupt late; some may never erupt.
   l. Voice somewhat husky; child has delayed speech and poor articulation.

2. Eyes/vision.
   a. Brushfield's spots (no clinical significance), hypoplasia of the iris.
   b. Eyes tend to slant upward (98%), with epicanthal folds; narrow palpebral fissures.
   c. Blepharitis and blocked tear ducts frequently observed.
   d. Strabismus, nystagmus, cataracts, and refractive errors commonly occur.

3. Ears/hearing.
   a. Small, low-set ears, with folded helix (margin of external ear).
   b. Narrow canals, cerumen impaction common.
   c. Susceptible to middle ear fluid and ear infections.
   d. Conductive, sensorineural, or mixed hearing loss.

4. Musculoskeletal.
   a. Moro's reflexes absent in newborn.
   b. Hypotonia common in newborn, improves with age.
   c. Short, broad neck with loose skin at nape.
   d. Little fingers are curved inward.
   e. Small, broadened hands and feet.
   f. Palms have single transverse crease, called *simian line.*
   g. Wide space between first and second toes; 96%; deep vertical crease on sole that runs between these two toes.
   h. Shorter than average.
   i. Atlantoaxial instability (AAI).

   j. Hyperflexibility.
   k. Patella dislocation.
   l. Hip subluxation.
5. Sexual.
   a. Male sex organs poorly developed.
   b. Females often have enlarged labia majora and clitoris and small breasts.
   c. Pelvic bone wide, flattened, and smaller.
   d. In males, sperm count is decreased and they are sterile; in females, start of menarche is usually within normal age range; recorded incidence of pregnancy is low; offspring have high risk of some abnormality.
6. Structural manifestations.
   a. Congenital heart defects, especially septal defects (40%-45%).
   b. Tracheoesophageal fistula.
   c. Esophageal atresia.
   d. Renal agenesis.
   e. Duodenal atresia/obstruction.
7. Other characteristics
   a. Prone to respiratory infections.
   b. Thyroid dysfunction (20%).
   c. Increased incidence of autoimmune disorders.
   d. Increased risk of developing acute leukemia (megakaryocytic is most common in younger children and requires special protocol for Down syndrome).
   e. Failure to thrive common in infancy; obesity may occur in adolescence.
   f. Diabetes mellitus.
   g. Hirschsprung disease.
   h. Increased incidence of autistic disorders.
IV. **Health Concerns/Emergencies**
   A. Children with congenital heart defects may require close observation and care:
      1. Watch for respiratory distress, cyanosis, failure to thrive, or signs of congestive heart failure.
      2. Children on digitalis may need their pulse rate monitored daily.
      3. When necessary, obtain instructions from physician for restrictions regarding activity.
   B. Tendency toward frequent otitis media and middle ear fluid necessitates frequent otological examinations and audiological and impedance audiometry screenings, along with referrals as necessary.
   C. Hearing loss is common; hearing aids may be necessary (70%-80% have hearing deficits; risk persists through adulthood).
   D. Upper respiratory tract infections (URTIs) may easily progress to involvement of bronchi and lungs.
   E. Susceptible to obstructive sleep apnea.
   F. Chronic constipation is common; consider Hirschsprung's disease.

V. Effects on Individual
  A. Hearing loss caused by frequent otitis media will affect language acquisition, emotional and social development, and educational progress.
  B. Surgical intervention for cardiac anomalies can be a frightening experience.
  C. May be isolated from others because of parents' fears of social rejection.
  D. In adolescence, the person's desire for independence may not be fulfilled, since parents may view person as a child.
  E. Parents may deny the individual's sexual maturation, which can cause inappropriate behavior and additional social isolation.
  F. Individual has predisposition to premature aging and seems more susceptible to diseases associated with older adults.
  G. Self-image and self-worth can be affected if relationship between the parents, caregiver, and their child is not positive.

VI. Management/Treatment
  A. Monitor hearing every 6 months until age 3 and annually thereafter.
  B. Vision evaluation by 6 months of age and annually thereafter.
  C. Monitor height and weight using Down syndrome charts and body mass index (BMI) (see Appendix A).
  D. Periodic otoscopic examination for children who tend to develop cerumen impaction.
  E. Mucus may have to be cleared from nose with bulb syringe because small, depressed nasal passages impede drainage.
  F. Myringotomy tubes may be placed; take precautions to ensure that fluid does not enter into middle ear by using earplugs during showering, swimming, or water play.
  G. Testing of thyroid function annually. Risk of hypothyroidism increases with age. Replacement therapy as needed.
  H. Radiographic screening for AAI is recommended between 3-5 years of age and/or before participation in sports, physically active exercise, or surgical procedures. Avoid activities involving strain or stress on neck (e.g., somersaults) until AAI is ruled out.
  I. Celiac disease screening between 2-3 years of age. Treatment is gluten-free diet.
  J. Cardiology evaluation in adolescence for possible valvular disease.

VII. Additional Information
  A. For *prenatal diagnosis,* amniocentesis is frequently recommended for women 35 or older at approximately 14 weeks gestation. For *postnatal diagnosis,* during the physical examination, the examiner notes signs commonly associated with the syndrome, extent of muscle hypotonia, any congenital defects, and adjustment of the infant to extrauterine life. Chromosome analysis confirms diagnosis.
  B. Developmental screening should begin as soon as possible and is necessary for planning and implementing special programs. The child with Down syndrome needs referral for an early stimulation program, with emphasis on language and speech development, large

and small muscle stimulation, enrollment in class best suited to their needs.

C. Development is frequently close to normal during the first 6 months of the child's life, causing parents to question the diagnosis. Affected individuals can vary widely in intellectual functioning; the majority are moderately retarded, whereas others may be borderline or severely retarded. A child with mosaic Down syndrome can have higher intellectual ability because there are some normal cells, as well as some misdivided cells.

D. With the translocation type, the chances of having a second child with Down syndrome is 10% if the carrier is the mother and 2% if the carrier is the father.

E. Approximately 15%-20% of individuals with Down syndrome have a displacement of the C1 vertebrae in relation to the C2 vertebrae. This condition is known as *AAI* and is generally asymptomatic. When symptomatic, there is risk of cord compression. Symptoms are deteriorating ambulatory skills, changes in bowel or bladder function, weakness in any of the extremities, limited neck movement, neck pain or weakness, changes in neck posturing, and neurological signs (e.g., hypertonicity, clonus of the ankles, hyperreflexia, extensor responses). Surgery may be required.

F. Cardiac defects may be asymptomatic, especially atrioventricular defects. Monitor closely for fatigue and failure to thrive, which may be subtle indicators.

G. Increased incidence of autoimmune thyroid disease; symptoms may be subtle; mood changes such as depression, abnormal menstrual cycles, and worsening of dry skin.

H. Alternative and complementary medicine are sought by some parents and may include: nutritional supplements/megavitamins, cell therapy, growth hormone, acupuncture, homeopathy, chiropractic manipulations, patterning, surgery for relief of midfacial hypoplasia/cosmetic reasons, and facilitated communication.

VIII. **Web Sites**

Down Syndrome
http://www.nas.com/downsyn
Down Syndrome: Health Issues
http://www.ds-health.com
National Association for Down Syndrome
http://www.nads.org/
National Down Syndrome Society
http://www.ndss.org/

EATING DISORDERS

I. **Definition**
A. *Anorexia nervosa:* Restriction of food intake as weight falls below ideal body weight from a fear of fatness and an unparalleled compulsion to be thin.
B. *Bulimia nervosa:* Patterns of binge eating exist while individual continues to manifest concern with body weight and shape. Overeating

and the fear of gaining weight is followed with purging by forced vomiting, fasting, laxative and/or diuretic use, and/or excessive exercise.

1. Prevalence in the United States is around 1% for anorexia and 2% for bulimia. Between 10% to 25% of female adolescents have some disorganized eating habits characterized by bingeing and self-forced vomiting.
2. Both disorders are observed more in the female population; males account for about 5% to 10% (Behrman et al, 1996) and occur most frequently when competing in sports with weight limitation, such as wrestling.
3. Age of onset for anorexia is bimodal; peaks at ages 13 to 14 and 17 to 18 years; childhood onset is reported between ages 7 to 11 years (Behrman et al, 1996). Onset of bulimia appears to occur during middle to late adolescence.
4. Eating disorders affect all socioeconomic and racial-ethnic groups.

II. Etiology

A. May involve biological, nutritional, psychological, and sociocultural factors. Eating disorders tend to run in families. Anorexia and bulimia are three times more common in relatives of eating-disordered individuals than in the general U.S. population.

B. Risk factors include dieting, obesity, family history of eating disorders, groups placing value on thinness (e.g., models, ballet dancers, figure skaters, gymnasts). Particular personal characteristics create an increased risk (e.g., low self-esteem, rigidity, compliance, dependency, competitiveness, impulsiveness, and/or perfectionism, difficulty with boundaries and self regulation). Comorbidity with psychiatric disorders is common and includes depression; with anorexia—social phobic, simple phobic, and obsessive-compulsive disorders; with bulimia—anxiety disorders and substance abuse.

C. American culture and other Western societies emphasize thinness, with role models observed on television, in movies, newspapers, and magazines, as well as in families. During adolescence, females are more conscious of their bodies; are prone to diets and restrictive food intake.

III. *Brain Findings*

A. Both disorders have abnormalities in the noradrenergic, dopamine, and serotonin systems of the brain but normalize with weight gain. This finding may contribute to why serotonin reuptake inhibitors are beneficial.

IV. Characteristics

A. Trigger factors include sexual abuse, traumatic loss, chronic dieting, family difficulties, peer pressure, sensitivity to teasing about body size and shape, and demands on performance from family and school staff.

B. Feeling of lack of control over eating.

C. Low frustration tolerance, poor self-esteem, suppressed anger, rebellion, hostility, and depression.

D. Bingeing/purging cycles or not purging with rigorous dieting, fasting, and/or rigorous exercise.
E. Anorexia: usually model child, obsessive-compulsive, high achiever, will deny illness, usually not sexually active.
F. Bulimia: often child who acts out, impulsive, loses self-control, fluctuating school performance, aware of illness, may be sexually active.

Table 4-6	Associated Symptoms of Eating Disorders	
Body System	**Anorexia Nervosa**	**Bulimia Nervosa**
General concerns	Excessively underweight Irritability, dizziness, syncope, confusion, sleep difficulties Lethargy, hyperactivity Hypothermia Amenorrhea, malnutrition Decreased growth parameters	Usually normal weight, or ranges from obese to extremely underweight Weakness, fatigue Irregular menses
Sensory system	Decreased concentration, drowsy, irritable, confused	—
Vital signs	Decreased temperature, pulse, blood pressure, and respiration	—
Dermatological	Hair dry, brittle, dull or hair loss, lanugo on body Skin dry, rough, yellowish or grayish, cracked	Ulcerations, scars/calluses on back of hand Skin dry, cracked, rough; sores on mucous membranes in mouth and around fingernails Face: edema, broken blood vessels
Extremities	Peripheral edema of feet/hands	Edema of feet and sometimes hands
Oral	—	Enamel erosion or discoloration of teeth, dental caries, parotid gland hypertrophy
Cardiovascular	Bradycardia, hypertension	Arrhythmia
Genitourinary	Thin, dry, pale, atrophic vaginal mucosa	—
Gastrointestinal	Decreased bowel sounds, constipation	Abdominal distension, epigastric tenderness, GER, diarrhea or constipation
Musculoskeletal	Decrease in bone mass (osteopenia), fractures	—
Neuromuscular	Muscle wasting/weakness Decreased deep tendon reflexes and decreased mass and definition, weakness	Muscle wasting/weakness with chronic use of ipecac

GER, Gastroesophageal reflux.
Individuals with both disorders can exhibit signs and symptoms of both diseases.

V. Health Concerns/Emergencies
A. Death related to cardiac arrhythmia, hypokalemia, suicide.
B. Osteoporosis.
C. Alcohol and drug abuse/addictions.
D. Growth retardation.
E. Dehydration.
F. Gynecological difficulties associated with prolonged amenorrhea.

VI. Effects on Individual
A. Guilt, depression, anxiety regarding bingeing behavior.
B. Fatigue and weakness.
C. Headaches.
D. Teasing, personal rejection by family or peers, and social stigma.
E. Family stress.

VII. Management/Treatment
A. Detailed history needs to be taken with student and include:
 1. Weight and dietary intake.
 2. Issues around being fat or thin.
 3. Perception of body image.
 4. Diet methods used.
 5. Exercise regimen.
 6. History of bingeing and purging.
 7. Symptoms or diagnosis of psychiatric disorders.
 8. Abuse of drugs or alcohol.
B. Management and treatment depend on the history, stage of illness, diagnosis of one or both eating disorders, presence of affective disorder or substance abuse, level of family support, and other indicators for referral and treatment. Many schools have nurses and/or counselors or individuals who are trained to work with this population for at-school supplemental counseling.
C. Referrals for physical examination, clinical assessment, nutritional counseling, individual and group psychotherapy, and family therapy. May require hospitalization for stabilization of electrolyte imbalance and nutrient intake, medications, and supplements (e.g., antidepressants, metoclopramide, estrogen, progesterone, and minerals [calcium, phosphate, zinc, potassium, iron]).

VIII. Web Sites
National Eating Disorders Association
206-382-3587
http://www.nationaleatingdisorders.org
Girl Power
1-800-729-6686
http://www.health.org/gpower
Harvard Eating Disorders Center (HEDC)
http://www.hedc.org
National Association of Anorexia Nervosa and Associated Disorders (ANAD)
http://www.anad.org/facts.htm

| **Box 4-6** | *DSM-IV Criteria: Anorexia Nervosa* |

1. Refusal to maintain body weight at or above a minimally normal weight for age and height (i.e., weight loss leading to maintenance of body weight <85% of that expected); or failure to make expected weight gain during period of growth, leading to body weight <85% of that expected.
2. Intense fear of gaining weight or becoming fat, even though underweight.
3. Disturbance in the way in which one's body weight or shape is experienced, undue influence of body weight or shape on self-evaluation, or denial of the seriousness of the current low body weight.
4. In postmenarchal females, amenorrhea (i.e., the absence of at least three consecutive menstrual cycles).

From *Diagnostic and statistical manual of mental disorders,* ed 4, revision, Washington, DC, 2000, American Psychiatric Association.

| **Box 4-7** | *DSM-IV Criteria: Bulimia Nervosa* |

1. Recurrent episodes of binge eating, characterized by both of the following: (a) eating an unusually large amount of food in a discrete period (within 2 hours) and (b) a sense of lack of control over eating during the episode.
2. Recurrent inappropriate compensatory behavior to prevent weight gain (e.g., self-induced vomiting; misuse of laxatives, diuretics, enemas, or other medications; fasting; excessive exercise).
3. Binge eating and compensatory behaviors both occur on average twice a week for 3 months.
4. Self-evaluation is unduly influenced by body shape and weight.
5. The disturbance does not occur exclusively during episodes of anorexia nervosa.

From *Diagnostic and statistical manual of mental disorders,* ed 4, revision, Washington, DC, 2000, American Psychiatric Association.

ENCOPRESIS (CHRONIC CONSTIPATION/RETENTION)

I. Definition

A. Encopresis is involuntary fecal soiling by a child beyond the usual age for toilet training. *Primary encopresis* is when a child has never achieved bowel control, and *secondary encopresis* occurs after bowel control has been established. The two subtypes of encopresis are with or without constipation and overflow incontinence. Organic pathology or illness is not present.

II. Etiology

A. Encopresis is believed to be psychogenic and/or physiological. It is associated with chronic constipation, fecal impaction, and overflow incontinence in about two thirds of cases and may progress to an enlarged colon. One cause may be the conscious or unconscious manipulation of the environment. Another cause is *chronic diarrhea* or *irritable bowel syndrome,* in which the child is incontinent as an apparent reaction to stress or emotional upset. Before age 4, chronic constipation occurs equally in the male and female; in the school-age child, encopresis affects around 1% of children and is more common in males.

III. **Characteristics**
  A. More prevalent in males; often unreported because of family embarrassment.
  B. Retention of stool for days or weeks.
  C. Abdominal pain.
  D. Palpable abdominal fecal mass.
  E. Poor appetite and lethargy.
  F. Often precipitated by upsetting or stressful event.
  G. Frequent refusal to defecate in the toilet.
  H. Often defecates in supine or standing position.
  I. Most accidents take place during the day.
  J. Frequent presence of fecal odor.
  K. Organic factors have been explored and ruled out.
  L. History of straining and constipation and intervention with laxatives and enemas.
  M. Retentive posturing.

IV. **Health Concerns/Emergencies**
  A. Organic factors need to be ruled out.
  B. Chronic megacolon from constipation.
  C. Anorexia.
  D. Lesions or perianal dermatitis may cause child to withhold stool.
  E. Fever and headache.
  F. Superficial fissures with bleeding may develop because of passage of large stool.
  G. Urinary tract infections and disease from obstruction of urinary tract are serious complications of chronic fecal retention; however, this rarely occurs.
  H. Ulceration with significant rectal hemorrhage is possible complication of constipation but uncommon.

V. **Effects on Individual**
  A. Irritable and avoids play.
  B. Embarrassed by soiling and fecal odor.
  C. Attempts to deny the problem exists.
  D. Abdominal discomfort and pain.
  E. Passage of a gigantic stool causes physical discomfort and fear.
  F. Detects disapproval of parents and peers; may affect self-esteem.
  G. Recipient of parental anger because of repeatedly clogged toilets and soiled clothing.
  H. May not want to attend school because of social difficulties that soiling may cause.

VI. **Management/Treatment**
   A. Listen to student to evaluate need for medical referral and/or psychologist counseling.
   B. Contact with parents, home visit when possible to lend support and educate regarding relationship between toileting and nutritional management.
   C. Combination of enemas, suppositories, dietary manipulation (increase/add fiber and fluids), and rewards.
   D. Enemas may be prescribed daily for 1 to 2 weeks, then gradually decreased; it is important that chosen enema is safe for repeated use and side effects watched for and controlled.
   E. Mineral oil may be used as a gentle laxative; however, nurse should educate parent regarding its use; mineral oil retards absorption of fat-soluble vitamins, so it should be administered 1 to 2 hours after meals or at bedtime.

VII. **Additional Information**
   A. Referral to a psychologist or psychiatrist may be the only means toward improvement. The nurse may be able to alleviate parental anxiety by explaining that the following common fears have *little* or *no scientific basis:*
      1. The colon ruptures if it accumulates too much stool.
      2. Retained waste substances will cause a toxic state; headache is directly caused by retention.
      3. A dilated rectosigmoid impedes defecation.
      4. The temporary anorexia preceding massive evacuation causes nutritional damage.

ENURESIS

I. **Definition**
   A. Enuresis is persistence of intentional or involuntary urination in the bed or clothing by a child beyond the age of being toilet trained. *Primary* enuresis is when control was never established, and *secondary* enuresis is present when child has been continent for at least 1 year. *Nocturnal* enuresis is voiding only at night, whereas *diurnal* enuresis is voiding while awake. The diagnosis is made when frequency of enuresis is twice a week for at least 3 consecutive months, or there is significant clinical distress or impairment in important functional areas of the child's life because of the incontinence.

II. **Etiology**
   A. Enuresis may be caused by an organic disorder, an emotional disturbance, or learning problems. Organic causes include structural disorder of the urinary tract, neurological deficits, infection, diabetes, spastic bladder, epilepsy, sickle cell disease, food allergies, or chronic renal failure. Organic factors account for such a small percent of urinary incontinence that the term enuresis is generally restricted to a disorder of inorganic origin. Emotional disturbances also account for only a relatively small percentage of the problem.

B. There is a genetic predisposition for nocturnal enuresis when *both parents* have a history of enuresis, since child has a 70% likelihood of having the disorder (Behrman, Kliegman, and Jenson, 2000). Nocturnal enuresis occurs more commonly in females and is rare after 9 years of age. Enuresis prevalence at age 5 years is 7% for males and 3% for females; age 10 is 3% for males and 2% for females; age 18 years, is 1% for males and rare in females (American Psychiatric Association, 1994).

III. **Characteristics**
   A. More common in boys than in girls.
   B. Family history of enuresis.
   C. Child may sleep more soundly than other children.
   D. Child has smaller functional bladder capacity.
   E. May have an abnormal level of antidiuretic hormone (ADH).

IV. **Health Concerns/Emergencies**
   A. Organic cause needs to be ruled out.
   B. Be aware of dosage and drug side effects, since antidepressants are most popular form of treatment, and children are more sensitive than adults to medication.
   C. Be alert to punitive techniques of control that may be used in the home.

V. **Effects on Individual**
   A. Suffers disapproval of parents and ridicule of peers, and self-esteem may be affected.
   B. May experience side effects of medications.
   C. If diurnal (daytime) wetting occurs, the child may resist going to school because of embarrassment.

VI. **Management/Treatment**
   A. Management depends on an understanding of underlying causative factors: physical, psychosocial, or both.
   B. Physical examination will determine if organic or inorganic cause and recommendations for treatment.
   C. History and a chart indicating date, time of incidents, and estimated volume may be helpful in diagnosis.
   D. Medications used include tricyclic antidepressants, antidiuretics, and antispasmodics.
   E. Imipramine (Tofranil) is an antidepressant frequently given to control enuresis; dosage should not exceed 2.5 mg/kg; given daily, 1 hour before bedtime.
   F. Desmopressin (DDAVP) is a fast-acting antidiuretic administered at bedtime and may be useful for overnights and other special occasions, but the relapse rate is high when medication is discontinued. Certain side effects are serious but rare (Behrman, Kliegman, and Jenson, 2000).
   G. If on medication, be aware of side effects.
   H. Additional forms of treatment and control:
      1. Bladder training.
      2. Withholding or restricting fluids after the evening meal.

3. Waking child during night to void.
4. Psychotherapy, hypnotherapy, and behavioral techniques.
5. Conditioning devices: bell and pad—wire pad is attached to bell or buzzer, occasionally a light; when urine touches pad, bell or buzzer is activated, waking child, goes to bathroom to finish emptying bladder; child then resets equipment and goes back to bed.
6. Be supportive and educate the child, family, and school staff regarding this phenomenon.

VII. Additional Information
   A. Usually a child is considered enuretic if daytime wetting occurs beyond the age of 3 or 4, although some experts set the age at 5 or 6. Most clinicians diagnose nocturnal enuresis if the child has a problem at age 4 or 5; others say 6 or 7 or older.

VIII. Web Sites
   National Kidney Foundation
   1-800-WAKE-DRY
   http://www.kidney.org/patients/bedwet.cfm

FETAL ALCOHOL SYNDROME AND EFFECTS

I. Definition
   A. *Fetal alcohol syndrome (FAS)* is used to describe a pattern of physical and mental birth defects. It is defined by four criteria; maternal alcohol use during pregnancy, a characteristic pattern of facial abnormalities, growth retardation, and brain damage.
   B. The term *alcohol-related neurodevelopmental disorder (ARND)* is used when signs of brain damage appear after fetal alcohol exposure without other indications of FAS. Those affected may have some or no facial anomalies and may exhibit difficulties in mental development and behavioral difficulties that impact learning and long-term development. The symptoms often are not apparent until in a school setting and vary in severity. Also referred to as *fetal alcohol effects (FAE)* and *alcohol-related birth defects (ARBD)*.

II. Etiology
   A. The syndrome is found in children whose mothers consumed alcohol during pregnancy. Alcohol is a teratogen that interferes with the ability of the fetus to receive adequate oxygen and nourishment for normal brain and body structural cell development. These alcohol-induced birth defects are the leading known cause of mental retardation in the United States and are preventable. FAS is a worldwide concern and is underreported. The incidence of FAS in an active South African study of first-grade students reported more than 40 in 1000 children among ages 5 to 9; a Washington state county survey yielded 3.1 per 1000 first-grade students; and a study reviewing birth records estimates a range from 0.33 to 3 per 1000 births (NIAAA, 2000).

III. *Brain Findings*
   A. Magnetic resonance imaging (MRI) studies demonstrate reduced overall brain size and structural or functional changes in the brain, which are reflected in behavioral and cognitive impairments in those with FAS. Decreased size of the cerebellum is noted, which is associated with balance, coordination, gait, and cognition. The changes noted in the basal ganglia can impair spatial memory and set-shifting (state rigidity) in animals and are known to impair cognitive processes in humans. The corpus callosum, which is a major communication link between the right and left hemispheres of the brain, is either absent or development is impaired (NIAAA, 2000).

IV. **Characteristics**
   A. Facial.
      1. Microcephaly.
      2. Short palpebral fissures, microphthalmia, hypertelorism, and ptosis.
      3. Epicanthal folds.
      4. Flattened midface.
      5. Low-set ears or poorly formed ears.
      6. Low nasal bridge; short, upturned nose.
      7. Hypoplastic philtrum.
      8. Smooth and thin upper lip.
      9. Small mouth with high-arched palate.
      10. Micrognathia or prognathia in adolescence.
   B. Growth retardation.
      1. Birth head (BH) size average 33 cm (normal full-term BH average 35 cm).
      2. Birth weight (BW) average 6 lb (normal full-term BW average 7 lb, 8 oz).
      3. Growth deficiencies usually continue postnatally.

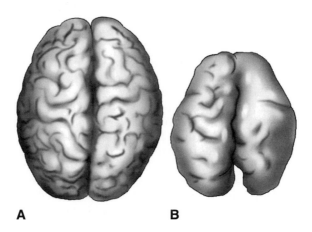

A   **B**

Figure 4-4 Normal brain **(A)** and fetal alcohol brain **(B)**.

C. Neurological.
   1. Microcephaly; defined in decreased head size and growth.
   2. Mental retardation; usually mild to moderate but can be severe.
   3. Motor retardation; poor coordination of body, hands, and fingers.
   4. Hypotonia.
   5. Hyperactivity.
   6. Hearing disorder.
D. Other.
   1. Cardiac defects, including ventricular septal defect (VSD) or atrial septal defect (ASD).
   2. Kidney abnormalities: hydronephrosis, horseshoe kidneys.
   3. Urinary defects.
   4. Increased risk of hearing loss, eighth nerve deafness, ear infections. Ears and kidneys form during the same time in utero, stressing the importance of diagnostic procedures of kidneys when ear anomalies are found.
   5. Small teeth with enamel hypoplasia, malocclusion.
   6. Myopia (nearsighted).
E. FAS and ARND cognitive and behavioral impairments.
   1. Attention: inappropriately referred to as *attention deficit-hyperactivity disorder (ADHD)*; however, these children are able to focus and maintain attention but display difficulty in shifting attention from one task to another; set shifting (transitioning).
   2. Executive functioning: perseveration, difficulty with set shifting, distractibility, and impulsivity contribute to attention and learning problems.
   3. Verbal learning: language and memory difficulties. They may have difficulty learning words (encoding, which is an initial stage of memory formation), but once they learn the task, they can recall the information.
   4. Visual-spatial learning: demonstrate poor performance on tasks that involve learning spatial relationship of objects.
   5. Reaction time: school-age children have been associated with slower, less-efficient processing of information.

V. **Health Concerns/Emergencies**
   A. Severity of health problems varies according to extent of involvement.
   B. Birth anomalies may be present that require additional care and medical intervention.
   C. Ethanol effects transferred through breast milk can produce motor delays in the baby and decrease prolactin hormone secretion, which is essential to maintain adequate lactation.
   D. Birth parent(s) may be alcoholic, and child is at risk for neglect and physical and emotional abuse.
   E. Lifelong health and learning disabilities may exist.

VI. **Effects on Individual**
   A. Frequently in out-of-home placement, and some have multiple placements, which can impair bonding and attachment, impact education achievement, and interfere with peer relationships.

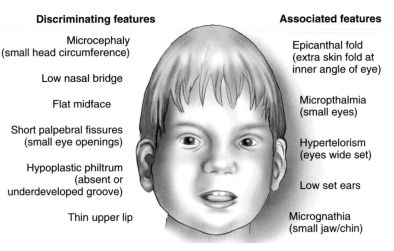

Discriminating features

Microcephaly
(small head circumference)

Low nasal bridge

Flat midface

Short palpebral fissures
(small eye openings)

Hypoplastic philtrum
(absent or
underdeveloped groove)

Thin upper lip

Associated features

Epicanthal fold
(extra skin fold at
inner angle of eye)

Micropthalmia
(small eyes)

Hypertelorism
(eyes wide set)

Low set ears

Micrognathia
(small jaw/chin)

FIGURE 4-5 Fetal alcohol syndrome features.

    B. Often petite and short, which can be detrimental for a male.
    C. May have feelings of academic inadequacies because of learning problems.
    D. May be self-conscious because of facial features.
    E. Often oversensitive to the environment, light, sound, touch, and in need of sensory integration.
    F. At risk for becoming alcoholic.
    G. When adopted or in a consistent placement at an early age, prognosis may be improved.

VII. Management/Treatment
    A. Early identification imperative for intervention to be most effective.
    B. Provide prompts and cues to facilitate transitioning.
    C. Monitor anthropometry.
    D. Monitor dental health, encourage good oral hygiene and frequent check-ups, and pursue fluoride sealant.
    E. Encourage fluids, and be alert for signs of possible urinary tract infection.
    F. Needs referral for special resources when having difficulty in academic achievement.
    G. Contact receiving school nurse, if student moving out of school district because of parental transfer or multiple home placements, to update health and educational concerns, provide smooth and consistent transition, and avoid gaps in services.

VIII. Additional Information
    A. The embryonic period, the first 2 to 8 weeks of gestation, is a time of great vulnerability to teratogenic effects of alcohol as evidenced by the structural symptoms of FAS. There are data that cessation of drinking in the third trimester, which is also a critical stage for brain development, can improve fetal outcome. Some studies suggest binge

drinking (large amounts at a given time) can be more dangerous to the fetus than drinking smaller amounts more frequently.

IX. **Web Sites**
National Organization on Fetal Alcohol Syndrome
http://www.nofas.org/main/what_is_FAS.htm

FRAGILE X SYNDROME

I. **Definition**
   A. Fragile X syndrome (FXS) is the most common genetically inherited disorder causing mental impairment. Down syndrome is more common but is not usually inherited. The incidence of FXS in males is 1 in 1250, and in females it is 1 in 2000. One in 259 females is a carrier. A spectrum of cognitive involvement ranges from normal to subtle learning disabilities to severe mental retardation. Disabilities are found in three major areas; cognitive, physical, and behavioral.

II. **Etiology**
   A. FXS is caused by a mutation of the X chromosome. The name is derived from the fragile site or break in the X gene (fragile X mental retardation 1 gene [FMR-1]). Males have one X and one Y chromosome, and females have two X chromosomes. An end section of the X chromosome normally contains between 6 and 50 repetitions of the genetic code CGG. When a code breakdown occurs, the number of CGG can increase. An increase of 50 to 200 CGG repeats, a permutation, causes few symptoms, but an increase of over 200 CGG repeats, a full mutation, results in FXS.
   B. Cognitive, physical, and behavioral problems are presumed to be caused by the lack of normal FMR-1 protein (FMR-P) production from the dysfunctional FMR-1 gene. This absence of adequate protein produces changes in brain structure, and therefore changes in neurotransmitter systems that can be improved by the use of medication. Executive function deficits are common (attention and organizational difficulties), which are a function of the temporal lobe.

III. **Characteristics**
   A. Male.
      1. Males are more severely affected than females.
      2. Long narrow face and large and/or prominent ears.
      3. Subtle features: prominent jaw and forehead, long palpebral fissures.
      4. Enlarged testicles (generally postpuberty).
      5. Connective tissue disorder manifestations: mitral valve prolapse, high arched palate, hyperextensible finger joints, flat feet, and hypotonia.
      6. Poor eye contact, fascination with spinning objects.
      7. Most males have IQ levels in mild-to-moderate range of mental retardation, with small percentage severely to profoundly retarded.
      8. Difficulty with mathematics, abstract reasoning, and attention.

9. ADHD or hyperactivity, impulsivity.
10. Delayed onset of speech and language.
11. Psychosocial deficits: anxiety, withdrawal, and depression.
12. Majority of males (especially younger) appear to have normal physical characteristics, but can exhibit perseverative behaviors and speech and language difficulties.
13. Hand biting or flapping.

B. Female.
1. Long narrow face.
2. Prominent forehead, ears, and jaw.
3. Hyperextensible finger joints, flat feet.
4. Generally higher cognition than males, occasional moderate to severe mental retardation.
5. Learning disabilities, poor attention and organizational skills.
6. Difficulty with mathematics, speech, and language concerns.
7. Poor eye contact, shyness, social emotional disturbances.
8. Perseveration in behaviors and speech.
9. Anxiety.

IV. Health Concerns/Emergencies

A. Health concerns depend on the state and level of involvement of the syndrome.
B. Visual concerns, strabismus (esotropia/exotropia) may be present and interfere with learning and physical activity. Occasional deficits: nystagmus, myopia, ptosis, hyperopia, astigmatism.
C. Recurrent otitis media, which may be caused by unusual angle or collapsibility of the eustachian tube and cause a conductive hearing loss and/or interfere with speech and language development.
D. Detection of murmur or click indicating cardiac involvement such as mitral valve prolapse, requiring a referral for cardiac evaluation.
E. High-arched palate, which can be associated with dental malocclusion.
F. Hypotonia, scoliosis, flat feet (pes planus), requiring adequate assessment and referral.
G. Seizures can include complex, partial, and generalized, which create a need for a school health emergency plan. Medications may be required during school day.
H. Autistic-like behaviors and sensory integration difficulties may create safety issues at school and home and decrease social opportunities with peers.
I. Infants often diagnosed as failure to thrive.
J. Obesity can be the result of obsessive compulsive behaviors such as food cravings, as well as hypothalamic dysfunction or sensory integration issues (e.g., food textures and consistencies). A school plan (exercise and diet) will need to be in place, support for the parent and counseling for the individual and/or family.
K. Masturbation and forms of self-stimulating behavior can be problematic for the adolescent and require family and/or individual counseling. Fertility is normal. Sex education needs to be provided at the individual's developmental level.

    L. Anxiety in social encounters; shy and withdrawn behavior may create abnormal social situations requiring intervention.

    M. Hypersensitive to touch; tactile defensiveness and environmental overstimulation caused by sensory integration issues can cause delay in early developmental milestones and later can produce a variety of behaviors, including temper outburst, aggression, and emotional instability.

V. Effects on Individual

    A. Depend on level of involvement.

    B. Developmental delays and vision and hearing manifestations may delay academic learning.

    C. Difficulties around eating, toileting, and inappropriate personal behaviors play an important role in making and keeping friends.

    D. May be teased because of physical appearance or behaviors and left out of recreational and social activities.

    E. Lack of confidence and self-esteem.

    F. Side effects from medication.

    G. Inability to screen out noises, lights, or confusion in their environment because of sensory integration issues.

    H. Visual learner more than auditory learner because of auditory processing problems.

    I. Sibling can have the same disorder.

VI. Management/Treatment

    A. Genetic counseling, including all family members.

    B. Complete school assessment for special educational needs and services as indicated.

    C. School treatment often includes special education, speech and language therapy, occupational therapy, sensory integration, and physical therapy.

    D. Assessment of hyperactivity, and appropriate treatment, including counseling and/or medication.

    E. Medications for hyperactivity and poor attention span include methylphenidate (Ritalin), pemoline (Cylert), and dextroamphetamine (Dexedrine). These medications work by stimulating both the dopamine and the norepinephrine neurotransmitter systems, which improves attention, hyperactivity, inhibition and visual motor coordination. Clonidine (Catapres) is better for calming down behavior (hyperactivity) and improvement of tics but does not work as well as stimulants for attention and concentration difficulties. Clonidine has also been used successfully with 3-year-olds and older. It works by lowering overall norepinephrine levels and can be used together with stimulants. Although controversial, folic acid has been used with prepubertal boys, with improvements noticed in attention, activity level, coping skills, and unusual mannerisms.

    F. Provide assessment of behavioral problems, aggression, anxiety, and mood instability and determine appropriate treatment with medication, counseling, or both. Carbamazepine (Tegretol) has been useful for those with mood disorders. Fluoxetine (Prozac) has been used with adolescents demonstrating aggression.

G. Obsessive thinking and compulsive behavior may be helped by serotonin agents, such as fluoxetine (Prozac) and sertraline (Zoloft) (both *selective serotonin reuptake inhibitors;* affect all of the serotonin receptors).

VII. **Additional Information**

A. FXS occurs in all racial and ethnic groups. The majority of families with FXS are unaware of its presence. Individuals with undiagnosed mental retardation or learning disabilities (LDs) and who exhibit several of the known characteristics should be considered for testing. A definitive diagnosis for carriers and those affected can be made by identification of the FMR-1 gene mutation. The test is performed on a blood sample with a direct DNA analysis. A diagnosis can be made prenatally by amniocentesis or CVS as early as 10 weeks and in the second trimester by percutaneous umbilical blood sampling (PUBS). However, a negative result for any of the intrauterine testing does not entirely rule out the syndrome.

B. *Affected* refers to those with FXS and mental retardation. *Permutation* refers to those with fewer CGG repeats and immediate alteration and are usually unaffected. *Full mutation* refers to those with FMR-1 repeats in the 200 and above range; males will have FXS, and about 50% of females will have intellectual and cognitive deficits and some level of LD. Females with normal IQs may also have LD. *Mosaic* refers to those with variability in number of working genes, showing a mosaic status and a range of symptoms less severe.

VIII. **Web Sites**

The National Fragile X Foundation
1-800-688-8765
http://www.fragileX.org/home.htm

HEMOPHILIA A, B, AND C

I. **Definition**

A. Hemophilia is a common hereditary disorder characterized by prolonged bleeding episodes that are either spontaneous or traumatically induced. There are three types of hemophilia: A (classic), B (Christmas disease), and C (Rosenthal's syndrome). Most hemophiliacs are type A; type B is the second most prevalent form. Hemophilia C is rare and is a milder disease.

II. **Etiology**

A. Each type of hemophilia is caused by a deficiency or abnormal functioning of specific clotting factors: factor VIII in type A, factor IX in type B, and factor XI in type C. Bleeding problems are related to the plasma level of activity of the affected factor, classified as mild, moderate, and severe hemophilia. A and B types of hemophilia are transmitted to the male by a carrier female, X-linked recessive gene. Type C is inherited as an autosomal dominant trait and affects both males and females. Hemophilia also occurs by spontaneous genetic mutation and about one third of children affected have no prior family history.

III. **Characteristics**
   A. *Mild hemophilia* (factor activity greater than 5%):
      1. May go undiagnosed until surgery or major trauma.
      2. First indication may be prolonged bleeding after a dental extraction.
   B. *Moderate hemophilia* (factor activity 1%-5%):
      1. Seldom spontaneous bleeding.
      2. Victims may suffer joint and muscle bleeds several times a year after minor injury.
      3. Additional factor replacements are necessary to stop bleeding after surgery or major injury.
   C. *Severe hemophilia* (factor activity 1% or less):
      1. Major category of hemophiliacs (60%).
      2. Usually diagnosed by 12-18 months of age, some identified at birth.
      3. Spontaneous bleeding can occur.
      4. Joints and muscles are most common bleeding sites (hemarthrosis).
   D. Bleeding is not harder or faster, just prolonged, and delayed bleeding is common.
   E. Minor cuts, scrapes, and bruises usually do not present a problem.
   F. Bleeding can occur anywhere in the body, internally or externally; the ankle is the most common joint bleed as the toddler learns to ambulate; hemarthroses of the elbows and knees are the most debilitating bleeds for the older child and adolescent.
   G. Signs of bleeding episode:
      1. Reported "tingling" or other sensation.
      2. Limb held in an abnormal position.
      3. Obvious signs of discomfort or pain.
      4. Area of bleeding warm, swollen, firm, and tender on palpation.
      5. Older student aware of early symptoms of joint bleeding; fluid accumulation and major swelling in the joint space.
      6. Restriction in range of motion indicates bleeding within joint.
      7. Hemorrhage in large muscle may produce pain with movement of joint or below muscle.
      8. Discoloration of skin is *not* a good indicator of bleeding.
   H. Common cause of death (25%) is intracranial bleed, and history of trauma found in only half of the individuals.
   I. Subcutaneous bleeding may extend over large portion of body; site of origin is indurated, raised, and purplish-black.
IV. **Health Concerns/Emergencies**
   A. Blow to head, abdomen, or throat can be particularly dangerous because bleeding may go unrecognized until serious complications occur.
   B. Even a suggestion of trauma to the head requires factor infusion and head scans to rule out hemorrhage.
   C. Bleeding in tongue, throat, or neck area may rapidly compromise airway; need immediate medical attention.

    D. Ocular bleeding needs treatment and evaluation for retinal detachment.

    E. Secondary complications of joint bleeds can occur (e.g., cartilage erosion, changes in joint space, chronic arthritis, fibrosis), which can lead to a disabling condition.

V. **Effects on Individual**

    A. Parents may be overprotective or overpermissive.

    B. Living with chronic health problem has imposed limitations, as with participation in contact sports.

    C. School life disrupted because of frequent absences; may become discouraged.

    D. May feel guilt because of family's enormous financial burden for medical care and the disruption of family life. Costs may exceed insurance limits.

    E. May become disabled if joint bleeds are not treated promptly and adequately.

    F. Possibility of early death can have emotional impact.

VI. **Management/Treatment**

    A. Schools should have medical and emergency information up to date and plan of action in place.

    B. Coordinate treatment plan with student's HCP and hemophilia treatment center (HTC).

    C. Encourage wearing medical alert identification.

    D. Teach parent(s), school personnel, child care providers, and other involved persons how to control bleeding:

        1. Using gloves, apply pressure to bleeding site for 10 to 15 minutes.

        2. Elevate affected part to heart level or above.

        3. Apply lightweight ice pack or cold compress.

        4. Contact parent or physician as needed.

    E. Treat bleeding episodes promptly to reduce secondary complications.

    F. Do not give aspirin or products containing aspirin because it decreases clotting time.

    G. Some antihistamines and ibuprofen can interfere with platelet action.

    H. Students may learn to self-administer factor concentrate by age 11-12.

    I. Factor concentrate may be kept refrigerated at school to facilitate rapid treatment in the emergency room or may be administered in school if appropriate plan is in place.

    J. Current treatments do not have threat of infection with HIV/AIDS or hepatitis.

    K. Routine intramuscular injections such as immunizations avoided because of possible muscle hemorrhage. Factor concentrate usually given before injection to reduce bleeding.

    L. Use protective helmet as needed for physical activity.

    M. Encourage regular exercise to strengthen muscles, which protects joints and decreases spontaneous bleeding.

    N. Resume activity gradually after injury.

    O. Excessive body weight increases strain on affected joints.

VII. **Additional Information**
   A. Prenatal diagnosis may be made as early as 8 to 12 weeks by CVS, at 13 to 18 weeks by amniocentesis, and at 18 to 29 weeks by fetal blood sampling. Bleeding symptoms can occur in the fetus or be present at birth. Some newborns may sustain intracranial hemorrhage, and about 30% of the males will bleed during circumcision (Behrman, Kliegman, and Jenson, 2000). Hepatitis B vaccine should be given during the neonatal period.
   B. Implanted venous access devices (IVAD) may be used for ease of infusion, but the frequency of line infections and clotting may outweigh the benefits.
   C. Carriers of hemophilia have lower-than-normal clotting factor, are susceptible to anemia, and may experience prolonged bleeding during menses and pregnancy. Occurs most frequently in factor IX carriers.
   D. Some children may develop an "inhibitor" or an "antibody" to the clotting factor and need a special plan of care. This usually develops between 5-10 years of age and makes management more difficult.
   E. Nosebleeds are usually not serious; oral medications (e.g., aminocaproic acid [Amicar], tranexamic acid [Cyclokapron]) are available to decrease the bleed by maintaining the clot.
   F. Gene therapy for hemophilia is promising because it is caused by the malfunctioning of a single gene, and just a slight increase in the clotting factor can provide substantial benefits. Human trials are in progress and are showing great potential for effective treatment. Cells have been removed from persons with hemophilia, genetically modified to produce factor VIII, and then reintroduced into the patient. The cells then began producing factor VIII. Gene therapy will not affect the inheritance of the defective gene.

VIII. **Web Sites**
   National Hemophilia Foundation
   1-800-424-2634
   http://www.hemophilia.org

HEPATITIS INFECTIONS A, B, C, D, E, AND G

I. **Definition**
   A. Six heterogeneous viruses are known to cause inflammation of the liver as part of their clinical manifestations and are designated hepatitis A, B, C, D, E, and **G**. Although similar in some ways, the infections caused by each virus differ in etiology, and in some features related to epidemiology, immunology, clinical characteristics, pathology, prevention, and control.

II. **Etiology**
   A. Hepatotropic infections are caused by viruses identified by their respective letters. For example, hepatitis B infection is caused by the hepatitis B virus (HBV).

III. Characteristics

A. Children often have few acute clinical symptoms.

B. Generally an insidious onset, except for type A (see Chapter 3 for further information on hepatitis A virus [HAV]).

C. Prodromal phase includes various combinations of slight or no fever; fatigue; malaise; anorexia; nausea; headache; vomiting; abdominal discomfort; myalgia (tenderness or pain in muscles); coryza (head cold); arthralgias (joint pain); rash; dark urine; and clay-colored stools approximately 1-5 days before jaundice.

D. Icteric phase (usually 1-2 weeks after onset of initial symptoms): jaundice; enlarged and tender liver; cervical adenopathy (swelling of lymph nodes in neck; pruritus may develop; other symptoms diminish).

E. Chronic stage: nonspecific symptoms of lethargy, malaise, fatigue, weight loss, abdominal pain, and enlarged liver.

IV. Health Concerns/Emergencies

A. Exposure to the virus during emergency care and clean-up during any bleeding episode is an immediate health concern.

B. Chronicity and ability to transmit virus to others.

C. Side effects or contraindications of medications.

V. Effects on Individual

A. Delayed or no identification of disease, since symptoms may be nonexistent, minimal, or confused with other causes of illness.

B. Feelings of guilt, shame, or need to place blame if contracted through drug abuse or sexual activity.

C. May have difficulty concentrating in class and diminished academic performance because of fatigue, general malaise, and arthralgia.

D. Loss of weight related to nausea, vomiting, and lack of appetite.

E. Self-conscious about appearance if rash and jaundice are noticeable.

F. Fear of living with a chronic disease, cirrhosis, liver cancer, or death.

VI. Management/Treatment

A. Treat symptomatically.

B. Allow student to return to school after acute clinical symptoms have subsided.

C. Contact local/state health department to determine action needed for health care and education of student, family, school staff, and other contacts.

D. Refer close contacts to their primary HCP for information regarding passive immunization with IG and hepatitis B immunoglobulin (HBIG) as soon as possible, preferably within 24 hours of exposure.

E. Teach student procedure for control of bleeding and clean-up of any body fluids so that they can assume control of their individual bodily needs.

F. Inform school staff (e.g., direct care providers, custodians, and bus transportation personnel), of any necessary cleaning or precautions.

G. The Occupational Safety and Health Administration (OSHA) requires annual training on bloodborne pathogens and an exposure control plan at each school site. See individual district/county or school site policy manual.

Table 4-7 Hepatotropic Viruses and Clinical Data

Virus	Hepatitis A Virus	Hepatitis B Virus	Hepatitis C Virus	Hepatitis D Virus	Hepatitis E Virus	Hepatitis G Virus
Incubation	15-50 days	45-160 (average: 60-120 days)	7-9 wk	2-4 mo	40 days	Unknown
Fecal-oral transmission	Common	No	No	No	Common	No
Percutaneous transmission	Rare	Common	Common	Common	No	Common
Sexual transmission	Rare	Common	Rare	Rare	Rare	Rare
Transplacental transmission	No	Common	Rare	No	Unknown	Rare
				Occurs as co-infection with HBV		
Chronic infection	No	Yes	Yes	Yes	No	Yes
Prophylactic	IVIG may be effective	HBIG effective	No	No	No	No
Vaccine	Yes	Yes	None	HVB vaccine prevents HDV	None	None
Rash	Rare	Common	Occasional	Similar to HBV	None	—
Jaundice	Occasional	Common	Common	Similar to HBV	Common	—
Fever	Common	Uncommon	Uncommon	Similar to HBV	Common	—
Dark urine, clay-colored stool	—	Common	—	Similar to HBV	Common	—
Joint pain	Rare	Common	Rare	Similar to HBV	—	—
Prodromal phase	Rare	Yes	Yes	Similar to HBV	—	—
Icteric phase	Yes	Yes	Yes	Similar to HBV	—	—
Mortality	Rare	Yes	Rare	Highest	Yes (pregnant women)	Rare

HBIG, Hepatitis B immunoglobulin; IVIG, intravenous immunoglobulin.

VII. Additional Information

A. Other viruses are known to cause hepatitis, including herpes simplex virus (HSV), CMV, varicella, rubella, HIV, Epstein-Barr virus (EBV), adenoviruses, enteroviruses, arboviruses, and parvovirus B19.

VIII. Web Sites

Nonprofit Organizations with Immunization and Hepatitis Resources
http://www.immunize.org/resources/noprofit.htm
Centers for Disease Control and Prevention (Viral Hepatitis)
http://www.cdc.gov/ncidod/diseases/hepatitis/index.htm
American Academy of Pediatrics
http://www.medem.com/MedLB/article_detaillb.cfm?article_ID=ZZZ9VB53R7C
&sub_cat=107
Centers for Disease Control: Protect Your Baby With Hepatitis B Shots
http://www.cdc.gov/ncidod/diseases/hepatitis/resource/hepbbaby.htm
Teenhealth: Hepatitis B
http://www.kidshealth.org/teen/infections/stds/std_hepatitis.html
National Foundation for Infectious Diseases, National Coalition for Adult Immunization: What every teen should know about Hepatitis B.
http://www.nfid.org/factsheets/hbagadol.html

HERPES SIMPLEX INFECTION TYPE 1

I. Definition

A. One of a group of acute infections occurring as a primary infection or recurring because of reactivation of a latent virus. *Herpes simplex virus type 1 (HSV-1)* usually is acquired in childhood and generally involves the oral cavity, lips, and face; also called a *cold sore* or *fever blister* when on the lips. HSV types 1 and 2 can overlap, and both types can reactivate throughout life.

II. Etiology

A. The infection is caused by human herpesvirus 1. Eye and digital herpetic infections generally are caused by HSV-1.

III. Characteristics

A. *Incubation period is 2 to 12 days after exposure. Period of communicability for HSV-1 is unknown but appears to be about 1 week.*

B. *Transmission is by infected oral secretions, by direct contact with infected genital secretions, and during both primary and recurring infections. Carriers can transmit the virus even though asymptomatic.*

1. Reactivation occurs after nonspecific internal or external disruptions to individual's system (e.g., cold, heat, stress).
2. It is a self-limiting infection.
3. It is usually acquired before age 5.
4. Complaints of pain, tingling, or burning in oral mucous membranes.
5. Starts as blisters, then changes to small spots with ulcerated centers surrounded by redness.
6. Primary infection may be found on gums, inner lips, cheeks, and tongue; reactivated infections usually involve lips and surrounding area.

    7. Usually accompanied by fever, hence the term *fever blister.*
    8. Infection may occur in other body areas (e.g., fingers, eyes, genitals).
    9. Activated by fever, menstruation, trauma, sunlight, tension, or physical and emotional stress.

IV. Health Concerns/Emergencies

  A. HSV-1 may infect the eye and cause herpetic keratitis, which is a significant cause of blindness. The inflammation results in a sensation of something in the eye, pain, sensitivity to light, and discharge. Without prompt treatment, the eye may be scarred.

  B. HSV-1 also can cause herpetic encephalitis, which affects the orbital portion of the frontal lobe and most commonly the temporal lobe. Severe and extensive disease may occur in immunosuppressed individuals, but it occurs primarily in infants.

V. Effects on Individual

  A. Self-conscious about facial lesions and may be teased about sores.

  B. Painful lesions may interfere with eating.

  C. Risk of decreased vision or blindness if lesion is in or around the eye.

VI. Management/Treatment

  A. Initial action varies greatly, depending on student's age, site of lesion, and circumstances.

  B. Good handwashing technique by staff and students.

  C. Use gloves when applying medicated ointment to any area.

  D. Isolate infected individual from newborns and those with eczema, burns, or compromised immune systems.

  E. Do not:
    1. Use sunscreen if sun is trigger factor; do not use sunscreen if lesions are present.
    2. Use common eating utensils when lesions are active.

  F. Avoid contact sports (e.g., wrestling) when there is a possibility of direct exposure with open active lesion (not transmitted through mats).

  G. Acyclovir (Zovirax) might be helpful during primary infection but is not necessary during reactivation. In primary infections and with immunocompromised individuals, as well as some particular individuals, medication can lessen the frequency of outbreaks and the severity of symptoms. Other medications include famciclovir (Famvir) and valacyclovir (Valtrex).

  H. Isolate towels, toys, and other items from others, and thoroughly clean and disinfect the articles if infant or toddler is in early intervention program or preschool.

  I. Children who have open blisters, mouth sores, or mouth toys that other children have access to should be excluded from school and cannot return until lesions are dry.

  J. Each exclusion should be evaluated on an individual basis (e.g., student's age, activity level, and circumstances).

HERPES SIMPLEX INFECTION TYPE 2

I. **Definition**
  A. One of a group of acute infections occurring as a primary infection or recurring because of reactivation of a latent virus. *HSV type 2 (HSV-2) infection is primarily found in the perineal and rectal area and is usually congenital or sexually acquired.* HSV types 1 and 2 can overlap, and both types can reactivate throughout life.

II. **Etiology**
  A. The infection is caused by human herpesvirus 2, which is a double-stranded DNA virus.

III. **Characteristics**
  A. *Incubation period for the primary infection is 2 to 20 days after exposure.*
  B. *Period of communicability is unknown but appears to be about 1 week.*
  C. *Transmission is by infected oral secretions, by direct contact with infected genital secretions, and during both primary and recurring infections. Carriers can transmit the virus even though asymptomatic.*
  D. Reactivation occurs after nonspecific internal or external disruptions to an individual's system (e.g., cold, heat, stress).
  E. It is a self-limiting infection.
  F. Primary infection begins with burning or tingling sensation.
  G. Painful lesions, which erupt and develop into fluid-filled blisters that spontaneously resolve or rupture and form shallow painful ulcers, which then scab and heal.
  H. In males, thin-walled blisters are usually located on the glans, prepuce, and shaft of the penis or on the anus; in females, lesions are usually located on the vulva, cervix, vagina, anus, or buttocks, and edema may be present.
  I. Burning sensation during urination, dysuria, and hesitancy during voiding.
  J. Lymph nodes in groin area may swell and become tender.
  K. Aching muscles.
  L. Fever, malaise, headache, and nausea are systemic symptoms.
  M. Initial infection may last 14 to 28 days.
  N. Women tend to have more discomfort than men, but infection of vagina or cervix does not always cause noticeable symptoms; cervix not sensitive to pain.
  O. Activated by menstruation, heat, systemic infection, emotional stress, fatigue, and pregnancy.

IV. **Health Concerns/Emergencies**
  A. HSV-2 complications include disseminated infections, encephalitis, pneumonia, and hepatitis.
  B. Predisposes woman to cervical cancer.
  C. Pregnant adolescent may transmit virus prenatally, perinatally, and postnatally; may result in CNS damage, disseminating encephalitis, resulting in death, risk of spontaneous abortion, or premature delivery.

V. Effects on Individual

A. May have localized pain and systemic symptoms, causing school absenteeism.

B. If sexually active, may be embarrassed to tell partner about sexually transmitted disease (STD).

C. May feel it is punishment for having sex.

D. If pregnant, individual has increased risk of premature delivery, spontaneous abortion; may affect newborn.

VI. Management/Treatment

A. Initial action varies greatly, depending on student's age, site of lesion, and circumstances.

B. Good handwashing technique by staff and students.

C. Isolate infected individual from newborns and those with eczema, burns, or compromised immune systems.

D. Use gloves when applying medicated ointment to any area.

E. Recurrent herpes can have viral shedding up to 4 to 5 days.

F. Lesion can be present for 7 to 10 days.

G. Acyclovir (Zovirax) might be helpful during primary infection but not necessary during reactivation. In primary infections and with immunocompromised individuals, as well as some particular individuals, medication can lessen the frequency of outbreaks and the severity of symptoms. Other medications include famciclovir (Famvir) and valacyclovir (Valtrex).

H. Younger child or developmentally delayed individual may have to be isolated.

I. Isolate towels, toys, and other items, and clean and disinfect thoroughly.

J. Exclude children from school who have open blisters, mouth sores, or who mouth toys that other children may use. If excluded, student cannot return to school until lesions are dry.

K. Each exclusion situation must be evaluated on individual basis (e.g., student's age, activity level, and circumstances).

HUMAN IMMUNODEFICIENCY VIRUS/ACQUIRED IMMUNODEFICIENCY SYNDROME

I. Definition

A. A deadly viral disease that leads to the destruction of the immune system by disabling and killing CD4$^+$ T-cells. Children under 13 years of age with acquired immunodeficiency syndrome (AIDS) are defined as having *pediatric AIDS*. Adolescents are classified as adults.

B. There are three sequential steps of development:

1. Stage I: A rapid viral replication occurs immediately after exposure. During this acute phase, high levels of plasma HIV ribonucleic acid (RNA) can be documented. Most people develop detectable antibodies within 30 to 50 days.

2. Stage II: A continuum from initial, asymptomatic/symptomatic HIV infection to AIDS diagnosis. Includes progressive damage to

the immune system. Referred to as *HIV disease* or *HIV/AIDS.* Asymptomatic HIV infection can last 10 years or more, making the individual unaware that he or she is infected.

   3. Stage III: Most severe manifestation of HIV disease, as evidenced by opportunistic infections and neoplasms of various organ systems, including the brain. Final clinical stage referred to as *AIDS.*

  C. The Centers for Disease Control and Prevention (CDC) continually clarify the definition and diagnostic criteria for HIV/AIDS (CDC, 2001).

II. Etiology

  A. HIV is a lentivirus from the subfamily of human retroviruses with two known serotypes: type 1 (HIV-1) and type 2 (HIV-2). *HIV-1* occurs in North and South America, Europe, sub-Saharan Africa and most other countries. *HIV-2* is serologically different from HIV-1. It occurs primarily in West Africa. Disease progression is slower than with HIV-1, but severe immunodeficiency can occur.

  B. HIV-2 is a rare cause of infection in children. It is most prevalent in western and southern Africa. HIV-2 infection is more difficult because the standard antibody assays are HIV-1-specific and may give indeterminate results in persons with HIV-2 infection.

III. Characteristics

  A. Three primary modes of transmission: sexual contact, exposure to blood, and perinatal transmission.

   1. Sexual contact:

    a. Unprotected sexual contact is the leading cause in the United States. It can occur during protected sexual contact with an infected person.

    b. Epidemiological studies support the correlation of advanced disease stage with increased likelihood of transmission to sexual partner(s).

    c. Semen and cervical secretions are implicated in transmission.

   2. Exposure to blood:

    a. Primary exposure is through injection drug use from sharing of needles or syringes.

    b. Transmission through blood transfusion or blood clotting factors is rare. Screening of the blood supply for HIV-1 was initiated in 1985; blood testing for HIV-2 began in 1992.

    c. Risk of HIV transmission through transfusion of screened blood has currently been estimated to be 1 in 200,000 to 1 in 2,000,000 per unit transfused in the United States.

    d. Transfusion of contaminated blood or blood factors accounts for 3% to 6% of all pediatric AIDS cases.

   3. Perinatal transmission:

    a. Vertical transmission of HIV from an infected woman to her infant can occur during gestation (in utero), at the time of delivery (intrapartum), or postpartum through breast-feeding.

  B. Other modes of transmission:

   1. Casual contact: Studies have examined the risk of transmission through casual contact by evaluating more than 1000 nonsexual

household contacts of both adults and children with HIV infection with no reported transmissions.

2. Saliva: HIV in saliva of infected persons has been found in very low concentrations. Therefore the probability of HIV-infected persons transmitting HIV through contact with saliva, either orally or genitally, is low but real. However, laboratory and epidemiological studies indicate extremely low-risk infectivity from saliva of infected persons through human bites. Multiple studies of household contacts have found no evidence of transmission through a human bite.

3. Pleural, cerebrospinal, synovial, peritoneal, pericardial, and amniotic fluid are potentially infectious. Also found in tears and sweat, but not to a level of infectivity.

C. Symptomatic HIV infection:

1. Acute syndrome occurs in 30% to 60% of individuals with primary HIV infection manifested by fever, malaise, lymphadenopathy, pharyngitis, headache, myalgia, and sometimes rash (CDC, 2001).

2. Persistent generalized lymphadenopathy; chronic lymph node enlargement.

3. Weight loss; caused by altered metabolism, poor absorption of nutrients, and decreased food intake.

4. Oral candidiasis; white patches on mucous membranes of the mouth or throat.

5. Oral hairy leukoplakia; painless, white, corrugated lesions appear on lateral surface of tongue but may spread; caused by EBV.

6. Vaginal candidiasis.

7. Diarrhea; two unformed stools daily for at least 30 days.

8. Fever; low-grade and intermittent.

9. Profound fatigue.

10. Disease in infants and children usually progresses faster because of the immaturity of the immune system; clinical manifestations unique to this group are failure to thrive, developmental delay, recurrent bacterial infections, lymphoid interstitial pneumonitis (LIP), parotitis, and recurrent fungal infections of the diaper area.

11. A small number of individuals do not manifest progression of the disease for a decade or more.

D. AIDS-defining symptoms:

1. *Pneumocystis carinii* pneumonia (PCP); most common life-threatening infection.

2. Cryptosporidiosis; a GI disease caused by a protozoan.

3. Toxoplasmosis; common parasitic infection and is major cause of AIDS encephalitis.

4. Esophageal candidiasis; a fungal infection.

5. Tuberculosis.

6. CMV.

7. Histoplasmosis; fungal infection manifested as pulmonary/lymph gland infection.

8. Cryptococcosis; a yeastlike fungus with lungs as the primary site of infection; may spread to meninges or CNS.
9. Kaposi's sarcoma (KS); can affect skin, mucous membranes, and/or internal organs.
10. Coccidioidomycosis; pulmonary infection caused by a fungus.
11. Disseminated *Mycobacterium avium-intracellulare* complex; caused by a bacterium.
12. Lymphomas.
13. Invasive cervical cancer.
14. HIV encephalopathy; often called *AIDS dementia complex (ADC)*.

IV. **Health Concerns/Emergencies**
    A. Conditions and functional level varies according to opportunistic infection involved.
    B. Remind staff of special precautions to prevent exposure to communicable disease. OSHA regulations and universal precautions should be in place and followed in all classrooms and throughout the school.
    C. Viral infections pose significant problems.
       1. Respiratory viruses may have prolonged symptoms. Most children will experience at least one episode of pneumonia. Recurrent ear and sinus infections are common.
       2. Chickenpox and measles are particularly significant to the individual with AIDS. Measles may occur despite immunization and may present without the typical rash. Student should be excluded temporarily during an outbreak; 3 weeks for chickenpox and 2 weeks for measles. Notify parent and health practitioner immediately if exposure occurs for administration of varicella-zoster immunoglobulin (VZIG) within 72 hours of exposure to chickenpox.
       3. Live virus vaccine immunizations are contraindicated. Most other vaccines are administered according to the American Academy of Pediatrics (AAP) or individual state guidelines. CDC recommends annual pneumococcal and influenza vaccines.
    D. GI problems are common, such as chronic or recurrent diarrhea with malabsorption, abdominal pain, dysphagia (difficulty swallowing), and failure to thrive.
    E. Be alert to and knowledgeable of signs and symptoms of illness, deterioration of condition, and side effects of medication.
       1. Skin eruptions may appear as an allergic reaction to drugs, especially if they are on sulfonamides.
       2. Student with HIV/AIDS should not be in school if there are weeping lesions or skin eruptions cannot be covered.
       3. Anemia caused by the chronic infection or as a side effect of drugs, so the child may appear disinterested, tire easily, or require periods of rest.
    F. CNS involvement in perinatally-infected children is 40% to 90%. Seizure activity is not common and usually indicates an additional pathological process, such as a tumor or other opportunistic infections.
    G. Elevated blood pressure may indicate renal disease.

H. If CNS involvement, seizure activity may occur, requiring assessment and communication with parent and HCP.

V. **Effects on Individual**

A. May feel various degrees of anxiety regarding condition and future.

B. May exhibit depression and social withdrawal.

C. Social contacts may be limited, and harmony with family may become disrupted.

D. May feel stress over the secretive nature of the disease or may feel guilt over exposing others to illness.

E. Fear of pain and death may be constant concern. HIV encephalopathy in a child infected perinatally may result in speech and language delays, cerebral palsy–like motor impairment, visual and auditory short-term memory problems, attention deficits, and compromised cognitive functioning.

F. Elevated blood pressure may indicate renal disease.

G. Sleep disturbances are common and may affect social, school, and family life.

H. Individual may be living with a parent or other family members with HIV infection or AIDS.

I. Frequent illness, neurological complications, medication, and treatment may negatively affect academic achievement.

VI. **Management/Treatment**

A. Care is supportive and depends on manifestations of virus.

B. Confidentiality is an ongoing concern; review school, county and/or state/federal policy and law.

NOTE: In some states (e.g., Illinois), the State Department of Health Services or the local health authority must notify the site principal within 3 days if a student with HIV/AIDS attends that school. They may disclose the information to the nurse, teacher, and others as needed. In other states (e.g., California), it is a misdemeanor to reveal the HIV status of an individual without written consent. Many states require written permission for disclosure of HIV status.

C. Maintain consistent communication regarding condition and recommendations of HCP.

D. Be available for dialogue and support with student and parent(s).

E. Maintain annual OSHA standard precautions and blood-borne pathogen inservice for all school staff, including transportation personnel and custodians.

F. Monitor pulmonary status, since majority of children with HIV disease develop lung disease.

1. Acute onset of respiratory symptoms requires immediate evaluation because it can progress to an emergency situation within hours.

2. Watch for episodes of gasping, deep inhalations or sighing, and prolonged coughing because they may indicate difficulty breathing, which may indicate impending respiratory distress.

G. Periodic hearing screening including impedance, since otitis media is one of the most common recurrent conditions.

H. Adequate nutrition is a concern; no special diet is needed, but a lactose-free diet may be beneficial for some.

I. Periodic dental screening; dental caries are a focus of infection and can become systemic. Fluoride and dental sealant may be helpful.

J. Live vaccines are generally contraindicated. Most vaccines are administered according to AAP or individual state guidelines. CDC recommends annual pneumococcal and influenza vaccines.

K. There are over 20 medications used, with the most common side effects listed as nausea, vomiting, fever, rash, anorexia, diarrhea, abdominal pain, and fatigue.

L. Adolescents may resist adherence to treatment protocol out of distrust of the medical system, lack of belief in medication, avoidance of side effects, or lack of understanding the need for medication when asymptomatic. When aware of an adolescent with an HIV/AIDS diagnosis, encourage medication compliance while discussing feelings and reactions of disease and process.

M. Review need for special education assessment because HIV encephalopathy in a perinatally infected child may result in speech and language delays, cerebral palsy–like motor impairment, visual and auditory short-term memory difficulties, attention deficits, and compromised cognitive functioning.

N. In adolescents with a fully developed nervous system, the neurological impact is not as pronounced and the deficits occur at a much slower rate.

O. Participation in sports should follow these general guidelines:
1. Participation should be determined by the ability of the individual to maintain the level of activity required.
2. All coaching staff should practice standard precautions for all participants during all sports activities, not only for sports at high risk for bleeding injuries (such as wrestling or football).
3. If a minor injury results in a laceration or puncture wound that bleeds or an abrasion that oozes fluid or blood, participation should be limited or discontinued if the wound cannot be covered adequately to prevent any fluid contact with another participant.

VII. **Additional Information**

A. Transmission to an infant born to an infected mother may occur in utero, during delivery by exposure to blood and vaginal secretions, or postpartum through infected breast milk. Administration of zidovudine (AZT) during pregnancy, labor, and to the newborn has resulted in reduction of perinatal infection rates from 25% to 8% (Stiehm et al, 1999). Recently developed techniques can diagnose HIV infections in most infants at 1 to 3 months of age.

B. No one has been identified as infected with HIV because of contact with environmental surfaces. HIV does not survive well in the environment, and HIV is not able to reproduce outside a living host. There are no reported cases of transmission in day care or school settings (Courville et al, 1998) or while participating in sports (CDC, 1998).

C. CDC recommends *HIV testing* for those at risk. Most people develop detectable antibodies within 3 months, with the average time being 25 days; however, it can take up to 6 months in rare cases. Therefore

CDC currently recommends testing 6 months after last exposure. In practice, most people are tested at 3 months. Enzyme immunoassay (EIA) is the most commonly used HIV antibody screening test; results are known in 1 to 2 weeks. A more expensive, rapid test has been approved by the FDA and is used in some settings. Results are available in 5 to 30 minutes. Both tests should be used in conjunction with a confirmatory test, such as the Western blot, before a diagnosis of infection is given. Testing is usually based on a sliding-fee scale, or the fee is waived in many cases.

D. Be aware of students who bite, scratch, or have self-abusive behavior that can potentiate transmission of the virus. CDC reports HIV transmission with severe trauma, extensive tissue tearing and damage, and presence of blood. Biting is not a common way of transmitting HIV infection (CDC, 2001).

E. Medications are usually given in combinations rather than as monotherapy to avoid developing drug resistance observed in some children taking only one drug. They delay progression of the disease, contribute to weight gain, diminish the effects of encephalopathy, and improve the immune system.

F. There are 3 classes of antiretroviral drugs:
  1. Protease inhibitors.
  2. Nucleoside reverse transcriptase inhibitors.
  3. Nonnucleoside reverse transcriptase inhibitors.

G. Combinations of drugs have been developed so that one pill can be given rather than many.

VIII. **Web Sites**
  Centers for Disease Control: HIV/AIDS
  http://www.cdc.gov/hiv
  CDC National AIDS Hotline (NAH)
  1-800-342-AIDS or 1-800-344-7432 in Spanish. Operated by trained information specialists 24 hours a day, 7 days a week.

HYDROCEPHALUS

I. **Definition**
  A. Hydrocephalus is a condition characterized by an imbalance in circulation, production, and absorption of cerebrospinal fluid (CSF) in the body, causing an abnormal increase of CSF within the intracranial cavities, leading to enlarged ventricles. The condition is often associated with myelomeningocele.

II. **Etiology**
  A. Hydrocephalus is usually caused by an obstruction in the normal circulation of CSF. The condition may be congenital or acquired by trauma, meningitis, neoplasms, or intracranial bleeding.
  B. In *nonobstructive* or *communicating hydrocephalus,* CSF passes freely between the ventricles and the subarachnoid space but is blocked from being absorbed into the subarachnoid space. The condition may result from spina bifida occulta, trauma, meningitis, or subarachnoid hemorrhage in premature infants. It may also be caused

by a prenatal maternal infection, such as toxoplasmosis, cytomegalic inclusion disease, or mumps.

C. In *obstructive* or *noncommunicating hydrocephalus,* CSF is blocked from leaving ventricles and entering the subarachnoid space. This may occur from congenital defects (e.g., Arnold-Chiari malformation), tumors, trauma, or prenatal maternal infections. The most common cause of obstruction is congenital stenosis of the aqueduct of Sylvius.

III. **Characteristics**

A. Manifestations depend on the child's age, whether fontanels have closed and cranial sutures have fused, and type and duration of hydrocephalus.

B. Symptoms develop slowly or very suddenly.

C. In infants, symptoms are:
   1. Abnormal increase in head size.
   2. Bulging fontanels or delayed closure.
   3. Intracranial pressure signs (listless and irritable, vomiting, loss of appetite, high-pitched shrill cry, change in vital signs, decreased pulse, decreased and irregular respirations, increased systolic blood pressure, coma).
   4. Motor function becomes impaired as head enlarges.
   5. Hyperactive reflexes.
   6. Spasticity of extremities.
   7. Forehead may become prominent.
   8. Scalp appears shiny, and scalp veins become prominent (transilluminated head).
   9. Increased visibility of sclera and iris (setting sun appearance).
   10. Impaired upgaze and other extraocular movements.

D. Children with closed sutures display symptoms indicative of increased intracranial pressure (ICP):
   1. Headache on awakening, which improves when sitting up or after vomiting.
   2. Papilledema.
   3. Lethargy, fatigue.
   4. Ataxia.
   5. Strabismus or pupillary changes.
   6. Separation of cranial sutures may be seen up to 10 years of age.
   7. Personality change.
   8. Change in vital signs similar to those seen in infants.
   9. Coma.

IV. **Health Concerns/Emergencies**

A. If no medical intervention, hydrocephalus causes brain damage and possible death.

B. Main health concerns center around proper function of shunt:
   1. Shunt infection; whenever child ill or running temperature, physician should be consulted.
   2. Malfunction of a shunt may occur; chronic or acute symptoms include:
      a. Vomiting.
      b. Irritability.

      c. Fever.

      d. Headache.

      e. Change in behavior.

   3. Holding infant in head-down position interferes with CSF flow.

   4. Increased risk of head injury because of poor head control.

   5. Precocious puberty, short stature, amenorrhea may occur secondary to endocrine dysfunction.

   6. Incidence of migraine headaches is twice that of peers. Risk of other headaches is three times greater than that of peers.

V. Effects on Individual

  A. There may be no obvious motor or educational problems.

  B. Brain damage may be present, resulting in motor (60%), language, perceptual, and/or intellectual disabilities. Verbal IQ is usually higher than performance and full-scale IQ.

  C. Memory functioning and reasoning skills may be affected.

  D. Areas frequently affected are math, reading, comprehension, and writing skills.

  E. Child may talk incessantly with meaningless chatter or be echolalic.

  F. Visual problems are common, including strabismus, optic atrophy, and decreased acuity.

  G. Hypersensitivity to noise.

  H. Problems with balance and spatial awareness affect performance in PE and on the playground.

  I. Low energy levels.

  J. Physical and social activities can be limited by parents' overprotection.

  K. Other children may laugh or make fun of individual's oversized head or ataxic gait, creating difficulties with peer relations and self-esteem.

  L. Limited intellect may affect ability to adequately deal with precocious puberty.

  M. Seizures may develop.

VI. Management/Treatment

  A. Monitor shunt functioning and refer if signs of ICP or infection are observed.

  B. Measure head circumference until sutures are fused; frequent, sometimes daily.

  C. Be alert to signs of complications that may cause pressure on the tubing in the peritoneal cavity (e.g., constipation, pregnancy).

  D. Screen vision annually.

  E. Provide early developmental screening for infants and toddlers.

  F. Wear helmet during activities with risk of falling (e.g., bicycling).

  G. Consider restriction of high-impact contact sports (e.g., football, wrestling, ice hockey).

  H. Encourage independence and taking responsibility. Emphasize optimistic prognosis.

  I. Support parents and provide information as they face the fear associated with multiple procedures and surgeries involving the brain.

  J. Note that medical treatment is primarily surgical: removal of obstruction, ventriculoperitoneal (VP) shunt, or ventriculoatrial (VA) shunt; rarely, medication is given to reduce production of CSF.

    K. Use of serial lumbar punctures are sometimes successful in premature infants to prevent need for a shunt.

VII. Additional Information

    A. Hydrocephalus can be detected in utero as early as 14 weeks. Although shunting can be done in utero, postnatal shunting is more successful.

    B. With a VP shunt, a radiopaque ventricular catheter is inserted into the ventricle and connected to a one-way valve that is threaded under the skin to the abdominal cavity. This procedure enables CSF to flow out of the brain into the peritoneal cavity and be absorbed by the blood vessels surrounding those organs. In a VA shunt, the tube is inserted into the heart instead of the peritoneal cavity. This procedure is only performed if abdominal problems prevent insertion of the VP shunt. Advances in neuroendoscopy and development of techniques make this surgery less invasive and more accurate in placement of shunts.

    C. Tubing is coiled in the peritoneum to allow for growth. The distal portion may need to be replaced in toddlerhood and before the adolescent growth spurt. If the shunt becomes unnecessary, it is usually left in place unless it becomes infected.

    D. New treatments are being developed. Third ventriculostomy is a new procedure done under general anesthesia by making a small hole in the third ventricle, which creates a natural opening for CSF to flow into the subarachnoid space. Recovery time is 1 or 2 days; occasionally the surgery is not successful and a traditional shunt will be placed. Medications to reduce production of CSF have been disappointing, but new medications are being researched.

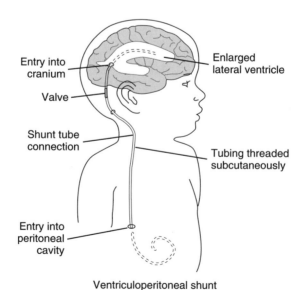

Ventriculoperitoneal shunt

FIGURE 4-6 Ventriculoperitoneal shunt.

VIII. **Web Sites**
   Hydrocephalus Association
   415-732-7040
   http://www.hydroassoc.org
   The Hydrocephalus Foundation, Inc.
   781-942-1161
   http://www.hydrocephalus.org

KLINEFELTER'S SYNDROME

   I. **Definition**
      A. Klinefelter's syndrome (KS) is a genetic disorder involving the sex chromosomes.
  II. **Etiology**
      A. Males with KS have one or more additional X chromosomes (usually only one extra X chromosome), described as 47 XXY rather than as 46 XY. KS is the most common single cause of hypogonadism and infertility. It affects approximately 1 in 500 to 1 in 1000 male births.
 III. **Characteristics**
      A. Has an extra female chromosome and atypically high levels of the female hormone.
      B. Spatial skills below the average male and may be about the same level as females.
      C. Lack of facial and body hair.
      D. Enlarged breasts, long limbs.
      E. Tendency to be taller than average and overweight.
      F. Mild elbow dysplasia.
      G. Fifth finger clinodactyly.
      H. Small penis and testes in childhood; continues into adulthood, where length of testes is 2.5 cm or less.
      I. Inadequate testosterone production, less than one half the normal.
      J. Usually infertile because of low sperm count; sexual dysfunction and impotence.
      K. At risk for autoimmune disorders.
      L. Wide range of IQ levels from low to above normal, mean full-scale IQ between 85 and 90, with performance IQ higher than verbal. IQ scores typically lower than those of siblings.
      M. Some are without noticeable learning problems in early school year, but these become more apparent as student progresses through school.
      N. Some may not speak before age 4 or 5.
      O. Problems with expressive language, auditory processing, and short-term auditory memory make reading and spelling difficult.
      P. May display immaturity, shyness, insecurity, poor judgment, and passivity.
      Q. Difficulty with peer relationships and psychosocial adjustments but no psychiatric difficulties.

IV. **Health Concerns/Emergencies**
   A. Risk of autoimmune disorders, such as thyroiditis, type 1 diabetes, breast cancer, and systemic lupus erythematosus (SLE).
   B. May need breast reduction because of gynecomastia (enlarged breast size).
   C. If not treated with testosterone, may have increased risk for developing osteoporosis.
   D. Poor gross motor coordination may affect balance and sports ability.

V. **Effects on Individual**
   A. May feel self-conscious and embarrassed when participating in gym class/showering.
   B. If lacking athletic ability, may become withdrawn and frustrated.
   C. Adolescents fatigue easily.
   D. The chromosomal abnormality may have an effect on the brain, producing a mild form of organic brain disorder.
   E. May have gender confusion because of gynecomastia, hypogenitals, and no or decreased body and facial hair.

VI. **Management/Treatment**
   A. May need special educational resources, especially for reading, spelling, and writing activities.
   B. May need adaptation for test taking (i.e., test verbally rather than in writing).
   C. May need social and emotional support.
   D. Provide education and ongoing support regarding disorder to student, parents, and staff.
   E. Testosterone injections and oral medication for delayed secondary sexual characteristics is available, but complete virilization is not usually achieved with oral replacement therapy.

VII. **Additional Information**
   A. There are other sex chromosomal variations (SCV) in which the cause is unclear but there is an abnormality in the egg or sperm cell. Individuals with SCVs have 47 chromosomes rather than the normal 46, with combinations XXX, XXY, or XYY. There is a mosaic condition in which manifestations are fewer, depending on the number of cells involved.

VIII. **Web Sites**
   Klinefelter's Syndrome and Associates
   http://www.genetic.org

LEAD POISONING

I. **Definition**
   A. Lead poisoning (plumbism) is caused by the absorption of lead or any of its salts into the body. It can be detected in blood, bones, and teeth; can interfere with CNS development; and can cause mental impairments such as cognitive disabilities and reading difficulties.
   B. It is a preventable, common, environmental and public health problem. Houses built before 1978 have internal and external surface ar-

eas painted with lead-based paint. Paint may chip, allowing children to eat or swallow chips or inhale lead-laden dust (ingestion or inhalation). Children of low-income families tend to have a higher rate of this condition. In 1991, CDC lowered the definition of plumbism blood lead levels to less than 10 μg/dl of whole blood and reported that significant adverse effects can occur even at this low level.

II. **Etiology**
A. Primary sources are lead-based paints and lead-contaminated dust found in interior and exterior paint (major source), drinking water, airborne dust, contaminated soil, folk remedies, cosmetics, and particular foods, and either exposure to or having hobbies known to include lead particles, such as ceramics and stained glass.
B. It is estimated that more than 12.8 million U.S. children born between 1972 and 1988 have blood lead levels in excess of 2.5 mg and have adverse affects from environmental lead exposure (Lanphear, 1998).

III. *Brain Findings*
A. Lead poisoning affects neurotransmitters and particular enzyme functions. It occurs when toxic effects interrupt hemoglobin formation and damage the nervous system.

IV. **Characteristics**
A. Often asymptomatic.
B. Mild-to-moderate exposure symptoms are nonspecific: abdominal discomfort, fatigue, anorexia, myalgias, headache, irritability, and paresthesias.
C. Continuous and high-level exposure symptoms:
   1. CNS: decreased hearing, lethargy, irritability, seizures, acute encephalopathy, coma (levels >100 μg/dl).
   2. GI: vomiting, constipation, and abdominal pain.
   3. Renal: hypertension, renal failure in affected adults.
D. Neurodevelopmental deficits in children: poor attention span and decreased school performance, behavior changes, cognitive deficits. Prenatally or postnatally lead-exposed children score lower on mental developmental scales. Severe prenatal exposure may cause congenital abnormalities.

V. **Health Concerns/Emergencies**
A. When individual is symptomatic, it is considered a medical emergency.
B. Children are at high risk because of considerable hand-to-mouth activity, pica behavior, and increased GI absorption of lead.
C. Anemia; iron deficiency accelerates lead absorption.
D. Young children absorb 50% to 60% of the lead they are exposed to, whereas adults only absorb 10%.

VI. **Effects on Individual**
A. Usually asymptomatic at low levels, which may be harmful.
B. May be pale secondary to anemia.
C. Can be irritable.
D. May have difficulty doing schoolwork.
E. May display cognitive deficits, learning disabilities, and behavior problems.

Table 4-8	*Blood Lead Measurements Recommendations*
Blood Levels	**Recommendations**
9 μg/dl	Not considered lead poisoning Retest according to universal protocol or if increased risk Treatment not required
10-14 μg/dl	6-35 mo of age: retest in 4 mo 37-72 mo of age: retest in 1 yr Conduct environmental investigation and provide remediation when needed Conduct nutritional assessment and correct any deficiencies Educate family/caregivers
15-19 μg/dl	Retest every 3-4 mo Provide medical evaluation, including nutritional status and correction of any deficiencies Conduct environmental assessment with remediation Educate family/caregivers Consider testing of other exposed children
20-44 μg/dl	Retest for confirmation Conduct environmental evaluation and remediation Complete medical examination, including nutritional status and correction of any deficiencies When blood level is 24-44 μg/dl, effectiveness of chelation treatment is not yet established Remove from lead source Educate family/caregivers Test other possibly exposed children
45-69 μg/dl	Complete medical evaluation and behavioral history; refer for chelation therapy Conduct nutritional assessment and correct deficiencies Conduct environmental assessment and remediation Remove from lead source
Greater than 70 μg/dl	Medical emergency; confirm immediately by retest Hospitalization recommended

Modified from National Centers for Disease Control and American Medical Association guidelines.

VII. **Management/Treatment**
   A. May display GI and neurological complaints in the nurse's office; teacher or staff may report learning difficulties (late sign).
   B. Rule out elevated blood lead levels if anemic, hyperactive, and/or has behavioral problems.
   C. Venous lead blood levels are the most accurate measurement of diagnosis. Fingersticks are adequate for screening.
   D. Chelating agents reduce the body's burden of lead. They may be given orally, intravenously, and intramuscularly, alone or in combination with other agents. Chelation therapy is necessary with all symptomatic exposures but cannot serve as a substitute for removing

the child from the source of exposure. Notable side effects of chelation therapy include transient transaminase elevations, GI upset, headaches, hypersensitivity reactions, renal damage, transient neutropenia, and mild conjunctivitis.

E. Be alert to environmental conditions of young child that can cause the disease, since they initially may be asymptomatic. Such conditions include children living or staying on a regular basis in a home, preschool, day care center, relative's/baby sitter's home built before 1978.

F. Radiography may indicate increased density (lead lines) of long bones.

G. Recommend routine screening between 1 and 2 years of age.

H. Educate parents, child care workers, and school staff about lead poisoning sources, symptoms, and complications and its learning and behavioral effects on children. Stress preventing or decreasing risk exposure (e.g., remodeling techniques, medicines for diarrhea from China and Mexico, glazed pottery from outside the United States). Encourage handwashing. Promote nutritious diet to decrease risk of anemia.

I. Notify public health officials; follow guidelines.

VIII. Web Sites

Centers for Disease Control and Prevention
http://www.cdc.gov/nceh/lead/lead.htm

MUSCULAR DYSTROPHY, DUCHENNE'S AND BECKER'S

I. Definition

A. Muscular dystrophies (MDs) are characterized by progressive degeneration of muscle cells that are replaced by fat and fibrous tissue. They are unrelated diseases, each transmitted by a different gene, each characterized by weakness and wasting of particular groups of skeletal muscles, and each differing in expression and clinical course. Duchenne's MD is the most common type and affects 1:3000 boys.

II. Etiology

A. Duchenne's MD *(pseudohypertrophic MD)* is inherited as an X-linked recessive trait. The X chromosome at the Xp21 locus carries the abnormal gene. The defective gene carried by the unaffected female affects all male offspring. Becker's MD is the same disease, but it follows a milder clinical course.

III. Characteristics

A. Infancy: may have no symptoms or manifest mild hypotonia and/or poor head control.

B. About age 2: mild hip girdle weakness and lordotic postures while standing may be observed.

C. Achieves developmental milestones at appropriate ages.

D. Walking on tiptoes is early sign.

E. Seems awkward and clumsy and has strange way of running.

F. By age 3, *Gowers' sign* may be observed. Child will get up from floor by "walking up" the legs with his or her hands.

G. Has difficulty ascending stairs and rising from squatting or sitting position on floor.
H. Age 5-6: Trendelenburg's gait or hip waddle appears.
I. Weakness progresses from lower to upper limbs.
J. Muscular enlargement because of fat replacing muscle.
K. Progression is rapid, with all voluntary muscles ultimately involved.
L. Calf enlargement is common because of wasting of thigh muscles *(pseudohypertrophy)*.
M. Can be confined to a wheelchair as early as 7 years of age. Most can walk up to age 10 but with increasing difficulty. Orthotic bracing, physiotherapy, and minor surgery (Achilles' tendon lengthening) can prolong ambulating up to age 12.
N. Often overweight or obese because of limited activity or wheel chair confinement.
O. Muscular atrophy, joint deformities, and contractures of the ankles, knees, hips, and elbows are common as disease progresses.
P. Scoliosis can develop because of trunk's muscle weakness and can be painful.
Q. Pharyngeal weakness can lead to nasal regurgitation of fluids, aspiration, and a nasal or airy voice quality.
R. Cardiomyopathy is noted.
S. Only 20% to 30% have an IQ less than 70. The majority have learning disabilities.
T. Mild mental retardation is common.
U. Life expectancy is around 18 years.

IV. **Health Concerns/Emergencies**
   A. URTIs are frequent because of weakness of respiratory muscles and resulting decrease in vital capacity.
   B. May show signs of cardiac failure because heart muscle has weakened.
   C. Osteoporosis.

V. **Effects on Individual**
   A. Choices and activities open to student are limited.
   B. Overprotective parent(s) may also restrict activities.
   C. Inappropriate behaviors may be condoned because of the parent(s)' sympathy or guilt.
   D. Health examinations and the knowledge that one is defective may generate feelings of shame and doubt.
   E. Social interaction with peers may be limited.
   F. May have to depend on others for help at school or social activities.
   G. As the disability progresses and becomes more severe, individual must face the uncertainty of the future.

VI. **Management/Treatment**
   A. Respiratory infections require prompt management and referral when indicated.
   B. Postural drainage may be necessary because of inability to cough and accumulation of secretions.
   C. Because of selective muscle involvement, contractures are common and physical therapy should be implemented; be aware of physical

therapy goals and instructions, proper positioning; work with physical therapist and assist family with range-of-motion exercises, stretching, or any suitable active exercises. Braces can help prevent contractures.

D. Muscles can atrophy if in bed for more than a few days (e.g., after surgery or from illness), and physical therapy or range-of-motion exercises needed to maintain muscle strength.

E. Surgery may correct lower limb deformities and prolong ability to stand erect and walk.

F. Education of family and student regarding proper dietary intake and needs may help to prevent and/or treat obesity.

G. Constipation can be a problem because of limited activity; increase in fluids and use of stool softeners can help.

H. As student becomes older, fatigue increases; teaching staff and others should be aware of possible need for rest period during school day and limited energy for learning.

I. Counseling can help individuals with MD deal with body changes and prognosis.

J. Boys with Becker's MD remain ambulatory until late adolescence or young adulthood. The onset of weakness is later, and learning disabilities are not as common. Life expectancy is mid-to-late 20s; less than half of the affected males are alive at age 40 but are severely disabled.

VII. **Additional Information**

A. MD is diagnosed by signs and symptoms: blood tests that show an elevated creatine phosphokinase (CPK) level, a muscle enzyme; electromyography (EMG); muscle biopsy; and echocardiography (ECG).

B. Other MDs include Emery-Dreifuss MD, myotonic MD; myotonic chondrodystrophy, myotonic congenita, limb-girdle MD, facioscapulohumeral MD, and congenital MD.

VIII. **Web Sites**

Muscular Dystrophy Association
http://www.mdausa.org
Parent Project Muscular Dystrophy
1-800-714-KIDS
http://www.parentdmd.org/

OBESITY

I. **Definition**

A. An increase in weight that is beyond the limitation of physical and skeletal requirement. For an adult, a body mass index (BMI) of 25 or higher is considered overweight and a BMI of above 30 is considered obese. For children 2 to 20 years old, the BMI classification has a broad range of healthy weights. For example, the child who reaches the ninety-fifth percentile is considered overweight and at risk. See Appendix A for BMI charts.

NOTE: BMI is a formula for determining overweight and underweight based on weight and height.

II. **Etiology**
   A. The results of excessive accumulation of fat in the body may occur in infancy, childhood, adolescence, or adulthood and may be caused by genetic susceptibility, hypothyroidism, overactivity of insulin secretion, hyperfunction of the adrenal cortex, hypofunction of the gonads, metabolic disorders, overeating, and/or inactivity. Rare mutations in the MC4-R gene account for 4% of extreme obesity (BMI greater than 40) cases (Vaisse, 2000).
      1. The primary (99%) cause of disordered eating is life situations or habits (e.g., demise of home cooking, increased television viewing, video games, and computers).
      2. Secondary (1%) causes include endocrine disorders (e.g., hypothyroidism, insulinemia, Cushing's syndrome, exogenous steroids, polycystic ovary syndrome, growth hormone deficiency, pseudohypoparathyroidism), CNS (e.g., after infections, trauma, tumor) and dysmorphic syndromes (e.g., Laurence-Moon-Biedel syndrome, Prader-Willi syndrome, Turner's syndrome).

III. *Brain Findings*
   A. In 1994 Dr. Jeffrey Friedman of Rockefeller University researchers discovered that mice lacking the hormone leptin have lower metabolism, eat more, and grow three times the weight of normal mice. This discovery led to the identification of numerous related molecules that form signaling pathways in the hypothalamus that help regulate appetite and energy expenditure in humans. Leptin helps the brain report on the state of the body's fat stores and may have aided mammalian evolution by preventing starvation.
   B. Research on mice is providing scientific understanding of key neurotransmitters that help govern eating. Discovery of one serotonic 2c receptor is very meaningful in regulating weight and is a target for serotonergic diet drugs (Norris, 2000).

IV. **Characteristics**
   A. Behaviors of eating more food, larger portions, and exercising less.
   B. Consumption of more processed foods and simple carbohydrates with associated increased obesity and incidence of diabetes.
   C. Excessive television viewing, computer use, and snacking.
   D. Eating fast food and junk food frequently.

V. **Health Concerns/Emergencies**
   A. Obese people are more likely to contract acute and chronic medical conditions such as diabetes, gallbladder disease, respiratory disease, and hypertension; they are at risk for arteriosclerosis, several types of cancer, gout, and arthritis, and in women, urinary incontinence and infertility.
   B. Obesity is the leading cause of sustained hypertension in children and adolescents.
   C. Some overweight children exhibit sleep apnea and fatty liver, which is a precursor to cirrhosis, type 2 diabetes, and elevated cholesterol.
   D. In diabetics, the inability to process glucose normally may cause damage to blood vessels, nerves, kidneys, and heart, which increases risk of death from heart attack, stroke, and kidney failure.

E. Obesity contributes to arthritis and back and foot pain.

F. If stressed and made to feel ashamed, obese individuals may develop dangerous eating disorders.

VI. **Effects on Individual**

A. Negative effect on social, emotional, and physical development and self-esteem.

B. Heavy adolescents tend to be heavy adults.

C. Orthopedic difficulties such as bowing of the tibia and a slipped femoral capital epiphysis (bone slippage at the head of the femur), which causes loss of range of motion, may manifest as knee pain.

D. More likely to experience aches and pains and impaired ability to perform daily tasks and exercise.

E. Experience educational, social, and economic disadvantages as obese adolescents and adults.

VII. **Management/Treatment**

A. Complete physical assessment.

B. Assessment of weight and height.

C. Complete history, including eating and activity patterns (television viewing, electronic games), emotional and social contributors (e.g., new in neighborhood, no friends, divorced family unit and missing one parent, depressed, having difficulty in school). Separate out possible factors to plan management strategies.

D. Discuss with parent(s). Success is usually related to parental involvement.

E. Focus on health not on appearance, on increased activity not on less food.

F. Form peer support group at school.

VIII. **Additional Information**

A. Many schools have reduced or eliminated physical education classes in an attempt to increase academic classes, which tend to be sedentary. This change may contribute to lack of exercise and weight gain. "Latch key" children and those living in families who fear violence or live in an unsafe neighborhood watch an inordinate amount of television, which also contributes to decreased exercise and increased weight. The greatest amount of advertising during children's television programming is for food products, which are usually high in salt, sugar, and fat.

Box 4-8	*Risk Factors for Obesity*

1. BMI above 30.
2. Weight for height above the eighty-fifth percentile.
3. Rate of weight gain exceeds rate of growth after age 3.
4. At least one obese parent.
5. Five or more hours of television viewing per day.

IX. **Web Sites**
 American Obesity Association
 1-800-986-2373
 http://www.obesity.org
 Child Obesity Resources for Health Professionals, Educators, and Families
 http://www.childobesity.com

SCOLIOSIS

I. **Definition**
 A. Scoliosis is an abnormal lateral deviation in the spine. It may or may not include deformity or rotation of the vertebrae. Idiopathic scoliosis results in a fixed rotation of the spine and is commonly observed and tested for in the school setting. It occurs more often in females than males. It usually develops during periods of active growth (10 to 16 years).
II. **Etiology**
 A. Because this particular type of scoliosis occurs without known cause, the term *idiopathic* is used. It is the most common type and typically occurs in the growth spurts of adolescence. There may be a genetic origin, and if a family history is noted, the risk is 7 times greater. See "Additional Information" for other classifications.
III. **Characteristics**
 A. Develops slowly.
 B. Usually painless; if there is pain, possible tumor or infection is indicated.
 C. Often not observed at home because individuals dress themselves and have developed feelings of modesty.
 D. Uncorrected torticollis or plagiocephaly (malformation of skull) may lead to scoliosis, monitor closely.
 E. Signs noted during screening procedure for scoliosis:
  1. Shoulder unequally elevated.
  2. Scapula prominence.
  3. Scapula elevation.
  4. Unilateral fullness of waist or extra folds.
  5. Iliac crest elevation.
  6. Lumbar or thoracic prominence while bending over (hump), but right thoracic is more common.
  7. Unequal rib prominence.
  8. Tufts of hair patches, dimple(s), skin discoloration at lower end of spine.
IV. **Health Concerns/Emergencies**
 A. Moderate to severe curvature, greater than 50 degrees, involving thoracic spine reduces efficiency of heart and lungs by creating chest deformity.
 B. Back pain seems to increase in adults.
 C. If individual is confined to wheelchair, neuromuscular scoliosis will prevent person from sitting upright without using hands to stabilize

torso; pressure sores can eventually develop from unequal pressure on buttocks.

V. **Effects on Individual**
   A. May feel self-conscious and develop problems of low self-esteem and self-worth.
   B. Bracing can be extremely uncomfortable.
   C. After surgical intervention, casting or some form of immobilization may be necessary and may limit socialization with peers and participation in school activities.
   D. Must deal with reactions of others to braces, casts, or other appliances.

VI. **Management/Treatment**
   A. Assessment per state/county/district requirements; usually screened at fifth or seventh grade at the latest.
   B. Referrals should be made when scoliometer is greater than 7 degrees or per individual school standards.
   C. Some curvatures will remain stable, requiring no treatment; others may increase for unknown reasons.
   D. When brace is prescribed, monitor for skin integrity.
   E. Mild curvature (less than 20 degrees).
      1. Periodic evaluation, observation, and x-rays to evaluate progression of curve.
      2. Not all curves are progressive.
      3. Mild exercise often prescribed but of questionable value.
      4. If curvature is less than 20 degrees but is secondary to another diagnosis, more aggressive treatment is initiated.
   F. Moderate curvature (20-40 degrees).
      1. Depends on age and cause.
      2. Bracing usual treatment; Boston brace-thoracolumbosacral orthosis (TLSO) (Boston Brace International, Avon, Massachusetts), Spine-Cor brace (Spinecorporation, Ltd, Sheffield, UK), and Milwaukee brace.
      3. Braces worn day and night until skeletal maturity attained, generally in 2 to 4 years.
      4. Bracing prevents progression, worn day and night.
   G. Severe curvature (40 degrees and greater).
      1. Treatment depends on age, cause, and previous therapy.
      2. Surgery considered, if curvature over 40 degrees, most likely in curves over 50 degrees; spinal fusion; anterior scoliosis correction by thoracoscopic surgery is less invasive, recovery is faster, with better cosmetic results; Harrington or Dwyer instrumentation (insertion of rod along spine to straighten) requires large incision, after spinal fusion, wearing of cast or an immobilizing jacket may be required and depends on type of surgery.

VII. **Additional Information**
   A. Scoliosis has five classifications based on etiology:
      1. Congenital.
      2. Idiopathic.
      3. Neuromuscular.
      4. Syndrome-related/mesenchymal.
      5. Other.

    B. Congenital form is caused by a vertebral anomaly that develops in utero, most likely during the third to fifth week.

    C. Idiopathic form is divided into three forms, depending on age at onset. Infantile form is birth to 3 years, juvenile is ages 4 to 9, and adolescent is from age 10 to skeletal maturity.

    D. Neuromuscular scoliosis may occur at any age and is secondary to disease and other disorders, such as muscular dystrophy, cerebral palsy, or myelomeningocele.

    E. Syndrome-related/mesenchymal is secondary to Marfan syndrome, Ehlers-Danlos syndrome, neurofibromatosis, or osteogenesis imperfecta.

    F. Other causes include tumors, fractures, rickets, and syringomyelia.

    G. Other malformations of the spine include kyphosis, lordosis, and kyphoscoliosis. In kyphosis (hunchback), there is an abnormally increased posterior convexity in the curvature of the thoracic spine as observed from the side. In lordosis (swayback), there is an abnormally increased concavity in the curvature of the lumbar spine as observed from the side. Mild kyphosis of the thoracic spine and mild lordosis of the lumbar spine is normal; scoliosis is never normal. Kyphoscoliosis is a combined abnormality.

VIII. **Web Sites**

    National Scoliosis Foundation
    1-800-673-6922
    http://www.scoliosis.org

SEIZURE DISORDER

  I. **Definition**

    A. A seizure is an atypical, sudden burst of excessive neuronal-electrical energy that can alter consciousness, motor activity, sensory phenomena, or appropriate behavior. A seizure disorder (epilepsy) is a condition of chronic, unprovoked recurring seizures. Classifications of seizures include *partial seizures* (simple or complex), which occur in specific areas of the brain, or *generalized seizures* (absence, myoclonic, clonic, tonic, tonic-clonic, atonic, and akinetic), which can affect nerve cells throughout the brain. There are also unclassified seizures and hybrids.

  II. **Etiology**

    A. Seizure disorder has numerous and varied causes based on genetic and acquired factors (e.g., congenital defects, brain injury, metabolic disorders, infectious diseases, tumors, exposure to toxins). Most seizures, however, are idiopathic. In children with existing neurological problems, taking melatonin has been found to cause seizures. Another documented etiology was particular patterns of rapidly flashing bright lights viewed on television in Japan, which triggered seizures in hundreds of children there (Sullivan, 1997). Up to 1% of the population have epilepsy, which makes this one of the most common neurological conditions (Purves et al, 1997).

III. *Brain Findings*
   A. With seizures, nerve cells in the brain may be damaged or difficulty may occur with the neurotransmitters, causing neuronal hyperactivity and a wide range of effects. The neurotransmitter gamma-aminobutyric acid (GABA) appears to be important in suppressing seizures, and it is suggested that a defect in the serotonin receptor may play a role in promoting seizures. Medications often act as agonists (activators) of the inhibitory transmitter GABA. Uncontrolled seizures can lead to degenerative brain alterations likely caused by excitotoxicity (consequences of oxygen deprivation).
   B. Juvenile myoclonic and absence seizures are heritable, and defective genes have been identified. Chromosome 22 has been implicated with absence.

IV. **Characteristics**
   A. Partial seizures (simple and complex):
      1. Simple partial seizures result from local cortical discharge; symptoms depend on area of brain involved and may be motor, sensory/somatosensory, autonomic, psychic, or combination of all types; no loss of consciousness occurs, and individual may verbalize during event. The average length is 10-20 seconds, and there is rarely a postictal phase.
         a. Motor: occurs in any part of the body; includes "Jacksonian march," which is an orderly sequential progression of clonic movements in foot, hand, or face as electrical impulses spread from irritable focus to indiscriminate regions of the cortex, often ending in a generalized seizure.
         b. Sensory/somatosensory: various sensations, such as visual, auditory, olfactory, gustatory (taste), and touch (e.g., paresthesias [numbness, tingling, prickling], or pain that originates in one area, such as face or extremities, and spreads to other parts of body).
         c. Autonomic: includes abdominal pain, headache, flushing of skin, rapid heart rate, perspiration, drop or rise in blood pressure, pupillary dilation, hair erection, laughing or crying.
         d. Psychic: disturbance of higher cerebral function (e.g. dreamy states, sense of time distorted, fear, hallucinations of music or scenes).
         e. Combinations of the above types.
      2. Complex partial seizures (psychomotor, temporal lobe): diffuse or focal discharges usually unilateral or bilateral discharges originating in temporal or frontal lobe; seizures may be preceded by aura, which indicates a focal onset; these seizures are the most difficult to recognize and are difficult to control.
         a. Period of altered behavior in which individual is amnesic and unable to respond to environment, which can be prolonged.
         b. Consciousness impaired during attack; children unable to articulate feelings or period of impairment makes it difficult to identify seizure.

    c. Automatisms are common in infants and children (50%-75%), including lip smacking, chewing, swallowing, picking at clothing, rubbing an object or walking/running in repetitive nondirective manner.

    d. Postictal drowsiness or sleep usually follows seizure.

    e. Sometimes complex sensory phenomena at beginning of seizure (e.g., odd smell, visual or auditory hallucinations).

    f. Variety of motor behavior patterns may be observed during attack; sometimes it is difficult to determine whether manifestations are related to seizure activity or nonconvulsive behavioral disturbance.

    g. Average length is 1-2 minutes.

B. Generalized seizures (involvement of both hemispheres):

  1. Absence (petit mal):

    a. Brief loss of consciousness or attention, 3 to 30 seconds, not associated with an aura or postictal state.

    b. Minimal or no alteration in muscle tone.

    c. May go unrecognized, since behavior is altered very little.

    d. Possibility of 20 or more attacks daily.

    e. Slight loss of muscle tone, which may cause individual to drop objects.

    f. Able to maintain postural control; person seldom falls.

    g. Frequently automatic movements (e.g., lip smacking, twitching of eyelids or face, slight hand movements).

    h. An attack is often mistaken for inattentiveness or daydreaming.

    i. Usually begins between ages of 5 to 12 years, is more common in girls, and often ceases at puberty.

  2. Myoclonic:

    a. Sudden, brief contractures of a muscle or muscle group.

    b. Occurs singly or repetitively without loss of consciousness or postictal state.

    c. Usually lasts less than 3 seconds.

    d. At least 5 subgroupings are known: benign myoclonus of infancy, typical myoclonic epilepsy of early childhood, complex myoclonic epilepsy (Lennox-Gastaut syndrome), juvenile myoclonic epilepsy, and progressive myoclonic epilepsy.

    e. Usually begins between ages 4 and 14 and may resolve by age 18.

  3. Clonic:

    a. Almost exclusively in early childhood.

    b. Begins with loss of or impaired consciousness associated with sudden decreased tone in skeletal muscles or brief generalized tonic spasm, followed by one to several minutes of bilateral jerks (often symmetrical) that may predominate in one limb.

    c. After seizure, there may be rapid recovery, prolonged confusion, or coma.

4. Tonic:
   a. Relatively rare and usually occurs between 1 and 7 years of age.
   b. Sudden increase in muscle tone produces number of characteristic postures or stiffening.
   c. Consciousness is usually partially or completely lost.
   d. Altered consciousness after seizure is usually brief but may last several minutes.
5. Tonic-clonic (grand mal):
   a. May be associated with an aura, indicating focal origin.
   b. Eyes roll upward.
   c. Immediate loss of consciousness; falls to floor or ground.
   d. Stiffening is generalized and symmetric tonic contraction of entire body musculature.
   e. Arms usually flexed, legs, head, and neck extended.
   f. May utter peculiar, piercing cry.
   g. Tonic rigidity replaced by jerking movements as trunk and extremities undergo rhythmic contraction and relaxation.
   h. May have increased secretions and be incontinent of urine and feces.
   i. Postictally, appears to relax but may stay semiconscious and be difficult to rouse or may waken in a few minutes but remain confused for several hours; will be poorly coordinated, with mildly impaired fine motor movements, and usually will sleep for several hours.
   j. Occasionally lips and fingernail beds are cyanotic; condition is not unusual and should subside in a short time; if not, emergency measures may be instituted.
   k. Series of seizures may occur at intervals too brief to regain consciousness between attacks; this is known as *status epilepticus* and requires emergency intervention because it can lead to exhaustion, respiratory failure, and death.
6. Atonic (drop attack):
   a. Loss of muscle tone.
   b. Nodding head, sudden brief dropping of head and neck, sagging at knees, and falling to the floor.
   c. Momentary or no loss of consciousness.
   d. Onset generally 2 to 5 years of age.
   e. Will get up and continue as if nothing happened.
   f. Often difficult to distinguish between atonic and akinetic seizures.
7. Akinetic:
   a. Lack of movement, muscle tone maintained.
   b. Freezes into position but does not fall.
   c. Impaired or momentary loss of consciousness.
8. Infantile spasms:
   a. Most commonly begin between 4-8 months of age; twice as common in males as in females.

      b. Consist of series of sudden, brief, and symmetrical muscular contractions.

      c. Seizure may be preceded or followed by cry or giggling.

      d. Possible loss of consciousness.

      e. Flushing, pallor, or cyanosis sometimes accompanies attack.

      f. May have numerous seizures during day.

      g. There are 3 types of spasms, which appear as momentary shocklike contractions of entire body: flexor, extensor, and mixed; flexor is sudden flexion of neck, arms, and legs occurring in clusters; extensor involves extension of trunk and extremities; mixed is combination of clusters of flexion and extension and is the most common.

      h. Research suggests a relationship to the sleep cycle, with underlying cause related to a particular phase of early brain development affecting neurotransmitter regulation.

V. Health Concerns/Emergencies

    A. Status epilepticus: continuous seizures or serial convulsions without return of consciousness, is an emergency situation because of risk of airway closure, aspiration, anoxia, metabolic acidosis, hypoglycemia, hyperkalemia, lactic acidosis, increased intracranial pressure, and death.

NOTE: Be alert to state, county, or district guidelines for calling emergency medical services (EMS) and individual student practitioner directives.

    B. Noncompliance issues with medication; discovery and experimentation with illicit drugs and alcohol during middle childhood and adolescence.

    C. Parents may need help understanding need for continuing medication even in the absence of seizures.

    D. Safety concerns during a seizure because of falling and potential injuries. May need to wear a helmet.

    E. Routine dental home care and office examinations may be difficult because of seizure activity, related disabilities, or compliance issues.

    F. Chronic use of the medications ethosuximide (Zarontin) and phenytoin (Dilantin) can cause lymphoid hyperplasia, which results in gum hypertrophy or enlargement of tonsillar and adenoidal tissue, causing partial airway obstruction and snoring. Gum massage and consistent dental care may reduce gum hypertrophy.

    G. Immunizations for pertussis and measles to be given to a child with seizures or a family history of seizures may need to be omitted or deferred if the child is not neurologically stable.

    H. School fire alarm systems with flashing lights and/or strobe lights in assembly programs may trigger seizures in predisposed individuals. Notification of health risks to school administrators is necessary.

VI. Effects on Individual

    A. Has to learn to live with the possibility that seizures may be lifelong.

    B. Apprehensive concerning the occurrence of seizures, helplessness, and care to be received during an episode and continued acceptance by peers, teachers, and others.

Box 4-9 *Guidelines for Seizure Management*

Protect individual during seizure and maintain airway by doing the following:

1. Make no attempt to halt seizure or restrain individual.
2. If standing or sitting in chair or wheelchair, ease down to floor immediately.
3. Do not force any object between teeth.
4. Loosen restrictive clothing.
5. Protect individual from hitting hard or sharp objects that might cause injury.
6. If salivation is excessive, turn onto side.
7. Cyanosis and cessation of breathing may occur briefly.
8. If individual appears in respiratory distress and skin is excessively blue, extend neck and gently pull on jaw; with infant, only slightly tilt head because overextension blocks airway; if breathing does not resume, start CPR and call for medical assistance.
9. Call EMS if seizure is followed by other seizures in rapid succession or if duration of seizure is excessive; duration about 10 min for known epileptics, 5 min if no history of seizures.
10. After episode, place individual on side and allow to sleep until he or she awakens.
11. Remain with individual until conscious and oriented

NOTE: Follow IECP or IHCP or adapt guidelines as needed.

CPR, Cardiopulmonary resuscitation; *EMS,* emergency medical services; *IECP,* individualized emergency care plan; *IHCP,* individualized health care plan.

Box 4-10 *Observational Notes*

During seizure, observe and document the following information on seizure log or health record and for diagnosis and management of disorder:

1. Significant preictal events, including aura and exposure to bright lights, noise, or excitement.
2. Movements before, during, and after attack.
3. Time seizure began and length of seizure.
4. Change in color/respiratory effort, profuse perspiration.
5. Where seizure movement began (e.g., legs, arms, head).
6. Change in facial expression, eye movements, muscle tone, and automatisms.
7. Involuntary urination or defecation.
8. Note length of postictal phase, confusion, orientation to time and person, impaired speech, report of headache or muscle soreness, and changes in motor ability and sensation.

C. Lack of confidence and low self-esteem because individual sees self as "different" from peers.
D. May be subjected to classmates' cruel remarks or left out of social recreational activities.
E. Feelings of dependence (e.g., must frequently visit the physician, needs daily medication, may need to rely on a stranger's help when a seizure occurs).

F. Embarrassed when consciousness regained after a seizure, especially if incontinent.
G. Children with a seizure disorder may have a lower-than-normal IQ.
H. Temporal lobe seizures can affect language and memory functioning, and partial seizures can impair attention span.
I. There is a greater incidence of psychiatric and behavioral problems and emotional disturbances in children with seizures.
J. Side effects from medication, or individual worries about the effects of prolonged use of seizure medication.
K. Difficulty obtaining a driver's license, and employment opportunities may be restricted.
L. Parents and school personnel can be overprotective, and child may be unnecessarily restricted from physical activity.
M. Safety at risk because of falling; may need to wear a helmet.
N. Caution while swimming; have person with lifesaving skills nearby.

VII. **Management/Treatment**
   A. During school:
      1. Treatment and management is both immediate and lifelong, involving medical, surgical, and dietary strategies and ongoing school assessments.
      2. Develop IHCP and/or IECP for individual student and train school staff regarding emergency procedures.
      3. Ongoing evaluations of vision, hearing, dental (alert to those on Dilantin and Zarontin for gum hyperplasia), blood pressure, hematocrit, urinalysis, and special diets.
      4. When student has complaints, be alert to symptoms related to medications, seizures, or diet, ruling out associations such as GER (vomiting), respiratory (apnea-breath holding), neurological (headache), and behavioral (short attention span, irritability) symptoms.
      5. Exercise good judgment before taking oral temperature of individual with history of seizures.
      6. Emphasize need to wear medical alert identification (e.g., bracelet).
      7. Oxygen may be prescribed and administered at school for children with severe seizure disorders.
      8. Seizure medications can be used alone or in combinations.
         a. Monitor compliance; abrupt withdrawal can precipitate status epilepticus.
         b. Anticonvulsants can modify the therapeutic level of birth control medication; higher doses of birth control should be considered.
         c. Illness, fatigue, and menstrual cycle can affect seizure threshold.
         d. OTC and prescription medications may alter seizure threshold or effectiveness of anticonvulsants.
         e. Blood levels, urinalysis, and liver function tests should be determined periodically for optimum dosage levels of anticonvulsive medications.

Text continued on p. 268

Table 4-9   *Common Anticonvulsant Drugs*

Drug	Action and Use	Side Effects	Considerations
Corticotropin	Inhibitory effect on excitability of developing brain only; not used in adults Infantile spasms Lennox-Gastaut	Increased weight or cushingoid appearance; hypertension, extreme irritability, GI distress, transient glycosuria, electrolyte disturbance **Infections, GI bleeding, sodium retention**	Given IM, usually few weeks-several months
Valproic acid (Depakene, Depakote) Usually adjunctive therapy Half-life 6-16 hr	Directly increases concentration of GABA Absence Tonic-clonic Myoclonic Partial Akinetic	Nausea, vomiting, diarrhea, irregular menses, tremor, indigestion, weight change, transient alopecia **Hepatotoxicity, thrombocytopenia**	Give with food if GI upset occurs; do not crush, break, or chew enteric coated tablets; teratogenic effects *Overdose:* somnolence, heart block, deep coma
Phenytoin (Dilantin) Half-life 7-42 hr, average 22 hr Hydantoin class	Decreases sustained repeated firing of single neurons by blocking sodium dependent channels and decreasing calcium uptake Tonic-clonic, simple partial, status epilepticus	Nausea, confusion, slurred speech, irritability, nystagmus, diplopia, gum hypertrophy, hirsutism, constipation **Hypersensitivity (rash, fever, lymphadenopathy); blood dyscrasias, osteomalacia caused by vitamin D deficiency; dizziness, ataxia, lethargy, rash**	Abrupt withdrawal may trigger status epilepticus; pregnancy risks may outweigh benefits (fetal hydantoin syndrome) May need vitamin D supplements

Modified from *Saunders nursing drug handbook*, Philadelphia, 2001, WB Saunders; *Physician's desk reference*, 2001.
NOTE: Drug names and adverse effects are listed in bold type.
NOTE: Pregnancy and breast-feeding risks are involved with many of the medications and warrant consideration for females of childbearing age.

Continued

Table 4-9 *Common Anticonvulsant Drugs—cont'd*

Drug	Action and Use	Side Effects	Considerations
Felbamate (Felbatol) Adjunctive therapy Half-life 7 to 9 hr	Action unknown Partial Lennox-Gastaut	Anorexia, weight loss, insomnia, nausea, vomiting; headache **Aplastic anemia, hepatic failure**	*PDR recommendation:* must have written informed consent of risk signed by parent(s) Not first-line anticonvulsant Not suggested for use under age 12
Tiagabine (Gabitril) Adjunctive therapy Half-life 18-50 hr	Blocks reuptake of GABA into glial and nerve cells Partial	Ataxia, dizziness, asthenia, tremor, headache, confusion, nervousness, somnolence	Take with food
Clonazepam (Klonopin) Benzodiazepine class Adjunctive and monotherapy Half-life 18-50 hr	Binds to specific GABA site that enhances opening frequency of chloride channel without changing duration Absence Myoclonic Simple partial Complex partial Akinetic Infantile spasms Lennox-Gastaut	Drowsiness, ataxia, Increased salivation **Behavioral changes (aggression, agitation, irritability), hyperactivity, cognitive dysfunction**	Abrupt withdrawal may result in striking restlessness, hand tremors, insomnia, status epilepticus, sweating Psychological or physical dependence may occur *Overdose:* somnolence, confusion, coma
Lamotrigine (Lamictal) Adjunctive therapy for Lennox-Gastaut and monotherapy for partial Half-life 12-59 hr	Inhibits voltage sensitive sodium channels, thus stabilizing neuronal membranes and regulating presynaptic transmitter release of excitatory amino acid, (e.g., glutamate) Lennox-Gastaut Partial	Nausea, vomiting, dizziness, headache, ataxia, somnolence, diplopia, blurred vision **Hypersensitivity: fever, rash, lymphadenopathy**	Can be used from age 2 and above

Drug	Action/Indications	Adverse Effects	Comments
Phenobarbital (Luminal) Barbiturate class Half-life 3-23 hr	Acts on GABA receptor to increase chloride channel opening time Tonic-clonic Complex partial Simple partial	Drowsiness, hyperactivity, irritability, interferes with motor speed and concentration, mood changes **Lethargy, learning difficulties, hepatic dysfunction, leukopenia**	Possibility of vitamin D and folic acid deficiency Dependence can occur with prolonged use of high dose; abrupt withdrawal may cause insomnia, tremor, delirium, status epilepticus *Overdose:* hypothermia, severe CNS depression, severe renal impairment Used for age 8 and older
Primidone (Mysoline) Half-life 5-7 hr	Action unknown Simple partial Complex partial Tonic-clonic	Drowsiness, dizziness, ataxia, hyperactivity, diplopia, loss of coordination **Behavioral disturbances, GI dysfunction**	
Gabapentin (Neurontin) Adjunctive therapy Half-life 5-7 hr	Action unknown Partial	Fatigue, dizziness, nystagmus, somnolence, ataxia **Mood/behavior changes**	Can be given with or without food No data on pediatric population; used for adults

Modified from *Saunders nursing drug handbook*, Philadelphia, 2001, WB Saunders; *Physician's desk reference*, 2001.
NOTE: Drug names and adverse effects are listed in bold type.
NOTE: Pregnancy and breast-feeding risks are involved with many of the medications and warrant consideration for females of childbearing age.

Continued

Table 4-9 *Common Anticonvulsant Drugs—cont'd*

Drug	Action and Use	Side Effects	Considerations
Vigabatrin (Sabril) Adjunctive therapy Half-life 5-7 hr	Binds to specific GABA receptor, increasing GABA levels Infantile spasms Tonic-clonic Complex partial	Appetite changes, drowsiness, sedation, abdominal pain, poor concentration **Behavior changes, visual field constriction, psychosis**	Not metabolized in liver like most antiseizure medications
Carbamazepine (Tegretol) Half-life 8-20 hr	Decreases sustained repetitive firing of neurons by blocking sodium channels and decreasing calcium uptake Tonic-clonic Simple partial Complex partial	Ataxia, drowsiness, dizziness, irritability, nausea/vomiting, visual abnormalities (spots before eyes, blurred vision, diplopia, difficulty focusing) **Rashes, movement disorders, hepatic dysfunction, bone marrow suppression, blood dyscrasias, CV disturbances**	Take with meals to decrease GI distress Abrupt withdrawal may precipitate status epilepticus Erythromycin and other antibiotics increase levels, causing toxicity and increased effects
Topiramate (Topamax) Half-life 21 hr	Blocks repetitive sustained firing of neurons by inhibiting sodium channels Tonic-clonic Partial Lennox-Gastaut	Somnolence, fatigue, dizziness, diplopia, anorexia, anemia, weight changes, impaired cognition, potential of CNS depression, malaise, psychomotor slowing, speech disorders, word-finding difficulty, abnormal sensation: burning or prickling, renal stones	Maintain adequate hydration to prevent renal stones; safety and effectiveness in children not established Trials in ages 4-17 yr

Drug	Action	Use	Adverse effects	Comments
Clorazepate dipotassium (Tranxene) Benzodiazepine class Half-life 48-96 hr Antianxiety, anticonvulsant	Enhances GABA neurotransmission and elevates seizure threshold in response to electrical/chemical stimulation when enhancing presynaptic inhibition	Partial	Drowsiness, dizziness, GI disturbances, irritability, nervousness, blurred vision, diplopia	Abrupt withdrawal may result in pronounced restlessness, irritability, insomnia, hand tremors, seizures *Overdose:* somnolence, confusion, coma
Ethosuximide (Zarontin) Half-life 60 hr	Blocks calcium channels linked with thalamocortical circulatory	Absence	Nausea, anorexia, gastric discomfort, headache, drowsiness, dizziness **Leukopenia, agranulocytosis**	Administer with food; may aggravate tonic-clonic seizures *Overdose:* nausea and vomiting, CNS depression

Modified from *Saunders nursing drug handbook*, Philadelphia, 2001, WB Saunders; *Physician's desk reference*, 2001.

CV, Cardiovascular.

NOTE: Drug names and adverse effects are listed in bold type.

NOTE: Pregnancy and breast-feeding risks are involved with many of the medications and warrant consideration for females of childbearing age.

B. Other medical care:
   1. A ketogenic diet is used with refractory complex myoclonic and tonic-clonic seizures.
      a. High in fats, low in proteins and carbohydrates, and sometimes used as treatment when control has not been achieved.
      b. Burning fat instead of carbohydrates causes ketosis, but exact mechanism of action is unknown.
      c. This is a strict diet with substantial risks and is initiated in the hospital to monitor metabolic and neurological changes.
      d. Families may have difficulty with the precise measurement of foods, and not all children can tolerate the food restrictions. Hypoglycemia and weight loss can occur.
      e. Studies indicate a 50% reduction in seizures in 40% of children, and 25% were seizure-free (Batchelor, Nance, and Short, 1997; McDonald, 1997).
      f. Diet may be discontinued when goal is achieved.
   2. Surgery is considered when seizures are uncontrolled by other methods. Regardless of the type of surgery performed, medication may still be needed for optimum control of seizures. Risks depend on type of surgery and include hemiparesis, language difficulties, and memory loss.
   3. There are 3 major surgical techniques: *resection, disconnection,* and *augmentation.*
      a. Resection includes lesionectomy, lobectomy, or hemispherectomy and is used for infants and young children with catastrophic seizures. Lesionectomy is performed for small brain tumors or abnormalities that cause seizures. Lobectomy is conducted when the focal point(s) is limited to one lobe; small portions or the entire lobe is removed (e.g., temporal or occipital lobe). Hemispherectomy is used for seizures associated with congenital hemiplegia, chronic encephalitis, hemimegalencephaly, Sturge-Weber syndrome, and when rampant epileptic discharges extend to the normal hemisphere.
      b. Disconnection examples are corpus callosotomy and subpial transection. Corpus callosotomy is used with generalized seizures and involves partial or total removal of the corpus callosum, the white matter connecting the two hemispheres. Subpial transection entails dividing the horizontal fibers of the motor cortex while sparing the vertical fibers, thus achieving a reduction in seizures while maintaining cerebral function.
      c. Augmentation is used for partial seizures and can reduce them by 20% to 42% (Brainconnection, 2000). Vagus nerve stimulation (VNS) is achieved by inserting a battery-powered device under the skin in the upper left chest with a lead attached to the vagus nerve in the lower part of the neck that provides automatic intermittent stimulation to the nerve. When seizures are preceded by an aura, the seizure activity may be aborted by

passing an external magnet over the implant to initiate VNS. In young children and those with disabilities, a responsible adult can apply the magnet. Older children and adolescents with normal cognitive functioning do well with the magnet, since it can be made to appear as a bracelet, and when a seizure is sensed, they simply move their hand across the chest area. Side effects include hoarseness, throat paresthesias, headache, and shortness of breath, which can be reduced or eliminated by adjusting the intensity of the stimulation.

VIII. Additional Information

    A. *Febrile seizures* are the most common seizure disorder in children; associated with rapidly rising fever (102 degrees or greater), generally brief, clonic, or tonic-clonic seizures with little postictal confusion. Usually in children from 9 months to 7 years of age with no long-lasting effects. Etiology is unclear, but genetic predisposition is supported by strong family histories and several gene markers have been identified. Treatment is usually limited to acute episode. Antipyretics may be used and diazepam (Valium) prescribed at the onset and for duration of a febrile illness. Prophylactic anticonvulsants are not recommended. Risk factors for developing seizure disorder are family history of epilepsy, prolonged or atypical febrile seizure, and initial febrile seizure before 9 months of age, abnormal neurological examination, and delayed developmental milestones.

    B. *Lennox-Gastaut syndrome* is refractory myoclonic and clonic seizure activity with specific electroencephalogram (EEG) patterns. It generally commences in the first year of life and has a poor prognosis. About 75% have mental retardation and behavioral problems. Seizure control is difficult to achieve with medication alone, and a ketogenic diet may be tried (see Table 4-9).

    C. Seizures can be triggered by daily events, including flashing or rotating lights, high-pitched sounds, and video or television's fast moving lights.

    D. Many well-known, intelligent people have had epilepsy, including Alexander the Great, Napoleon, Julius Caesar, and Vincent Van Gogh.

    E. Anticonvulsant drugs:

        1. Three new drugs are FDA-approved but not listed in the 2001 *Physician's Desk Reference* (PDR). Oxcarbazepine (Trileptal) is adjunctive therapy for partial seizures in children as young as 4 years and monotherapy for older students. Zonisamide (Zonegran) is adjunctive therapy for partial seizure in older ages. Levetiracetam (Keppra) is the fastest FDA-approved antiseizure drug to date.

NOTE: Abrupt discontinuation of any antiseizure medication is not recommended.

    IX. Web Sites

        Epilepsy Foundation
        http://www.epilepsyfoundation.org

SPINA BIFIDA/MYELODYSPLASIA

I. **Definition**
  A. Neural tube defects are anomalies of the spinal column, spinal cord, and skin that develop early, around the third to fourth weeks of embryonic development. There are two common forms of neural tube malformations: spina bifida occulta and spina bifida cystica.
  B. With *spina bifida occulta,* no abnormalities of the spinal cord or meninges exist. The vertebral defect is covered by skin.
  C. *Spina bifida cystica* involves two major malformations. With *meningocele,* the meninges pouch out because of a defect in a vertebra of the spine, forming a saclike membrane containing CSF. The area is covered by skin. It does not involve the spinal cord. Hydrocephalus is associated with this diagnosis.
  D. In *meningomyelocele* or *myelomeningocele,* the membranes, a portion of the spinal cord, and the nerves protrude through a defect in the vertebra. The sac is covered with a thin membrane, and hydrocephalus is common when the defect is in the lower vertebral area.

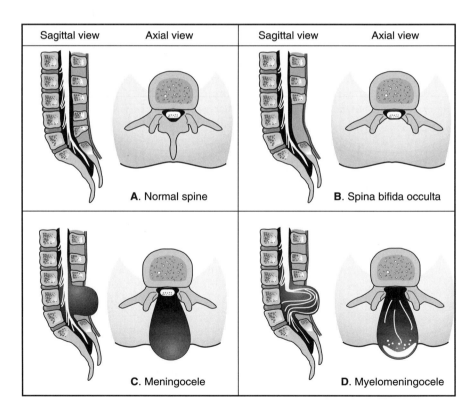

| Sagittal view | Axial view | Sagittal view | Axial view |

A. Normal spine

B. Spina bifida occulta

C. Meningocele

D. Myelomeningocele

FIGURE 4-7 Forms of spina bifida. **A,** Normal. **B,** Spina bifida occulta. **C,** Meningocele. **D,** Myelomeningocele.

II. **Etiology**
   A. The exact cause of spina bifida is unknown. There is a genetic pre-disposition, however, and nutritional and environmental factors play a role in the etiology. Research studies provide evidence that folic acid deficiencies are associated with neural tube defects, and an adequate intake of folic acid can reduce the incidence by 50% to 70%. Particular drugs can also increase the risk for malformations, such as valproic acid.

III. **Characteristics**
   A. Spina bifida occulta:
      1. Many individuals have no symptoms.
      2. May display superficial manifestations; these signs may occur alone, together, or in combinations.
         a. May be noticed as a depression or dimpling over the malformed vertebrae, which may mark the site of a dermoid sinus.
         b. Abnormal tufts of hair may be present.
         c. Telangiectasia, small red lesion comprised of dilated capillaries.
         d. Subcutaneous lipomas (fatty tumors) present.
      3. Spinal cord and meninges are normal.
      4. Defect is covered by skin and may go unnoticed unless there are associated manifestations:
         a. Gait abnormalities become progressive.
         b. Bowel or bladder difficulties.
      5. Generally occurs at L5 and S1 levels but may affect any area of the spinal column.
   B. Spina bifida cystica:
      1. Symptoms and prognosis depend on level and type of lesion, presence of hydrocephalus, or secondary complications (e.g. meningitis).
   C. Meningocele:
      1. Sac containing meninges and CSF protrudes through vertebral defect.
      2. Cord and nerve roots generally are not involved.
      3. May occur anywhere along spinal column.
      4. Generally no bowel or bladder involvement.
      5. Lower extremities usually not involved.
      6. Hydrocephalus is associated.
      7. Defects above thorax are usually meningoceles.
      8. Females may have genital tract anomalies such as vaginal septa and rectovaginal fistula.
   D. Meningomyelocele:
      1. Most common form of open spine defect.
      2. Occurs anywhere along the neuraxis, but usually in the lumbosacral area.
      3. Sac contains meninges, spinal fluid, portion of spinal cord, and its nerves.

4. Leak in utero of sac or rupture after birth causes CSF drainage and makes the newborn susceptible to meningitis.
5. Surgical intervention should be within the first few days after birth unless a CSF leakage is present.
6. Neurological, orthopedic, and urological and bowel difficulties are associated conditions.
   a. Neurological factors:
      (1) Extent of paralysis depends on location of defect.
      (2) Loss of sensation below level of lesions.
      (3) Hydrocephaly occurs in most of the children.
      (4) Arnold-Chiari malformation is usually associated with hydrocephalus. Associated symptoms occur from a medulla and cerebellar compression through the foramen magnum (where the spinal cord enters the spinal column) and include feeding difficulties, choking, stridor, hoarse cry, vocal cord paralysis, apnea, and spasticity of the upper extremities.
   b. Orthopedic factors:
      (1) Dislocation of hips.
      (2) Equinovarus (clubfoot) often associated anomaly.
      (3) Scoliosis, lordosis, or kyphosis in later years.
      (4) Contractures of feet, ankles, or knees usually occur.
      (5) Prone to fractures of lower extremities.
      (6) Ambulation may or may not occur; canes and braces may be required.
   c. Urological and bowel factors:
      (1) Neurogenic bladder and bowel.
      (2) Increased susceptibility to urinary tract infections because of stasis of urine.
      (3) Poor bowel musculature or paralysis.
      (4) No bowel sensation present.

IV. **Health Concerns/Emergencies**
   A. Medical concerns depend on state and extent of lesion and generally are associated with meningomyelocele.
   B. Loss of sensation puts individual at risk for decubiti, abrasions, and burns.
   C. If shunted for hydrocephalus, awareness of signs of increased intracranial pressure or shunt failure is necessary: irritability, restlessness, vomiting, complaints of headache, possible seizures, change in vital signs, and pupillary changes.
   D. Buttocks and areas around braces and shoes are prone to skin breakdown and must be checked frequently for rubbing and redness.
   E. Obesity can result from inactivity, inappropriate dietary management, or both.
   F. Fecal incontinence and lack of bladder control cause skin breakdown and make toilet training difficult.
   G. High risk for latex allergies.

V. Effects on Individual

A. This condition is associated with neurodevelopmental deficits that interfere with school performance, such as visual conditions (e.g., astigmatism), memory deficits, poor organizational skills, visual-perceptual problems, impaired eye-hand coordination, and hand-writing difficulties.

B. Numerous medical appointments, surgery, and hospitalization take the student away from home and out of school for extended periods, interfering with academic achievement.

C. Child may be obese from low activity level.

D. Some limitations and inconvenience imposed by confinement to a wheelchair (e.g., certain routes may take longer to get to a class).

E. How student is treated and viewed by parent(s) affects his or her self-esteem and feelings of competence or incompetence (e.g., fostering independence or being overprotective).

VI. Management/Treatment

A. Treatment and management is both immediate and lifelong.

B. Develop IHCP or IECP to address urgent issues (e.g., VP shunt obstruction, injuries). If student is receiving special education, write nurse assessment report for IEP and attend meeting as appropriate.

C. Monitor vision and hearing.

D. Be alert for latex allergies. Reactions from latex exposure can extend from rashes to anaphylaxis. Latex products include gloves, pacifiers, balloons, diapers, wheelchair cushions and padding, blood pressure cuff and tubing, and stethoscope tubing. The protein in certain foods may potentiate this allergy and includes bananas, kiwi, avocado, tomatoes, potatoes, and chestnuts.

E. As with all children, allergy identification should be available, such as a bracelet or necklace.

F. Be aware of all medication and their side effects taken at school.

G. Teach designated school staff how to give emergency medication; check for guidelines in school/state policy and Nurse Practice Act.

H. Catheterization or Credé's method may need to be taught to child or staff performing procedure. Check Nurse Practice Act for guidelines related to delegation of care.

I. Evaluate and teach designated school staff to observe periodically for skin breakdown caused by immobility, bracing or rubbing of appliances, and high-fiber diet, and encourage fluids to decrease urinary problems.

J. Assess wheelchair for good working order and appropriate size.

K. Evaluate usability and safety of school routine and pathways via wheelchair. Emergency evacuation plans should be in place.

L. Be available to share and discuss health and psychosocial concerns that may interfere with friendships, family relationships and life satisfaction both with student and parent(s).

M. Be knowledgeable about local resources for child and/or family counseling.

VII. **Additional Information**
   A. Prenatal diagnosis may be possible between the sixteenth to eighteenth weeks of gestation. An elevated alpha-fetoprotein (AFP) indicates a risk, and an ultrasound of the uterus may be able to detect an open neural tube defect.
   B. Folic acid supplements, 4 mg daily, are now recommended for all women of childbearing age (CDC, 2001). Supplements are absolutely essential before conception and at least through the first 12 weeks of gestation, when neurulation development is complete (Behrman, Kliegman, and Jenson, 2000). This intervention should decrease the incidence of neural tube defects, which is currently 0.7 to 1.0 for every 1000 live births each year (McComb, 1998).
   C. Abnormal adhesion of the spinal cord to a bony structure to the area of malformation results in a tethered cord. Manifestations include altered gait pattern, foot weakness, back pain, and problems with bowel and bladder control. These symptoms may not be seen for years or unless a child has the ability to walk or be toilet trained. Surgical intervention is based on level of involvement. May occur with both spina bifida occulta and spina bifida cystica.
   D. Management of a neurogenic bladder beyond catheterization may include drug therapy with anticholinergic medication to relax the bladder and tighten the urinary sphincter or surgery including bladder augmentation, implantation of artificial urinary sphincter, or construction of continent ileostomy for catheterization. Reducing intake in the evening may prevent nighttime incontinence.

VIII. **Web Sites**
   Association for Spina Bifida and Hydrocephalus
   1-800-621-3141
   http://www.asbah.org
   March of Dimes Birth Defects Foundation
   1-888-MODIMES (663-4637)
   http://www.modimes.org
   National Institute of Neurological Disorders and Stroke
   http://www.ninds.nih.gov/health_and_medical/disorders/spina_bifida.htm

TURNER'S SYNDROME

I. **Definition**
   A. Turner's syndrome is an X chromosomal disorder in which females have only one X chromosome instead of two. It is also known as *XO syndrome* and is called *Ullrich-Turner syndrome* in Europe.
II. **Etiology**
   A. Turner's syndrome results from complete or partial monosomy of the short arm on the X chromosome. Risk does not increase with maternal age but does increase with paternal age (Finberg, 1998). The syndrome occurs in about 1 in 1500 to 1 in 2500 female births. More than 99% of the fetuses are lost to spontaneous abortion in early or middle trimester.

III. **Characteristics**
  A. Symptoms recognized at birth include edema of the dorsa of the hands and feet, loose skinfolds at the nape of the neck (nuchal folds), epicanthal folds, low-set ears, small mandible, low birth weight, decreased length, and left-sided cardiac anomalies.
  B. School-age child: webbing of the neck, micrognathia (small jaw), high-arched palate, rotated or protruding ears, low hairline in back of head.
  C. Hypoplastic, hyperconvex fingernails, short metacarpals or metatarsals.
  D. Primary hypertension.
  E. Pectus excavatum, coarctation of the aorta, and other cardiovascular abnormalities.
  F. Absent kidney or renal abnormalities.
  G. Hashimoto's thyroiditis (autoimmune thyroid disorder).
  H. Susceptible to GI bleeding because of abnormal vascular development of the bowel.
  I. Primary amenorrhea, sterility.
  J. No ovaries, so do not produce any male hormones.
  K. Impaired vision and hearing.
  L. Visual spatial processing, visual memory and visual motor integration difficulties; rarely associated with decreased IQ levels.

IV. **Health Concerns/Emergencies**
  A. Otitis media is the most common illness and is caused by anatomical distortions.
  B. Cardiac and kidney problems can contribute to absences from school and therefore learning difficulties.

V. **Effects on Individual**
  A. Rarely fertile.
  B. May grieve lack of fertility; begin discussion before adolescence.
  C. Self-conscious of appearance when epicanthal folds, protruding ears, and webbed neck are prominent.

VI. **Management/Treatment**
  A. Evaluate hearing and vision.
  B. Assess blood pressure frequently.
  C. Monitor anthropometry when receiving hormone replacement therapy.
  D. Be aware of parent/student consideration of plastic surgery for epicanthal folds, protruding ears, and webbed neck.

VII. **Additional Information**
  A. Can be diagnosed prenatally by CVS or amniocentesis. Associated with polyhydramnios, oligohydramnios, unexplained anemia, or preeclampsia.

VIII. **Web Sites**
  Turner's Syndrome of the United States
  http://www.turner-syndrome-us.org/resource/
  eMedicine
  http://www.emedicine.com/ped/topic2330.htm

BIBLIOGRAPHY

American Academy of Pediatrics Committee on Genetics: Health supervision for children with sickle cell diseases and their families, *Pediatrics* 98(3):467-472, 1996.

American Diabetes Association: *Diabetes 1996 vital statistics,* Alexandria, Va, 1996, The Association.

American Medical Association: Report 6 of the Council on Scientific Affairs (1-94), *Lead poisoning among children,* July 6, 2000, Available online: http://www.amaassn.org/ama/pub/article/2036-2556.html. Accessed on Nov 24, 2000.

American Psychiatric Association: *Diagnostic and statistical manual of mental disorders, fourth edition,* Washington, DC, 1994, The Association.

Anderson K, editor: *Mosby's medical, nursing, and allied health dictionary,* ed 5, St Louis, 1998, Mosby.

Anshel J: *Smart medicine for your eyes: a guide to safe and effective relief of common eye disorders,* Garden City Park, NY, 1999, Avery Publishing Group.

Arthritis Foundation: *Children and arthritis, juvenile arthritis: a national response,* 2001, Available online: http://www.arthritis.org/advocacy/priorities/priorities_children.asp. Accessed on Sep 14, 2001.

Batchelor L, Nance J, Short B: An interdisciplinary team approach to implementing the ketogenic diet for the treatment of seizures, *Pediatric Nurs* 23(5):465-473, 1997.

Behrman RE, Kliegman RM, Jenson HB: *Nelson textbook of pediatrics,* ed 16, Philadelphia, 2000, WB Saunders.

Biederman J, Faraone SV, Monuteaux MC, et al: Patterns of alcohol and drug use in adolescents can be predicted by parental substance use disorders, *Pediatrics* 106(4):792-797, 2000.

Bowden VR, Dickey SB, Greenberg CS: *Children and their families: the continuum of care,* Philadelphia, 1998, WB Saunders.

Burns CE et al: *Pediatric primary care: a handbook for nurse practitioners,* ed 2, Philadelphia, 2000, WB Saunders.

Burson J: Klinefelter's syndrome, *Am J Nurs* 98(12):16AAA-16BBB, 1998.

Calli J, Farrington E: Vigabatrin, *Pediatr Nurs* 24(4):357-361, 1998.

Catlin A: Ethical commentary on gender reassignment: a complex and provocative modern issue, *Pediatr Nurs* 24(1):63-65, 1998.

Centers for Disease Control and Prevention: Division of HIV/AIDS Prevention, *HIV and its transmission,* Jan 31, 2001, Available online: http://www.cdc.gov/hiv. Accessed on July 7, 2001.

Centers for Disease Control and Prevention: Division of HIV/AIDS Prevention, *Frequently asked questions,* Nov 30, 1998, Available online: http://www.cdc.gov/hiv. Accessed on July 7, 2001.

Centers for Disease Control and Prevention: *Strategic plan for the elimination of childhood lead poisoning,* Atlanta, 1991, U.S. Department of Health and Human Services, Public Health and Human Service.

Chasnoff IJ: *The nature of nurture: biology environment and the drug-exposed child,* Chicago, 2001, National Training Institute.

Christensen D: Sobering work: unraveling alcohol's affects on the developing brain, *Science News* 158(2):28-29, 2000.

Christian BJ, D'Auria JP, Fox LC: Gaining freedom: self-responsibility in adolescents with diabetes, *Pediatr Nurs* 45(3):255-260, 1999.

Cohen WI: Health care guidelines for individuals with Down syndrome: 1999 revision, *Down Syndrome Q* 4(3):1-16, 1999.

Courville T, Caldwell B, Brunell P: Lack of evidence of transmission of HIV-I to family contacts of HIV-I infected children, *Clin Pediatr (Phila)* 37:175-178, 1998.

Cronister A, Schreiner R, Hittenberger M, et al: The heterozygous fragile X female: historical, physical, cognitive, and cytogenetic features, *Am J Med Genet* 38:269-274, 1991.

Dietz WH: Health consequences of obesity in youth: childhood predictors of adult disease, *Pediatrics* 101(3):518-524, 1998.

Edwards P et al: *Pediatric rehabilitation nursing,* Philadelphia, 1999, WB Saunders.

Eicher PS, Batshaw ML: Cerebral palsy, *Pediatr Clin North Am* 40(3):540-543, 1993.

Environmental Protection Agency: Document #800-B-92-0002, *Lead poisoning and your children,* Nov 9, 2000, Available online: http://www.epa.gov/iaq/pubs/lead.html. Accessed on Dec 1, 2000.

Faro B: The effect of diabetes on adolescents' quality of life, *Pediatr Nurs* 45(3):247-253, 1999.

Finberg L: *Saunders manual of pediatric practice,* Philadelphia, 1998, WB Saunders.

Fisher A, Vessey J: Prevention lead poisoning and its consequences, *Pediatr Nurs* 24(4):348-350, 1998.

Fryns JP, Haspeslagh M, Dereymaeker AM, et al: A peculiar subphenotype in the fragile X syndrome: extreme obesity, short stature, stubby hands and feet, diffuse hyperpigmentation. Further evidence of disturbed hypothalamic function in the fragile X syndrome? *Clin Genet* 32(6):388-392, 1987.

Gersh E: What is cerebral palsy? In Geralis E, editor: *Children with cerebral palsy: a parents' guide,* ed 2, Bethesda, Md, 1998, Woodbind House.

Gradow KD, Poling AG: *Pharmacotherapy and mental retardation,* Boston, 1988, College Hill Press.

Hagerman RJ: *Medication intervention in fragile X syndrome,* May 16, 2000, The National Fragile X Foundation, Available online: http://www.fragileX.org/html/medication.htm. Accessed on May 20, 2000.

Hagerman RJ: Fragile X syndrome, *Curr Probl Pediatr* 17:621-674, 1987.

Hagerman RJ, Amiri K, Cronister A: The fragile X checklist, *Am J Med Genet* 38:283-287, 1991.

Hagerman RJ et al: Fluoxetine therapy in fragile X syndrome, *Brain Res Dev Brain Res* 7:155-164, 1994.

Hagerman RJ et al: Institutional screening for the fragile X syndrome, *Am J Dis Children* 142:1216-1221, 1988.

Hagerman RJ, Kemper M, Hudson M: Learning disabilities and attentional problems in boys with the fragile X syndrome, *Am J Dis Children* 139:674-678, 1985.

Hodgson BB, Kizior RJ: *Saunders nursing drug handbook 2001,* Philadelphia, 2001, WB Saunders.

Jackson PL, Vessey JA: *Primary care of the child with a chronic condition,* ed 3, St Louis, 2000, Mosby.

Jones K: *Smith's recognizable patterns of human malformation,* ed 5, Philadelphia, 1997, WB Saunders.

King RA, Hagerman RJ, Houghton M: Ocular findings in fragile X syndrome, *Dev Brain Dis* 8:121-126, 1995.

Kuehr J, Frischer T, Meinert R, et al: Sensitization to mite allergens is a risk factor for early and late onset of asthma and for persistence of asthma in children, *J Clin Immunol* 95(3):655-662, 1995.

Lanphear BP et al: Community characteristics associated with elevated blood levels in children, *Pediatrics* 101(2):264-271, 1998.

Lewis KD: *Prenatal drug exposure: assessing risk,* Unpublished doctoral dissertation, 1998, University of California–San Francisco.

Lewis KD: *Infants and children with prenatal alcohol exposure: a guide to identification and intervention,* North Branch, Minn, 1995, Sunrise Press.

Luckman J: *Saunders manual of nursing care,* Philadelphia, 1997, WB Saunders.

Mahony DL, Murphy JM: Neonatal drug exposure: assessing a specific population and services provided by visiting nurses, *Pediatr Nurs* 25(1):27-36, 1999.

Maino DM, Schlange D, Maino JH, et al: Ocular anomalies in fragile X syndrome, *J Am Optom Assoc* 61:316-323, 1990.

Martinez FD, Wright AL, Taussig LM, et al: Asthma and wheezing in the first six years of life, The Group Health Medical Associates, *N Engl J Med* 332(3):133-138, 1995.

Mazzocco MM, Pennington BF, Hagerman RJ: The neurocognitive phenotype of female carriers of fragile X: additional evidence for specificity, *J Dev Behav Pediatr* 14:328-335, 1993.

McDonald M: Use of the ketogenic diet in treating children with seizures, *Pediatr Nurs* 23(5):461-464, 1997.

McDonough PG: Gonadal dysgenesis. In Quilligan EJ, Zuspan FP, editors: *Current therapy in obstetrics and gynecology,* vol 3, Philadelphia, 1990, WB Saunders.

Minear WL: A classification of cerebral palsy, *Pediatrics* 18(5):841-852, 1956.

Moore K, Persaud T: *The developing human,* Philadelphia, 1993, WB Saunders.

Mott S, James S, Sperhac M: *Nursing care of children and families,* ed 2, Menlo Park, Calif, 1990, Addison Wesley.

National Fragile X Foundation: *What is fragile X?* May 16, 2000, Available online: http://www.fragileX.org. Accessed on May 20, 2000.

National Asthma Education and Prevention Program: *Expert panel report 2: guidelines for the diagnosis and management of asthma,* NIH Pub No 97-4051, Bethesda, Md, 1997, National Heart, Lung, and Blood Institute (NHLBI), Available online: http://www.nhlbi.nih.gov/guidelines/asthma/asthgdln.htm. Accessed on July 20, 2001.

National Institute on Alcohol Abuse and Alcoholism: Fetal alcohol exposure and the brain, *Alcohol Alert* 50:1-4, 2000.

Nimmagadda S, Evans R: Allergy: etiology and epidemiology, *Pediatr Rev* 20(4):111-115, 1999.

Norris J: Weighing in on obesity, *UCSF Magazine,* Sept:32-63, 2000.

Nussbaum E: A question of gender, *Discover* 21(2):92-99, 2000.

O'Sullivan B: Asthma. In Roberts KB, editor: *Manual of clinical problems in pediatrics,* Philadelphia, 2001, Lippincott Williams & Wilkins.

O'Toole M, editor: *Miller-Keane encyclopedia and dictionary of medicine, nursing, and allied health,* ed 6, Philadelphia, 1997, WB Saunders.

Oberle I, Rousseau F, Heitz D, et al: Instability of a 550-base pair DNA segment and abnormal methylation in fragile X syndrome, *Science* 252(5010):1097-1102, 1991.

Partington MW: The fragile X syndrome: preliminary data on growth and development in males, *Am J Med Genet* 17:175-194, 1984.

Phelps L: *Health-related disorders in children and adolescents: a compilation of 96 rare and common disorders,* Washington, DC, 1999, American Psychological Association.

Purves D, Augustine G, Fitzpatrick D, et al, editors: *Neuroscience,* Sunderland, Mass, 1997, Sinauer Associates.

Rakel R: *Saunders manual of medical practice,* Philadelphia, 1996, WB Saunders.

Richardson GA, Day NL, Goldschmidt L: Prenatal alcohol, marijuana, and tobacco use: infant mental and motor development, *Neurotoxicol Teratol* 17:479-487, 1995.

Robinson TN: Reducing children's television viewing to prevent obesity: a randomized controlled trial, *JAMA* 282(16):1561-1567, 1999.

Rossiter K, Diehl S: Gender reassignment in children: ethical conflicts in surrogate decision making, *Pediatr Nurs* 24(1):59-62, 1998.

Rousseau F, Rouillard P, Morel ML, et al: Prevalence of carriers of permutation-size alleles of the FMRI gene—and implications for the population genetics of the fragile X syndrome, *Am J Hum Genet* 57(5):1006-1018, 1995.

Rudkin CL: Vegetarian planning for adolescents with diabetes, *Pediatr Nurs* 45(3):262-266, 1999.

Rutgers JL: Advances in the pathology of intersex conditions, *Hum Pathol* 22:884, 1991.

Scharfenaker S, Hickman L, Braden M: An integrated approach to intervention with fragile X individuals. In Hagerman RJ, Silverman AC, editors: *Fragile X syndrome: diagnosis, treatment, and research,* Baltimore, 1991, Johns Hopkins University Press.

Scharfenaker S, Schreiner R: Cognitive and speech language characteristics of the fragile X syndrome, *Rocky Mountain Journal of Communication Disorders* 4:25-27, 1989.

Schopmeyer BB, Lowe F, editors: *The fragile X child,* San Diego, 1992, Singular Publishing Group.

Sheldon SH: Pro-convulsant effects of oral melatonin in neurologically disabled children, *Lancet* 351:1254, 1998.

Siberry G, Iannone R, editors: *The Harriet Lane handbook,* ed 15, St Louis, 2000, Mosby.

Sifton DW, editor: *Physician's desk reference,* Montvale, NJ, 2000, Medical Economics.

Sobesky WE, Pennington BF, Porter D, et al: Emotional and neurocognitive deficits in fragile X, *Am J Med Genet* 51(4):378-384, 1994.

Stiehm ER, Lambert JS, Mofenson LM, et al: Efficacy of zidovudine and human immunodeficiency virus (HIV) transmission from HIV-infected women with advanced disease: results of pediatric AIDS clinical trials group protocol 185, *J Infect Dis* 179(3):567-575, 1999.

Sullivan K: Japan's cartoon violence: TV networks criticized after children's seizures, *Washington Post Foreign Service,* p D01, Dec 17, 1997.

Turk J: Fragile X syndrome and folic acid. In Hagerman RJ, McKenzie P, editors: *International fragile X conference proceedings,* Dillon, Colo, 1992, The National Fragile X Foundation and Spectra Publishing.

Troiano RP, Flegal K: Overweight children and adolescence: description, epidemiology, and demographics, *Pediatrics* 101(3):497-504, 1998.

United States Center for Health Statistics: *Overweight prevalence,* July 10, 2001, Available online: http://www.cdc.gov/nchs/fastats/overwt.htm. Accessed on Aug 10, 2001.

United States Department of Health and Human Services, Public Health Service: Identifying the needs of drug-affected children: public policy issues, *Office for Substance Abuse and Prevention Monograph 11,* Rockville, Md, 1992, Office for Substance Abuse and Prevention.

Vaisse C, Clement K, Durand E, et a1: Melanocortin-4 receptor mutations are a frequent and heterogenous cause of morbid obesity, *J Clin Invest* 106(2):253-262, 2000.

Verkerk AJ, Pieretti M, Sutcliffe JS, et a1: Identification of a gene (FMR-I) containing a CGG repeat coincident with a breakpoint cluster region exhibiting length variation in fragile X syndrome, *Cell* 65(5):905-914, 1991.

Walters MC, Patience M, Leisenring W, et al: Bone marrow transplantation for sickle cell disease, *N Engl J Med* 335(6):369-376, 1996.

Williams JO, Achterberg C, Sylvester G: *Prevention, treatment of childhood obesity,* New York, 1995, River Press.

Wong DL, Hockenberry-Eaton M, Wilson D, et al: *Nursing care of infants and children,* ed 6, St Louis, 1999, Mosby.

Yu S, Pritchard M, Kremer E, et al: Fragile X genotype characterized by an unstable region of DNA, *Science* 252(5010):1179-1181, 1991.

CHAPTER 5

Affective and Behavioral Disorders

*A*ffective and behavioral disorders have a significant impact on cognitive and perceptional abilities such as decision making, language, memory, concentration, impulse control, prosocial behavior, and self-esteem. Disabilities in any of these areas can affect the school performance and school life of a child or adolescent. Current brain research provides data regarding the areas of brain involved and the association to learning as it relates to these disorders.

Assessment and knowledge of the various domains that condition the learning process, such as perceptual, cognitive, sensory, neurological, psychosocial, and moral, are essential to nursing intervention that provides an optimal educational experience for the student. Child-centered nursing interventions realistically accept the genetic and predisposing conditions that cause these disorders, but nurturing, socialization, education, and acculturation in the educational context also are important. The school nurse plays a vital role in the assessment, diagnosis, educational planning, and remediation of learning problems caused by these disorders present at school.

ATTENTION DEFICIT HYPERACTIVITY DISORDER

I. **Definition**
  A. Attention deficit hyperactivity disorder (ADHD) is one of the most common childhood disorders, occurring in approximately 3% to 10% of children (Barkley, 1990, 1997; Goldman et al, 1998).
  B. They lack sustained attention and may be overactive and impulsive. ADHD is more common in males and generally is diagnosed before age 7. *Diagnostic and Statistical Manual of Mental Disorders,* 4th edition (DSM-IV) diagnosis requires at least 6 symptoms of inattention and at least 6 symptoms of hyperactivity/impulsivity of more than 6 months' duration in two settings. Prior terminology includes minimal brain damage (MBD), minimal brain dysfunction, and hyperactivity.

II. **Etiology**
  A. ADHD has been associated with genetic factors and neuroanatomical abnormalities in the brain that are known to regulate motor and attention behaviors. Psychosocial, emotional, and environmental-exacerbating factors include depression, anxiety, coercive discipline, lack of consistency, exposure to media violence, parental unsociable behaviors or marital conflict, abuse, and neglect. Symptoms of hyperactivity or inattention can be secondary to medications (e.g., theophylline, albuterol, phenobarbital).

III. *Brain Findings*
  A. ADHD is associated with poor regulation of the neurotransmitters dopamine and norepinephrine in the frontal lobe and basal ganglia.

These two areas have been reported to be 10% smaller in children with ADHD and are associated with focusing attention, inhibiting behaviors, and blocking distractions.

IV. **Characteristics**
   A. Inattention and distractibility: difficulty in organizing, tendency to lose things, makes careless mistakes, does not understand instructions or follow instructions that require mental effort.
   B. Selective attention: focuses on something he or she wants or enjoys.
   C. Hyperactive: squirms and fidgets in seat, climbs and moves about when inappropriate, talks excessively.
   D. Impulsive: interrupts conversation, difficulty taking turns, blurts out answers, talks or acts without thinking.
   E. One third have specific learning disorders, one third have conduct problems, and others may have poor self-esteem, depression, and anxiety.
   F. Associated symptoms may include motor coordination difficulties, disruptive sleep, susceptible to multiple accidents, and poisoning.

V. **Effects on Individual**
   A. Difficulty maintaining friendships, social immaturity.
   B. Poor academic performance may result in grade retention and potential school dropout.
   C. Accident-prone because of impulsivity.
   D. World is confusing because of multiple sensory distractions.
   E. Engages in socially unacceptable behaviors.
   F. Poor self-esteem because of lack of success and rewards caused by inappropriate behaviors.
   G. Frequent daydreaming and excessive boredom.
   H. Difficulty achieving long-term goals.
   I. Strained family and peer relationships.
   J. Problems with driving (e.g., impulsivity combined with poor judgment, resulting in more than average traffic citations, especially speeding and accidents).
   K. Susceptible to drug abuse.

VI. **Health Concerns/Emergencies**
   A. Frequent visits to school nurse office with psychosomatic complaints.
   B. Poor weight gain, with or without stimulant medications.
   C. Higher risk for accidents or poisonings.

VII. **Management/Treatment**
   A. Rule out hearing loss or visual impairment.
   B. Address psychosocial stressors that contribute to physical symptoms (e.g., parental relationship, conflicts).
   C. When weight gain is slow, encourage increased caloric intake.
   D. Various diets and nutritional supplements are advocated by family or practitioners, but research on effectiveness is inconclusive.
   E. Monitor growth patterns every 6 months when taking medications that may suppress appetite and growth.
   F. Pharmacological management effective in 70%-75% of children.

G. Liaison with parents and physician regarding effectiveness and side effects of medications.

H. Provide listening, nonjudgmental ear to parents.

I. Screen for and address learning disorders, which are present in one third of children with ADHD.

J. Focus on positive behaviors and find ways to increase child's motivation.

K. Ensure proper supervision.

VIII. **Additional Information**

A. In 1991, ADHD was recognized as a qualifying disability for special education services by Part B of the Individuals with Disabilities Education Act (IDEA) and/or Section 504.

B. Progressive or static neurological disease is ruled out before diagnosis (e.g., Tourette's syndrome, absence seizures, fragile X syndrome). Treatment usually is multimodal and may include behavioral modifications using positive reinforcements, anger management and social skills training, and sensory integration therapy. Less validated modalities include vision therapy, electroencephalographic (EEG) biofeedback or neurofeedback (i.e., training the brain to increase the type of brain activity associated with sustained attention). Restricted diets (e.g., Feingold) may be used. Most common diet restrictions are sugars, additives, and preservatives to eliminate possible allergens. Works best in children younger than 5 years and those with food or food additive allergies. Nutritional supplements include liquid calcium and vitamin B complex to calm the nervous system or choline, which may improve memory and attention span.

C. Generally, ADHD persists into adulthood. The prognosis is negatively affected by family history of ADHD, children raised in a disruptive family environment, and a comorbid condition (e.g., conduct disorders, anxiety, mood disorders). Adolescents with ADHD taking stimulant medication cannot enlist in the armed services without a medical waiver even if the medications have been discontinued. Career choices generally are not affected by ADHD, and many adults are successful in their chosen occupation.

IX. **Web Sites**

Attention Deficit Disorder Association (ADDA)
1-800-487-2282
http://www.add.org
Children and Adults with Attention Deficit Disorder (CHADD)
1-800-233-4050
http://www.chadd.org

OPPOSITIONAL DEFIANT DISORDER

I. **Definition**

A. Oppositional defiant disorder (ODD) is a negative, hostile, defiant, disobedient pattern of behavior lasting at least 6 months and includes 4 of the following symptoms: frequent loss of temper; arguments with

Table 5-1   Medications for Attention Deficit Hyperactivity Disorder/Hyperactivity

Drug	Action	Side Effects	Considerations
Methylphenidate (Ritalin) Ritalin SR Methylphenidate (Concerta)	Mild CNS stimulant Duration: 3½-4 hr Duration: 6-8 hr Duration: 12 hr Uses osmotic pressure to release immediate dose from outer layer; inner layer sustains effect throughout school day Technologically controlled dose rate	Anorexia, insomnia, weight loss, reduced growth rate, nervousness, headache, palpitations, angina, tachycardia, dermatitis, thrombocytopenia, increased tics and seizures, Tourette's syndrome, seizure, possibility of psychological addiction Increased levels of TCAs Additional side effects for Concerta: URTI, increased cough, sore throat, sinusitis, vomiting, dizziness	Avoid decongestants, drinks containing caffeine Better when taken after lunch than before lunch Advise not to chew or cut sustained-release tablets Monitor blood pressure, pulse, height, and weight
Pemoline (Cylert)	CNS stimulant, structurally different than Ritalin Duration: 6-8 hr	Acute hepatic failure, insomnia, Tourette's syndrome, seizures, aplastic anemia, long-term growth retardation	Take 6 hr before bedtime May lower seizure threshold Liver function studies before starting and every 6 mo
Dextroamphetamine (Dexedrine) tablets, elixir, spansules (sustained-release) Methamphetamine (Desoxyn) 4 amphetamine salts (Adderall)	CNS stimulants Duration: 6-8 hr	Nervousness, tics, anorexia, weight loss, insomnia, dysphoria, tremor, dizziness, headache, chills, dry mouth, GI disturbances, urticaria, addiction (only in those with predisposition)	Take 6 hr before bedtime Avoid caffeine Risk of abuse Monitor blood pressure, pulse, height, and weight Report signs of excessive stimulation

Continued

CNS, Central nervous system; GI, gastrointestinal; TCA, tricyclic antidepressant; URTI, upper respiratory tract infection.
NOTE: Some medications used to treat children are not approved for child/adolescent psychiatry by the FDA. However, some are being tried in ADHD and Tourette's syndrome (Zito et al, 2000). Some drugs are used to treat comorbid conditions (e.g., depression, oppositional and conduct disorders). Effects of long-term use of psychotropic drugs on the developing brain of a child are unknown; thus caution in their use is critical.

Table 5-1   *Medications for Attention Deficit Hyperactivity Disorder/Hyperactivity—cont'd*

Drug	Action	Side Effects	Considerations
Methylphenidate (Methylin)	CNS stimulant Presumed to activate arousal system and cortex, which produces stimulant effect	Anorexia, insomnia, weight loss, reduced growth rate, nervousness, headache, palpitations, angina, tachycardia, dermatitis, thrombocytopenia, increased tics, seizures, possibility of psychological addiction	Take before meals Monitor blood pressure, pulse, height, and weight Prolonged therapy requires routine CBC, differential, and platelet counts
Imipramine (Tofranil) Desipramine (Norpramin) Nortriptyline (Aventyl)	Increases amount of norepinephrine, serotonin, or both in CNS by blocking reuptake by presynaptic neurons (TCAs)	Increased levels of TCAs Cardiac arrhythmias, especially with overdose Dizziness, sedation, blurred vision, difficult urination, dry mouth, constipation, urine retention, diaphoresis, seizures Flulike illness if stopped suddenly	ECGs before and during treatment Blood levels when applicable Suicide risk Reduce dosage in adolescence Do not stop abruptly Discontinue before surgery Photosensitivity (use sunblock)
Clonidine (Catapres)	Antihypertension Duration: 4-6 hr	Sedation, dry mouth, drowsiness, dizziness, weakness, rebound hypertension if abruptly stopped, constipation	Monitor blood pressure, pulse If given with stimulants, Ritalin, associated with cardiac problems in children
Bupropion (Wellbutrin)	Weak inhibitor of dopamine, serotonin, and norepinephrine reuptake Antidepressant	Headache, seizures, confusion, insomnia, sedation, tremors, dizziness, fatigue, dry mouth, blurred vision, constipation, tachycardia and arrhythmias, auditory disturbances, agitation, irritability	Monitor pulse Generally avoid if seizures present, bulimic, or if positive family history of seizures

CBC, Complete blood cell count; *CNS,* central nervous system; *ECG,* electrocardiogram; *TCA,* tricyclic antidepressant.

adults; deliberate annoyance, active defiance, or refusal of adult requests; spiteful or vindictive manner; touchy and easily annoyed; anger and resentment and blaming of others (American Psychiatric Association, 1994). Comorbid conditions include learning problems, depressed moods, hyperactivity, and addictive behaviors.

II. Etiology

A. Common in families with mood disorders, serious marital discord, history of child physical or sexual maltreatment and harsh or inconsistent discipline, or succession of multiple caregivers. Often observed before age 8. More common among boys before puberty, but gender distribution is fairly equal thereafter. Some also may have a conduct disorder (e.g., pattern of acts against people or social rules).

III. *Brain Findings*

A. Studies suggest dopamine, serotonin, and noradrenaline play a role in ODD, with the most significant impact caused by noradrenaline. Research is lacking in comparison of the number of children with this disorder.

IV. Characteristics

A. Difficulty being comforted or soothed and high motor reactivity during early childhood.

B. Defiant, annoying, spiteful, vindictive, resentful, argumentative behaviors lasting more than 6 months.

C. Stubbornness, resistance to directions, unwillingness to compromise, testing of limits, and usually unable to accept blame.

D. Oppositional behaviors tend to increase with age.

E. Symptoms same in both genders, but male students have more persistent symptoms and confrontational behaviors.

F. Aggression generally verbal rather than physical for conduct disorder.

G. Behaviors usually manifest in the home and may not be observed in the school or community.

H. Often is present in association with other conditions (e.g., ADHD, depression, anxiety).

V. Effects on Individual

A. Affects school achievement and social success.

B. Peer rejection leading to social isolation.

C. Negative appearance to parents and teachers, thereby stigmatizing student.

D. Possible precursor to conduct disorder and later antisocial personality, delinquency, and potential future criminality.

E. Risk indicator of potential school dropout.

F. Possibility of strained family relationships.

VI. Health Concerns and Emergencies

A. Dependent on severity of symptoms.

B. Monitoring of medication for hyperactivity or other symptoms.

C. Child abuse potential by parents, staff, or both; includes both verbal and physical abuse.

D. Sustained high cortisol levels (stress hormones) contribute to compromised immune system, with resultant vulnerability to infections.

VII. Management/Treatment

A. Rule out hearing loss as cause for failure to follow directions.

B. Monitor blood pressure, pulse, and weight.

C. Observe for depression or other comorbid conditions.

D. Set limits and be consistent during any interactions.

E. Clear limits and consequences are difficult because these children are affected more by the emotion of the moment and do not seem to care about the consequences.

F. Reinforce socially acceptable behaviors.

G. Provide staff education regarding disorder and behavior management.

H. Support limiting television viewing and video and CD use that includes violence.

I. Encourage positive parenting and behavioral approach.

TIC DISORDERS AND TOURETTE'S DISORDER

I. Definition

A. Tics are the most common childhood movement disorder; various muscle groups are affected. Tics often are classified according to age of onset, duration and severity of symptoms, and presence of vocal and motor tics. Tourette's disorder is a hereditary, neurological movement disorder characterized by repetitive, uncontrolled vocal and motor tics. It is usually first observed between the ages of 2 and 10. Comorbid conditions are behavioral and learning disabilities (e.g., ADHD, depression, anxiety, mood swings, obsessive-compulsive traits or disorders). Tics can occur sporadically, change in character, and often are changed by the person into something that appears like a "real" thing (e.g., a head touch into a hair twirl, a guttural noise into a swear word).

II. Etiology

A. Tics can be genetic or occur as a result of brain insult, long-term use of antipsychotic drugs, and disease processes (e.g., encephalitis). Tics occur in up to 24% of children (Erenberg, 1998). Tourette's disorder is inherited and occurs in 4 to 5 of 10,000; ratio is 4:1 male/female (American Psychiatric Association, 1994).

III. *Brain Findings*

A. Tic disorders and Tourette's disorder are associated with abnormalities in the genes that affect the metabolism of the neurotransmitters, primarily dopamine, serotonin, and norepinephrine. Usually occurs in the area of the basal ganglia (with increased activity of dopamine receptors in the caudate nucleus). The caudate nucleus is an area in the brain that inhibits purposeless movements. The cells may either produce too much or release excess dopamine or are oversensitive to the neurotransmitters, which results in release of inhibited urges or tics. The exact mechanisms of this process are unknown.

IV. Characteristics

A. Symptoms may wax or wane over time, making diagnosis difficult.

B. Motor tics are both simple (e.g., eye twitches or blinks, grimaces, head jerk, shoulder shrug) and complex (e.g., smelling objects, mimicking movements of another person [echopraxia], such as head shaking, repeated kicking movements). The activities appear purposeful and coordinated but are involuntary.

C. Vocal tics include clearing the throat, grunting or barking noises, outbursts of nonsensical sounds or obscene words (coprolalia, 5%), repetition of words said by others (echolalia), and repetition of one's own words (papilalia). Vocal tics may be simple (throat clearing and grunting, vocal sounds) or complex (stammering, stuttering, swearing, more words).

D. Rare symptoms include lip and cheek biting, head banging, and other self-abusive behaviors.

E. Tics are increased by fatigue and physical and mental stress, but in some people manifest more when in a relaxed state.

F. Reduced or absent during sleep.

G. Tics may be suppressed for a brief period but eventually escape.

H. Tics can be exacerbated by seasonal or life changes (e.g., holidays) but tend to decrease with age.

I. Tics generally improve after puberty; 20%-30% are symptom-free by their 20s.

J. Associated traits include obsession, compulsion, hyperactivity, impulsivity, inattentiveness, anxiety, depression, and learning disability. These neuropsychiatric symptoms may increase with age.

K. Treating one disorder may worsen another (e.g., stimulant for hyperactivity may increase tics).

L. Intelligence is not impaired.

M. Found in all ethnic groups or races but is rare in African Americans.

V. **Effects on Individual**

A. Social stigma, embarrassment and shame, self-consciousness, low self-esteem, feelings of peer rejection, social isolation.

B. If severe, can interfere with daily activities (e.g., reading, writing, classroom concentration).

C. Side effects of medication create resistance to medication compliance.

D. Some side effects, such as muscular rigidity, drooling, tremors, slow movement, and restlessness, interfere with class participation and peer acceptance.

E. Possibility of strained family relationships.

F. Some individuals with most involved symptomatology can achieve outstanding social, vocational, and academic success.

VI. **Health Concerns/Emergencies**

A. Vary according to involvement and medications.

B. Complex medication management creates possibility of negative drug interactions.

C. Medications for one symptom can create or exacerbate other symptoms.

D. Weight gain secondary to medication.

VII. **Management/Treatment**

A. Identification of severe stressors to minimize impact whenever possible.

B. Awareness of medications, side effects, and contraindications.

C. Medications used most frequently include haloperidol (Haldol), pimozide (Orap), clonazepam (Klonopin), fluphenazine (Prolixin), clonidine (Catapres), and thiothixene (Navane). Often medicated for ADHD, obsessive-compulsive disorder (OCD), anxiety, or depression. Be aware of side effects and contraindications.

D. Monitoring of height and weight.

E. Classroom and staff teaching important to develop peer and adult knowledge, understanding, and support.

F. Distinguish between student misbehavior and disorder symptoms and manage appropriately.

G. Extended time and privacy may be needed during testing.

H. If student's movements are disruptive, nurse should consider that they are involuntary; use strategies for the moment; be calm to reduce student's stress and decrease tics.

I. Psychotherapy, especially cognitive behavioral therapy, may be helpful.

VIII. **Additional Information**

A. Transient tic disorder.

1. Transient tics usually do not last more than a year; recurrent episodes over the course of a few years are not uncommon. They last only weeks or months and usually are not associated with learning or behavioral problems. Transient tic symptoms include eye blinking, nose puckering, grimacing, and squinting. Vocalizations are less common and include humming or other mouth or throat sounds. Other bizarre behaviors occur (e.g., poking and pinching of the genitals, palm licking).

B. Chronic motor or vocal tic disorder.

1. Chronic tics are motor or vocal but not both. Tics may be single or multiple and last more than a year without more than 3 consecutive tic-free months.

SCHOOL AVOIDANCE AND SCHOOL PHOBIA

I. **Definition**

A. A generalized anxiety or a fixed fear associated with attending an educational facility. The school fear can be a transient, situational problem (school avoidance) or intransient pervasive disorder (school phobia). School avoidance is a developmental challenge for a preschooler leaving home for kindergarten and a social challenge for an adolescent who becomes school phobic. By definition, *truancy* (absence from school) generally is a behavioral problem, not a phobia (see "Additional Information").

II. **Etiology**

A. A multitude of causes and conditions exist for these fearful or phobic behaviors. For the elementary-age child, the psychosocial issues may be separation anxiety from a caregiver, apprehension about new surroundings and strangers, or dislike of a problem person such as a peer bully or an overly harsh or strict teacher. Often the young student has an avoidant reaction to school arising from dependency on an overprotective and possessive parent.

B. School phobia in adolescence is more likely associated with a social withdrawal syndrome, an underlying depressive disorder, or both factors. School phobia may lead to social isolation in reaction to peer ostracism or radical nonconformity to peer norms.

C. School phobia is more common for students 10 years of age and older. The onset is usually sudden and precipitated by a school-related incident. Occurrence is rare, affecting approximately 2% of the school population (Martin, Waltman-Greenwood, and Novotny, 1995).

III. **Characteristics**

A. Lack of social skills.

B. Major life change (e.g., family grief, acute medical illness, divorce, loss of peer playmate or companion).

C. Expression of shyness may be a precursor to a social phobia.

D. Conduct disordered youth experiencing peer rejection.

E. Fixed learning disabilities evidenced by chronic frustration and underachievement that represent failure or avoidance.

F. Unrealistic parental standards for the student's academic and social standing, leading to feelings of inadequacy.

IV. **Effects on Individual**

A. Stress symptoms such as anxiety, panic states, and psychosomatic illness (e.g., nausea, vomiting, diarrhea, dizziness, headache, abdominal pain).

B. Behavioral regression to lower development.

C. Overreliance on parents or adult caregivers.

D. Diminished self-confidence and ability to take risks.

E. School absenteeism.

F. Development of perfectionist attitudes and procrastinating habits.

G. Educational underachievement.

H. Social isolation.

I. School dropout.

V. **Health Concerns/Emergencies**

A. An acute health problem or emergency at home may not result in immediate medical care (e.g., drug or medication overdose).

B. While at home, student may overeat, have lack of exercise, loss of educational knowledge, fall behind academically; all are secondary complications leading to medical and social problems.

VI. **Management/Treatment**

A. Assess for underlying physical problems (e.g., vision, hearing, undetected or untreated physical injury or illness, fatigue related to nutritional deficiency, sleep deprivation).

B. Assess for psychosocial, emotional, and mental problems (e.g., depression, drug and alcohol abuse).

C. Evaluate familial/home issues (e.g., Munchausen's syndrome by proxy, parental depression, parental criminal behaviors, child abuse, lack of parental motivation).

D. Parental guidance related to dependence/independence issues.
E. Discern/differentiate stress symptoms requiring assurance and tender loving care (TLC) versus medical model treatment, such as rest and medication.
F. Referral for appropriate follow-up (e.g., psychosocial or emotional intervention, grief counseling, evaluation of learning disabilities, treatment with antianxiety medications).
G. Help child gain a sense of control and problem-solving skills for personal development.
H. Reprogramming of irrational fears and desensitization training.
I. Make school friendly, positive, and rewarding for student (e.g., by assigning duties in health office or making peer counseling referral).

VII. **Additional Information**
A. No formal DSM-IV diagnostic category exists for school phobia. However, associated diagnoses include separation anxiety disorder, adjustment disorders, social phobia, ODD, and early-onset dysthymia.
B. School truancy is a choice of the student to be noncompliant with requirements to attend school (e.g., willful disobedience, conduct disorder, antisocial behavior).
C. School avoidance is an absence caused by evasion or self-perceived barriers for school attendance by the student (e.g., not being safe, being bullied in school). School avoidance may lead to school phobia.
D. School phobia is an absence from school because of a fixed, chronic, focal fear.
E. Delineation of the above categories or differential diagnosis depends on the severity of the problem, secondary complications, and length of absenteeism.

PERVASIVE DEVELOPMENTAL DISORDERS

AUTISM

I. **Definition**
A. Autism is a disorder involving impairments in language, social communication, social interactions, and repetitive and stereotyped behaviors that manifests in one of these areas before age 3 as defined by the DSM-IV. The distinguishing behavior is relative lack of interest in other persons.

II. **Etiology**
A. This disorder is elusive; however, strong evidence exists for a genetic component, organic cause, or both. The prevalence rate is 4-50 in 10,000. More boys are affected than girls, generally reported to be a 4:1 ratio. Autism is associated with fragile X syndrome with tuberous sclerosis and a family history of similar disorders, depression, and OCD. Chromosomes 7 and 15 have been implicated as causative factors. Hoxa 1 (a gene) is lacking in chromosome 7, which plays a central role in the development of the brainstem, which is shorter in these children. Gamma-aminobutyric acid (GABA) research found that the chromosome 15 gene recognizes this chemical signal and is associated with one type of autism (Rodier, 2000).

III. *Brain Findings*
   A. Although the following findings vary in their level of replicated certainty, they offer compelling hypothesis about the nature of autism spectrum disorders. Unusually high levels of four specific proteins associated with brain development have been reported in children with autism, whereas these levels were normal in the control group. Parts of the frontal lobe are thicker than normal; this region controls decision making and planning. Neuron cells in the limbic system where emotions are processed are plentiful but are one third smaller than normal and immature with incomplete connections. Cerebellum cells are reduced by 30%-50%, affecting the cerebellum's ability to assist in making predictions of ensuing thoughts, emotions, and motor movements. Purkinje's cells, which are essential to the wiring of the cerebellum, are 10% to 40% of normal number in persons with autism. These cells inhibit action of other neurons.

IV. Characteristics
   A. Social communication.
      1. Delayed onset of intentional communication, both verbal and nonverbal (e.g., babbling, gesturing, head nods), poor eye contact. Some never gain useful communicative skills.
      2. Unusual language if acquired (e.g., echolalia, pronoun reversal, literal or concrete use of words, peculiar voice intonation [monotone or singsong]).
   B. Social interactions.
      1. Inability or significant difficulty in developing relationships; inability to recognize and respond to social cues; aversion to touch and cuddling; flat affect; persistent tantrums.
      2. Inability or great difficulty using facial expressions or gestures for regulation of social interactions.
   C. Restricted and repetitive behaviors and interests.
      1. Insistence on routine and sameness, narrow range of interests, bizarre attachment and inappropriate use of objects, intense preoccupation with activity or object.
      2. Motor disturbances, arm flapping, whirling, rocking, toe walking, repetitive hand and finger mannerisms, and head banging.
      3. Atypical responses to sensory stimuli (e.g., sound, pain, cold, heat).
   D. Other.
      1. Symptoms vary considerably in severity. A few children have exceptional skills in specific areas (e.g., memory, calendar calculation, solving puzzles, art, music) and are called *savants*. Other high-functioning children may do well in regular classrooms with support.
      2. Approximately 75% function at retarded level (American Psychiatric Association, 1994).
      3. Difficulty in generalizing knowledge/skills, reasoning or symbolic thinking, verbal concept formation, and integration skills.
      4. Strengths in visuospatial processing, rote learning, and memory skills.

V. Effects on Individual

    A. Negative or impaired family relationships.

    B. Few if any peer relationships because of indifference, oblivious social behavior, or inability to empathize. Interactive or parallel play almost nonexistent.

    C. Actions inadvertently may provoke anger in others.

    D. Social isolation and ostracism, vulnerable to peer harassment and bullying.

    E. Difficulty in learning because of lack of imitation and unresponsiveness to social reinforcement.

    F. Personal safety at risk because of impulsive, disorganized motor activity.

    G. Overwhelmed by own nervous system, resulting in heightened sensitivity to stimuli and uncontrollable repetitive actions.

    H. Sleep disorders.

VI. Health Concerns/Emergencies

    A. Seizures occur in 15%-35%. Peak of onset in early childhood and again in adolescence.

    B. Hyposensitivity or hypersensitivity to pain, noise, touch, and so forth.

    C. Poor nutrition because of limited food preferences. May ingest inedible substances.

    D. May express affection but indiscriminately, leading to potential child abuse.

    E. Often medicated with sedatives or tranquilizers.

VII. Management/Treatment

    A. Rule out hearing loss.

    B. Behavioral management as part of daily routine; use simple language, provide visual and verbal cues when making transitions, be mindful of child's sensory profile, especially hypersensitivity to sound or touch.

    C. Monitor medications and side effects. Selective serotonin reuptake inhibitors (SSRIs), such as fluoxetine (Prozac), sertraline (Zoloft), clomipramine (Anafranil), fluvoxamine (Luvox), and citalopram (Celexa), are used to treat children with stereotypical behaviors but are not approved by the Food and Drug Administration (FDA) for autism. SSRI medications inhibit reuptake of serotonin, which promotes increased serotonin activity and benefits some children by improving behaviors. Ritalin and other stimulants are used for hyperactivity; vitamin B_6 with magnesium may be used to stimulate brain activity but studies are inconclusive; antipsychotics also are used.

    D. Monitor injuries or self-abuse because of high pain threshold.

    E. Monitor weight.

    F. Monitor nutrition and diet; vitamins and food supplements may be needed because of strong but limited food preferences. Monitor lead levels because children with autism are known to eat inedible items, such as paint chips.

G. Data reveal a reduction of the amino acid tryptophan, a precursor to serotonin, which may interfere with serotonin synthesis. Serotonin is produced in the brain, thyroid gland, and gastrointestinal (GI) tract and affects mood, aggressive behavior, anxiety, memory, neural development, pain, repetitive behaviors, and sleep. Tryptophan is found in certain foods (e.g., beef, chicken, turkey, broccoli, brussel sprouts, eggs, fish, milk, nuts, fennel).

H. Diagnosis usually is made by taking a careful history, doing a communication assessment, and performing a psychological evaluation with tests not highly dependent on verbal abilities.

VIII. **Additional Information**

A. Much of the outcome data were collected before the 1980s when fewer services were available and intervention usually was not started until school years. Long-term outcome may improve with earlier identification and mandated services. Early risk indicators include no babbling or gesturing by 12 months, no single words by 16 months, no two-word spontaneous phrases by 24 months, and any loss of any language or social skills at any age. Assessments for autism are provided later in this text (see Chapter 9).

B. The educational focus for children with autism is to decrease unacceptable behaviors and increase social awareness and verbal communication. Important elements in the classroom include predictability and routine, assistance with transition, and family involvement. Multiple treatment approaches are used, including behavioral modification, which focuses on learning specific behaviors through repetition; teaching of more global behaviors that will affect a wide range of other behaviors (pivotal behaviors); interactive play with adults or peers; and provision of sensory integration or sensory processing therapy.

C. Examples of educational intervention techniques include Treatment and Education of Autistic and Communication Handicapped Children (TEACCH); Floor Time/Interactive Play Therapy; Facilitated Developmentally Integrated Free Play; Applied Behavioral Analysis/Discrete Trials; Pivotal Response Training; Sensory Integration/Sensory Processing; Picture Exchange Communication System (PECS).

IX. **Web Sites**

Autism Society of America
1-800-3-AUTISM
http://www.autism-society.org
Cure Autism Now (CAN)
1-888-8-AUTISM
http://www.canfoundation.org
Center for Study of Autism
http://www.autism.org
Child Development Institute
714-998-8617
http://www.cdipage.com

Box 5-1   *DSM-IV Criteria: Autistic Disorder*

A. Total of six or more items from 1, 2, and 3, with at least two from 1, and one each from 2 and 3:
1. Qualitative impairment in social interaction, as manifested by at least two of the following:
   a. Marked impairment in the use of multiple nonverbal behaviors, such as eye-to-eye-gaze, facial expression, body postures, and gestures to regulate social interaction.
   b. Failure to develop peer relationships appropriate to developmental level.
   c. A lack of spontaneous seeking to share enjoyment, interests, or achievements with other people (e.g., by a lack of showing, bringing, or pointing out objects of interest).
   d. Lack of social emotional reciprocity.
2. Qualitative impairments in communication as manifested by at least one of the following:
   a. Delay in, or total lack of, the development of spoken language (not accompanied by an attempt to compensate through alternative modes of communication such as gestures or mime).
   b. In individuals with adequate speech, marked impairment in the ability to initiate or sustain a conversation with others.
   c. Stereotyped and repetitive use of language or idiosyncratic language.
   d. Lack of varied, spontaneous make-believe play or social imitative play appropriate to developmental level.
3. Restricted repetitive and stereotyped pattern of behavior, interests, and activities, as manifested by at least one of the following:
   a. Encompassing preoccupation with one or more stereotyped patterns of interest that is abnormal either in intensity or focus.
   b. Apparently inflexible adherence to specific, nonfunctional routines or rituals.
   c. Stereotyped and repetitive motor mannerisms (e.g., hand or finger flapping or twisting, or complex whole-body movements).
   d. Persistent preoccupation with parts of objects.
B. Delays or abnormal functioning in at least one of the following areas, with onset before age 3 years:
1. Social interaction
2. Language as used in social communication
3. Symbolic or imaginative play
C. The disturbance is not better accounted for by Rett syndrome or childhood disintegrative disorder.
1. Qualitative impairment in social interaction (e.g., impairment in nonverbal behaviors, failure to develop peer relationships, lack of social or emotional reciprocity).
2. Qualitative impairments in communication (e.g., delay or lack of spoken language, inability to initiate or sustain a conversation, stereotyped and repetitive use of language, lack of varied make-believe play).
3. Restricted, repetitive, and stereotyped patterns of behavior, interests, and activities, including motor stereotypes and mannerisms.
D. The disturbance is not better accounted for by another specific pervasive developmental disorder or by schizophrenia.

From the *Diagnostic and statistical manual of mental disorders,* ed 4, revision, Washington, DC, 1994, American Psychiatric Association.

ASPERGER'S SYNDROME

I. Definition
  A. Asperger's syndrome is considered a form of high-functioning autism, and individuals generally display a full range of intellect. Deficits in social interaction and unusual repetitive, stereotyped patterns and behaviors are observed.

II. Etiology
  A. Asperger's syndrome is believed to be hereditary because many families report an "odd" relative or two. Onset may occur later than in autism. The condition is more frequent in males.

III. Characteristics
  A. Exhibits repetitive, atypical patterns and behaviors and focuses on special interests.
  B. Shows interest in social relationships but often is unable to facilitate.
  C. Pedantic speech, absorption in circumscribed subjects (e.g., baseball scores, weather).
  D. Often verbal but tends to be egocentric in conversation, repeats words or phrases, perseveration.
  E. Poor nonverbal communication and eye contact.
  F. Frequently repetitive and stilted speech with monotone emotionless voice; vocabulary and grammar generally very good.
  G. Awkward and clumsy movements, fine and gross motor deficits.
  H. No significant delays in cognitive or language development, adaptive behavior, or self-help skills.
  I. May have dyslexia and difficulty with writing and math, history of hyperlexia, (i.e., reading without thought of meaning at a precocious age).
  J. Depression and bipolar disorder (mood instability) occurs.

IV. Effects on Individual
  A. Socially isolated with limited friendships, vulnerable to bullying.
  B. Possibility of strained family relationships.
  C. Behavior problems may develop because of rejection by others.
  D. Awkward motor abilities.
  E. Limited interests and routines.

V. Health Concerns/Emergencies
  A. Accident-prone.
  B. Depression and mood instability/bipolar disorder.

VI. Management/Treatment
  A. Treat symptomatically.
  B. Antidepressants and antianxiety medications as needed.
  C. Monitor medications and side effects.
  D. Psychosocial intervention for depression.
  E. Occupational therapy and physical therapy as needed.
  F. Facilitated and protected social intervention in class, especially on the playground.

VII. Additional Information
  A. Often lead productive lives in adulthood, with independent living, having a family, and job satisfaction.

| **Box 5-2** | ***DSM-IV Criteria: Asperger's Syndrome*** |

A. Qualitative impairment in social interaction, as manifested by at least two of the following:
  1. Marked impairment in the use of multiple nonverbal behaviors, such as eye-to-eye gaze, facial expression, body postures, and gestures, to regulate social interaction.
  2. Failure to develop peer relationships appropriate to developmental level.
  3. A lack of spontaneous seeking to share enjoyment, interests, or achievements with other people (e.g., by a lack of showing, bringing, or pointing out objects of interest to other people).
  4. Lack of social or emotional reciprocity.
B. Restricted repetitive and stereotyped patterns of behavior, interests, and activities, as manifested by at least one of the following:
  1. Encompassing preoccupation with one or more stereotyped and re-stricted patterns of interest that is abnormal either in intensity or focus.
  2. Apparently inflexible adherence to specific, nonfunctional routines or rituals.
  3. Stereotyped and repetitive motor mannerisms (e.g., hand or finger flapping or twisting, or complex whole-body movements).
  4. Persistent preoccupation with parts of objects.
C. The disturbance causes clinically significant impairment in social, occupational, or other areas of functioning.
D. There is no clinically significant delay in language (e.g., single words used by age 2 years, communicative phrases used by age 3 years).
E. There is no clinically significant delay in cognitive development or in the development of age-appropriate self-help skills, adaptive behavior (other than in social interaction), and curiosity about the environment in childhood.
F. Criteria are not met for another specific pervasive developmental disorder or schizophrenia.

From the *Diagnostic and statistical manual of mental disorders,* ed 4, revision, Washington, DC, 1994, American Psychiatric Association.

VIII. Web Sites
  Center for Study of Autism
  http://www.autism.org
  Asperger Syndrome with Tony Attwood
  http://www.tonyattwood.com

RETT SYNDROME

  I. Definition
      A. Rett syndrome is a rare neurodegenerative disorder reported only in females. Affected males die shortly after birth of a severe brain disorder. Although present at birth, symptoms do not manifest until 6-18 months of age or later. Rett syndrome is similar to autism in social and language delays. Girls may live into adulthood but never regain their ability for speech or use of hands.

II. Etiology

A. Rett syndrome is a genetic disorder caused by mutation of a single gene, MeCP2, located on one of the two X chromosomes that determine sex. MeCP2 makes methyl cytosine–binding protein, and the mutation results in excessive amounts. Rett syndrome may be misdiagnosed as autism, cerebral palsy, or nonspecific delay. Diagnosis is based on symptoms and chromosome studies, but not all individuals have the abnormal gene. Genetic testing is available.

III. Characteristics

A. Normal development until 6-18 months.

B. Purposeful hand movements replaced by repetitive hand movements—hand wringing, licking, or clapping.

C. Loss of acquired speech.

D. Head circumference growth decelerates—cerebral atrophy.

E. Growth retardation, diminished body fat and muscle mass.

F. Unsteady, stiff-legged gait, small feet.

G. Disruptive sleep patterns.

H. Irritability and agitation.

I. Loss of interest in people and decreased interpersonal contact occur, but eye contact is maintained.

J. Mental deficiency—severe to profound.

K. Hypoactivity and diminished mobility with age.

IV. Effects on Individual

A. Dependent on extent of involvement and age.

B. Activities of daily living become difficult or impossible.

C. Behavioral problems develop because of rejection by others.

D. Limited recreation and social outlets.

V. Health Concerns/Emergencies

A. Breathing pattern irregularities, including breath holding, hyperventilation, apnea, and air swallowing.

B. Abnormal EEG, clinical seizures in 80%.

C. Scoliosis.

D. Bruxism and difficulty chewing and swallowing.

E. Gastroesophageal reflux, constipation, malabsorption.

F. Reduced circulation to legs and feet.

G. Instability of trunk and sometimes limb involvement.

H. Muscle rigidity/spasticity/joint contractures.

I. At risk for injury because of motoric degeneration.

VI. Management/Treatment

A. Dependent on age, extent of involvement, and degree of disability.

B. Includes pharmacological and psychosocial interventions.

C. Monitor medication and side effects.

D. Rule out hearing loss.

E. Monitor for seizure activity.

F. Observe for breathing problems, development of contractures; monitor skin integrity on the lower extremities.

| Box 5-3 | *DSM-IV Criteria: Rett Syndrome* |

A. All of the following:
   1. Apparently normal prenatal and perinatal development.
   2. Apparently normal psychomotor development through the first 5 months after birth.
   3. Normal head circumference at birth.
B. Onset of all of the following after a period of normal development.
   1. Deceleration of head growth between ages 5 and 48 months.
   2. Loss of previously acquired purposeful hand skills between ages 5 and 30 months with the subsequent development of stereotyped hand movements (e.g., hand wringing or hand washing).
   3. Loss of social engagement early in the course (although often social interaction develops later).
   4. Appearance of poorly coordinated gait or trunk movements.
   5. Severely impaired expressive and receptive language development with severe psychomotor retardation.

From the *Diagnostic and statistical manual of mental disorders,* ed 4, revision, Washington, DC, 1994, American Psychiatric Association.

VII. **Additional Information**
   A. Not every female with Rett syndrome displays all of the symptoms, and individual symptoms may vary in severity. Autistic-like behaviors usually disappear after preschool years. Deterioration is rapid, usually within a year.
VIII. **Web Sites**
   Rett Syndrome Research Foundation (RSRF)
   http://www.rsrf.org

PERVASIVE DEVELOPMENTAL DISORDER—NOT OTHERWISE SPECIFIED

Pervasive Developmental Disorder—Not Otherwise Specified (PDD-NOS) is a diagnosis by exclusion when a child has some, but not all, of the characteristics of autism. Diagnosis is made when the child exhibits significant, pervasive "autistic-like" impairment in communication, social, and behavioral skills, yet does not meet criteria for a specific pervasive developmental disorder (American Psychiatric Association, 1994). Also called *atypical autism.*

This category should be used when a severe and pervasive impairment exists in the development of reciprocal social interaction or verbal and nonverbal communication skills, or when stereotyped behavior, interests, and activities are present, but the criteria are not met for a specific pervasive developmental disorder, schizophrenia, schizotypal personality disorder, or avoidant personality disorder. For example, this category includes atypical autism—presentations that do not meet the criteria for autistic disorder because of late age of onset, atypical symptomatology, subthreshold symptomatology, or all of these.

   I. **Web Sites**
   Child Development Institute
   714-998-8617
   http://www.cdipage.com

BIBLIOGRAPHY

American Psychiatric Association: Disorders usually first diagnosed in infancy, childhood, or adolescence. In *Diagnostic and statistical manual of mental disorders,* ed 4, Washington, DC, 1994, The Association.

Barkley R: *ADHD and the nature of self control,* New York, 1997, Guilford Press.

Barkley R: *Attention-deficit hyperactivity disorder: a handbook for diagnosis and treatment,* New York, 1990, Guilford Press.

Carlucci D: Brain wiring in autism, *ADVANCE for Speech-Language Pathologists and Audiologists* 9(1):6-9, 1999.

Centers for Disease Control and Prevention: *Autism,* July 1, 2001, Centers for Disease Control, National Immunization Program, Available online: http://www.cdc.gov/nip/vacsafe/concerns/autism/autism-facts.htm. Accessed on July 6, 2001.

Comings DE, Gade-Andavolu R, Gonzalez N, et al: Comparison of the role of dopamine, serotonin, and noradrenaline genes in ADHD, ODD, and conduct disorder: multivariate regression analysis of 20 genes, *Clin Genet* 57(3):178-196, 2000.

Cook EH Jr, Courchesne R, Lord C, et al: Evidence of linkage between the serotonin transporter and autistic disorder, *Mol Psychiatry* 2(3):247-250, 1997.

Cook EH, Leventhal BL: The serotonin system in autism, *Curr Opin Pediatr* 8(4):348-354, 1996.

Dychkowski L: Helping school nurses recognize student behaviors that may indicate PDD and other autism-related symptoms, *School Nurse News* 17(3):3-6, 2000.

Erenberg G: Movement disorders. In Finberg L, editor: *Saunders manual of pediatric practice,* Philadelphia, 1998, WB Saunders.

Fisher E, Van Dyke D, Sears L, et al: Recent research on the etiologies of autism, *Infants Young Child* 11(3):1-8, 1999.

Ford JD, Racousin R, Daviss WB, et al: Trauma exposure among children with oppositional defiant disorder and attention deficit-hyperactivity disorder, *J Consult Clin Psychol* 67(5):786-789, 1999.

Goldman LS, Genel M, Bezman RJ, et al: Diagnosis and treatment of attention deficit/hyperactivity disorder in children and adolescents, Council on Scientific Affairs, American Medical Association, *JAMA* 279(14):1100-1107, 1998.

Jackson PL, Vessey JA: *Child with a chronic condition,* ed 3, St Louis, 2000, Mosby.

Koenig K, Rubin E, Klin A, et al: Autism and the pervasive developmental disorders. In Zeanah CH, editor: *Handbook of infant mental health,* New York, 2000, Guilford Press.

Kronenberger WG, Meyer RG: *The child clinician's handbook,* Boston, 1996, Allyn and Bacon.

Martin M, Waltman-Greenwood C, Novotny PP: *School phobia: solve your child's school-related problems,* New York, 1995, Harper Perennial.

Parker S, Zuckerman B, editors: *Behavioral and developmental pediatrics: a handbook for primary care,* Boston, 1995, Little, Brown & Co.

Rodier PM: The early origins of autism, *Sci Am* 282(2):56-63, 2000.

Vayda W: *Mood foods,* Berkeley, Calif, 1995, Ulysses Press.

Wong DL, Whaley LF, Wilson D, et al, editors: *Whaley and Wong's nursing care of infants and children,* ed 6, St Louis, 1999, Mosby.

Zand J, Walton R, Rountree B: *Smart medicine for a healthier child,* Garden City Park, NY, 1994, Avery.

Zelazo P: Infant-toddler information processing assessment for children with pervasive developmental disorder and autism. Part I, *Infants Young Child* 10(1):1-14, 1997.

Zelazo P: Infant-toddler information processing assessment for children with pervasive developmental disorder and autism. Part II, *Infants Young Child* 10(2):1-13, 1997.

Zito JM, Safer DJ, dosReis S, et al: Trends in the prescribing of psychotropic medications to preschoolers, *JAMA* 283(8):1025-1030, 2000.

CHAPTER 6

Substance Abuse

Clinicians are becoming increasingly aware of the staggering numbers of social and health problems created by substance abuse (SA). Much more is known about how drugs affect the brain, body, and behavior. Those who work with children and adolescents are responsible not only for understanding and teaching these facts but also must accept the challenge of identifying and preventing abuse. Effective intervention requires realistic, practical solutions for personal emotions, peer affiliations, and self-defeating behaviors that can lead to SA.

SA is a major concern in our society. Not only is it prevalent among adolescents, but many more elementary-age children now are involved in substance abuse. Temporary or permanent changes in the chemistry of brain cells, associated health problems, loss of productivity, and suicide are only four of the possible devastating effects of substance abuse. The nurse can be a key person in initiating steps to remedy the problem.

The information in this chapter enables the nurse to understand the devastating effects that occur, identify at-risk students, and engage in effective interventions with drug-related health concerns and emergencies. The latest information on chemical interactions in the brain is presented. The various categories of drugs are presented, but because alcohol is extensively abused, socially acceptable, and easily accessible, an entire section is devoted to this abused substance.

SA prevention programs are widespread in schools through health education and Safe and Drug-Free School programs. Although school nurses are important partners in such prevention efforts, they are crucial when individual students show symptoms of SA or when an overdose occurs. Thus this chapter focuses on providing basic information about drugs that are abused and defines the role of nurses in assisting individual students.

THE NEUROBIOLOGY OF REINFORCEMENT AND DRUG ADDICTION

Reinforcement and drug addiction are closely linked because they share a common brain pathway. Reinforcement is anything that increases the likelihood of a future recurrence of a given behavior. The basic neural pathway for reinforcement involves the projection from the ventral tegmental area (VTA) of the brain to the nucleus accumbens. The VTA sends fibers along a pathway called the *medial forebrain bundle*. When neurons in the VTA increase their activity, the neurotransmitter dopamine is released into cells in the nucleus accumbens. This activity is primarily responsible for reinforcement. Therefore any behavior that causes a release of dopamine in the nucleus accumbens is more likely to occur in the future. A variety of behaviors can cause a release of dopamine, and these behaviors vary among individuals. For example, sky

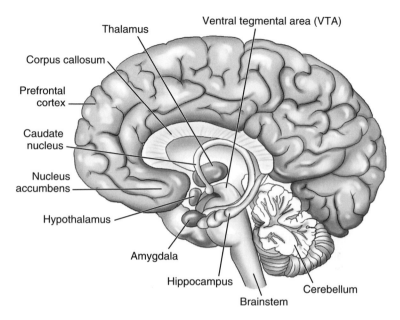

FIGURE 6-1 Brain structures involved with substance abuse.

diving, jogging, weight lifting, or even reading could cause a release of dopamine, depending on the individual. When this happens, the individual tends to continue that particular behavior because it is reinforced. Many forms of drug addiction work in a similar manner. For example, cocaine, amphetamines, nicotine, and alcohol consumption all cause a release of dopamine in the nucleus accumbens. Therefore the behaviors that are responsible for the delivery of the drug (e.g., snorting cocaine, smoking cigarettes, drinking alcohol) are reinforced. This reinforcement can be so powerful that the individual continues to engage in these behaviors even when they become destructive. In essence, this drug addiction is not an addiction to the drug but to the behavior of administering the drug. This addiction occurs because the drug causes a release of dopamine in the nucleus accumbens.

ILLICIT SUBSTANCES

UNDERSTANDING ABUSED SUBSTANCES

SA is the self-administered misuse of a chemical or toxic material to the extent that the individual's health or ability to function responsibly is adversely affected and compromised. SA may be referred to as *substance use disorder.*

The physical, cognitive, behavioral, and emotional effects on individuals vary according to the substance used, age of youth, and body mass. Teenage substance abusers often lag behind peers in accomplishing the adolescent tasks necessary to attain psychosocial maturity. Judgment, evaluative thinking, perception, and general function usually are impaired. Impulse control is diminished, and sleep time is interrupted. These abrupt personality and behavioral changes may threaten relationships with peers, parents or caregivers, and teachers.

Although SA is not understood completely, improved technology and research continuously provide new data about genetics, the brain, and human motivation. These data indicate that SA is the interaction among three basic factors: the individual, the environment, and the substance; each factor contributes to the SA problem in varying degrees.

COMMON RISK INDICATORS FOR SUBSTANCE ABUSE

1. Genetic predisposition
2. SA in the family of origin
3. Affective and mood disorders
4. Antisocial youth subculture affiliation
5. Inadequate coping with traumatic life experiences

SYMPTOMS OF SUBSTANCE ABUSE

1. Change in choice of friends and companions
2. Change in dress, appearance, and hygienic practices
3. Change in eating or sleeping habits
4. Frequent unexplained arguments or violent actions
5. Skipping school and absenteeism
6. Failing classes and educational underachievement
7. Delinquent and runaway behavior
8. Deteriorating relationship with family
9. Severe mood swings, apathy
10. Affective disorders, depression
11. Suicide attempts
12. Legal problems

STIMULANTS

Stimulants are drugs that stimulate the central nervous system (CNS) and can have neurotoxic effects. These drugs are used by the individual for weight control, pain control, and for alertness and feelings of calmness. Users risk a high potential for psychological dependence as tolerance develops. Commonly used stimulants are *caffeine,* such as coffee, tea, cocoa, and cola drinks; *nicotine* in cigarettes, cigars, pipe tobacco, chewing tobacco, and snuff; *amphetamines,* such as benzedrine, dextroamphetamine (Dexedrine), and dextroamphetamine with amobarbital (Dexamyl); and *cocaine.*

   I. Caffeine
   A. Found in at least 60 plants, including kola nuts, tea leaves, and cacao and coffee beans. It potentiates the release of cortisol and influences effects similar to arousal caused by stress. The effect comes by blocking the neurotransmitter sedative adenosine, a calming chemical. In moderate amounts, caffeine appears to stimulate nerve cell activity, temporarily boosting concentration, memory, and alertness. This alertness may occur in the more primitive limbic section but not in areas managing higher-level reasoning, which seem unaffected.

Table 6-1   *Drug Neurotoxic Effects*

Substance	Mental Status	Pupils	Respiratory Rate	Heart Rate	Additional Information
Stimulants	Agitation to paranoid psychosis	Mild to moderate dilation	Increased	Increased	Irritability, seizures, arrhythmias, death
Hallucinogens	Variable psychosis, coma, decreased awareness, paranoia	Mild to moderate dilation Nystagmus	Increased	Increased	Flashbacks, muscular rigidity, cardiovascular collapse
Narcotics (Opiates)	Lethargy, coma	Constricted with intoxication Dilated with anoxia or withdrawal	Decreased	Decreased	Shock, pulmonary or cerebral edema, respiratory failure
Inhalants	Disorientation, hallucinations, coma	Possible dilation Vertical and horizontal nystagmus	—	Increased Irregular heart rate	Panic, slurred speech, vomiting, cardiac arrhythmia, brain and liver damage, death
Depressants	Irritability to stupor-coma	Barbiturates: constricted Sedatives: dilated	Decreased and shallow	Decreased	Combative, violent, CNS depression, coma, psychosis
Alcohol	Drunklike to stupor-coma	Normal or dilated	Decreased	Decreased	Slurred speech, ataxia, stupor, coma, death

NOTE: Hyperthermia may be exhibited with use of Ecstasy, PCP, and some inhalants.

Table 6-2   *Stimulant Effects*

Physical and Behavioral Symptoms	Toxic Effects
General: Euphoria, exaggerated sense of well-being Increased energy and alertness Blurred vision Dizziness Talkativeness Restlessness Sleeplessness Anxiety and panic attacks Reduced appetite Insomnia Dilated pupils Increased perspiration when injected Increased blood pressure, heart rate, respiration Elevated body temperature Poor body care Amphetamine: jerky, flailing, writhing movements, extreme nervousness plus general listed symptoms	Tremors Cardiac abnormalities, some fatal Seizures, some fatal Deficient immune system, malnutrition, fatal kidney, heart and lung disorders, brain and liver damage Depression, hallucinations, violent and aggressive behaviors, panic, paranoia, formication (feelings of insects crawling on skin) Learning deficits: attention, concentration, verbal and visual memory, word production, visual motor integration Nicotine and chemicals: increased risk of miscarriages and lower–birth-weight babies, decreased sense of smell and taste; changes in DNA lead to cancer, heart and lung disease; chewing and snuff can cause cancer of throat, mouth, cheek, gums, and tongue Amphetamine: can result in stroke, high fever, sudden heart failure Amphetamine/cocaine psychosis: hallucinations, delusions, paranoia

Table 6-3   *Stimulant Withdrawal Symptoms*

Caffeine	Nicotine	Amphetamines	Cocaine
Headaches Anxiety Dizziness Unusual tiredness Nervousness Irritability Depression Nausea and vomiting	Headaches Fatigue Depression Anxiety Increased appetite Loss of concentration Loss of energy Difficulty with stress, mood control	Depression Severe abdominal cramping or pain Nausea and vomiting Trembling Unusual tiredness, weakness Anxiety Suicidal thoughts or actions	Irritability Depression: exhaustion, weakness Poor thinking ability Restless sleep Decreased appetite Aches and pains

II. Nicotine

A. A poisonous, colorless, oily fluid, with a bitter, burning taste; obtained from tobacco leaves or produced synthetically. Nicotine disrupts the flow of oxygen to the brain that results in decreased metabolism of glucose, which affects memory and lowers mental output. It also elevates cortisol levels, a stress hormone. It is used in veterinary medicine, as an external parasiticide, and as an agricultural insecticide spray.

B. Chemicals in cigarette smoke are toxic and with other substances cause changes in deoxyribonucleic acid (DNA) that can lead to cancer and heart and lung disease. Passive smokers, nonsmokers who inhale cigarette smoke, are exposed to the same tar and nicotine as smokers and have the same health-related concerns.

C. Smokeless forms of tobacco, such as chewing tobacco and snuff, include the same chemicals as cigarettes and have the same addictive qualities but also lead to an increased risk of leukoplakia (precancer) and throat and mouth cancers. Chewing tobacco also can lead to cancer of the cheek, gums, and tongue. Chewing tobacco is put between the cheek and gum, and when chewed, it releases the nicotine juices that mix with saliva. Smokeless tobacco, snuff, is ground tobacco that can be chewed but usually is inhaled through the nose.

D. Nicotine, like other drugs, alters neuronal communications, specifically acetylcholine, either by increasing or decreasing the neurotransmitters. This neurotransmitter targets release of other reward system chemicals and feelings of pleasure, followed by feelings of increased mental alertness and acuity. The receptors become increasingly less sensitive with chronic use and habituate, a chemical basis of addiction.

E. Dopamine neurons also are activated by the nicotine, mimicking or copying the effect by binding to receptors in the cells' membrane; this process inhibits the reuptake of dopamine. Chronic smoking causes the brain to produce additional nicotinic receptor sites that increase nicotine craving. This biochemical demand is relieved only by more smoking. Students with attention deficit hyperactivity disorder (ADHD), depression, and schizophrenia are more likely to smoke because it may be a way to self-medicate.

III. **Amphetamines**

A. This class of stimulants includes methamphetamine and dextroamphetamine. These drugs can be smoked, snorted, taken orally, or injected and can be made in a laboratory or at home. Chemicals similar in pharmacological qualities also are abused, such as amphetamine-like drugs used to treat ADHD (methylphenidate), narcolepsy (methylphenidate and dextroamphetamine), and over-the-counter (OTC) medications for congestion (pseudoephedrine). When taken in therapeutic dosages, these drugs are helpful and do not cause brain damage. When abused, underactivity in the temporal parietal and frontal areas has been noted (see "Learning deficits" in Table 6-2).

B. Amphetamines have a similar but more powerful effect than cocaine on the neurotransmitters noradrenaline and dopamine by prevention of their reabsorption into neurons. This effect is noted in the continuous body movements and distractibility exhibited by the user.

IV. **Cocaine**

A. A natural alkaloid derived from the *Erythroxylon coca* plant grown in South America. It is used medically as a local anesthetic and appetite suppressant. Cocaine is found in different forms and can be inhaled, smoked, injected, and absorbed intraanally and intravaginally. Crack is a potent form that is smoked, producing a rapid high with intense addictive qualities.

B. The National Institute of Drug Abuse (NIDA) reports that repeated microscopic strokes occur that lead to dead spots in the brain's nerve circuitry (NIDA, 1998).

C. Three important neurotransmitters are disturbed with cocaine use and abuse: norepinephrine, serotonin, and dopamine. Cocaine blocks the reuptake of dopamine from the synapse. This results in dopamine remaining in the synapse for longer periods where it can stimulate receptors to a greater extent, resulting in an extreme feeling of well-being.

D. *Prenatal cocaine exposure* has been documented as having subtle effects on motor skills, irritability, attention span, alertness, and intelligence quotient (IQ) level in some children. It also can alter neural systems that are crucial to behavior and response to stimuli. A few systems are seriously damaged. Prenatal effects are not as dramatic as previously reported but are significant when coupled with the environment of the child. Cocaine abuse has a financial impact related to the special education resources needed to support the children through school to succeed in their chosen endeavors.

HALLUCINOGENS

Hallucinogens are drugs that act primarily on the CNS and profoundly alter sensory perception. Individuals see images, hear sounds, and feel sensations that do not exist but seem very real. Rapid and intense emotional swings occur, and changes in feelings and thoughts are exaggerated and magnified. Hallucinogens usually are taken orally. Effects of these drugs vary greatly from person to person and from one episode of drug use to another episode, making "bad trips" unpredictable. Users develop psychological dependence and can develop tolerance. No withdrawal symptoms for hallucinogens have been documented. Effects can last for 12 hours. Currently no accepted medical use for these drugs exists. Commonly abused hallucinogens are *lysergic acid diethylamide (LSD)*, derived from a fungus; *psilocybin* (mushroom, found in 90 species); *mescaline* (peyote, a cactus); *cannabis* (marijuana, hashish); and *methylenedioxymethamphetamine (MDMA), Ecstasy,* and *methylenedioxyamphetamine (MDA)*.

This group of drugs disrupts the interaction of nerve cells and the neurotransmitter serotonin to produce their effects. Serotonin is found throughout the brain and spinal cord and is associated with the control of the regulatory, perceptual, and behavioral systems.

Dissociative drugs include *phencyclidine (PCP)* and *ketamine*. These two drugs originally were used as anesthetics—general (PCP) and veterinarian (ketamine). They affect many neurotransmitter systems, including norepinephrine and dopamine. They also alter or affect the distribution of the neurotransmitter glutamate. Glutamate is involved in memory, responses to the environment, and the perception of pain, specifically reducing sensations, and leads to a sense of detachment or dissociation; hence the term *dissociative drugs,* not hallucinogens. PCP can be taken orally, injected, or smoked. Long-term abusers often exhibit lack of motivation, feelings of burnout, aggressive behavior, and violence. Large doses can lead to coma and death. PCP is considered to have

Table 6-4	*Hallucinogen Effects*
Physical and Behavioral Symptoms	**Toxic Effects**
Increased heart rate and blood pressure	Decreased awareness to touch and
Sleep disturbance, sweating, dizziness,	pain
tremors	Seizures
Sparse and incoherent speech	Flashbacks, leading to unpredictable
Disturbances in body heat regulation,	behaviors, accidents, panic, and
loss of appetite	suicide
Lethargy, fatigue	Behavior similar to schizophrenic
Inability to feel pleasure	psychosis
Changes in perception, feelings, and	Catatonic syndrome: mute, lethargic,
thoughts	disoriented; repetitive, meaningless
Decreased motivation, personality	movements
change, memory impairment, sense	Kidney and cardiovascular failure
of distance	
Confusion, suspicion, and loss of control	
Depression, anxiety, and paranoia	
Violent behavior	

the most pervasive, complex effects on the brain of any of the abused drugs. Chronic users appear to have neuronal impairment leading to lack of motivation, extreme apathy, and a severe burnout that does not return to normal even after abstinence.

  I. **Ketamine**

    A. Called *K, special K,* or *vitamin K,* this drug is used as a liquid applied to marijuana or tobacco items or as a white powder that is snorted. High doses can cause delirium, amnesia, impaired motor function, and occasional fatal respiratory arrest. It is one of the emerging *date rape drugs.* Ketamine is related to PCP and affects glutamate by blocking receptors for glutamate. Ketamine, like PCP, blocks N-methyl-D-aspartate (NMDA) receptors, which are located on the nerve cells and normally are stimulated (activated) by glutamate. Thus ketamine interferes with normal glutamate signal transmission.

  II. **Marijuana**

    A. Marijuana is a product of the hemp plant, flowers, and leaves; contains approximately 42 chemicals. The prime mind-altering chemical is delta-9-tetrahydrocannabinol (THC) with an average concentration of 3% THC. Marijuana is an example of a fat-soluble abused drug and contains up to 50% more tar and cancer-causing chemicals than cigarette smoke. Different types and potencies are found in various parts of the world. Sinsemilla is a mixture of the buds and flowers of the female plant with an average concentration of 7.5%. Hashish is the sticky resin from the flowers of the female plant with an average concentration of 3.6% THC. Marijuana is generally rolled into a homemade cigarette. Effects are longer when ingested (5-12 hours) versus smoking (2-4 hours). Users develop psychological dependency.

    B. Marijuana smoking affects the brain and leads to impaired short-term memory, perception, judgment, and motor skills. It can impair the immune system and cause dysmenorrhea and lower sperm production. Chronic heavy use is associated with risk for developing the amotivational syndrome, which includes symptoms such as general apathy; passivity; loss of interest, motivation, energy, and personal grooming and hygiene care; and decreased frustration tolerance. Marijuana affects skills required for driving a car, such as alertness, coordination, reaction time, and the ability to concentrate for up to 24 hours after smoking. These impaired skills can make it difficult for a driver of a car to react to signals, road sounds, and judge distances.

    C. Studies have shown that THC is passed to the baby in breast milk. Maternal breast milk is more concentrated than THC in the maternal blood.

III. LSD

    A. Called *acid* and *sugar,* LSD is a powerful, synthetic, cheap hallucinogen. It was originally considered helpful in the treatment of mental illness. Its effects can last 8 to 12 hours. It generally is taken orally, on squares of blotter paper, sugar cubes, or pills that have absorbed the liquid drug.

    B. LSD disrupts and mimics serotonin and activates areas in the temporal lobe, causing hallucinations. The most common mental symptoms are perceptual distortions and visual hallucinations. Its effects are unpredictable and range from euphoria to psychotic reactions, panic and depression; flashbacks can occur weeks or months after the last use.

IV. MDMA, Ecstasy, and MDA

    A. MDMA, Ecstasy (called *X-TC* or *X*), and MDA are synthetic drugs that are hallucinogens when taken in high dosages but in low dosages produce effects similar to those of amphetamines. MDMA is taken orally as a tablet and causes increased heart rate and blood pressure that may elevate body temperature, causing cardiovascular and kidney failure. When used with alcohol, it can be dangerous and sometimes fatal (NIDA, 2000a). Common side effects are jitteriness, jaw clenching, and anxiety.

    B. Higher doses can cause panic and paranoia reactions and with long-term use, exhaustion, depression, fatigue, and numbness. Long-term-use symptoms are attributed to serotonin deficiencies and long-lasting neurotoxic effects in the brain. Ecstasy is called a sensual drug rather than sexual, since males report decreased orgasm and females report sexual arousal. MDA is often called the *love drug.*

    C. Ecstasy affects numerous brain neurotransmitter systems. As a serotonin agonist, it causes excessive release of serotonin and then stops its reuptake; the long-term effect of use is serotonin depletion in the brain. Whether damaged serotonin-producing neurons regenerate is unclear. Other documented long-term effects are residual problems of verbal and visual memory and congenital abnormalities associated with prenatal drug exposure (National Institute on Drug Abuse, 1999a).

V. Gamma-Hydroxybutyrate (GHB)

A. GHB, also called *liquid Ecstasy, Georgia Home Boy,* and *G,* is a CNS depressant, steroidlike substance. GHB is known to diminish inhibitions and enhance sexual experiences and has been associated with overdoses, poisonings, and *date rape.* It is a clear, odorless liquid that also is found in tablet or capsule form. An overdose can lead quickly to loss of consciousness, coma, and death. The purity and strength of each dose can vary greatly, making overdoses more likely.

OPIATES

Opiates are a group of toxic substances originally derived from the opium poppy-opiates (codeine, morphine, heroin). Synthetic opiates also have been produced (e.g., methadone, meperidine [Demerol], oxycodone with aspirin [Percodan]). Opiates have pain-relieving properties, induce sleep, and are effective for diarrhea, cough, and agitation. They act primarily on the central and parasympathetic nervous system. They can be taken by injection, orally, or through smoking. Abusers develop physical and psychological dependence; tolerance develops. Chronic users may have noticeable needle marks on their arms and legs.

Opiates are compounds that act on opiate receptors and block the reuptake of the natural neurotransmitters. Synthetic chemicals have been developed to block the opiate receptor sites, thus eliminating the high produced by these drugs in addicts. These synthetic chemicals are narcotic antagonists used to treat addiction.

I. Heroin

A. Heroin is a white powder derived from morphine that is highly addictive. It is injected intravenously but can be smoked or taken by mouth. This drug is illegal in the United States and many other countries. Street names include *smack, H, skag, junk, Mexican black tar,* and *bomb.*

Table 6-5 *Opiate Effects*	
Physical and Behavioral Symptoms	**Toxic Effects**
Constricted pupils, watery eyes, itching	Slow, shallow breathing, clammy
Drowsiness	skin, sedation, seizures
Early use: nausea, vomiting	Overdose: respiratory depression,
Slows bowel function	coma, death
Reduced sex, hunger, and aggressive drives	
Feeling of warmth and detachment	
Euphoria	
Suppression of pain and distress	
Clouded mental functioning	
Heroin: infectious diseases, AIDS, hepatitis B and C, collapsed veins, abscesses, bacterial infections, infections of heart lining and valves, arthritis and other rheumatological problems, spontaneous abortion	

AIDS, Acquired immunodeficiency syndrome.

Box 6-1	*Withdrawal Symptoms of Opiates*

Similar to flu: aches, rhinorrhea	Restlessness, irritability
Sweating, chills	Elevated blood pressure, pulse,
Tremors or jerks	respirations, temperature
Anorexia	Severe drug craving
Diarrhea, chronic nausea	Muscle spasm
Insomnia	Seizures
Muscle and abdominal cramps	Coma
Hypersensitivity to pain	Possible death

B. Heroin and morphine mimic natural endorphins and related pain-killing hormones. The drugs travel quickly to the brain, stimulating dopamine-containing neurons to fire and releasing the neurotransmitter into the nucleus accumbens. The drugs bind to the opiate receptor on the receiving terminal, sending a signal to release more dopamine.

C. Prenatal heroin exposure.

1. During pregnancy, heroin addiction places the fetus at severe risk and potential death. Complications associated with prenatal heroin exposure include preterm labor and birth, growth retardation, and a withdrawal syndrome after birth. The abstinence syndrome manifestations include irritability, gastrointestinal (GI) dysfunction, respiratory difficulties, tremulousness, high-pitched cry, poor feeding, increased tone, and seizures. Human immunodeficiency virus (HIV) and hepatitis B are also risks related to the intravenous route of abuse. If pregnancy is known, heroin-addicted women usually are maintained on methadone during the pregnancy to reduce perinatal complications. Methadone helps to satisfy the physical cravings without the psychological high associated with heroin abuse.

II. **Methadone**

A. Street name *Meth;* is used to control opiate withdrawal symptoms. It is taken orally once a day, producing a steady, unrewarding blood and brain level of the opiate. If misused and injected, it produces intense, short-term euphoria similar to that of heroin. A heroin addict receiving maintenance methadone treatment is not intoxicated or impaired because of the complete tolerance to opiate effects and the steady blood levels of the daily drug.

III. **L-alpha-acetylmethadol (LAAM)**

A. LAAM is a longer-acting methadone-like medication used in addiction treatment clinics. It is taken 3 times a week, thus reducing take-home abuse. When taken orally, LAAM works the same way as methadone, permitting the individual to live a more normal life by reducing cravings and preventing withdrawal symptoms.

INHALANTS

Inhalants are legal chemicals that include a variety of agents that are inhaled to produce psychoactive effects or an alcoholic-like intoxication. They are sniffed or huffed and can cause physical and emotional problems; even a one-time use can result in death. Most common abusers of these chemicals range in age from 7 to 17 years. Long-term inhalant use can cause blood chemistry disorders, fatigue, muscle fatigue, and weight loss. Deeply inhaled vapors or high concentrations of inhalants may result in disorientation, unconsciousness, or death. Users develop psychological dependency, and tolerance develops. Street names include *glue, laughing gas, poppers,* and *snappers.*

Inhalants can be divided into two classifications: organic solvents and abusable gases. Solvents that contain inhalant fumes include glue, quick-drying plastic cement, paint thinner, lacquer, gasoline, cleaning fluids, lighter fluid, marker pen, typewriter correction fluid, dry cleaning fluids, nail polish remover, hair spray, room deodorizers, and food products (vegetable cooking spray and dessert whipped cream spray).

Gases include nitrous oxide, amyl nitrite, and butyl nitrite. Nitrous oxide is known as "laughing gas" and is an anesthetic used for minor dental surgery. The effects of these gases are short, lasting only a few minutes, and are perceived as "safe." However, they increase the heart rate and decrease blood pressure so that the user feels light-headed and dizzy. Long or continual use can cause fainting and lead to coma. The cardiac arrhythmias caused by inhaled gases can be fatal.

A single prolonged session of inhalant use can cause heart failure and death—"sudden sniffing death." Chronic use may cause long-term CNS damage, resulting in learning, movement, vision, and hearing impairments. Damage to the heart, kidneys, lungs, and liver may be permanent.

Inhalants quickly enter the bloodstream and then the brain after inhalation. Inhalants produce a variety of deleterious effects—reduced vision and hearing, impaired movement, and lowered cognitive ability—and sometimes strip the protective myelin sheath from brain fibers, with resulting apparent dementia. Solvents are fat soluble and affect the neuron membrane, which is composed of fat. Neuronal transmission is increased in low doses, whereas inhalation of large amounts inhibits neuronal transmission, causing brain dysfunction, paralysis, and death.

DEPRESSANTS

Depressants produce an inhibitory, constricted effect on the CNS. These drugs are used for relief of insomnia, anxiety, and pain. The three main categories are barbiturates, nonbarbiturates, and tranquilizers. Chronic users risk a high potential for both physical and psychological dependence; tolerance develops.

Commonly used *barbiturates* are phenobarbital (Nembutal), secobarbital (Seconal), amobarbital-secobarbital (Tuinal), and amobarbital (Amytal). Commonly used *nonbarbiturates* are glutethimide (Doriden), methyprylon (Notudar), ethchlorvynol (Placidyl), and methaqualone (Quaalude). Commonly used *tranquilizers* are diazepam (Valium), chlordiazepoxide (Librium), meprobamate (Miltown, Equanil), lorazepam (Ativan), chlorpromazine (Thorazine), alprazolam (Xanax), paroxetine (Paxil), hydroxyzine (Atarax), and oxazepam (Serax).

Table 6-6   *Symptoms and Toxic Effects of Inhalants*

Physical and Behavioral Symptoms	Toxic Effects
Solvents	
Euphoria, belligerence, dizziness	CNS system depression
Alcohol-like effects: interfere with coordination, thoughts, perceptions	Panic, disorientation, severe tissue damage, hallucinations, coma, respiratory arrest
Moderate amount: exhilaration, lessening of inhibitions	
Large amount: drowsiness, memory loss, mental confusion, physiological symptoms; slurred speech, dizziness, nausea, vomiting, tremors	
Gases	
Dizziness, light-headedness	Irregular heartbeat, fainting, coma, respiratory arrest
Increased heart rate	
Decreased blood pressure	
General	
Nausea and nosebleeds	Liver, lung, kidney impairment
	Irreversible brain damage
	Nervous system damage
	Chemical imbalances

Table 6-7   *Depressant Effects*

Physical and Behavioral Symptoms	Toxic Effects
Slurred speech	CNS depression, decreased respirations, blood pressure
Unsteadiness	
Loss of balance and falling	Hepatic damage
Difficulty in thinking and faulty judgment	Respiratory arrest
Quarrelsome disposition	Unconsciousness
Loss of inhibitions	Coma
Emotional instability	Possible death
Drowsiness or sleep	Psychosis
Irritability, hostility	
Tranquilizers: symptoms/behaviors the same but with less intensity	

I. Rohypnol

    A. Flunitrazepam (Rohypnol) is implicated in sexual assaults (i.e., *rape*). It was developed as a benzodiazepine sedative to treat insomnia and as a presurgery anesthetic. It is used in 60 countries but is not approved for prescription in the United States. It is taken orally in tablet form and dissolves quickly in carbonated beverages; snorting also has been

Table 6-8	*Depressant Withdrawal Symptoms*	
Barbiturates	**Nonbarbiturates**	**Tranquilizers**
Restlessness, weakness	Anxiety	Anxiety
Anxiety, nervousness	Ataxia	Muscle twitching
Nose twitching, tremors	Tremors	Tremors
Abdominal cramps	Memory loss	Weakness
Headaches	Slurred speech	Abdominal and muscle
Insomnia	Perceptual distortions	cramps
Nausea and vomiting	Irritability	Seizures
Grand mal seizures	Agitation	Psychosis
Hallucinations	Delirium	Delirium
Mental exhaustion, confusion,	Insomnia	
and delirium	Nausea and vomiting	

reported. It is tasteless and odorless, and its sedative and toxic effects are enhanced by alcohol. Even a small dose of Rohypnol can impair the individual for 8 to 12 hours. Profound amnesia can occur after use; the individual may not be able to remember events experienced while under the effects of the drug. Side effects include decreased blood pressure, drowsiness, dizziness, confusion, visual disturbances, GI disturbances, and urinary retention.

CLUB DRUGS

Club drugs are an ambiguous term to describe illicit drugs used at bars, clubs, or all-night dance parties called *raves* or *trances*. They are used as mood enhancers and to increase energy for dancing. Drugs used can be stimulants, depressants, hallucinogens, or a combination. The common use of these drugs at a party is not perceived as a risk among users; however, club drugs do cause toxic and chronic effects. For example, Ecstasy can produce hyperthermia and mask thirst, which has been reported to cause acute dehydration and death after dancing for an extended time. Six substances identified as club drugs are Ecstasy, GHB, ketamine, Rohypnol, methamphetamine, and LSD. GHB, ketamine, and Rohypnol are identified as emerging *date rape drugs*.

THE WIDESPREAD PROBLEM OF ALCOHOL ABUSE AND DEPENDENCY

Alcohol abuse refers to the degree of drinking that interferes with an individual's normal functioning and is both a biological and psychosocial disease. Alcohol dependence or alcoholism is characterized by the loss in control of drinking and a dependency on alcohol. It is a CNS depressant.

The cause of alcohol abuse and dependency now is better understood. Several causative factors have been implicated: environmental influences, lifestyle choices, and genetic factors. Genetic research is focused on more than one gene. Children of alcoholics are four times more likely to become addicted to drink than those whose parents are not alcoholics. Approximately 50%-60% of alcoholics have a genetic predisposition, and it is presumed that they are unable to produce adequate dopamine. The U.S. Substance Abuse and Mental Health Services Administration's National Household Survey on Drug Abuse (1999) found that almost 7 million youths between 12 and 20 years of age binge drink at least once a month. Of those individuals who drink, one in nine become alcoholic.

Brain imaging techniques allow real-time visualization of the changes in the structure of the brain with chronic alcohol use. Initially, alcohol stimulates the pleasure center, which prompts repetition of the action. Alcohol eventually can turn this pleasant feeling into intense cravings and destructive behavior. Long-term drinking makes new pathways to the areas in the brain that are associated with attention and judgment. Alcohol increases levels of dopamine in the nucleus accumbens, which are associated with motivation, although the exact role of this process is unknown.

Alcohol decreases neural activity through action on GABA neurons. All drugs that block the receptors reduce the pleasure of drinking and therefore are effective in the treatment of alcoholism.

I. **Health Concerns/Emergencies**
   A. Alcohol abuse can lower an adolescent's resistance to infection, impair reflexes, and stunt emotional growth.
   B. An adolescent's brain appears susceptible to damage in the limbic system, prefrontal cortex, and hippocampus, which may impair personality development and sound decision making.
   C. Binge drinking damages the prefrontal cortex and associated areas more than other areas.
   D. The greatest brain damage occurs during withdrawal from alcohol.
   E. Combined use of alcohol and another substance (polysubstance abuse) intensifies the effect of each substance and may be extremely dangerous, causing physical or mental impairment or death.
   F. Impairment of the CNS by alcohol produces changes in vision, hearing, muscular control, and judgment; these changes may cause bodily harm (e.g., automobile accidents).
   G. Alcohol overdose involves a greater risk of suicide and death.
   H. A pregnant minor who abuses alcohol increases the chance of damage to the developing fetus (see Chapter 4: Fetal Alcohol Syndrome/Fetal Alcohol Effects).
   I. When alcohol intake interferes with an adolescent's normal dietary requirement, nutritional deficiencies can occur:
      1. Depressed appetite.
      2. Alcohol becomes a substitute for normal caloric intake.
      3. Vitamin and mineral deficiencies, particularly B vitamins (niacin and thiamin), magnesium, potassium, iron, and folic acid.
   J. Possible consequences of long-term excessive use of alcohol:
      1. Liver disease (cirrhosis, alcoholic hepatitis, cancer of the liver).
      2. Cancer of the mouth, esophagus, or abdominal organs.
      3. Peripheral neuropathy and brain damage.

II. **Effects on Individual**
   A. A 10% difference was found in brain power between the alcohol abuser and the healthy teenager. This effect may be the difference between passing and failing a test, a class, or a grade.

B. Frequent absenteeism and failure to complete assignments can cause academic failure, expulsion, and dropping out. In addition, career goals and opportunities become limited.

C. Alcohol abuse/dependency may prevent an adolescent's emotional growth, thereby interfering with daily functioning with significant others.

D. Alcohol-induced lack of judgment may lead to unsafe sex, unwanted pregnancy, and early marriage.

E. Arrests, loss of driver's license, and other altercations with law enforcement can affect the family and attainment of future vocational goals.

F. Alcohol dependence causes carelessness in appearance and personal hygiene.

III. Management/Treatment

A. Some students who exhibit signs of depression do not feel successful in school or friendships, experience more headaches or stomachaches, fight with parents, and generally do not feel good about themselves; may be abusing substances.

B. Many students frequently in the nursing office have difficulties in the above areas, live in difficult family environments, or both, and need a friendly word, smile, or compliment that may promote self-esteem.

C. Formation of close bonds with students for talk time, empathic listening, and positive support may activate natural reward pathways in the brain.

D. Special education students are more at risk for SA.

E. Consider need for peer counseling.

F. Long-term dependency involves medical intervention:
  1. Special diet and vitamin supplements for nutritional deficiencies.
  2. Treatment of any underlying disorders caused by alcoholism.
  3. Medication:
     a. Naltrexone (ReVia) is a pure antagonist that blocks endogenous opioids in the brain that reinforce the effects of alcohol. Naltrexone may reduce cravings and prevent relapse. It has recently been approved by the FDA, and two other drugs are in clinical trials.
     b. Psychotherapy and psychopharmacology are recommended as treatments of choice.
     c. Medication may be prescribed to reduce anxiety and restlessness during withdrawal.
     d. Antabuse may be prescribed to discourage relapse.
  4. The symptoms of alcohol withdrawal are tremors, fever, perspiration, nausea, vomiting, anorexia, restlessness, hallucinations, and delirium tremens.

DRUG ACTIONS ON THE BRAIN

Positron emission tomography (PET), functional magnetic resonance imaging (fMRI), and single photon emission computed tomography (SPECT) imaging scans allow scientists to view the brain and learn how drugs affect neuronal activity. Drugs are carried to the brain through the bloodstream. They stimulate a region of the brain that releases neurotransmitters, such as dopamine, that are normally released in response to pleasurable experiences. Drug molecules with similar shapes to the neurotransmitter either block or activate a particular neurotransmitter's receptors. Through various means, drugs of abuse increase the concentration of dopamine in cells located in the brain's pleasure and reward system in the limbic area. Many scientists believe this process is the basis of all addiction. Two key areas in the management of the pleasure circuit are the nucleus accumbens and the VTA. The pleasure circuit is connected closely to the pathways and nuclei that manage pain, fear, and anger and houses gratification of hunger, thirst, and sex. Because this circuit is considered a part of the brain's control center of behavior, it also is connected to the frontal cortex and areas that assist movement. Addictive drugs produce their rewarding action by increasing dopamine in the nucleus accumbens and the VTA. Two other neurotransmitters play a role in drug abuse: endorphins and norepinephrine. The basal ganglia, which manages movements and repetitive tasks and plays a role in compulsion, and the amygdala, which helps the body to respond to stress, also are believed by neuroscientists to be involved with addiction (see Figure 6-1).

Toxic substances found in illicit drugs and pharmaceuticals have mind-altering effects and can cause cell damage and death. Technology has allowed discovery of those neurotransmitters in the brain that are affected by these substances. A basic knowledge of the function of these chemical transmitters is necessary to understand the role of drugs in addiction, drug dependence, tolerance, and withdrawal.

Figure 6-2 illustrates the influence of different chemicals on brain function. All brain activity is a result of communication between neurons. This communication is accomplished by transmitters that are released from a neuron and change the activity of another neuron by stimulating a receptor on that neuron. Stimulation of a receptor by the transmitter requires the transmitter to have the correct shape (i.e., chemical makeup). The transmitter fits neatly into the receptor. When the transmitter fits into the receptor, a process known as *binding,* it stimulates the receptor and thus allows one neuron to influence another neuron. Some drugs block this activity. A blocker can bind to the receptor but is not similar enough in shape to stimulate the receptor. However, because it is bound to the receptor, the blocker prevents the neurotransmitter from attaching to the receptor and thus influences normal brain activity. Other drugs are similar enough to bind to a receptor and activate the receptor. These activators influence normal brain activity because they stimulate receptors in the absence of regular transmitters.

All neurotransmitters except acetylcholine can be classified in one of three categories: (1) amino acids—chemical compounds that form the building blocks of protein, (2) amines—derived from amino acids (occasionally called *neuromodulators*), and (3) peptides—a chain of two or more amino acids.

Addiction is a molecular process and physiological/behavioral dependence produced by neuronal changes. *Physical dependence* means that the body de-

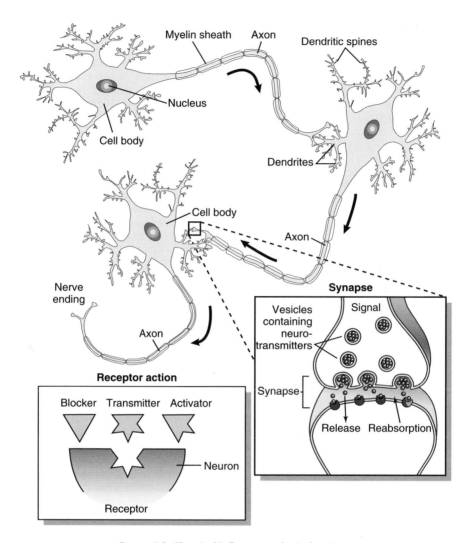

FIGURE 6-2 Chemical influence on brain function.

velops a dependence on the continued presence of a substance and reacts negatively when the drug is removed. This process is known as the *withdrawal syndrome*. *Psychological dependence* prompts a persistent desire or even undeniable compulsion to obtain and take a substance to experience satisfaction and pleasure or avoid discomfort. The body develops resistance to the effects of a substance by requiring progressively larger doses to produce the same desired effect. This *drug tolerance* develops as the result of chronic drug abuse.

| **Box 6-2** | *Neurotransmitters and Actions Involved* |

Acetylcholine

The transmitter responsible for controlling all skeletal muscle activity. At the neuromuscular junction, acetylcholine is excitatory. However, it is inhibitory on the muscle fibers in the heart. This illustrates an important principle: the effect of a transmitter on a postsynaptic cell is not determined by the transmitter but by the postsynaptic receptors. In the brain, acetylcholine is strongly related to learning and memory and in controlling REM sleep.

Dopamine

Primarily inhibitory catecholamine. It is an important part of the brain's reward and pleasure system, causing feelings of euphoria; has many roles, including regulation of conscious movement and mood, and affects management of hormonal balance and the immune system (via the pituitary gland). Degeneration of dopamine-producing neurons is associated with Parkinson's disease.

Endorphins

Peptide. The broad class of endorphins that are the brain's natural morphine. The system modulates pain and pleasure and manages reactions to stress. They act not only as neurotransmitters but also as neurohormones and neuromodulators.

Gamma-Aminobutyric Acid (GABA)

Inhibitory-amino acid. GABA is found in the brain and other major organs and quiets the system. Because the brain is highly interconnected, any excitatory activity would quickly result in a massive chain reaction of activity without the influences of inhibitory neurons, which stabilize brain activity. Low levels are associated with a tendency toward violence.

Glutamate

Principal excitatory amino acid of the brain. Involved in memory, responses to the environment, and perception of pain, specifically reducing sensations, and leads to a sense of detachment or dissociation.

Norepinephrine, Noradrenaline

Amines. Released by the sympathetic nervous system (not subject to voluntary control). Serve as vasoconstrictors, relax the muscle walls, increase blood pressure, and dilate eyes; initiate the fight-or-flight response, anger, or fear, energy, pain reduction, and mental focus. Low levels are associated with anxiety.

Serotonin (5-HT)

Primarily an inhibitory monoamine. Plays a role in the regulation of mood, control of eating, arousal, perception of pain, and sleep. Appears to be related to dreaming. Many hallucinations result from the stimulation of serotonin receptors, an effect that could be described as dreaming while awake.

SCHOOL NURSING ROLE

I. **Health Concerns/Emergencies**
   A. Nurses' assessment skills are necessary for prevention and intervention with students who use illicit substances. Important observation and assessment tasks for examination of the student in the school setting are listed in Table 6-9.
   B. Assessment of emergencies in school settings.
      1. Assessment of substance use emergencies and action vary depending on student, circumstances, and medical condition.

Table 6-9 Substance Abuse Assessment Procedures

Nursing Assessment	Procedure	Observation or Documentation	Normal
General observations	Observation of physical, behavioral, and cognitive changes	Facial sweating, flushed or pale appearance, tense, itching, burn areas on thumb and index finger, confusion, muscle rigidity, tremors, chemical or alcohol breath, rapid or slurred speech, loss of time perception, or any of signs listed below	Normal is ability to follow simple, sequential directions, coherent Rule out disease, infectious process, or injury that can confuse observations
Pulse	Take while seated and at rest when possible May use radial, brachial, or carotid pulse Student may be anxious, causing increased pulse; therefore check pulse twice more, at midway and at end of examination	Concern if consistently above 90 or less than 60 beats/min Physically active students may have lower heart rates	Normal pulse is 60-90 beats/min
Gaze nystagmus (horizontal)	Observe while student follows finger or pen 12-15 in from face, moving slowly from center to extreme right of nose Hold 3 sec at maximum deviation, then move slowly to left side and back to center position Rapid movement of object can result in false nystagmus	Observe for: Jerky, quivering, or smooth pursuit Nystagmus at maximum deviation Angle of onset, angle at which nystagmus is noted—in degrees of 5 (e.g., 35-40-45 or none)	Normal is smooth pursuit

Modified from California Department of Justice (DOJ), Sacramento, Calif, 1998, Advanced Training Center.

Continued

Table 6-9 *Substance Abuse Assessment Procedures—cont'd*

Nursing Assessment	Procedure	Observation or Documentation	Normal
Gaze: nystagmus (vertical)	Assess by moving finger or pen from center of nose up, hold in position 3 sec; move down, hold 3 sec; repeat	Observe for eye bounce	Normal is smooth pursuit at all angles When positive, may indicate high blood alcohol levels
Non/convergence of eyes	Do circular movement with finger or pen 12-15 in away from face; bring stimulus slowly to bridge of nose; hold 3 sec	Observe for any failure of eyes to follow stimulus, inability to cross eyes	Normally, both eyes follow stimuli to point of convergence Rule out any physical condition affecting ability to do testing
Pulse, second	Take while seated	See Pulse	See Pulse
Pupillary size	Pupil size can be done in various settings, room light, near total darkness, or indirect/direct light Pupillary meter is available for use Size more noticeable if performed in darkened room	Observe pupillary size; note size in mm, right and left, and setting of test	Normal pupillary range is 3.0-6.5 mm, but normal adolescents may be outside this range
Pupillary reaction to light	Check reaction while checking pupil size Use penlight to evaluate pupil reaction	Note if slow, sluggish, or nonreactive and setting of test	Pupils normally constrict within 1 sec; slow or sluggish is more than 1 sec Inquire about any current medications because can influence assessment With diabetes, pupils do not dilate even in darkness Congenital anomalies can prevent dilation

Hippus	In direct light (penlight) observe for hippus (e.g., pulsating of pupil) May occur with or without stimulus	Observe for exaggerated rhythmical constriction and dilation of pupil (pulsating) under direct light	Normal is no pulsating Certain drugs produce hippus (e.g., opiate withdrawal) Should not dilate under direct light
Rebound dilation	Use penlight to illicit constriction of pupil Check both eyes	Observe for inability of pupil to remain constricted Positive results if pupils dilate 1 mm or more with continued direct light	Occurs with marijuana, certain hallucinogens
Romberg	Student stands erect with hands at side and feet together Tell student to wait for your instructions Cue to start, ask to tilt head slightly backward, close eyes, and hold position for 30 sec Stop task at 90 sec if not stopped earlier	Note amount of time passed when student indicates 30 sec Observe ability to maintain position	Normally holds position and can estimate sec Under influence of stimulants, will call time rapidly, influence of opiates will slow call Swaying noted with alcohol use
Pulse, third Ingestion-method examination	Take while seated Examine nasal cavity for irritation/inflammation and debris and oral cavities for discoloration and debris Examine limbs and trunk for injection sites	See Pulse Note if white coating on the tongue, blackened lips/gums, or debris, irritation/inflammation in nasal passages Note track marks on skin	See Pulse No evidence of substance use Rhinitis from snorting Marijuana may leave green coating or debris on tongue
Eyes	Observe for: Droopy eyelids (e.g., upper lid touches pupil) Retracted eyelids (e.g., bug-eyed—see white sclera above iris) Swollen eyelids Reddened sclera Watering/tearing Glazed eye appearance	Note droopy, retracted, swollen eyelids Reddened sclera, tearing, or glazing	Rule out familial or physical conditions (e.g., ptosis or conjunctivitis)

Modified from California Department of Justice (DOJ), Sacramento, Calif, 1998, Advanced Training Center.

2. Evaluate for need to call 911; call if any concern regarding:
   a. Decreased or increased pulse.
   b. Decreased respiration.
   c. Hyperthermia with increased thirst and suspected use of inhalants, PCP, or Ecstasy.
   d. Extreme agitation, delirium, seizures.
   e. Any combinations of neurotoxic effects.
3. Eliminate documented or undiagnosed medical condition (e.g., diabetes). Note any prescribed medications.
4. Identify substance whenever possible and gather information from teachers, other staff, peers, and parents.
5. Notify school site administrators, parents, and site and local law enforcement officer as soon as possible.
6. Follow up and coordinate with other team members (e.g., teacher, counselor, school social worker, psychologist).
7. Document according to educational and health requirements.

C. School nurse interventions.
   1. Provide information for staff and parents through several methods (e.g., school meetings and mandated in-service sessions, Parent-Teacher Association meetings, classroom teaching [role playing], newsletters, postings in staff restrooms).
   2. Alcohol and drug education with students, especially pregnant minors, regarding SA is an important tool.
   3. One-on-one counseling with at-risk or abusing student.
   4. Referral for peer counseling.
   5. Awareness of special school and community resources.
   6. Encourage teachers, coaches, and all school staff to take time to listen and support students, which may initiate a natural high on a daily basis.
   7. Encourage mentoring and bonding to a positive role model, either a peer or an adult. Often a former drug user is the preferred helper.
   8. Help student to explore personal capabilities and determine ways to become resilient for contributing to school and family system.

D. Long-term treatment/management.
   1. Be aware of personal biases, prejudices, and personal value conflicts that could be a barrier to fair and humane interventions.
   2. Most adolescents deny their substance use; acceptance of the problem and motivation for change is the beginning focus of treatment.
   3. A continuum of services exists for adolescent substance use disorder: intervention, rehabilitation, and maintenance.
   4. Twelve-step–based treatment program.
   5. Treatment in an adolescent therapeutic community.
   6. Family therapy.

II. **Legal Requirements for School Nurses**
   A. No legal requirement for mandatory reporting as exists for child abuse.
   B. Federal and state law surrounding SA usually is interpreted by individual county or district offices of education. Nurses need a working knowledge of these policies and procedures (e.g., Education Code).

C. Local law enforcement and school administration may have memorandums of understanding.
D. Be knowledgeable regarding state Nurse Practice Act.
E. Use best practices to prevent and intervene with substance abuse patterns.
  1. Opportunities can be provided in school settings for:
     a. Students to learn and practice skills necessary to promote wellness, healthy choices, ability to cope with personal struggles and adversity, and achieve academic success.
     b. Both individual and group counseling, peer counseling and support groups for adolescents trying to achieve and maintain SA abstinence.
     c. Families to participate in educational SA workshops, support groups, and network with community agencies.
     d. Student-centered activities that attract those with various personal interests and capabilities.

WEB SITES

National Institute of Drug Abuse
   http://www.nida.nih.gov
   http://www.clubdrugs.org
National Institute on Alcohol Abuse and Alcoholism
   http://www.niaaa.nih.gov
The Center for Alcohol and Addiction Students
   http://center.butler.brown.edu
Substance Abuse and Mental Health Services Administration
   http://www.samhsa.gov
UCLA Center for Mental Health in Schools
   http://www.smhp.psych.ucla.edu
Al-Anon and Alateen Family Group Headquarters
   212-302-7240
   1-800-356-9996
   http://www.al-anon.alateen.org
Alcoholics Anonymous World Service, Inc.
   212-870-3400
   http://www.aa.org
Inhalant Prevention Coalition
   1-800-269-4237
   http://www.inhalants.org
Families Anonymous
   818-989-7841
   1-800-736-9805
   http://www.familiesanonymous.org

BIBLIOGRAPHY

Allard-Hendren R: Alcohol use and adolescent pregnancy, *Maternal Child Nurs* 25(3): 159-162, 2000.
Anderson K, editor: *Mosby's medical, nursing, and allied health dictionary,* ed 5, St Louis, 1998, Mosby.

Biederman J, Farone VS, Monteaux MC, et al: Patterns of alcohol and drug use in adolescents can be predicted by parental substance use disorders, *Pediatrics* 106(4):792-797, 2000.

Bradley A, Miller D: *Naltrexone approved for alcoholism treatment,* National Institute on Alcohol Abuse and Alcoholism, January 17, 1995, updated October, 2000, U.S. Department of Health and Human Services, Available online: http://www.niaaa.nih.gov/press/1995/naltre-text.htm. Accessed on May 18, 2001.

Brink S: Alcohol: a new understanding of how alcohol alters brain chemistry may transform treatment of the disease, *US News* & *World Report,* pp 51-57, May 7, 2001.

California Department of Justice: *The biochemistry of drugs,* Sacramento, 1998, California Department of Justice Advanced Training Center.

Carper J: *Your miracle brain,* New York, 2000, HarperCollins.

Carter R: *Beneath the surface: mapping the mind,* Berkeley, 1999, University of California Press.

Christensen D: Sobering work: unraveling alcohol's affect on the developing brain, *Science News* 158(2):28-29, 2000.

Ciccetti D, Rogosch FA: Psychopathology as risk for adolescent substance use disorders: a developmental psychopathology perspective, *J Clin Child Psychol* 28:355-365, 1999.

Dupont RL: *The selfish brain: learning from addiction,* Center City, Minn, 2000, Hazelden.

Glantz MD, Hartel CR, editors: *Drug abuse: origins and interventions,* Washington, DC, 1999, American Psychological Association.

Glenmullen J: *Prozac backlash: overcoming the dangers of Prozac, Zoloft, Paxil, and other antidepressants with safe, effective alternatives,* New York, 2000, Simon & Schuster.

Goldstein A: *Addiction: from biology to drug policy,* ed 2, New York, 2001, Oxford University Press.

Heischober BS, Hofmann AD: Substance abuse. In Hofmann AD, Greydanus DE, editors: *Adolescent medicine,* ed 3, Stamford, Conn, 1997, Appleton & Lange.

Horn KA, Maniar SD, Dino GA, et al: Coaches' attitudes toward smokeless tobacco and intentions to intervene with athletes, *J Sch Health* 70(3):89-94, 2000.

Hurt H, Brodsky NL, Betancourt L, et al: Cocaine-exposed children: follow-up through 30 months, *J Dev Behav Pediatr* 16(1):29-36, 1995.

Institute of Medicine: *Pathways of addiction: opportunities for drug abuse research,* Washington, DC, 1996, National Academy Press.

Lewis KD: *Prenatal drug exposure: assessing risk,* doctoral dissertation, San Francisco, 1998, University of California–San Francisco.

Lewis KD: *Infants and children with prenatal alcohol exposure: a guide to identification and intervention,* North Branch, Minn, 1995, Sunrise Press.

Limbird L, Hardman J: *Goodman and Gilman's the pharmacological basis of therapeutics,* ed 10, New York, 2001, McGraw-Hill.

Lindsay GB, Rainey J: Psychosocial and pharmacological explanations of nicotine's "gateway drug" function, *J Sch Health* 67(4):123-126, 1997.

Loveland-Cheery CJ, Leech S, Laetz VB, et al: Correlates of alcohol use and misuse in fourth-grade children: psychosocial, peer, parental, and family factors, *Health Educ Q* 23:497-511, 1998.

Lowry R, Cohen LR, Modzeleski W, et al: School violence, substance use, and availability of illegal drugs on school property among U.S. high school students, *J Sch Health* 69(4):347-355, 1999.

Mahony DL, Murphy JM: Neonatal drug exposure: assessing a specific population and services provided by visiting nurses, *Pediatr Nurs* 25(1):27-36, 1999.

National Institute on Alcohol Abuse and Alcoholism: Fetal alcohol exposure and the brain, *Alcohol Alert* 50:1-4, 2000.

National Institute on Drug Abuse: Maternal smoking during pregnancy associated with negative toddler behavior and early smoking experimentation (NIH Pub No 01-3478), *NIDA Notes* 16(1):1-5, 2001.

National Institute on Drug Abuse: Methamphetamine brain damage in mice more extensive than previously thought (NIH Pub No 00-3478), *NIDA Notes* 15(4):1, 10-11, 2000a.

National Institute on Drug Abuse: NIDA launches initiative to combat club drugs (NIH Pub No 99-3478), *NIDA Notes* 14(6):1-4, 2000b.

National Institute on Drug Abuse: *Community drug alert bulletin,* (NIH Pub No 00-4723), Bethesda, Md, 1999a, The Institute, Available online: http://165.112.78.61/ClubAlert/ClubdrugAlert.html.

National Institute on Drug Abuse: NIDA studies clarify developmental effects of prenatal cocaine exposure (NIH Pub No 00-3478), *NIDA Notes* 14(3):5-7, 1999b.

National Institute on Drug Abuse: Twin studies help define the role of genes in vulnerability to drug abuse (NIH Pub No 99-3478), *NIDA Notes* 14(4):1, 5, 1999c.

National Institute on Drug Abuse: Cocaine abuse may lead to strokes and mental deficits, *NIDA Notes* 14(3):1-3, 1998.

National Institute on Drug Abuse Research Report: *Hallucinogens and dissociative drugs* (NIH Pub No 01-4209), 2001, Available online: http://165.112.78.61/Research Reports/Hallucinogens/Hallucinogens.html.

National Institute on Drug Abuse Research Report: *Heroin abuse and addiction* (NIH Pub No 00-4165), 2000, Available online: http://165.112.78.61/ResearchReports/Heroin/Heroin.html.

Nevins J, editor: Society for neuroscience annual meeting, *Brain Work: The Neuroscience Newsletter,* 11(1):5-6, 2001.

Nicotine and the brain, *Brain Briefings,* Oct 1998, Society of Neuroscience, Available online: http://www.sfn.org/content/Publications/BrainBriefings/nicotine.html. Accessed March 30, 2001.

Petraitis J, Flay BR: Reviewing theories of adolescent substance use: organizing pieces of the puzzle, *Psychol Bull* 117:67-86, 1995.

Pope HG, Yurgelun-Todd D: The residual cognitive effects of heavy marijuana use in college students, *JAMA* 275(7):521-527, 1996.

Richardson GA, Day NL, Goldschmidt L: Prenatal alcohol, marijuana, and tobacco use: infant mental and motor development, *Neurotoxicol Teratol* 17:479-487, 1995.

Rodriguez de Fonseca F, Carrera MR, Navarro M, et al: Activation of corticotropin-releasing factor in the limbic system during cannabinoid withdrawal, *Science* 276:923-925, 1997.

Scattergood P, Dash K, Epstein J, et al: *Applying effective strategies to prevent or reduce substance abuse, violence, and disruptive behavior among youth,* Newton, Mass, 1998, Educational Development Center.

Smith-DiJulio K: People who depend upon substances of abuse. In Varcolis EM, editor: *Foundations of psychiatric mental health nursing,* ed 3, Philadelphia, 1998, WB Saunders.

Substance Abuse and Mental Health Services Administration, Center for Substance Abuse Treatment: *Treatment of adolescents with substance use disorders. Treatment Improvement Protocol (TIP) Series,* Rockville, Md, 1999, The Administration.

Substance Abuse and Mental Health Services Administration, National Advisory Council: *Improving services for individuals at risk of, or with, co-occurring substance-related and mental health disorders,* Rockville, Md, 1997, The Administration.

Tronick EZ, Frank DA, Cabral H, et al: Late dose-response effects of prenatal cocaine exposure on newborn neurobehavioral performance, *Pediatrics* 98(1):76-83, 1996.

U.S. Department of Health and Human Services, Public Health Service: *Summary of findings from the 1998 household survey on drug abuse,* Rockville, Md, 1999, Substance Abuse and Mental Health Services Administration, Office of Applied Studies.

U.S. Department of Health and Human Services, Public Health Service: *Identifying the needs of drug-affected children: public policy issues,* Office for Substance Abuse and Prevention [OSAP] Monograph 11, Rockville, Md, 1992, OSAP.

Weinberg NZ, Glanz MD: Child psychopathology risk factors for drug abuse: overview, *J Clin Child Psychol* 28:290-297, 1999.

Wolfe P: *Brain matters: translating brain research to classroom practice,* Alexandria, Va, 2001, Association of Supervision and Curriculum Development.

Wong DL: Behavioral health problems of adolescence. In Wong DL, Hockenberry-Eaton M, Wilson D, et al, editors: *Whaley & Wong's nursing care of infants and children,* ed 6, St Louis, 1999, Mosby.

Wuethrich B: Getting stupid, *Discover* 22(3):56-63, 2001.

Yazigi RA, Odem R, Polakoski KL: Demonstration of specific binding of cocaine to human spermatozoa, *JAMA* 159(4):163-167, 1991.

CHAPTER 7

Violence

N urses cannot escape the consequences of violent acts toward and by the school-age population. Health problems resulting from the violence, both physical and emotional, can be lifelong and the disabilities extensive. These events occur in schools, homes, and communities. This chapter focuses on *violence toward self* (self-mutilation and suicide), sexual *violence toward others* (rape, date rape), *violence in the home* (physical, emotional, sexual abuse, and neglect), and *violence in schools* (peer harassment and bullying, physical aggression and assault, life threats and homicides, and gangs).

Suicide, or *violence toward self*, increased 100% among children ages 10 to 14 from 1980 to 1996; among 15- to 19-year-olds it increased 14% during the same time period (U.S. Public Health Service, 2000). Public awareness of early subtle and overt signs must be expanded, intervention services and programs require improvement, and research is needed to broaden the knowledge base and develop additional strategies for suicide prevention in all children. Self-mutilation is a pathological yet complex behavior of youth that commonly is expressed as cutting or injury to the body for personal comfort or relief from emotional pain.

Rape is a display of sexual *violence toward another person*. Three relational categories are defined within adolescent rape: stranger, non-stranger (date or acquaintance rape), and incest. All can be detrimental to the victim's health and have serious, long-lasting consequences. These categories are unique in three ways: (1) how the victim processes the event determines his or her prevailing cognitive and psychological behaviors, (2) how the health professional is affected by the incident and how he or she sorts through the salient issues, and (3) the techniques and methods used for treatment. In 1998, 2.7 of every 1000 females suffered a sexual assault compared with 0.2 of every 1000 males (U.S. Department of Justice, 1998).

Violence in the home is defined as physical, sexual, and emotional abuse and neglect of the child or adolescent. Observations of domestic violence and sibling and elder abuse also are considered child abuse. Persons who work with children are responsible for identification of abuse but also are aware that one fourth of all substantiated abuse and neglect reports receive no follow-up by Child Protection Services or other community service system professionals (Wang and Daro, 1997). Often the school nurse is the first person who is aware of the incident and is most likely to report suspected abuse. When the nurse can identify poor relationships and stressors that place an individual or family member at high risk for child abuse, intervention strategies can be implemented.

Violence in schools occurs for all students at each level of elementary and secondary education. Students experience peer conflict and aggression on a daily basis that may lead to interpersonal violence, and an increasing number of students become victims of juvenile crime. The most common types of school violence in U.S. schools are peer harassment and bullying behavior. Assault and bodily injury are less common but still frequent. During the 1990s, documented incidences of peer threats to student life security and safety and homicide on school campuses increased.

Gangs are peer and reference groups organized for both social and antisocial purposes, including peer violence. Gangs have been part of American culture since the colonial era, but the nature of the group has changed. The environment creates the need for violence and antisocial behavior. Participation in gangs may facilitate accomplishment of developmental tasks even if they are counterproductive and harmful to gang members themselves and society. For example, the need for independence is provided by the structure and acceptance of the gang, allowing *emancipation* from the family. The need for *intimacy* is met by peer support within the group, allowing members to redefine their gender role. Security of the gang provides the confidence to pursue intimate relationships. The gang provides acceptance, significance, and protection, allowing the cognitive and social freedom to explore various roles away from the family, thus meeting the adolescent's need for *identity.*

Brain Findings

Numerous studies of human and nonhuman primates provide data on genetic, biological, and environmental keys to aggression and violence. A biochemical link indicating an interaction between defective genes and the environment produces abnormal levels of two mood-altering neurotransmitters, serotonin and noradrenaline. Serotonin plays a key role in regulation of emotions, including control of aggression. Noradrenaline organizes the brain's response to danger. Researchers suggest serotonin has an effect on regulation of self-esteem. High levels of serotonin are associated with high self-esteem and social status and low levels with low self-esteem and status, which can lead to aggression, impulsivity, and suicidal and violent behavior (Fuller, 1995; Kotulak, 1996; Wright, 1995).

Research suggests that the orbitofrontal cortex, located in the prefrontal cortex of the brain, and interconnected structures are associated with self-regulation, social intelligence, impulse control, and attention. In violence-prone individuals, this area appears to be dysfunctional (Davidson, Putnam, and Larson, 2000). This phenomenon occurs not only in overt expressions of aggression but also during everyday demonstrations of failed self-regulation, such as a child's temper tantrums, teenage driving with excessive speed, and parental emotional outbursts.

The most common cause of disruption of self-regulation circuitry is not heredity or trauma but the lack of a nurturing, emotionally consistent living environment during the infant and young child's developing years. Research suggests that the primary caregiver's emotional interactions with the infant are the major influence on biochemical and physiological development of the brain circuitry responsible for emotional and behavioral self-regulation (Davidson, Putnam, and Larson, 2000).

VIOLENCE TOWARD SELF

SELF-MUTILATION

Intentional injury or harm to one's own body is regarded as *self-abuse.* Many terms refer to the problem of self-abuse, including *self-injury, self-inflicted injury, self-destructive behavior, self-defeating behavior,* and *self-mutilation.* In the broadest sense, affected individuals are regarded as those who engage in body modification, self-punishment, or both practices.

I. Definition

A. A useful definition of self-mutilation that incorporates all the variables from different studies is "a direct socially unacceptable, repeated behavior that causes minor to moderate physical injury" (Suyemoto and Kountz, 2000, p 1). This behavior is regarded as pathological and differs from socially acceptable bodily modifications such as body piercing and tattooing. It also differs from indirect, risk-taking self-harm such as driving while drinking. Furthermore, it is not regarded as a suicide attempt in that the motivation for the self-mutilator is to inflict injury or cause suffering but not cause death.

B. Estimates of self-mutilation in the general population range from 14 to 600 per 100,000 annually. Most researchers believe it is underreported. In psychiatric populations, a higher percentage is reported, ranging from 4.3% to 20% for inpatients. Rates among adolescent inpatients range from 40% to 61%. A survey of outpatient therapists showed that 47% had known one self-mutilating adolescent (Suyemoto and Kountz, 2000). This behavior is contagious among adolescents and is more frequent in institutional settings, such as detention facilities, hospitals, and jails.

II. Etiology

A. Youth who self-mutilate have been studied in the medical and psychiatric literature for more than 40 years. Clinicians and researchers differ on the actual diagnosis for self-mutilators, but the consensus is that the practice is related to borderline personality disorder, which has "self-mutilating" behavior as one of its criteria (American Psychiatric Association, 1994). Some authorities associate self-mutilation with bulimia nervosa, and others document co-occurrence with dissociative identity disorder and obsessive compulsive disorder. Youths who are mentally retarded or autistic engage in self-mutilation, but these individuals are not classified in the same manner as self-mutilators.

III. Characteristics

A. Self-cutting is the most common form of self-mutilation. The cuts often are made by razor blades and inflict injury to the wrist and forearms. Girls represent the large majority of self-mutilators; the first incident usually occurs in middle to late adolescence. Occurrence does not vary according to ethnicity, race, or class. Self-cutting usually is a secretive behavior, but scars and wounds often are visible if uncovered. Because of the shame and self-repulsion, affected individuals are socially isolated and selective in their social relationships. Substance abuse frequently is associated with self-mutilation. As many as three fourths of youths describe violence, abuse, and family disruptions as common in their family of origin. They can have severe bodily injury, resulting in hospitalization and need for institutionalization as a means of self-protection. Some studies indicate that as many as 25% of adolescent self-mutilators have never sought medical advice regarding their self-abuse (Suyemoto and Kountz, 2000). Medication is not the treatment of choice except to treat underlying associated disorders (e.g., depression, obsessive-compulsive behavior).

B. Episodes of self-mutilation usually are less than an hour in duration and are a part of a recurring cycle in response to stress triggers that can be seen largely as unconscious, automatic processes of cognition distortion, negative feelings, and critical self-talk.

IV. Effects on Individual

A. Common themes among youths are that self-injury helps them feel physical pain on the outside, instead of emotional pain on the inside; self-injury is a way to gain attention or have someone care about them; or they can manipulate situations and have a sense of power or control for themselves. Usually the emotional incentive to mutilate is fear, hurt, anger and/or perceived rejection or abandonment by others. Obviously, volatile and exaggerated responses can trigger events, but these youths learn to relieve overwhelming emotions by self-injury. Most youths report feeling calm, relief, or more contentment after the injury.

V. Management/Treatment

A. Health care interventions for self-mutilators are similar to those for eating disorders and include the following:
1. A nonjudgmental, hopeful acceptance of the youth.
2. Provision of immediate first aid and medical treatment for cuts/wounds.
3. Understanding of the variance in personal triggers and usual episodes of self-mutilation for each youth.
4. Clarification of negative emotions and identification of cognitive distortions.
5. Teaching of alternative strategies for self-comfort/soothing (e.g., rocking, massage, cold pack/warm bath).
6. Development of personal care contracts with some youths.
7. Referral for intensive psychotherapy or group support services.
8. Further research in this area, which nurses are ideally suited to perform.

VI. Web Sites

Self-Injury: You are not the only one
http://www.palace.net/~llama/psych/injury.html

SUICIDE

I. Definition

A. Deliberate violence toward self or self-destruction, with the intent of taking one's own life, resulting in death.

B. Nationwide, 19.3% of students have seriously considered suicide. *Suicide is the third leading cause of death* among students ages 10 to 24 years; in many states it ranks as the second leading cause of death in students ages 15 to 19 years (U.S. Public Health Service, 2000). The incidence is greatest among white males, with a 105% increase among black males from 1980 to 1996. Males outnumber females 5:1 in ages 15 to 19. Between 1952 and 1995, the prevalence of suicide for adolescents and young adults nearly tripled (U.S. Public Health Service, 2000).

II. Etiology

A. Suicide is multicausal. Causes of *childhood suicide* may include escape from physical or sexual abuse, chaotic family situations, feelings of being unloved, constant criticism, depression, loss of significant relationships, humiliation, potential or actual failure in school, or intent to punish friends or family. Professionals who work with these students report a high prevalence rate of suicidal thoughts among adolescents.

B. Causes of *adolescent suicide* (in addition to the causes listed previously) may include difficulties or lack of meaningful relationships, perfectionist expectations, serious problems with parents, sexual issues, or fight with a close friend. In some cases, "copy-cat" suicide occurs to gain attention or identify with a peer who has completed suicide. Suicide and attempted suicide are more prevalent among youth in cults, homosexual youth, high-risk youth (i.e., those using drugs and alcohol), and Hispanic students. Teenage girls attempt suicide more frequently, whereas teenage boys have a higher rate of completed suicides. Girls more often use less violent methods of suicide (e.g., pills), and boys use guns more frequently.

III. Characteristics

A. Elementary-age student, kindergarten through sixth grade.
   1. *Verbal cues:* somatic complaints about headaches and stomachaches. Comments indicating loneliness, isolation, and not being loved.
   2. *Behavioral cues:* poor school performance, withdrawal from play and leisure interests, apathy, listlessness, erratic appetite, and sleep disturbance. Sometimes are careless and destructive toward property—both their own and others.
   3. *Affective cues:* feelings of sadness, irritability, lack of empathy, tend not to be carefree or engage in spontaneous laughter. Change in routine of doing chores (i.e., cleaning their room, caring for animals).

B. Adolescent student, junior and senior high school.
   1. *Verbal cues:* students may make subtle or obvious comments about suicide (e.g., "Will you miss me when I am not here?" or "I won't be bothering you anymore.").
   2. *Behavioral cues:* may stockpile pills, obtain a weapon, withdraw from activities and friends, abuse drugs or alcohol, neglect appearance and self-care, dispose of personal belongings, change sleep patterns, listen to suggestive music, suddenly receive different academic grades, change friends and relationships, engage in promiscuous sex, change appetite, or report sleep problems.

3. *Affective cues:* decreased self-gratification, feelings of hopelessness and guilt, sadness, lack of empathy, boredom, and chronic or acute depression.

IV. Health Concerns/Emergencies
A. Physical health issues (e.g., appetite, sleep, hygiene).
B. Acute or recurrent depression, mood swings, or other psychiatric problems.
C. Pattern of repeated suicide attempts missed by adults.
D. Failed suicide attempts, resulting in temporary or permanent handicap.
E. "Copy-cat" behaviors of friends and other students.
F. Mental health disorder, with need for suicide watch or placement in a more restrictive setting for self-protection.

V. Effects on Individual
A. Temporary or permanent handicap caused by failed suicide attempt.
B. Emotional trauma related to repeated attempts.
C. Depression or recurrent depression.
D. Feeling of loss with sadness, grief, guilt, and disbelief by family, friends, and school peers despite whether suicide is successful.

VI. Management/Treatment
A. Be alert to warning signs to intervene early to prevent attempts or completion. Never ignore a warning or threat and do not be afraid to ask the question.
B. Address drug and alcohol use that contributes to depression.
C. Support and teach student and others about stress, depression, sadness, coping with loss, and academic, social, and athletic challenges that may put the student at greater risk for suicide attempts or completion. This may be a component of the School Crisis Team or non-crisis intervention and prevention.
D. Refer for intensive counseling and treatment.
E. Treat underlying mental health disorders.
F. Provide counseling to intervene for affective, behavioral, and self-esteem issues. Suicide attempts should always be professionally evaluated.
G. Interventions centering around family support system, including listening to child, being needed and respected by family, high but realistic expectations of student, caring and nurturing, spiritual/religious involvement, and perceiving school staff as supportive.
H. If not in place, establish School Crisis Team with emergency guidelines and mechanism of referral for at-risk students manifesting depressive behaviors, suicidal characteristics, or both features.
I. Counseling and referral to a survivor's support group for classmates after the incident and at the anniversary of event.
J. Knowledge and skill in interviewing techniques, including the use of a suicidal lethality checklist.

VII. Additional Information
A. More people are killed by suicide than by homicide (U.S. Public Health Service, 2000). The actual rate may be higher than reported

rates because suicide deaths sometimes are concealed because of stigma, uncollectible insurance, and incidence of some accidents as actually suicides. More than 75% of youth suicide is associated with a diagnosable mental or substance abuse disorder. With constant media exposure to violence and homicidal behavior, youth may become desensitized to life-threatening behavior and increase feelings of omnipotence or invulnerability to death. Suicide attempts may be a nonverbal cry for help. Gender identity issues related to sexual orientation and behavior increase the risk for depression and subsequent suicide attempts and completions.

B. The nurse should be familiar with and knowledgeable of the landmark document, *National Strategy for Suicide Prevention: Goals and Objectives for Action,* spearheaded in 2001 by Dr. David Satcher, U.S. Surgeon General (U.S. Public Health Service, 2000).

VIII. Web Sites

The American Association of Suicidology (AAS)
http://www.suicidology.org
The American Foundation for Suicide Prevention (AFSP)
212-363-3500
1-888-333-2377
http://www.afsp.org

VIOLENCE TOWARD OTHERS

RAPE

I. Definition

A. Rape is unwanted sexual acts involving force, threats, violence, or inability to give consent (e.g., mental illness, intoxication, date-rape drugs such as gamma-hydroxy butyrate [GHB] or Ecstasy). Definition of rape now includes all forms of sexual victimization, including vaginal or anal penetration and oral sex, and it includes both male and female victims. The Bureau of Justice (1995) states the crime of rape only requires slight penile penetration; full penetration and ejaculation are not necessary for rape to occur. Definitions may vary from state to state.

B. Family members or acquaintances commit 74% of rapes, of these 48% are date rapes; 26% by strangers; highest percentages occur in summer on weekends and at night; more than 50% of victims are younger than 18 years old (U.S. Department of Justice, 1998). These statistics reflect the need for heightened awareness among school nurses and others working with this population. Incidents of rape among youth are underreported.

II. Etiology

A. Rape reflects antisocial and relational problems of the perpetrator and is not something the victim provoked. It is usually a violent expression of power and control rather than sexuality.

III. *Brain Findings*

A. The hormones cortisol and corticotropin are neurotransmitters released during stress. Repeated release of these neurotransmitters during early childhood abuse causes physical changes in brain structures that make the individual subject to increased sensitivity to minimal stress in adulthood.

B. These relatively permanent brain changes caused by physical and sexual abuse of young girls can affect later life experiences, resulting in more emotional and physical difficulties (e.g., depression, anxiety disorders, gastrointestinal problems) (Heim et al, 2000).

IV. Characteristics

A. *Rape trauma syndrome,* or the acute stage of disorganization and longer stage of reorganization for the victim's life adjustments after sexual assault, is used by the North American Nursing Diagnosis Association (NANDA) (NANDA, 1994), but it is referred to as *posttraumatic stress disorder (PTSD)* by mental health practitioners.

   1. Acute stage:
      a. *Somatic responses:* genitourinary discomfort or pain, pruritus; muscle spasms and pain related to tension; gastrointestinal disorders, nausea, vomiting, and anorexia.
      b. *Psychological responses:* denial, shock, hysteria or stoicism, panic, nightmares, anger, guilt, and fear.
      c. *Sexual responses:* mistrust of males, change in sexual behavior.

   2. Long-term stage:
      a. *Psychological responses:* phobias, nightmares or sleep disturbances, anxiety (chest pain, palpitation, and diaphoresis), or depression, suicidal thoughts; may appear normal; may deny or suppress; mistrust of men and friends or withdrawal; reliving the event through flashbacks or intrusive thoughts; avoidance of experiences previously enjoyed; difficulty with memory and concentration; avoidance of situations or place where assault occurred.
      b. Victimized adolescents can be more resilient with supportive parents who are not abusive, and when their negative feelings and thoughts of the event are countered by an enduring self-integrity.

V. Health Concerns/Emergencies

NOTE: State laws may vary regarding time of reporting, evidence required, and consents needed for reporting.

A. Evidence must be gathered within 72 hours by health care professionals with special training and equipment.

B. Individual should not shower, brush teeth, or urinate if possible.

C. Victims need time to express feelings; proceed slowly with the process.

D. Advise regarding transmission of sexually transmitted diseases (STDs), including human immunodeficiency virus (HIV)/acquired immunodeficiency syndrome (AIDS).

E. Victim may have vaginal or anal lacerations, bruising, bleeding, and possibility of pregnancy.

F. Rape trauma syndrome or PTSD is not unusual.

VI. Effects on Individual

A. Fear of contracting STDs, including HIV/AIDS; fear may last for months.

B. Somatic complaints often increase in frequency.

C. Individual may experience lack of trust, feelings of loss of control, and victimization.

D. Rape is one of life's most devastating experiences, with recurrent flashbacks and recall in long-term memory.

E. Older youth may experience lack of sexual desire and intimacy fears.

F. Male sexual abuse is uncommon but is usually unreported because of embarrassment about homosexual implications.

G. Males are more likely to experience rape trauma syndrome.

VII. **Management/Treatment**

A. Postcrisis support system development and counseling should be in place for the student for at least 1 year after trauma.

B. Facilitate support in the victim's social networks (e.g., school, church, and other places).

C. Protect the victim from accusations and blame by the perpetrator for the rape action.

D. Maintain strict confidentiality so as not to humiliate the victim.

E. When treating the victim, be aware that different responses in recovery exist, depending on different developmental stages.

F. Provide continuity of care for the victim, who likely will suffer from PTSD.

G. Nurses should be aware of their own thoughts and feelings about rape as an influence on how they respond to the victim.

H. Crisis intervention: victim needs time to express feelings and receive emotional support; help victim with approaches and methods to increase sense of safety.

I. Victim assistance funds are available in most states for provision of physical and mental health services.

J. When providing services to parents and family members, be concerned and sensitive to anger, guilt, blame of the victim, and self-blame.

VIII. **Additional Information**

A. Prevention teaching can be conducted in schools as early as the elementary years through discussions of respect, cooperation, consideration, and other life skills necessary for healthy social relationships.

B. Factors significant in adolescent rape can be discussed and role-played with older youth, including alcohol and drug use; interactions with older males or with acquaintances or strangers in unsupervised settings; accepting rides from strangers; staying out extremely late; physical, mental, or emotional deficits; homelessness.

C. A health care professional with special training and equipment should gather *evidence* regarding the rape. Most metropolitan cities in the United States and Canada have Sexual Assault Nurse Examiner/Sexual Assault Response Teams (SANE/SART) available; if not, the emergency room physician performs the examination.

1. Victim service/rape victim advocate is called before examination to stay with the victim through the assessment phase and will bring a complete set of clean clothing because personal clothing may be

collected for evidence. Each step in the examination is explained before performing it. When desired, a companion is supportive for the victim during history taking and examination.

2. Follow rape assessment protocol for individual state for proper chain of evidence; procedures for each may differ in requirements for examination process.

3. When doing an *evidentiary sexual assault* examination, the following may be done:

   a. Detailed history of alleged assault, after which examination is performed according to victim's reported history. May include examination of genitalia, perineum, anus, rectum, and pharynx; colposcopy photographs (a magnifying lens for the purpose of examination of the cervix and vaginal areas; for rape victims, a camera is mounted for photographs to detect trauma).

   b. Sample collection of vaginal, anal, and oral secretions.

   c. Photographs of trauma, or if provided, use of diagrams of the body to indicate findings such as bruises, abrasions, lacerations, or scars.

   d. Use of Wood's light to detect dried secretions on body.

   e. Wet mount of vaginal secretions; slides for sperm motility.

   f. Collection of foreign hair.

   g. Pubic hair and blood for typing and swabs of perianal area and rectum only if history indicates.

   h. Serum human chorionic gonadotropin (HCG) hormone is used to determine pregnancy before giving morning-after pill.

   i. Treatment of acute trauma.

   j. Provision of other at-home testing and care and recommendation for appointment with primary care provider for follow-up and supervision of trauma event.

DATE RAPE

Date rape is the most common rape event in adolescence and is underreported because the victim may feel guilt and responsibility for the event. Girls usually do not define rape that occurs during a date as a reportable offense. Drugs and alcohol frequently are associated.

Several illicit drugs can be used by the perpetrator—Rohypnol, GHB (liquid Ecstasy), and ketamine. When it is mixed with a liquid, soda, alcohol, or water, Rohypnol dissolves instantly and is effective within 20 to 30 minutes. It is colorless, odorless, tasteless, and virtually undetectable.

Educational programs are an important component for prevention. The definition of rape and date sex refusal skills (to reduce risk) should be included. These can also be discussed by the nurse with individual students as needed.

I. Web Sites
   International Society for Traumatic Stress Study
   847-480-9028
   http://www.istss.org

VIOLENCE IN THE HOME

PHYSICAL, EMOTIONAL, AND SEXUAL ABUSE AND NEGLECT

I. Definition
   A. *Child abuse* is any situation in which a child suffers mistreatment or serious injury by other than accidental means. Child abuse encompasses physical, emotional, and sexual harm and neglect. The abuser can be a parent, sibling, custodian, or guardian.
   B. *Physical* abuse is any damage to the skin, bones, and internal and external organs or structures. *Emotional* abuse is a nonphysical, usually verbal, form of assault. The child does not experience the usual feelings of love, security, and worthiness. *Sexual* abuse is the use of a child for sexual gratification by an adult or a person who is significantly chronologically or developmentally older than the victim. Sexual abuse includes molestation, exploitation for prostitution, incest, or use of the child for pornographic materials. *Neglect* is the failure, over a long time, to provide the child with basic needs, such as food, clothing, home cleanliness and safety, medical care, supervision, and education. Infants and young children are those most often neglected.
   C. It is estimated that more than 3 million children in the United States were reported as victims of child abuse or neglect, or approximately 45 per 1000 children (Peddle and Wang, 2001).

II. Etiology
   A. Child abuse is seldom the result of any single factor; it is a combination of various factors: environment, circumstances, parenting skills, coping mechanisms, and stress factors.

III. *Brain Findings*
   A. Research suggests an increase of stress hormones during childhood abuse produces sharper hormonal and physical responses to minor stress events in adulthood. These findings in adult women are consistent with numerous animal studies (Heim et al, 2000).

IV. Characteristics
   A. *Physical abuse.*
      1. Ecchymosis (bruises).
         a. May be multiple and in various stages of healing and discoloration.
         b. Often seen in places where bruising does not commonly occur as result of normal childhood activity.
         c. Marks from belts and rulers are frequently seen patterns.
      2. Burns of questionable origin.
         a. Recognizable by shape (e.g., iron, grill of electric heater),
         b. Indication of immersion into hot water is glovelike or socklike appearance on hands and feet or doughnut-shaped scald on buttocks.
         c. Burns caused by hot running water form a zebra-striped pattern on the body (creases on abdomen and folds of upper legs remain clear) and occur when the child is held by hands and legs.

     d. Cigarette burns are usually multiple and found on palms and soles.

     e. Rope burns generally are found around wrists or ankles.

  3. Abrasions and lacerations.

     a. May be found on any area of body, including mouth, lips, ears, eyes, and external genitalia.

     b. Frenulum is torn from jabbing spoon into mouth during feeding.

     c. Injury to oral mucosa or frontal dental ridge from poking a bottle into mouth.

  4. Intracranial trauma.

     a. Lethargy, stupor, confusion, coma, or other signs of altered mental state.

     b. Nausea, vomiting, irritability.

     c. Seizures.

     d. Papilledema.

     e. Bulging fontanel in infant.

     f. Prominent veins.

  5. Damage to internal organs.

     a. Shock.

     b. Blood in urine or stool.

     c. Increased pulse rate.

     d. Abdominal pain or distention.

  6. Skeletal damage: fractures.

     a. Commonly skull, nose, and other facial structures involved; "spiral" fractures result from twisting of arms or legs.

     b. Rib fractures.

     c. Old fractures evident with x-ray films.

     d. Dislocations.

  7. Behavior of child.

     a. Unpleasant, demanding, disobedient, and difficult to get along with.

     b. Reports injury by parents.

     c. Extremely aggressive or extremely withdrawn.

     d. Frequently comes to school late or often absent.

     e. May linger around school after dismissal.

     f. Avoids physical contact with others.

     g. Wears concealing clothing (e.g., long sleeves) to hide injuries.

     h. Child's explanation does not fit type or seriousness of injury.

     i. Child appears frightened of parents or shows little or no distress at separation from parents.

     j. Eager to please or placate an angry adult to avoid injury.

     k. Indiscriminately seeks affection from any adult.

     l. Demonstrates poor self-concept.

B. *Emotional abuse.*

  1. Signs not as obvious as with other forms of abuse.

  2. Best indication is behavior.

     a. Apathetic, withdrawn, passive, depressed, and shows lack of positive self-image

     b. Antisocial behavior (e.g., stealing, destructiveness).

      c. Signs of emotional turmoil (e.g., rocking, biting, enuresis, encopresis).

      d. Problems in school: developmental delays, excessive activity, behavior problem, failure.

      e. Assumes inappropriate adult roles and responsibility, such as those of parent.

      f. Difficulty making friends.

      g. Fearful, prone to nightmares, anxious.

      h. Compulsively conforms to adults' instructions.

      i. Anxious when faced with new situations or people.

      j. Excessive fantasizing.

      k. Sadistic behavior.

C. *Sexual abuse.*

  1. Signs.

      a. Stained or bloody underwear.

      b. STD of eyes, mouth, genitalia, or anus.

      c. Lacerations, bleeding, or bruising of genitalia, vaginal or anal area, mouth, or throat.

      d. Early awareness of sexuality.

      e. Dysuria, edema, or itching in genital area.

      f. Vaginal or penile discharge.

      g. Pregnancy.

  2. Behavior of child.

      a. Informs nurse or other adult of sexual assaults.

      b. Withdrawn, preoccupied with fantasy, or may appear retarded.

      c. Infantile behavior or acts like adult instead of child.

      d. Poor relationships with peers.

      e. Displays early seductive behavior or knowledge of sex inappropriate for age.

      f. Unwilling or hesitant to participate in physical activities.

      g. Poor academic performance, engages in delinquent acts or runs away from home.

D. *Neglect.*

  1. Signs.

      a. Failure to thrive.

      b. Malnutrition.

      c. Does not receive necessary medical or dental care, immunizations, or medication.

      d. Dirty clothing or dressed unsuitably for weather.

      e. Frequently unwashed, body odors, and poor oral hygiene.

      f. Often left unattended for long periods.

      g. Often hungry, has not eaten breakfast, and has no money for lunch.

      h. Child under 14 years left alone or unsupervised.

  2. Behavior of child.

      a. Constantly fatigued or sleepy.

      b. Steals food.

      c. Frequent absences from school or comes early and stays late.

d. Few friends, seeks refuge in siblings.

e. Uses alcohol or drugs.

f. Engages in vandalism or sexual misconduct.

V. Differential Diagnosis

A. Cultural practices: traditional healing practices may be confused with physical abuse.

1. Cupping, which is a Chinese practice for headaches or abdominal pain.

2. Coining, a Vietnamese health practice used for minor aliments. Both of these practices are used by other cultures.

3. Native Americans have various healing rituals that may seem to delay seeking appropriate care.

4. Homeopathic remedies are gaining wide support cross-culturally and when not effective can delay other care or treatment.

B. Health conditions.

1. Mongolian spots can be confused with bruising.

2. Dermatological conditions have been confused with abuse because they may resemble burns from cigarettes or scalding water (e.g., epidermolysis bullosa, bullous impetigo).

VI. Health Concerns/Emergencies

A. Long-term handicapping sequelae of physical abuse require multidisciplinary services (i.e., neurological, orthopedic, surgical, nursing, rehabilitation, and social welfare services).

B. Subtle signs of head injury may be manifest after trauma and must be identified.

C. Frequent colds, bronchitis, and pneumonia commonly are related to physical neglect.

D. When immunizations have not been given because of neglect, child lacks protection from a number of serious diseases and their medical consequences.

E. Children with poor hygiene and unsanitary living situations have frequent skin conditions (e.g., impetigo, scabies, severe diaper rash, boils); dental and periodontal problems also are common.

F. Lacerations, punctures, and burns may become infected.

G. STD, pregnancy, poor sphincter control, and other results of sexual abuse require immediate medical care and ongoing emotional support.

H. *Inorganic failure to thrive* is often a consequence of neglect or inadequate parenting skills.

1. Height and weight are under third percentile; decreased weight reflects acute malnutrition; depressed height is indicative of cumulative effects of chronic malnutrition.

2. Unresponsiveness and withdrawal.

3. Little smiling.

4. Developmental delays.

5. Feeding difficulties.

6. Delayed dentition.

7. Delayed speech and social skills.

I. *Munchausen syndrome by proxy* is a cluster of signs and symptoms in which illness in a child is simulated, faked, or produced by a caregiver, resulting in numerous medical appointments or procedures and frequent school absenteeism. Acute symptoms decrease or stop when separated from the caregiver. *Munchausen syndrome by proxy* encompasses both physical and emotional abuse. This is seen as a spectrum of medical child abuse from parental hypervigilance, parent fabrication, or induced illness/injury, resulting in unnecessary medical treatment.

J. *Shaken baby syndrome* is violent shaking of a child that causes intracranial trauma that can result in brain damage, visual impairment, or death.

K. *Maternal deprivation syndrome* (infants) and *psychosocial dwarfism* (children) are defined as growth failure in infants and children caused by growth hormone secretory impairment. This syndrome results from living in an environment of severe emotional deprivation.

L. Abuse of all forms causes emotional damage and frequently requires professional intervention and support of those closely associated with student.

VII. **Effects on Individual**
   A. Development of self-concept suffers.
   B. Difficulties in school and in making friends.
   C. Delinquency, drug abuse, alcoholism, and obesity can develop during adolescence.
   D. Lessons of violence learned in childhood frequently are used by the abused against their own children and society in general.
   E. Young child may undergo delays in cognitive, social, and motor development.
   F. As adults, the abused have difficulty maintaining relationships and choosing a good mate.
   G. Adults who have been abused as children frequently seek love and acceptance from those who are unable to meet their expectations, and as parents they have an exceptional need for love from their children.
   H. Female victims of incest have been shown to be at high risk for suicide and eating disorders.
   I. Often victims of sexual abuse become prostitutes, both male and female.
   J. Greater risk for suicide attempts or completion.

VIII. **Management/Treatment**
   A. Treatment of child's physical injuries is initial concern.
   B. Report *all* cases of suspected child abuse to child protective services. Teachers and others require education regarding the importance of early detection and mandated reporting of suspected child abuse.
   C. Damage and other long-term handicapping sequelae must be identified and services provided (e.g., schooling, rehabilitation, counseling, physical therapy).
   D. Entire family should be part of program that uses multidisciplinary team approach in meeting both physical and psychological needs.

E. Psychological counseling is vital for abuser and victim.

F. Parents and victim may benefit from participation in support groups.

G. Many community resources are available to families; these resources provide needed support (e.g., public health nurses, day care centers, child abuse hotlines, volunteer organizations, mental health agencies, safe houses or shelters).

H. Be alert for parents who show a potential for child abuse and, when possible, direct them to needed resources, such as parent groups, hotlines, and counseling services.

I. Be available and empathetic when the parent and child need someone who can provide practical assistance and resources.

J. Be aware of personal feelings or bias regarding those who committed or allowed the abuse to occur.

K. See "Additional Information" for preventive measures.

IX. **Additional Information**

A. Observed effects of domestic violence vary according to a student's age. *Infants* through age 5 may display signs of health problems, including loss of weight, feeding problems, and inconsolable crying. *Preschoolers* may appear anxious or sad, be clingy or aggressive with peers, or regress in toilet training. *Ages 6 to 12* may be depressed, fearful, demonstrate aggressive behavior, or have low self-esteem. May appear socially isolated because of restricted social activity from embarrassment of family violence. *Adolescents* may act out by running away from home, using drugs and alcohol, becoming withdrawn or depressed, leading to suicide attempts or completions. Others may assume parenting roles while caring for younger siblings and not attend school. Many are argumentative and verbally abusive to parents and may have a strong fear of parental breakup and divorce. They usually have internal conflict and ambiguous feelings about taking sides, preferring a neutral and aloof demeanor.

B. Statutes now exist in all 50 states regarding the reporting of suspected cases of child abuse and neglect. In all states, anyone can report a case of suspected child abuse and neglect; however, states differ regarding who is *mandated* to make a report. Certain states mandate everyone to report suspected child abuse and neglect (i.e., doctors , nurses, teachers, social workers, and police officers). Physicians are mandated in every state to make a report. All states provide the reporter with immunity from civil and criminal liability provided the report is made in good faith.

C. Preventive measures.

1. Promote prenatal classes to help the expectant mother and her partner prepare for parenting and the changes a child will bring to their lives.

2. Develop high school parenting classes to prepare the adolescent for the physical and emotional care of a child and the enormous responsibilities of parenting.

3. Educate nurses, teachers, and society in general regarding detection, prevention, and reporting of suspected child abuse.

4. Initiate parent groups, hotlines, respite services, day care centers, and other parental support systems if they are not available in the community.
5. Remove the child from the home to prevent further abuse when intervention methods have failed.
6. Involved agencies should follow up with the family after the child has returned to the home and should provide ongoing counseling and services as needed.
7. Refer high-risk parents for services. The high-risk parent may display any one or a combination of the following:
   a. Low self-esteem.
   b. History of being abused and no parenting role models.
   c. Coping problems with daily activities.
   d. Unrealistic expectations and attitudes toward the child.
   e. No friends or distrust of others.
   f. Weak coping skills when faced with a crisis.
   g. Personal needs are lacking, such as food, housing, and employment.
   h. Significant illness or the birth or presence of a child with special needs.
   i. Little or no support from spouse.
   j. Inadequate financial resources.

X. **Web Sites**
   Prevent Child Abuse America
   312-663-3520
   http://www.preventchildabuse.org
   Child Welfare League of America
   202-638-2952
   http://www.cwla.org/
   National Clearinghouse on Child Abuse and Neglect Information
   1-800-394-3366
   http://www.calib.com/nccanch/

VIOLENCE IN THE SCHOOLS

PEER HARASSMENT AND BULLYING

Peer competition, aggression, and conflict commonly is expressed in the form of teasing, taunting, name calling, rumor mongering, scapegoating, threats, intimidation, and minor nonverbal actions, such as scowls, negative finger movements, and physical isolation or social ostracism. Students who are the most likely victims for peer harassment and bullying (PH&B) are those who are small of stature, overweight, handicapped or disabled, passive and quiet, socially isolated or nonconformist, new or transient, and ethnic or racially diverse students. Studies have indicated that students at low risk include those who are from intact families, popular, high achieving, and academically proficient, and those recognized, rewarded, and liked by school staff.

Research concludes that male students are more likely to bully or be bullied; bullies have higher rates of tobacco and alcohol use; peer verbal abuse is a frequent antecedent to physical harm and assault; peer pressure prohibits reporting of incidences to adults; student absenteeism and truancy increase by student victim; victims develop internalizing disorders such as acute anxiety (fears, phobias, and panic attacks), depression, and psychosomatic illness (headaches, stomachaches, and muscle aliments). A nationwide study reports that bullying behavior in American schools affects 1 in every 3 children and teenagers. U.S. government officials have declared that bullying in schools is a major, compelling public health problem today (Nansel et al, 2001).

Because bullying has been common in public and private schools for generations, school staff have not given the necessary attention for prevention, intervention, and postvention. The recent alarming research has been a "wake-up call" for educators, counselors, and nurses to design and manage a positive, proactive, school-wide culture of cooperation and care for all students. As the health care member of the school staff, the nurse can initiate and collaborate with the following practices:

1. Target health history taking on PH&B.
2. Solicit relevant self-report regarding PH&B when providing health care.
3. Provide timely and appropriate intervention when cruelty or discrimination is observed.
4. Prepare and distribute critical incident report to parents and school staff.
5. Assist in follow-up counseling, discipline, and sanctions for the bully.

PHYSICAL AGGRESSION AND ASSAULT

Another category of school violence is the occurrence of hurt or harm from one student to another by pushing, shoving, hitting, kicking, biting, and pinching that leads to bodily injury and personal humiliation. Physical assaults with weapons such as sticks, furniture, eating utensils, knives, and guns result in abrasions, lacerations, contusions, concussions, fractures, severe bleeding wounds, or loss of consciousness; some of these injuries are beyond nursing care at the school site. This level of school violence leads to administrative action, school security intervention, primary health care provider service, or emergency medicine, paramedic, and emergency room care.

Epidemiological studies and research have documented the increasing incidence of school violence, especially for inner-city schools and high schools. A national school survey of more than 12,000 middle and high school students revealed that one fourth reported that they had been victims of violence (Resnick et al, 1997). Urban schools reported the following acts of violence: (1) 93% of the districts reported student assaults, (2) 91% of districts reported student possession of weapons, (3) 40% reported shootings and stabbings in schools, (4) 25% reported drive-by shootings, and (5) 19% reported rape on the school grounds (NASB, 1993). All these statistics have increased with the availability of firearms so that injuries have led to fatalities. Regarding violent crime, 21% of all public high schools and 19% of all public middle schools reported at least one serious violent crime to the police or other law enforcement (Pratt and Greydanus, 2000).

Students who are victims or who witness violent behaviors develop specific emotional and psychosocial distress symptoms, including pervasive fear, feelings of vulnerability, traumatic memories, and sleep disorders. Exposure to violence also has been associated with truancy, school avoidance, phobias, hypervigilance, inability to concentrate or learn, and school dropout. Frequent or severe student violence creates an atmosphere of insecurity and mistrust that lowers student body morale and motivation for academic achievement (Warner and Weist, 1996). Posttraumatic reactions are common for student victims.

School nurse interventions for physical aggression and assaults are the same as those listed for PH&B. Other effective violence prevention practices and policies adopted countrywide for school sites include the following:

1. Vigilant adult supervision of the student body throughout school day, especially in high-risk areas (e.g., restrooms, playgrounds, stairways, before and after school, and during transitions).
2. Staff development and training in critical incident management and crisis intervention.
3. Classroom training in anger management and conflict resolution.
4. Increased use of peer mediation, peer counselors, and helpers.
5. Additional uniformed security guards and supervisory staff on playgrounds and after school hours.
6. Hallway and classroom camera surveillance, better lighting, more open spaces.
7. Intensive mental health services for perpetrators and victims.
8. Zero tolerance for student violence, leading to suspensions, mandated counseling services, and expulsion, with referral to daily educational and psychosocial treatment services.

LIFE THREATS AND HOMICIDES

The most serious and apprehensive student violence consists of threats to human life and limb and actual incidences of homicides. Overall, *homicide is the second leading cause of death* for persons 15 to 24 years of age and is the leading cause of death for black and Hispanic males ages 15 to 24. At schools, homicide has increased in frequency over the last two decades, with 194 school-related deaths reported between July 1994 and June 1998. Crime statistics show that 28% of fatal injuries happen in school buildings, slightly more than one third occurred on the school campus, and 25% occurred off campus (Pratt and Greydanus, 2000).

Recent high-profile school shootings throughout the country that have led to injuries and deaths among students have resulted in the identification of high-risk youth who perpetrate violence. The following factors are common among high-risk youth:

1. Male students and older students.
2. Victims of physical or sexual abuse, or both, and neglect in their backgrounds.
3. Antisocial or delinquent histories.
4. Unpopular students and victims of bullying.
5. History of poor school relationships and academic failure.
6. History of substance abuse and access to firearms.
7. Depression and/or personality disorders (e.g., antisocial personality).
8. Those who threaten or resort to intimidation for control or power.
9. Heavy exposure to violence in the media.
10. Member of a hate group or cult.

Additional *violence prevention/intervention practices and policies* for homicides include the following:
1. Quick prosecution and sentencing of perpetrators of juvenile violence/crime.
2. Early detection and treatment for high-profile students.
3. Threat-appraisal teams and intervention services.
4. Available crisis intervention teams and posttraumatic support services.
5. Gun control enforcement, limited access to weapons.
6. Timely school day cancellations for threats and campus-wide lock-down during violent episodes.

In development of effective and cost-efficient intervention strategies, no easy answers or certain solutions exist to prevent violence in the schools (Lamberg, 1998). Research has concluded that positive policies and practices are more effective than those that are punitive (Dusenbury et al, 1997). However, children and youths are still safer at schools than in their homes or communities. School nurses should be careful not to generalize from past dramatic and sensational school violence episodes with catastrophic predictions and an ominous perspective. Nurses should join with other responsible school adults, concerned parents, and prosocial students to provide a protective shield and a caring ethos at the school setting.

GANG ACTIVITY

I. **Definition**
   A. Group of individuals (usually peers) bound together by camaraderie, loyalty, common sense of purpose, and common clothing or colors. Gangs are cliques and groups with social and antisocial objectives. Recent studies estimate about 400,000 U.S. youths are in gangs.

II. **Etiology**
   A. Multiple long-term factors are involved; can include poor parenting or lack of parental involvement and supervision and support, low self-esteem and confidence, antisocial or aggressive behaviors with rejection by peers, poor school achievement, and increased school truancy. Alcohol consumption, drug abuse, gambling, or a combination of these factors are common among gang members. Gangs are more common in inner-city schools. Onset may occur in the elementary school years.

III. **Characteristics**
   A. Informal social groups with unusual names.
   B. Signing, display of gestures.
   C. Representation by clothing, mannerisms, display of actions on one side of body (i.e., bandanna on one arm, cut on one eyebrow).
   D. Wearing of colors to display allegiance (e.g., red, blue, black, silver, gold).
   E. Possession of unexplained cash and material items.
   F. Breaks curfews, rules, and laws.
   G. Sacrifices morals and feelings for those of the gang.
   H. Developmental needs and goals are no different than those of youth who are not gang members.
   I. Gang is structured, secure, and protective.

J. Most members drop out of gangs by age 20.

K. Antisocial outcome factors associated with gang activity include drug availability in or near school; graffiti or tagging, which marks particular gang territory as a warning; increased use of beepers, pagers, and cellular telephones; presence of weapons; drive-by shootings; daytime burglaries; and number of racial incidences.

IV. Health Concerns/Emergencies

A. Homicide.

B. Bodily injury from violence, including rape.

C. Disfigurement and risk of infections and disease (e.g., hepatitis B from tattoos and piercing).

D. Incarcerations.

E. Drug and alcohol use.

F. Sexual activity.

V. Effects on Individual

A. Lack of personal or academic success, school failure.

B. Sense of belonging and purpose, although not socially acceptable.

C. Negative peer pressure related to association with gangs or unpopular reference groups.

D. Radical peer orientation contrary to parental bonding and family association.

E. Change in personality and preference for nickname or street name.

F. Outcomes can include violence recidivism, criminality, incarceration, and premature death.

G. Effects extend to the community and society in general (e.g., increased financial liability, impact on criminal justice system, decreased individual safety and freedom, loss of life and productivity).

VI. Management/Treatment

A. Must start intervention early in life. Early prevention and intervention techniques include support techniques for good parenting skills, appropriate social and emotional support; referrals to centers for child care and management of behavioral, aggressive, and violence problems.

B. School-age intervention: school staff can be more tolerant of students who have different personal styles and behaviors; all children "need to be needed" (i.e., tasks can be assigned in the school setting [school nurse assistant, runner for secretary] to increase self-esteem and provide sense of accomplishment, acceptance, and feelings of belonging).

C. School security may profile known gang members and provide additional monitoring of these students.

VII. Additional Information

A. Incarcerated youths have higher incidences of physical abuse, learning disabilities, psychiatric illness, lead toxicity, and early sexual activity; access juvenile diversion programs.

B. Much attention has been directed to school violence, including the use of guns and weapons by students on school sites across the country. News stories are dramatic and shocking, but national incidences should not lead the school nurse to postulate that schools are unsafe places for students. Less than 1% of all homicides and suicides occur in or around school campuses (Barrios, 2000).

VIII. Web Sites
National Youth Gang Center
850-385-0600
http://www.iir.com/nygc/
National Criminal Justice Reference Center
http://www.ncjrs.org
Keep Schools Safe.com
http://www.startcolorado.com/safe/
Youth Crime Watch of America
http://www.ycwa.org
Center for Mental Health Services
http://www.mentalhealth.org/

BIBLIOGRAPHY

American Psychiatric Association: *Diagnostic and statistical manual of mental disorders,* ed 4, Washington, DC, 1994, The Association.
Barrios L: Federal activities addressing violence in schools, *J Sch Health* 70(4):119-121, 2000.
Behrman R, Larner M, Stevenson C: Protecting children from abuse and neglect: analysis and recommendations, *The Future of Children,* 8(1), 1998, Packard Foundation.
Bureau of Justice Statistics: *Violence against women: estimates from the redesigned survey,* Washington, DC, 1995, U.S. Department of Justice.
Carpenito L: *Nursing diagnosis: application to clinical practice,* ed 8, Philadelphia, 2000, Lippincott Williams & Wilkins.
Coupey S: *Primary care of adolescent girls,* Philadelphia, 2000, Hanley & Belfus.
Crime and Violence Prevention Center: *Child abuse prevention handbook and intervention guide,* Sacramento, 2000, California Attorney General's Office.
Davidson R, Putnam K, Larson C: Dysfunction in the neural circuitry of emotion regulation: a possible prelude to violence, *Science* 289:591-594, 2000. Available online: http://www.sciencemag.org.
Dusenbury L, Falco M, Lake A, et al: Nine critical elements of promising violence prevention programs, *J Sch Health* 67(10):409-414, 1997.
Enserink M: Searching for the mark of Cain, *Science* 289:575-579, 2000.
Farrington DP, Loeber R: Epidemiology of juvenile violence. In Lewis DO, Yeager CA, editors: *Child and adolescent psychiatric clinics,* Philadelphia, 2000, WB Saunders.
Federal Bureau of Investigation: *Uniform crime reports: crime in the United States,* Washington, DC, 1997, U.S. Government Printing Office.
Finberg L: *Saunders manual of pediatric practice,* Philadelphia, 1998, WB Saunders.
Fuller R: Neural functions of serotonin, *Sci Med* 2(4):48-57, 1995.
Garrity C, Jens K, Porter W, et al: Bullyproofing your school, *Intervention in School and Clinic* 32(4):235-243, 1997.
Girardin BW, Faugno DK, Seneski PC, et al, editors: *Color atlas of sexual assault,* St Louis, 1997, Mosby.
Heim C, Newport DJ, Heit S, et al: Pituitary-adrenal and autonomic responses to stress in women after sexual and physical abuse in childhood, *JAMA* 284(5):592-597, 2000.
Kotulak R: *Inside the brain: revolutionary discoveries of how the mind works,* Kansas City, Mo, 1996, Andrews & McMeel.
Lamberg L: Preventing school violence: no easy answers, *JAMA* 280(5):404-407, 1998.
Martin M, Waltman-Greenwood CW, editors: *Solve your child's school-related problems,* Washington, DC, 1995, Harper Collins.

Nansel TR, Overpeck M, Pilla RS, et al: Bullying behaviors among U.S. youth: prevalence and association with psychosocial adjustment, *JAMA* 285(16):2131-2132, 2001.

National Centers for Disease Control and Prevention: *Youth risk behavior surveillance—United States 1999*, Washington, DC, 2000, U.S. Government Printing Office.

National School Boards Association: *Violence in the schools: how America's school boards are safeguarding our children*, Alexandria, Va, 1993, The Association.

Niehoff D: *The biology of violence: how understanding the brain, behavior, and environment can break the vicious circle of aggression*, New York, 1999, Free Press.

North American Nursing Diagnosis Association: *NANDA nursing diagnoses: definitions & classifications 1995-1996*, Philadelphia, 1994, NANDA.

Olweus D: *Bullies at school: what we know and what we can do*, Cambridge, Mass, 1993, Blackwell.

Peddle N, Wang C: *Current trends in child abuse preventing and reporting fatalities: the 50-state survey*, 2001, Available online: http://www.preventchildabuse.org/learn_more/research_docs/1999_50_survey.pdf.

Perry BD, Azad I: Posttraumatic stress disorders in children and adolescents, *Curr Opin Pediatr* 11(4):310-316, 1999.

Pfefferbaum B, Allen JR: Stress in children exposed to violence: reenactment and rage, *Child Adolesc Psychiatr Clin N Am* 7(1):121-135, 1998.

Pollak SD, Cicchetti D, Hornung K, et al: Recognizing emotion in faces: developmental effects of child abuse and neglect, *Dev Psychol* 35(5):679-688, 2000.

Pratt HD, Greydanus DE: Adolescent violence: concepts for a new millennium, *Adolesc Med* 11(1):103-125, 2000.

Reece R: *Child abuse: medical diagnosis and management*, Philadelphia, 1994, Lea & Febiger.

Resnick MD, Bearman PS, Blum RW, et al: Protecting adolescents from harm: findings from the National Longitudinal Study on Adolescent Health, *JAMA* 278(10):823-832, 1997.

Riner M: Stopping school violence in its tracks, *Nurse Week* Nov:16-17, 1999.

Schafran LH: Topics for our times: rape is a major public health issue, *Am J Public Health* 86:15-16, 1996.

Smith-DiJulio K: Evidence of maladaptive responses to crisis: rape. In Varcolis E, editor: *Foundations of psychiatric-mental health nursing*, ed 5, Philadelphia, 1995, WB Saunders.

Suyemoto K, Kountz X: Self-mutilation, *Prevention Researcher* 6(94):1-11, 2000.

Sylwester R: The neurobiology of self-esteem and aggression, *Educational Leadership* Feb:75-79, 1997.

U.S. Department of Health and Human Services, Centers for Disease Control and Prevention: Youth risk behavior surveillance, 1999, *MMWR Morb Mortal Wkly Rep* 49(SS05):1-96, 2000, Available online: http://www.cdc.gov/mmwr/preview/mmwrhtml/ss4905a1.htm.

U.S. Department of Justice: *National crime victimization survey*, Washington, DC, 1998, Bureau of Statistics, Available online: www.ojp.usdoj.gov/bjs/pub/ascii/cv98.txt.

U.S. Public Health Service: *The surgeon general's call to action to prevent suicide*, 2000, Available online: http://www.mentalhealth.org/suicideprevention/calltoaction.asp. Accessed on July 7, 2001.

Wang C, Daro D: *Current trends in child abuse reporting and fatalities: results of 1996 annual 50-state survey*, Chicago, 1997, National Community to Prevent Child Abuse.

Warner BS, Weist MD: Urban youth as witnesses to violence: beginning assessments and treatment efforts, *J Youth Adolesc* 25:361-377, 1996.

Wong DL: *Whaley and Wong's nursing care of infants and children*, ed 6, St Louis, 1995, Mosby.

Wright R: The biology of violence, *The New Yorker*, pp 68-77, Mar 13, 1995.

CHAPTER 8

Adolescent and Gender-Specific Issues

*P*roviding comprehensive care to adolescents with an emphasis on preventive and proactive health care services is a strategic and challenging role for school nurses. Adolescents are an at-risk population for accidents, illness, and inconsistent health care. Adolescents generally have a challenging lifestyle, often with inadequate nutrition, sleep deprivation, and poor physical fitness habits. Because they live "for the moment," they take their health for granted, unaware of the long-term implications of poor health habits. Subject to peer pressure that promotes experimentation with technology, toxic substances, and sexuality, they often become victims of accidents, illness, and addictions.

Nurses who work with middle school and high school adolescents need resources to consistently and creatively provide health information. Health screening, diagnosis, management, and treatment of diseases should be accessible to adolescents, and the confidentiality provided by state laws should be followed.

Adolescents are peer oriented; therefore interventions centralized among teens as helpers and trainers result in optimal outcomes for adolescent compliance or practice. The nurse should support and oversee programs such as peer tutoring, peer counseling, antidrug dramas and plays, safe-sex peer psychoeducational programs, and Teens Against Drunk Driving.

School health clinics on high school campuses throughout the United States have been standard educational services since the late 1980s. These services often are staffed by school nurses, school nurse practitioners, or nurse practitioners with a specialty in adolescent medicine. Other health care staff may include adolescent primary care physicians, mental health practitioners, and other public health providers.

Every nurse requires up-to-date, reliable reference guides and manuals to access best practices for adolescent health care. This chapter addresses general health issues, gender-specific issues, sexually transmitted infections (STIs), and breast and testicular self-examinations. Some controversial and basic adolescent concerns are presented, such as tattooing, body piercing, steroid use, cosmetic-related skin care concerns, and oral health care. Other adolescent health issues are covered elsewhere in the manual, including eating disorders, obesity, depression, rape, herpes I and II infections, and suicide. The bibliography at the end of the chapter lists useful resources.

General guidelines and recommended frames of reference for school nurses serving adolescent students in middle schools and high schools include the following:
• Adolescence is a time of change, experimentation, and risk taking.
• Adolescents need a basic positive, proactive lifestyle based on healthy choices regarding self-care and personal health.

- School nurses should affirm the decision-making and problem-solving capacities of the adolescent for self-determination in the context of confidential delivery of service.
- Adolescents have a great capacity for individual responsibility and can be supported and strengthened by personal grievance and treatment contracts with school nurses, teachers, and parents.
- Health care providers (HCPs) should access the protective factors and risk factors to maximize the resiliency of the vulnerable adolescent.
- Given the effect of peer orientation on the adolescent, preventive health care efforts should promote a positive peer culture whereby teenagers assume responsibility for the well-being of each other.
- Every effort should be made to strengthen the adolescent's resources within the family and from parents or parent surrogates, such as foster parents and group home staff.
- The stage of adolescence is fundamental to the formation of attitudes and personal habits regarding health that have long-range prognostic implications for quality of life and onset of diseases and disabilities.
  The nurse should:
- Be skilled at using health history and high-risk inventories.
- Provide anticipatory guidance in social, sexual, peer pressure, nutrition, exercise, substance abuse, and risk-taking behavioral issues.
- Be aware of important mental health issues.

GENERAL CONDITIONS

ACNE VULGARIS

I. Definition
  A. Chronic skin condition of the pilosebaceous units (well-developed sebaceous glands with miniature hairs) usually located on the face, neck, upper chest, shoulders, and upper back. Acne is the result of an interaction between keratin, sebum, and sometimes bacteria (comedo). When the opening of the follicle is tight, it appears to be white (whitehead); when the pore is open to the air, it appears black (blackhead). The black color probably is due to the melanin pigment in the skin and does not represent dirt.

II. Etiology
  A. The causes of acne include a strong genetic predisposition; increased secretion of hormones, specifically androgens, which trigger production of oil (sebum) on the skin; and plugged oil ducts that allow bacteria on the skin (keratin) to multiply and produce redness and swelling. The exact mechanisms of acne are unknown.
  B. Many adolescents (85%) develop some degree of acne. No scientific link has been identified between diet and acne.

III. Characteristics
  A. Most common skin problem seen by HCPs.
  B. Usually observed between the ages of 12 and 17, but it can begin as early as age 8 and can last for 10-15 years.

C. Boys have more severe acne that lasts a shorter time, and girls have milder acne that lasts a longer time.

D. Whiteheads may resolve spontaneously or rupture, resulting in an inflamed pustule.

E. Inflammation, redness, and swelling can occur and may result in pustules, papules, nodules, and cysts, some of which may cause scars.

F. Inflammation, slow healing, and possible scar formation may occur as a result of trauma (e.g., picking, wearing athletic gear).

G. Hormonal triggers such as premenstrual flares occur in about 70% of female adolescents.

H. Acne is aggravated and intensified by emotional stress or nervous tension.

I. Oil-based cosmetics may increase production of comedones; adolescents should avoid occlusive products such as cocoa butter and vitamin E oil.

J. Acne is exacerbated by some medications (e.g., androgenic oral contraceptives [e.g., Lo-Ovral, Nordette], barbiturates, hydantoin [Dilantin], corticotropin, and oral and topical steroids).

K. Acne can be exacerbated by environmental factors at work (e.g., exposure to cooking oils in fast-food facilities, grease in auto repair shops).

IV. **Health Concerns/Emergencies**

A. Excoriée des filles or picker's acne is a superficial type of acne caused by compulsive picking of trivial facial lesions, which causes secondary damage and often leads to scarring.

B. Acne fulminans is rare but occurs in adolescent boys and manifests with inflammatory nodules and plaques, which lead to severe pustules and leave large ulcerations. Onset is abrupt with fever, weight loss, anemia, and polyarthritis.

C. Differential diagnosis.

1. Flat warts: skin-colored papules that spread with trauma.

2. Rosacea, milia, folliculitis, and cosmetic, environmental, mechanical or drug-induced acne. Acne clears with removal of causative factors.

V. **Management/Treatment**

A. Preventive teaching during early sex education and family education classes.

B. Student education should include the following:

1. Wash face with mild soap such as Neutrogena bid; harsh and frequent scrubbing may irritate the skin.

2. Do not pick, scrub, or squeeze acne.

3. Identify aggravating agents, such as oil-based cosmetics, face creams, hair spray, or mousse.

4. Discuss lack of documentation that cola, chocolate, nuts, or french fries cause acne; emphasize importance of well-balanced diet for healthy skin.

5. Discuss psychosocial concerns.

6. Encourage compliance to treatment regimen, since it takes months to clear acne; some teenagers believe particular foods are related to a flare-up; recommend avoidance of those foods.

7. Avoid sun when using tretinoin (Retin-A), or antibiotics (e.g., tetracycline [Achromycin], minocycline).
8. If acne does not resolve, referral to a dermatologist for prescription medication is indicated.
C. Monitor side effects of medications.
D. Medications include topical agents (e.g., tretinoin, benzoyl peroxide); systemic therapy to clear eruptions and prevent recurrence (e.g., tetracycline, clindamycin, minocycline, erythromycin); acne surgery, extractions of comedones, or incision and drainage; and peeling treatments, cryotherapy with liquid nitrogen (removes superficial skin). Usually 6-8 weeks is required before significant improvement is noted with antibiotic treatment.
E. Isotretinoin (Accutane) is an important prescriptive antiacne treatment for severe nodulocystic acne. It is a major teratogenic drug in males and females and *must not be taken during pregnancy or lactation.* A pregnancy test must be performed before use by all females, and they must sign a patient consent form regarding birth defects and Accutane.
F. Warnings for adolescents taking prescribed medications include the following:
1. Girls taking oral contraceptives should use a backup method of contraception for the first 2 weeks they take systemic antibiotics.
2. Effective contraception must be used 1 month before, during, and 1 month after therapy with isotretinoin for sexually active adolescents.
3. Sun exposure should be avoided, particularly with certain medications (e.g., tetracycline, tretinoin, isotretinoin).

VI. Web Sites
American Academy of Dermatology: Acne
http://www.aad.org/pamphlets/acnepamp.html
MedlinePlus: Acne
http://www.nlm.nih.gov/medlineplus/acne.html

COSMETIC-RELATED SKIN CARE CONCERNS

I. Definition
A. The regular use of products, specifically with teenage girls, to cleanse, enhance, beautify, or alter appearance that contribute to irritations, infections, and physical health problems.

II. Etiology
A. Cosmetic-related skin care concerns may be associated with the integrity of the skin, nails, and predisposition or family genetics. The type of product, amount used, frequency, and lack of adherence to recommended use also may contribute to skin care concerns. Product ingredients, such as fragrances and preservatives, may cause contact dermatitis and allergic reactions.

III. Characteristics
A. Part of many students' daily grooming habits.
B. Health concerns usually develop within the first few applications of a cosmetic or skin care product but may develop after continual use.

C. Reaction depends on the skin condition and the immune system.

D. Open skin lesion that is irritated or an allergic reaction.

E. Overly dry, sensitive skin or oily skin that obstructs pores.

F. Burning, itching, stinging, and redness are indicators of irritation.

G. Sunlight may potentiate the allergen or irritant in the product.

IV. **Health Concerns/Emergencies**

  A. *Irritant contact dermatitis* may be caused by many products, including antiperspirants, bath soaps, detergents, eye cosmetics, moisturizers, shampoos, and permanent hair wave solutions. Water is known to irritate very dry skin.

  B. *Allergic contact dermatitis* may be caused by cosmetic ingredients, such as *fragrances and preservatives.*

  1. More than 5000 known additive fragrances are used in skin care products; hypoallergenic fragrances are available. By law, hypoallergenic products must be labeled, so users should *check label* for *fragrance-free* or *without perfume* notations. Unscented does not mean fragrance-free because an additive may be used to disguise the chemical odor. Users *must* also check labels of products advertising natural ingredients to avoid plant or animal allergens.

  2. The second most common cause is *preservatives* added to skin products. These agents are added to preserve the products from light and oxygen damage and prevent bacterial and fungal growth that causes skin reactions. Preservatives must be added if a cosmetic contains water. Not all students will react to every preservative. Reaction to one preservative does not apply to all preservatives. Preservatives include dimethol dimethyl (DMDM) hydantoin, formaldehyde, imidazolidinyl urea, methylchloroisothiazolinone, phenoxyethanol, and quaternium-15.

  C. *Acne cosmetica* may be caused by the use of heavy, oil-based products. Check the product label for the term *noncomedogenic* or *nonacnegenic;* this means the product will not clog pores or cause acne.

V. **Management/Treatment**

  A. Discuss and problem solve with the student to determine the cause and available solutions.

  B. Washing hands and using the small scoop included with a product before applying cosmetics or performing skin care decreases contamination of skin and products. Bacteria in the products can contribute to skin irritations and decrease the effectiveness of the product.

  C. Use of products developed to maintain healthy skin, such as astringents, moisturizers, and sunscreens, may minimize potential concerns but also has risks:

  1. Astringents may cause drying, itching, burning skin.

  2. Users may be allergic to some ingredients in moisturizers and sunscreens.

  D. Discuss proper use of cosmetics and skin care products:

  1. Makeup should be discarded if color or odor changes.

  2. Liquid should never be added unless indicated in instructions.

3. Container should be stored away from sunlight and tightly closed to maintain active preservatives.
4. Eye makeup should never be used if wearer has an active eye infection (e.g., conjunctivitis).
5. Contaminated products should be discarded.

VI. Web Sites

American Academy of Dermatology: Solving Problems Related to the Use of Cosmetics & Skin Care Products
http://www.aad.org/pamphlets/cosmetic.html
American Academy of Dermatology: Your Skin and Your Dermatologist
http://www.aad.org/pamphlets/yourskin.html
U.S. Food and Drug Administration: On the Teen Scene: Cosmetics and Reality
http://www.cfsan.fda.gov/~dms/cos-teen.html
U.S. Food and Drug Administration: Cosmetic Safety: More Complex Than at First Blush
http://www.cfsan.fda.gov/~dms/cos-safe.html

Table 8-1 *Potential Risks of Cosmetic Products*

Products	Risks	Comments
Artificial nails	Fungal infection may lead to permanent nail loss Nail may peel and crack with methacrylate-free glue Methacrylate is an allergen	May be avoided when complete seal is made between natural and artificial nail Avoid methacrylate-free glue
Nail polish	May cause rash on other parts of body that have been exposed before drying (face, eyelids, neck, fingers)	Avoid touching body parts or try hypoallergenic polish
Hair dye	Semipermanent and permanent dyes may cause contact dermatitis or immediate reaction of hives and/or wheezing	Be aware of personal allergens and avoid ingredients Temporary dyes usually are nonallergenic
Hair shampoo	May irritate and dry skin/scalp	Change product brand
Hair permanents	Can damage hair and cause brittle, dry hair and scalp irritation	Do not use more frequently than every 3 mo; do not use on damaged or dyed hair without corrective products Always follow instructions
Aerosol sprays	Risk of fire Contamination of food Inhalation may cause lung damage	Avoid use while smoking, near heat or fire Keep away from foods Avoid inhaling product or do not use
Powders	Inhalation may cause lung damage	Avoid when possible or apply gently to decrease airborne inhalation

HOMOSEXUALITY

I. Definition
   A. Homosexuality is the persistent attraction to a member of the same sex. Same-sex attractions have their onset in late elementary and early adolescence and may involve some homosexual experimentation.

II. Etiology
   A. The etiology of homosexuality is unknown. Several theories are associated with the cause of homosexuality: *genetic* (gene and twin studies), *hormonal* (prenatal effects of sex hormones on the brain), *psychosocial circumstances* (learned behavior, lack of heterosexual exposure), *neurological* (prenatal development of brain structures and genitalia), and *combinations* (complex interplay of many theories).

III. Characteristics
   A. Sexual identity is formed gradually over time and is more dominant in late adolescence and young adulthood.
   B. Feeling of being different.
   C. Acknowledgment of same-sex attraction.
   D. Guilt and embarrassment regarding feelings.
   E. Strives to change feelings by adapting behaviors and thoughts.
   F. Unable to alter sexual preference.
   G. Exploration of homosexual lifestyle.
   H. May experiment with both sexes until preference or orientation is established.
   I. Commitment to a lifestyle and pursuit of a positive image.

IV. Health Concerns/Emergencies
   A. At risk for STIs; traumatic injuries related to intercourse should be assessed by sexual behavior, not sexual orientation.
   B. At risk for hepatitis A, B, and C and human immunodeficiency virus (HIV).
   C. May have psychosocial problems adjusting to identity.
   D. Suicide risk: 25% of homosexual and bisexual youth have attempted suicide (USHHS, 1989).
   E. Increased concerns for depression, substance abuse, and suicide.
   F. Health care may not be adequate because some health care professionals will not treat homosexuals since the acquired immunodeficiency syndrome (AIDS) epidemic.
   G. Documentation could jeopardize confidentiality and ability to obtain insurance and certain jobs.
   H. Concern for physical danger because of homophobia.

V. Management/Treatment
   A. Listen and encourage adolescents to articulate concerns and fears about sexual orientation.
   B. Screen and immunize for hepatitis A and B.
   C. Recommend yearly testing for gonorrhea, syphilis, and chlamydia and periodic HIV testing if sexually active or substance abusers; discuss safe-sex practices.
   D. Listen to and support parents; provide contacts for local chapter of Parents, Family, and Friends of Lesbians and Gays (PFLAG) when appropriate.

VI. Additional Information

A. Some heterosexual teens will engage in homosexual activity in particular environments (e.g., incarceration facilities, summer camps, military, boarding schools) but revert to heterosexual activities when environment changes. These experiences may lead to confusion and panic, especially when the teenager enjoys the activity.

B. Decisions made related to a child with ambiguous genitalia may have been incorrect. Genitalia, genes, internal gender structures, and feelings may not match sexual assignment of individual, causing inner confusion, guilt, and discontent (see "Ambiguous Genitalia" in Chapter 4).

C. Bisexual students are attracted to both sexes and engage in both heterosexual and homosexual behaviors. They may have masculine and feminine characteristics, which place them at increased risk for STI/HIV.

VII. Web Sites

Sex, etc: A web site by teens for teens
http://www.sxetc.org/
Jacksonville Area Sexual Minority Youth Network: GLBTQ Youth On-line Resources
http://www.jasmyn.org/links.htm

DENTAL CARIES

I. Definition

A. Dental caries is the progressive loss of tooth mineral caused by a bacterial infection, particularly *Streptococcus mutans*. It is the most common health problem of the school-age child.

II. Etiology

A. Formation of dental caries depends on dietary sucrose or fermentable carbohydrates that are broken down into sugar in the mouth. Bacteria in plaque feed on the sugar-producing organic acids, which demineralize the tooth.

III. Characteristics

A. Caries may begin in toddlers with bedtime bottle use and frequent intake of sugary drinks and food.

B. Cavity-causing bacteria, *S. mutans,* may be spread from person to person (e.g., a mother or father with cavities may pass the bacteria to the baby through kissing).

C. Children's early cavities begin as white spots, demineralization, on the four upper front teeth.

D. Left untreated, cavities progress and cause pain, infection, and tooth loss.

IV. Health Concerns/Emergencies

A. Large holes in teeth, pain, inflammation with or without fistulas, or draining abscesses on gums in root area of teeth.

B. Premature loss of primary teeth can affect nutrition, speech, self-esteem, and crowding of permanent teeth.

V. Management/Treatment

A. Refer for dental checkups beginning at age 1.

B. Biannual dental examinations.

C. Provide fluoride supplements in areas with nonfluoridated water supply up to age 18.
D. Brush twice a day and floss between teeth daily.
E. Limit intake of sweet, sticky foods and drinks, especially at snack time; provide fruits and vegetables.
F. Use small pea-sized amount of fluoride toothpaste daily as early as age 1 and larger pea-sized amount for adolescents.
G. Apply sealants on permanent molars when they erupt: age 6 for first molars and 12 for second molars (see Appendix C).

VI. Web Sites
American Dental Association: Teens Oral Health
http://www.ada.org/public/topics/teens/teens.html

MALOCCLUSION, ORTHODONTIA, AND BRACES

I. Definition
A. Orthodontia is concerned with the diagnosis, prevention, and correction of malocclusion and irregularities of the teeth. Orthodontic appliances modify teeth positions and move or keep teeth in correct position for an extended period of time; most exert continuous pressure. A variety of appliances are used, including fixed, removable, intraoral, and extraoral devices.

II. Etiology
A. A common cause of malocclusion is genetics, but thumb sucking, tongue thrusting, trauma, dental disease, or early loss of primary or permanent teeth may be contributory factors.

III. Characteristics
A. Malocclusion.
1. Malocclusions include overbite, underbite, crossbite, rotated or twisted teeth, or overcrowded mouth.
2. Self-consciousness or embarrassment because of appearance of teeth.
3. Mastication may be painful and ineffective.
4. May interfere with speech.
5. Predisposition to dental disease.
B. Orthodontic appliances.
1. May be uncomfortable, especially after initial placement and adjustments.
2. Braces may be metal attached with adhesives; clear and attached to outside surfaces; ceramic, appearing like natural teeth; mini-braces; or invisible, which are fixed to the inside of the teeth.
3. Head or neck gear is ordered when extra tension outside the mouth is needed; it is worn during the day or at night or evening.
4. Appliances may be needed from 6 months to 2 years or longer.

IV. Health Concerns/Emergencies
A. Dental disease caused by inability to brush teeth well.
B. Orthodontic wires may come loose and harm oral tissue.

V. Management/Treatment
   A. Assessment of pain for medication or referral to orthodontist.
   B. Analgesics: ibuprofen (Motrin) or acetaminophen (Tylenol) may be needed to relieve discomfort and pain. Never place medication directly on gums.
   C. Encourage wearing of orthodontic devices during lengthy treatment regimen and after treatment if wearing retainer devices.
   D. First aid for broken braces and wires.
      1. If the damaged appliance can be removed, take it out.
      2. If unable to remove, cover sharp/protruding point with cotton balls, gauze, or chewing gum.
      3. If wire is stuck in the gums, cheek, or tongue, do not remove; immediately refer student to a dentist or orthodontist.
      4. Broken or loose appliance: if not bothering student, usually does not need immediate attention.

VI. Additional Information
   A. After appliances are removed, the teeth are cleaned thoroughly, and more x-ray films and impressions of the teeth may be taken. Monitor growth of wisdom teeth for possible extraction. Retention treatment may be needed to maintain teeth position and prevent shifting and moving of teeth until gums, bones, and muscles adapt to the change. Retainers may be ordered to be worn on a daily basis for a few months up to several years. Retainers prevent shifting of teeth back to prior position.

VII. Web Sites
   Kidshealth.org: All About Orthodontia
   http://www.kidshealth.org/teen/your_body/medical_care/braces.html
   American Dental Association: Braces and Orthodontics
   http://www.ada.org/public/faq/braces.html

PERIODONTAL DISEASE

I. Definition
   A. Periodontal disease, often called *gum disease,* refers to a pathological condition of the tissues surrounding and supporting the teeth.

II. Etiology
   A. Periodontal disease usually is caused by plaque, a sticky film of bacteria, which continuously forms on teeth. When the plaque is not removed, gums become irritated, inflamed, and begin detaching from teeth to form pockets where bacteria can be harbored. When untreated, this process can destroy bone and other important tooth-supportive tissues, eventually leading to tooth loss.

III. Characteristics
   A. Early stage.
      1. Called *gingivitis.*
      2. Red, swollen, and gums bleed easily.
      3. Normally easily reversible by better brushing and flossing and routine professional cleanings.

B. Late stage.
   1. Called *periodontitis.*
   2. Gums and bone that are supportive structures of the teeth are seriously damaged; pockets form, and gums recede or pull away from teeth.
   3. Teeth become loose and fall out or need to be extracted.
C. Warning signs.
   1. Bleeding of gums while brushing.
   2. Tender, red, or swollen gums.
   3. Pulling away of gum from teeth.
   4. Separating or loose teeth.
   5. Pus between gums and teeth.
   6. Changes in the way teeth fit together when biting.
   7. Pain usually is not present.
   8. Persistent bad breath.

IV. **Health Concerns/Emergencies**
   A. Inflammatory process can destroy bone and healthy tissue in and around the teeth.
   B. Plaque or bacteria create toxins that can damage gums.
   C. Bacteria or the inflammatory response from gum disease may be associated with systemic problems (e.g., bacterial pneumonia, cardiovascular problems, or stroke).
   D. Loss of teeth.

V. **Management/Treatment**
   A. Brushing and flossing twice a day and use of proximal brush between teeth daily.
   B. Routine dental assessments.
   C. Avoidance of tobacco.
   D. Eating a balanced diet.

VI. **Additional Information**
   A. When plaque hardens, it become a porous, rough deposit called *tartar* or *calculus.* When hardened, plaque can be removed only by a dentist or dental hygienist. An instrument called a periodontal probe is used to measure the gingival sulcus depth around each tooth and the space between the gums and teeth to determine whether pockets are present. The normal depth between healthy gums and teeth is 3 mm or less.

VII. **Web Sites**
   American Dental Association: Periodontal Disease
   http://www.ada.org/public/topics/gum.html

TATTOOING AND BODY PIERCING

I. **Definition**
   A. *Tattoos* are permanent body designs by insertion of a needle containing pigment into the dermal layer of the skin. This includes permanent facial makeup, such as eyebrow and lid lining and lip augmentation.
   B. *Body piercing* is a creation of a hole anywhere in the body for placement of adornments. May include ears, eyebrows, nose, lip, tongue, breasts, navel, and genitalia on both males and females. Both tattoos and body piercing are considered body art.

II. Etiology

A. Tattoos may express commitment to a significant other, be an expression of individuality, or beauty enhancement. They also may be symbols of loyalty to a particular group membership (e.g., gangs, motorcyclists, military affiliation). Body piercing is an expression of enhanced beauty, individuality, and/or loyalty.

III. Characteristics

A. May be observed on various body areas.

B. Both procedures present a risk for infection.

C. Piercing is less permanent than tattooing.

D. Average age of first tattoo is 14 years; for first body piercing, average age is 15 years, but does occur at younger ages.

E. Some states ban tattooing of minors.

F. Teenagers may like the shock value of tattooing or piercing in unusual places.

G. Swelling, inflammation, crusting, or scabs at tattoo or piercing site.

IV. Health Concerns/Emergencies

A. Improper follow-up care by students.

B. Infections and hygienic concerns.

C. Allergic reaction to tattoo dye.

D. Should not donate blood for a year after receiving a tattoo or any body piercing.

E. Possibility of serious infection from unsterile needle injection and piercing equipment. May include tetanus, hepatitis, and HIV infection.

F. Potential complications can occur with piercing, including excessive bleeding, development of keloids, nerve and soft tissue damage, or speech impediment.

G. Typically done by unlicensed personnel; permanent facial makeup usually is done by licensed personnel.

V. Management/Treatment

A. Discuss with adolescents the possible health risks, the stigma attached to piercing and tattooing particular body parts, and the fact that adolescents are doing these procedures.

B. Suggest with adolescents that they:
  1. Talk with peers who have tattoos or body piercing.
  2. Discuss expense, healing time, pain, and complications.
  3. Consider individuality and independent decision making.
  4. Can always delay or change decision.

C. If a decision to proceed is made, follow up with how to select a professional tattoo artist or body piercer. Suggest they:
  1. Use recommendations from peers or family.
  2. Visit shops to observe room lighting, cleanliness of the area, techniques for sterilization of equipment, and talk with the body piercer or tattooer.
  3. Observe for handwashing, use of gloves, use of unopened ink container, and sterile packaged equipment.
  4. Use stainless steel, niobium, titanium, or 14K gold jewelry immediately after piercing procedure.

Box 8-1 *New Tattoo*

- Leave dressing on for 2-12 hours or overnight; remove by gently soaking or showering.
- Clean with antibacterial or mild soap and pat dry.
- Do not use alcohol (drying) or hydrogen peroxide (cytotoxic) for cleaning.
- Do not use petroleum jelly; may cause heavy scabbing and will dull the tattoo.
- Apply antibiotic (i.e., Bacitracin) ointment for around 5 days unless allergic reaction occurs.
- Do not disturb scab when applying antibiotic ointment.
- Application of cream/ointment can promote the healing process and help preserve color.
- Avoid sun exposure; approximately 4 weeks.
- Do not use tanning bed during healing.
- Avoid soaking in spa, swimming, or taking hot baths for about 1 week or until peeling has stopped.

Box 8-2 *New Body Piercing*

- Requires routine wound care.
- Wash at least twice daily; some oozing and edema are anticipated; if scabbing occurs, remove with wet swab.
- Do not use alcohol (drying) or hydrogen peroxide (cytotoxic) for cleaning.
- *Navel piercing:* Do not wear tight clothing over area; slowest site to heal.
- *Tongue piercing:* Rinse mouth after all meals and snacks with antibacterial mouthwash without alcohol. If bad breath occurs or tongue color changes are seen, the natural mouth bacteria may have been destroyed; change to salt water rinses.
- *Tongue piercing:* Ice reduces swelling; once healed, avoid smoking and use dental dams for dental work.

Box 8-3 *Potential Risks of Piercing and Tattooing*

General:

Bloodborne pathogen transmission.
Risk of tetanus.
Severe inflammation and swelling.

Piercing Only:

Allergic reaction to jewelry.
Nerve and/or soft tissue damage, keloids.
Dental fracture, speech impediments.
Swelling of tongue and airway occlusion.

Jewelry may cause pain or impair healing when too small or too big.
Aspiration of jewelry—*oral piercing.*
Prolonged bleeding—*tongue piercing.*
Easily infected—*navel or oral piercing.*

Tattooing Only:

Severe allergic reaction to dyes.
Sarcoidlike granuloma.
Magnetic resonance imaging (MRI) scanning complications; rare; short-term effects.

Table 8-2	*Healing Times for Body Piercing*	
	Site and Tissue	Healing Time
	Ear cartilage	4-12 mo
	Ear lobe	6-8 wk
	Eyebrow	6-8 wk
	Nostril	1-4 mo
	Nasal septum	6-8 mo
	Lip	2-3 mo
	Tongue	4-8 wk
	Nipple	2-6 mo
	Navel	4-12 mo
	Female genitalia	3-10 wk
	Male genitalia	1-6 mo

5. Do not allow a piercing gun to be used for the procedure because of potential tissue damage and lack of adequate sterilization that could lead to infections.
   D. Treatment of infections includes use of dicloxacillin (Diclox) or cephalexin (Keflex).
   E. Check date of last tetanus injection.
VI. Additional Information
   A. Many notable historical figures and celebrities who serve as role models for teenagers have tattoos and body piercing. Body embellishment has been a tradition in many cultures. Late-nineteenth-century Victorian royalty preferred nipple and genital piercing, and Lady Randolph Churchill had a snake tattooed around her wrist. Most types of body adornment sought by adolescents have been done previously.
   B. The adolescent may use *fake body jewelry* on the eyebrow, nose, tongue, eyelid, and other areas. This practice allows for the appearance of piercing with the advantage of easy removal in certain social situations not accepting of this practice.
   C. *Tattoo removal* usually is possible but can be very expensive and is done over a long period. A laser is used and in some cases may cause permanent discoloration.
VII. Web Sites
   American Dental Association: Oral Piercing
   http://www.ada.org/public/topics/piercing.html
   Virtual Hospital: Iowa Health Book: Dermatology Tattooing and Body Piercing: Decision Making for Teens
   http://www.vh.org/Patients/IHB/Derm/Tattoo/

STEROID ABUSE

I. Definition
   A. Anabolic-androgenic steroids are synthetic substances related to male hormone androgens. These drugs promote skeletal muscle growth and androgenic effects that influence development of male sexual charac-

teristics. Some athletes and others seeking to improve physical appearance and increase performance abuse them. These are illegal uses of the drug and are known to cause numerous health hazards.

II. **Etiology**
   A. Steroids are derived from the male hormone testosterone. Steroid abuse is lower in females than males but is increasing. A 1999 study estimated that 2.7% of eighth and tenth graders and 2.9% of twelfth graders have used anabolic steroids at least once. More than 500,000 eighth and tenth grade students use steroids, and many high school seniors believe they are not risky drugs (NIDA, 2000a).

III. *Brain Findings*
   A. Anabolic steroid action is in the limbic system. Impaired learning and memory have been demonstrated in animals. A new term, *roid rages,* describes a sudden outburst of severe rage. Testosterone production is controlled by neurons in the hypothalamus, which controls appetite, blood pressure, moods, and reproduction. Steroids can disrupt normal hormone functioning within the brain, causing somatic changes, including loss of scalp hair in the male and facial hair in the female; these changes are believed to be irreversible (NIDA, 2001).

IV. **Characteristics**
   A. Illegal in the United States unless through prescription.
   B. Used by prescription to treat delayed puberty, impotence, and body wasting in those with AIDS and other diseases.
   C. Obtained illegally from clandestine laboratories or by smuggling.
   D. Substances sold illegally as anabolic steroids are diluted and contaminated.
   E. Used illegally by some adolescents, athletes, and competitive body builders to increase strength and body mass, reduce body fat, and improve sports performance.
   F. The International Olympic Committee has 20 anabolic steroids and related compounds on its list of banned anabolic drugs.
   G. Steroid abuse is higher among males than females.
   H. Abuse can cause trembling, fluid retention, aching joints, severe acne, hypertension, lower high-density lipoprotein (HDL) levels, jaundice, and liver tumors.
   I. Withdrawal syndrome includes clinical depression, which can contribute to dependence for these drugs.
   J. Steroids can be taken orally as tablets or capsules, by injection directly into muscles, or as creams or gels applied to the skin.
   K. "Stacking" is a practice in which the abuser mixes oral, injectable, or both forms of anabolic steroids.
   L. "Pyramid" is a practice in which the abuser stacks compounds in cycles of 6 to 12 weeks, gradually increasing the dose followed by slowly decreasing to none.
   M. The abuser believes that stacking and pyramiding produce larger muscles while simultaneously helping the body to adjust from the high doses of synthetic steroids.
   N. Over-the-counter drugs include androstenedione and androstenediol. These oral products are advertised as less toxic, and adolescents and

Table 8-3   *Effects of Anabolic Steroid Abuse*

Side Effects	Men	Women	Adolescents	General Population
Behavioral				Aggressive and combative behavior more frequent with high doses; homicidal rage, mania, delusions
Cardiovascular				Cholesterol modifications, heart disease; hypertension; enlargement of left ventricle; strokes; anaphylactic shock
Hormonal disruptions	Shrinking of testicles; reduced sperm count; baldness; irreversible breast enlargement; impotence	Growth of facial hair; deepened voice; decreased body fat and breast size; change in or cessation of menstrual cycle; enlarged clitoris	Irreversible breast enlargement in male; growth halted prematurely through accelerated pubertal changes; premature skeletal maturation	
Infections				Hepatitis B and C; HIV/AIDS; infective endocarditis if injected
Skin diseases				Acne and cysts
Liver diseases				Cysts and cancer
Musculoskeletal system			Premature and permanent termination of growth	
Withdrawal				Depression, mood swings, fatigue, loss of appetite, restlessness, reduced sex drive, more when use stops

Modified from National Institute on Drug Abuse: *Research report: steroid abuse and addiction*, Revision April 2000b, Available online: http://www.nida.nih.gov/ResearchReports/Steroids/AnabolicSteroids.html. Accessed on Oct 10, 2001.

older students use these products. They currently are not classified as anabolic and are not regulated; their use is controversial.

O. Many men's magazines (e.g., *Men's Health, Exercise for Men Only*) stress the use of compounds that include small doses of steroids to improve performance and to "bulk up."

V. Health Concerns/Emergencies

A. In the male: baldness, breast development, shrunken testicles, reduced sperm count, impotence, infertility, difficulty or pain in urination, and prostate enlargement.

B. In the female: growth of facial hair, deeper voice, smaller breasts, enlargement of the clitoris, changes in or cessation of the menstrual cycle.

C. In adolescents: premature skeletal maturation and accelerated puberty that leads to stunted growth.

D. Can cause emotional lability and wide mood swings with uncontrolled anger and aggression, which can induce violent episodes.

E. Other side effects include paranoid jealousy, extreme irritability, delusions, and impaired judgment.

F. Increased risk of heart attacks and stroke.

VI. Management/Treatment

A. Present a balanced overall picture of both the adverse and beneficial effects of steroids.

B. Educate coaches, trainers, school staff, and parents of adolescents with the same information presented to the student.

C. Be aware of signs and symptoms of anabolic steroid use in this population of students.

D. Drugs abused can be up to 100 times more potent than the prescribed drug for a medical condition.

VII. Web Sites

The National Clearinghouse for Alcohol and Drug Information
http://www.health.org/govpubs/phd726/
The National Institute of Drug Abuse
http://www.steroidabuse.org

GENDER-SPECIFIC CONDITIONS

AMENORRHEA

I. Definition

A. *Primary amenorrhea* is failure to start menstruation by age 17; a medical examination is recommended if no secondary characteristics develop by age 15 or if menarche does not occur within 2 years of development of secondary sexual characteristics. *Secondary amenorrhea* is the absence of menses for 6 months or 3 cycles after menarche has been established and pregnancy is ruled out.

II. Etiology

A. The cause of *primary amenorrhea* may be genetic (e.g., Turner's syndrome, structural abnormal X); caused by dysfunction of the hypothalamus, pituitary gland, ovary, or uterus, or the congenital absence,

malformation, or surgical removal of the uterus or both ovaries; or caused by medication.
   B. Use of drugs, such as marijuana, cocaine, heroin, tricyclic antidepressants, metoclopramide, cimetidine, and contraceptive methods, can cause amenorrhea.
   C. *Secondary amenorrhea* is the cessation of an established menstrual cycle caused by extreme weight loss or gain, systemic illness, extreme physical activity, or increased stress.

III. **Characteristics**
   A. *Primary amenorrhea.*
      1. Absence of menses by age 15, absence of breast bud development by age 13, absence of menses more than 4 years after breast bud development, height and weight below 3% for age, cyclic lower abdominal pain without menses.
   B. *Secondary amenorrhea.*
      1. Abrupt cessation of menstrual cycles, oligomenorrhea (scant, infrequent periods), or pregnancy symptoms.

IV. **Management/Treatment**
   A. Complete reproductive history, including the following:
      1. Age of menarche, frequency and length of periods, amount of flow, presence of cramps, use of tampons or pads, last menstrual period (LMP).
      2. Family history: dysmenorrhea and gynecological problems.
      3. Past medical history: hospitalizations or surgery, chronic illnesses, bleeding disorders.
      4. Medication: medications, contraceptives, substance abuse.
      5. Related health issues: weight changes, nutrition, exercise, sports, emotional symptoms, and eating disorders.
   B. Counsel student regarding extreme exercise, workouts, and diet as appropriate. Supplementation such as calcium and protein may be considered.
   C. Referral for endocrinology evaluation, which may include bone age, determination of follicle-stimulating hormone (FSH), luteinizing hormone (LH) levels, and karyotyping.
   D. Oral contraceptives may be used to treat secondary amenorrhea to establish normal ovulatory cycles.

V. **Web Sites**
   Children's Hospital, Boston, Center for Young Women's Health: Sports and Menstrual Periods—The Female Athlete Triad
   http://www.youngwomenshealth.org/triad.html
   TeensHealth: Coping with Common Period Problems
   http://www.kidshealth.org/teen/sexual_health/girls/menstrual_problems.html
   Nutricize: Athletic Amenorrhea Is Not Healthy—Period
   http://www.efit.com/servlet/article/womenshealth/28265.html

DYSMENORRHEA

I. **Definition**
   A. Dysmenorrhea is cramping and lower abdominal pain during menses. Primary dysmenorrhea incapacitates females for 1 to 3 days, whereas

secondary dysmenorrhea varies depending on the etiology; this is the most common cause of short-term school absenteeism for girls.

II. **Etiology**

   A. *Primary dysmenorrhea* occurs when no evidence of a pelvic pathological condition exists; however, a familiar factor is associated. An increased release of prostaglandin leads to strong uterine contractions and pain. *Secondary dysmenorrhea* is caused by an underlying pathological condition such as pelvic inflammatory disease (PID), endometriosis, uterine fibroids, or polyps or anatomical abnormalities. A higher level of prostaglandin release results in pain.

   B. For both types of dysmenorrhea, a cultural and/or family behavioral component influences the nature and extent of the adolescent response to menstrual discomfort.

III. **Characteristics**

   A. *Primary dysmenorrhea.*

      1. Pain is crampy or spasmodic, bilateral, symmetrical, localized to the lower back and/or anterior thighs, and may be accompanied by nausea, vomiting, and diarrhea.

      2. Depression and anxiety may intensify pain.

      3. Obesity, longer menstrual periods, and use of intrauterine devices (copper) may contribute to increased dysmenorrhea.

      4. Pain lasts from a few hours to 3 days before and during start of menses.

   B. *Secondary dysmenorrhea.*

      1. Pain may be dull and constant, accompanied by nausea, vomiting, and diarrhea.

      2. Dyspareunia.

      3. Pain may occur at menarche, or onset may be 3 or more years later.

      4. History of abnormal discharge, infection, intermenstrual bleeding, or menorrhagia.

IV. **Management/Treatment**

   A. Complete reproductive history, including the following:

      1. Age of menarche, frequency and length of periods, amount of flow, presence of cramps, use of tampons or pads, LMP.

      2. Family history: dysmenorrhea and gynecological problems.

      3. Past medical history: hospitalizations or surgery, chronic illnesses, bleeding disorders.

      4. Medications: contraceptives, medications, substance abuse.

      5. Related health issues: weight changes, nutrition, exercise, sports, emotional symptoms, eating disorders.

      6. Sexual history: sexual activity, method of contraception, STIs, number of sexual partners, age of first coitus, types of sexual contact, sexual abuse.

   B. *Primary dysmenorrhea.*

      1. Assure adolescent that pain is a normal occurrence with primary dysmenorrhea.

      2. Primary palliative treatment: use of pads instead of tampons, application of mild heat to abdomen, warm herbal teas, avoidance of salt, increased exercise to increase endorphins.

3. Muscle relaxation may be enhanced with use of supplements such as magnesium (400-500 mg/day) and calcium (1000 mg/day).

4. Fluid retention may be reduced by vitamin B_6 (400-600 mg/day).

5. Mild pain may be treated with nonsteroidal antiinflammatory drugs (NSAIDs) such as ibuprofen (Motrin), naproxen (Naprosyn), or ketoprofen (Orudis). NSAIDs inhibit prostaglandin and provide relief for some women if their use is started 1 to 3 days before menstruation and continued through the first few days of menses.

6. More severe pain may be treated with oral contraceptives, which are 90% effective in controlling pain.

7. Complementary treatments include use of transcutaneous electrical nerve stimulation (TENS), a battery-powered device that reduces pain by transmitting an electrical impulse to underlying nerves.

8. Primary dysmenorrhea generally decreases with age and after childbirth.

C. Secondary dysmenorrhea.

1. Symptomatic treatment is the same as for primary dysmenorrhea.

2. Refer for evaluation and treatment of underlying cause.

V. **Additional Information**

A. General health may have an effect on dysmenorrhea. Encourage exercise, proper nutrition, no smoking, and weight loss if indicated.

VI. **Web Sites**

TeensHealth: Dysmenorrhea

http://www.kidshealth.org/teen/sexual_health/girls/menstrual_problems_p9.html

WebMD.com: Dysmenorrhea in the adolescent

http://www.webmd.lycos.com/content/article/1680.51123

ENDOMETRIOSIS

I. **Definition**

A. *Endometriosis* is the implantation and growth of endometrial tissue on pelvic and abdominal organs, such as the uterus, bladder, ovaries, fallopian tubes, and ligaments that support the uterus; the lining of the pelvic cavity; and the internal area between the vagina and rectum.

II. **Etiology**

A. Endometriosis is rare but occurs in one half of adolescents with refractory dysmenorrhea or chronic pelvic pain. The condition is believed to be familial.

B. Endometriosis affects about 5 million women, preadolescents, and adolescents in the United States. Often it is misdiagnosed in the teenage years.

III. **Characteristics**

A. Complicated by increased prostaglandin release by the endometrium and endometrial implants, resulting in severe dysmenorrhea.

B. Ectopic implants become larger with each cycle, and pain increases over time.

C. Severe pelvic pain (lower abdominal area).

D. May be occasional, constant, or be associated with menses.

E. Heavy period, constipation, or diarrhea.

    F. Often misses school, social, and/or sports activities because of pain.

    G. Pain may increase during exercise or during sexual activity.

IV. Management/Treatment

    A. Refer student/parent to HCP.

    B. Complete reproductive history, including the following:

        1. Age of menarche, frequency and length of periods, amount of flow, presence of cramps, use of tampons or pads, LMP.

        2. Family history: dysmenorrhea and gynecological problems.

        3. Past medical history: hospitalizations or surgery, chronic illnesses, bleeding disorders.

        4. Medication: medications, contraceptives, substance abuse.

        5. Related health issues: weight changes, nutrition, exercise, sports, emotional symptoms, and eating disorders.

    C. Discuss type of pain experienced (location, duration, intensity) and whether anything is used to treat pain.

    D. Suggest keeping a diary of symptoms.

    E. Avoidance of sugar, wheat, dairy products, and caffeine may reduce discomfort.

    F. Use of over-the-counter pain relievers may be helpful.

    G. Oral contraceptives may be prescribed; these are known to reduce painful menstrual periods.

V. Additional Information

    A. A confirming diagnosis is made by laparoscopy. Endometriosis can cause infertility and chronic pelvic pain. Medical and surgical options are available, but recurrence is common and may occur from 6 months to years later.

VI. Web Sites

Endometriosis Association

http://www.endometriosisassn.org/index.html

MEDLINEPlus: Endometriosis

http://www.nlm.nih.gov/medlineplus/ency/article/000915.htm

DYSFUNCTIONAL UTERINE BLEEDING

I. Definition

    A. *Dysfunctional uterine bleeding (DUB)* is described as abnormal uterine bleeding that occurs in the absence of a pathological condition or disease. DUB is a diagnosis of exclusion and should be considered only after other causes have been ruled out.

II. Etiology

    A. DUB usually occurs at the beginning and end of a woman's reproductive years. The most severe DUB occurs shortly after the onset of menstruation. Adolescents with sustained anovulation, which includes those with eating disorders, chronic illness, endocrine disorders, or competitive athletes, have a higher incidence of DUB. Anovulatory DUB is caused by an imbalance in hormones. Approximately 90% of DUB is caused by anovulation, but anovulation does not always lead to DUB.

    B. When a woman does not ovulate, the ovaries do not receive the signal to produce progesterone. Without progesterone, the endometrium continues to grow until it breaks down and is rejected in a very heavy period. Irregular or prolonged bleeding occurs when the endometrium is shed irregularly and incompletely.

III. **Characteristics**
  A. DUB may be mild, moderate, or severe and usually is painless.
  B. DUB can result in a variety of menstrual patterns, including the following:
    1. Hypermenorrhea: exceptionally heavy bleeding during a normal-length period; synonymous with menorrhagia.
    2. Metrorrhagia: periods that occur at irregular intervals, or frequent bleeding of varying amounts but not heavy.
    3. Menometrorrhagia: frequent, excessive, and prolonged bleeding that occurs during menses and at irregular intervals.
    4. Oligomenorrhea: menstrual intervals of more than 5 weeks for longer than a 6-month period.
    5. Polymenorrhea: frequent, regular periods that occur more often than every 21 days.
  C. DUB is common in overweight girls who have increased endogenous estrogen from both peripheral conversion of androgens to estrogens and fat storage.

IV. **Management/Treatment**
  A. Treatment depends on the underlying mechanism.
  B. Initially, concern is for the amount of blood loss and symptoms; observe student and reassure her.
  C. Obtain a complete reproductive history (see "Amenorrhea").
  D. Assess orthostatic blood pressure, pulse changes, height and weight changes, hirsutism, and thyroid enlargement or nodules.
  E. Assess number of pads or tampons saturated in current 24-hour period, which may or may not be typical, and history of previous three menstrual cycles.
  F. Refer to parent for HCP assessment.
  G. Treatment consists of bleeding control, prevention of endometrial hyperplasia and recurrence, and prevention and treatment of anemia.
  H. Treatment is based on the intensity and timing of the bleeding.
  I. Hormonal regulation is 90% effective among those with anovulatory bleeding.

V. **Additional Information**
  A. Most unusually heavy uterine bleeding has no underlying anatomical cause and is considered DUB. However, many possible underlying problems could cause the same symptoms. Diagnosis of DUB usually involves elimination of more serious causes.

VI. **Web Sites**
  American Academy of Family Physicians: When you have abnormal uterine bleeding (handout)
    http://www.aafp.org/afp/991001ap/991001a.html
  MEDLINEPlus: Dysfunctional Uterine Bleeding
    http://www.nlm.nih.gov/medlineplus/ency/article/000903.htm

PREMENSTRUAL SYNDROME

I. Definition

    A. Premenstrual syndrome (PMS) is a pattern of symptoms that occur in the second half of the menstrual cycle, usually appearing after ovulation (day 14) and resolving with the onset of menses. Symptoms disrupt daily living and must be present for at least two to three cycles to establish diagnosis.

II. Etiology

    A. The cause of PMS is unknown, but research links the symptoms to an unusual response to normal hormonal changes (Rubinow and Schmidt, 2001). Recent research also has demonstrated a connection between PMS and low levels of serotonin. Approximately 40% of women who menstruate have some symptoms of PMS, but only 3% to 7% have symptoms severe enough to interfere with school, work, and social life.

III. Characteristics

    A. Symptoms are cyclical, appearing and resolving about the same time every month.

    B. Discomfort starts about the middle of the cycle and intensifies in the last days before menses.

    C. Rapid relief occurs with start of menses.

    D. Days 4-12 of cycle are symptom-free.

    E. More than 150 physical and emotional symptoms are linked to PMS; they may be mild, moderate, or severe.

    F. Physical symptoms:

        1. Abdominal bloating and swollen breasts, hands, and feet.

        2. Backache, lower abdominal pain, headache.

        3. Joint or muscle pain.

        4. Exhaustion.

        5. Upset stomach, constipation followed by diarrhea.

        6. Increased appetite or anorexia.

        7. Acne.

    G. Emotional/behavioral symptoms:

        1. Mood swings, anxiety, depression, irritability.

        2. Tearfulness, withdrawal from usual activities.

        3. Changes in sexual desire.

        4. Difficulty in concentrating and handling stress.

        5. Feelings of being out of control.

IV. Management/Treatment

    A. Complete reproductive history, including the following:

        1. Age of menarche, frequency and length of periods, amount of flow, presence of cramps, use of tampons or pads, LMP.

        2. Family history: dysmenorrhea and gynecological problems.

        3. Past medical history: hospitalizations or surgery, chronic illnesses, bleeding disorders.

        4. Medication: medications, contraceptives, substance abuse.

        5. Related health issues: weight changes, nutrition, exercise, sports, emotional symptoms, and eating disorders.

B. Establish pattern by keeping a diary or calendar of symptoms.

C. Eliminate common offending foods and substances:
1. Sugars, including honey, syrup, fructose, and sucrose.
2. Artificial sweeteners.
3. Caffeine (chocolate, coffee, and colas).
4. Cigarettes and alcohol.

D. Avoid foods that may exaggerate symptoms:
1. Salty or smoked foods.
2. Dairy products.

E. Increase intake of foods that will diminish symptoms of PMS:
1. Whole grains (e.g., bread, pasta, brown rice).
2. Dried beans and nuts.
3. Fresh fruits and vegetables (especially spinach).

F. Establish rigorous exercise routine; aerobic exercise is especially helpful.

G. Practice stress reduction (e.g., deep breathing, meditation, naps, walking, hot baths, massage).

H. Consider using supplements, discuss with HCP.
1. Multivitamin with vitamins B_6 and E, calcium, and magnesium.
2. Evening primrose oil (available in health food stores).
3. L-tryptophan, an amino acid.

V. **Additional Information**

A. Treatment is symptomatic; antidepressants (selective serotonin reuptake inhibitors [SSRIs] and tricyclics) have been helpful in relieving emotional symptoms. Other pharmacological treatments include diuretics, oral contraceptives, progesterone, thyroid hormone, and prostaglandin inhibitors.

VI. **Web Sites**

Arnot Ogden Medical Center: Premenstrual Syndrome
http://www.aomc.org/HOD2/general/general-PREMENST.html

VAGINITIS, VULVITIS, AND VULVOVAGINITIS

I. **Definition**

A. *Vaginitis* refers to a discharge with irritation and pruritus of the vagina. *Vulvitis* refers to erythema and pruritus of the vulva. *Vulvovaginitis* refers to inflammation, generally with a discharge, from infection or irritating substances that involve the vulva and vagina.

II. **Etiology**

A. An infection in the vagina caused by an overcolonization of bacteria normally found in the vaginal flora or the introduction of pathological organisms. A small amount of vaginal mucus, which is usually clear, is normal; mucus production in adolescent girls generally increases during ovulation and before the onset of menses. This normally does not cause discomfort.

III. **Additional Information**

A. This is an opportunity for health teaching about *personal hygiene:* correct toileting habits of wiping from front to back, changing underclothes daily, and washing hands frequently; *protective measures:* avoiding bubble baths, perfumed powder, lotions or soap, shampoo in

Table 8-4   *Vaginitis and Vulvitis: Types and Clinical Information*

Type	Etiology	Characteristics	Discharge	Treatment and Care
Bacterial	*Streptococcus, Escherichia coli, Shigella, Staphylococcus,* or other bacteria; usually sexually transmitted	Often asymptomatic	Green, possible bleeding, malodorous	Penicillin, erythromycin, broad-spectrum antibiotic; concurrent treatment of sexual partner
Candidiasis	Diabetes, pregnancy, recent antibiotic, contraceptive, or systemic corticosteroid use or depressed immunity	Abrupt onset Severe itching, erythema, edematous, dysuria, dyspareunia	Thick, white, cottage cheese–like, except in pregnancy; odorless	Miconazole (Monistat) or clotrimazole (Gyne-Lotrimin) cream nightly for 1 week or ketoconazole orally or single-dose fluconazole (Diflucan); oil-based preparations may weaken condoms or diaphragms
Chemical/ irritant	Bubble bath, lotion, perfumed soap, tampons, deodorant pads, sand or dirt, tight-fitting clothing	Erythema, itching, vulva inflammation, dysuria	White to yellow, small amount	Topical steroids, removal of irritant
Gardnerella	Gram-negative bacteria G; vaginalis; nonspecific; sexually transmitted; most common contagious bacterial STI	No itching or symptom or mucosal irritation	Thin, gray, fishy odor discharge	Metronidazole (Flagyl), clindamycin (Cleocin) may be taken orally or as topical cream; concurrent treatment of sexual partner
Nonspecific	Poor hygiene, irritating substances	Itching and burning, dysuria, varied vulvitis	Foul smell, scant to copious, mucoid, brown to green in color	Topical antibiotics or estrogen, removal of irritating substances
Trichomonas	*Trichomonas vaginalis,* a parasitic protozoan, usually sexually transmitted	Often asymptomatic, self-limiting in males; vulvovaginal soreness, dysuria	Vaginal discharge	Metronidazole, 500 mg bid for 7 days or single dose, which is best for adolescent; concurrent treatment of sexual partner

Bid, Twice a day.

bath water, bleach and fabric softener in clothes during laundry; using mild soaps (Neutrogena, Dove, Basis); and double rinsing clothes during laundering. *Development and sexuality,* including the importance of an evaluation when vaginal discharge occurs, is also part of health teaching.

IV. **Web Sites**

MEDLINEPlus: Vaginal Discharge

http://www.nlm.nih.gov/medlineplus/ency/article/003158.htm

Southeast Missouri Hospital Adolescent Medicine: Vaginitis

http://www.southeastmissourihospital.com/health/kids/adoles/vgnts.htm

Southeast Missouri Hospital Adolescent Medicine: Vulvitis

http://www.southeastmissourihospital.com/health/kids/adoles/vvts.htm

MEDLINEPlus: Vulvitis

http://www.nlm.nih.gov/medlineplus/ency/article/001445.htm

CERVICAL CANCER

I. **Definition**

A. Cancer of the uterine cervix is a neoplasm that can be detected in early developmental stages. The Papanicolaou (Pap) smear is a diagnostic test to detect and diagnose early-stage cancers of the cervix and other organ tissues. It usually is performed at an annual routine pelvic examination, beginning at 18 years of age or younger if sexually active.

II. **Etiology**

A. Risk factors for cancer of the cervix include young age at first coitus, multiple sex partners or partners who have had sex with someone who has had cervical cancer, human papillomavirus (HPV) infection, exposure to diethylstilbestrol (DES), and possibly smoking and oral contraceptive use. Current data are unclear why these risk factors may cause cancer. Some research suggests that sexually transmitted viruses cause cervical cells to begin the developmental changes that can result in cancer.

III. **Characteristics**

A. Cervical cancer usually is asymptomatic and develops slowly.

B. Vaginal bleeding.

C. Abnormal-appearing cervix.

IV. **Management/Treatment**

A. Complete reproductive history, including the following:

1. Age of menarche, frequency and length of periods, amount of flow, presence of cramps, use of tampons or pads, LMP.

2. Family history: dysmenorrhea and gynecological problems.

3. Past medical history: hospitalizations or surgery, chronic illnesses, bleeding disorders.

4. Medications: contraceptives, medications, substance abuse.

5. Related health issues: weight changes, nutrition, exercise, sports, emotional symptoms, eating disorders.

6. Sexual history: sexual activity, method of contraception, STIs, number of sexual partners, last sexual contact, types of sexual contact, sexual abuse.

B. Assess for risk factors.
C. Discuss the need for a yearly Pap smear if the adolescent is or has ever been sexually active.
D. Yearly chlamydia and gonorrhea testing if adolescent is sexually active.
E. Treatment options are individualized based on the adolescent's history and likelihood of continuous follow-up.
F. Pap smear findings are grouped descriptively into classes:
    1. Class I: only normal cells seen.
    2. Class II: atypical cells consistent with inflammation.
    3. Class III: mild dysplasia.
    4. Class IV: severe dysplasia, suspicious cells.
    5. Class V: carcinoma cells seen.
V. **Web Sites**
MEDLINEPlus: Pap Smear
http://www.nlm.nih.gov/medlineplus/ency/article/003911.htm
Reproductive Health Outlook: Cervical Cancer
http://www.rho.org/html/cxca_keyissues.htm
Women's Health Queensland: Student Fact Sheet: Cervical Cancer
http://www.womhealth.org.au/factshts/cvcancer.htm

UNDESCENDED TESTIS (CRYPTORCHIDISM)

I. **Definition**
    A. Undescended testis *(cryptorchidism)* that does not enter and cannot be manipulated into the scrotum; can be unilateral or bilateral.
II. **Etiology**
    A. The testes usually descend into the scrotum by the eighth month of fetal life; less than 1% have not descended by the ninth month of life. Undescended testis also can be a result of retractile testes or anorchia (absence of testes). Anorchia is categorized according to location: abdominal, canalicular, or ectopic.
III. **Characteristics**
    A. Fertility is severely affected if cryptorchidism is bilateral and not corrected by age 6.
    B. Between 5% and 12% of testicular cancers occur in men with a history of undescended testes. Cancer is more common with an intraabdominal testis.
    C. Testes undescended into scrotum.
    D. Rarely cause discomfort.
    E. All or one side of scrotum appears smaller than normal with incomplete development.
    F. Undescended testis usually is softer and smaller than descended one.
    G. Retractile testes can be manipulated back into the scrotum, usually bilateral.
    H. Distinction between a lymph node and an undescended testis is made by its elastic nature. A testis can be manipulated down into the scrotum but will spring back into the inguinal canal.
    I. No evidence exists that testes will descend with puberty, unless they are retractile and not truly undescended.

IV. **Management/Treatment**
   A. Refer to parent for HCP assessment.
   B. Hormone therapy trial may be initiated.
   C. Corrective surgery between 1 and 2 years of age.
   D. Teach testicular self-examination to adolescent students.
V. **Web Sites**
   MEDLINEPlus: Undescended testicle
   http://www.nlm.nih.gov/medlineplus/ency/article/000973.htm

TESTICULAR CANCER

I. **Definition**
   A. Development of a malignant neoplasm in the testicle. Testicular cancer occurs most frequently in the 15- to 34-year-old age group. It can occur anytime after age 14.
II. **Etiology**
   A. The cause of testicular cancer is unknown, but a tenfold to fortyfold greater risk exists with a history of ectopic or undescended testes, even if the testes have been descended surgically. Most solid tumors in males younger than age 30 are testicular tumors and may be benign or malignant, but most testicular masses in adolescents are malignant. Testicular cancer is the cause of one in seven deaths among late adolescent and young adult males. It is approximately five times more common in white American men than in African American men, and white men have twice the risk of Asian American men (Gottlieb, 2001).
III. **Characteristics**
   A. Risk factors include the following:
      1. Late descended testes or undescended testes, even if they were corrected surgically.
      2. Family history of testicular cancer.
      3. Abnormal testicular development.
      4. Inguinal hernia.
      5. Klinefelter's syndrome.
   B. Usually asymptomatic, although localized pain or a dull ache may be present in the back or lower abdomen, or a sudden collection of fluid may occur in the scrotum.
   C. Detected as a heavy, hard, unilateral lump usually about the size of a pea but may be as large as an egg. Palpable on the anterior or lateral part of the testis (see "Testicular Self-Examination").
   D. May be found after an injury, but injury is not believed to be a causative factor. Pain and tenderness may be due to hemorrhage into the tumor.
   E. Develops more commonly in the right testicle. Involved testis often hangs lower.
   F. Mass does not transilluminate unless associated with a hydrocele, which is present in 10% of malignancies.
   G. May metastasize to lymph nodes, liver, or lungs before detection.
   H. Later stages include pulmonary symptoms, ureteral obstruction, gynecomastia (enlarged breasts), or an abdominal mass.

I. Early discovery and treatment leads to a 95% survival rate. Approximately 70% of men with advanced testicular cancer can be cured, according to the National Cancer Institute.

IV. **Management/Treatment**
   A. Depends on type of tumor and the stage. Three stages of testicular cancer exist.
      1. Stage 1: Malignancy is confined to the testicle.
      2. Stage 2: Disease has spread to retroperitoneal lymph nodes.
      3. Stage 3: Cancer has spread to remote sites in the body such as the lungs and liver.
   B. First line of treatment is orchiectomy of the affected testicle.
   C. Radiation, chemotherapy, and bone marrow transplantation are other treatments.
   D. The Food and Drug Administration (FDA) has approved several drugs for testicular cancer, including ifosfamide (Ifex), bleomycin sulfate (Blenoxane), vinblastine sulfate (Velban), cisplatin (Platinol), and etoposide (VePesid). The drugs may be given in combination after surgery and radiation.
   E. Sexual function and fertility usually are unaffected, since the remaining testicle can produce sperm. More extensive surgery may cause infertility but does not affect ability to have erections or orgasms. A prosthesis can be inserted to provide a normal appearance.
   F. Teach testicular self-examination in early adolescence.

V. **Web Sites**
   National Cancer Institute: Testicular Cancer
   http://www.cancer.gov/cancer_information/cancer_type/testicular/
   MEDLINEPlus: Testicular Cancer
   http://www.nlm.nih.gov/medlineplus/ency/article/001288.htm

SEXUALLY TRANSMITTED INFECTIONS

The role of the school nurse in meeting with students with suspected or confirmed STIs involves the following:

1. Discuss safe-sex practices, including abstinence, condoms, spermicidal barriers, and risk of multiple partners.
2. Complete reproductive history assessment:
   - Age of menarche, frequency and length of periods, amount of flow, presence of cramps, use of tampons or pads, LMP.
   - Family history: dysmenorrhea and gynecological problems.
   - Past medical history: hospitalizations or surgery, chronic illnesses, bleeding disorders.
   - Medication: medications, contraceptives, substance abuse.
   - Related health issues: weight changes, nutrition, exercise, sports, emotional symptoms, and eating disorders.
   - Sexual history: sexual activity, method of contraception, STIs, number of sexual partners, last sexual contact, types of sexual contact, sexual abuse.
3. Collect data regarding physical health and social, emotional and sexual developmental history, include Tanner stages of development (see Appendix D).

4. Maintain student confidentiality and awareness of state laws. The American Academy of Pediatrics (AAP) has a policy statement on confidentiality and adolescence health care.

CHLAMYDIA

I. **Definition**
   A. Chlamydia is the most common bacterial STI and the fastest spreading STI in the United States.
II. **Etiology**
   A. *Chlamydia trachomatis* is a gram-negative bacterium contracted through vaginal sex, oral-genital contact, and perinatally. *C. trachomatis* infection may occur in the eye with exposure to contaminated body fluid. Approximately 15% to 37% of sexually active adolescent girls and 3% of males have chlamydia (Hofmann and Greydanus, 1997).
III. **Characteristics**
   A. The *incubation period* is poorly defined but probably is 7-14 days or longer.
   B. Chlamydia often is asymptomatic, thus making this STI difficult to diagnosis.
   C. Symptoms:
      1. Females may have a white or yellowish vaginal discharge, dysuria, burning or itching from vagina, dyspareunia, and pelvic or abdominal pain.
      2. Males may have discharge from penis, urethra pain, dysuria, swollen testicles, and may be able to express discharge from the urethral meatus; rectal infections usually are asymptomatic.
   D. Reiter's syndrome (conjunctivitis, disseminated arthritis, and dermatitis).
   E. Untreated chlamydia can cause infection of the urethra, inflammation of the cervix, or DUB and PID, which can lead to infertility.
IV. **Additional Information**
   A. Newborns can be infected in the birth canal; ophthalmic prophylaxis is used after birth.
V. **Web Sites**
   MEDLINEPlus: Chlamydia
   http://www.nlm.nih.gov/medlineplus/ency/article/001345.htm
   Planned Parenthood: Chlamydia Fact Sheet
   http://www.plannedparenthood.org/library/STI/Chlamydia_fact.html
   TeensHealth: Chlamydia
   http://www.kidshealth.org/teen/sexual_health/stds/std_chlamydia.html

GONORRHEA

I. **Definition**
   A. *Neisseria gonorrhoeae,* or gonorrhea (GC), is a bacterial infection of the urethra and genital tract. It is the most frequently reported communicable disease in the United States.
II. **Etiology**
   A. *N. gonorrhoeae* is a gram-negative coccus that is contracted through oral, vaginal, or anal sexual contact and perinatally.

III. Characteristics
  A. The *incubation period* varies between men and women; infection usually occurs in 2-14 days in men and 7-21 days in women.
  B. GC may be asymptomatic in the female but often symptomatic in the male.
  C. Symptoms:
    1. Females may have a yellowish green vaginal discharge and pelvic pain; other symptoms include burning or itching around the vagina, odor from vagina, DUB, dyspareunia, or dysuria. Females often exhibit no symptoms but learn about presence of STI from their partner.
    2. Males have urethral pain, dysuria, and a thick, greenish, purulent discharge from the penis.
    3. Occasionally pharyngitis, conjunctivitis, or perihepatitis occurs.
  D. Untreated infection increases risk for damaged heart valves, chronic infection of the genital tract, and disseminated arthritis-dermatitis syndrome (fever, chills, arthritis, skin lesions), meningitis, and peritonitis.
  E. GC can cause PID.
IV. Additional Information
  A. Guidelines from the Centers for Disease Control and Prevention (CDC) recommend treatment by single dose of two 200-mg tablets of cefixime (Suprax) unless cervical motion tenderness is present. The treatment of choice formerly was penicillin, but many strains of GC have become resistant. Other antibiotics are used, including spectinomycin (Trobicin) or ceftriaxone (Rocephin), which are single-dose injections. Some antibiotics are available in one-dose oral preparations. Concurrent treatment for chlamydia is recommended.
  B. Newborns can be infected in the birth canal. Ophthalmic prophylaxis is used after birth.
V. Web Sites
  eMedicine.com: Gonorrhea
  http://www.emedicine.com/ped/topic886.htm
  TeensHealth: Gonorrhea
  http://www.kidshealth.org/teen/sexual_health/stds/std_gonorrhea.html

HUMAN PAPILLOMAVIRUS

  I. Definition
  A. HPV causes a variety of distinct-appearing *warts*. The most common HPV is condyloma accuminata.
  II. Etiology
  A. HPV infection is spread by sexual activity. The warts are found on any part of the female and male genitalia. It presents as single or multiple, soft, generally painless growths. To date, 70 different genotypes have been identified.
  III. Characteristics
  A. The *incubation period* is usually 2 weeks to 9 months.
  B. In females, the warty lesions are commonly found on the vulva, cervix, vagina, or rectum.

C. In males, the lesions usually occur on the shaft of the penis but also appear on the meatus, scrotum, rectum, or anus.

D. Condom use can decrease transmission.

E. Condyloma acuminata warts are described as cauliflower-like in appearance.

F. Untreated lesions grow larger and multiply; when condyloma affects the cervix, it can lead to cervical cancer.

G. Large warts can obstruct the birth canal.

H. Newborns can develop warts on larynx from exposure in the birth canal.

IV. **Additional Information**

A. The treatment goal is to decrease transmission to partners and alleviate symptoms; no cure exists. Treatment includes laser therapy, cryotherapy (liquid nitrogen), catheterization, and surgical excision. Chemical agents (topical ointment) are used to treat low-level lesions of the cervix; these agents should not be applied to healthy tissue.

B. Females should have annual pelvic examinations and Pap smears when atypical warts are observed to eliminate cancer.

V. **Web Sites**

MEDLINEPlus: Genital Warts
http://www.nlm.nih.gov/medlineplus/ency/article/000886.htm
Planned Parenthood: HPV and Genital Warts
http://www.plannedparenthood.org/STI/hpv.htm

PELVIC INFLAMMATORY DISEASE

I. **Definition**

A. PID is an acute, progressive, infection of the upper genital tract (endometrium, fallopian tubes, or surrounding structures) that usually is caused by ascending microorganisms from the vagina or endocervix.

II. **Etiology**

A. PID usually is a result of polymicrobial infections, mainly GC and chlamydia. It is more common in females under age 25.

III. **Characteristics**

A. Lower abdominal tenderness or pain, DUB.

B. Fever, chills, gastrointestinal (GI) symptoms (e.g., nausea, vomiting, anorexia).

C. Lower-quadrant pain that worsens with movement or sexual intercourse.

D. Foul-smelling vaginal discharge.

E. Malaise, weakness, and dizziness.

IV. **Additional Information**

A. *Hospitalization is necessary whenever possible* when cervical motion tenderness is present but absolutely with strong suspicion of appendicitis, ectopic pregnancy, adnexal mass, severe illness, pregnancy, lack of response to outpatient medications, or if the adolescent is unreliable for follow-up and treatment. Outpatient treatment generally consists of broad-spectrum antibiotics and bed rest.

V. Web Sites

MEDLINEPlus: Pelvic Inflammatory Disease
http://www.nlm.nih.gov/medlineplus/ency/article/000888.htm
National Institute of Allergy and Infectious Disease Fact Sheet
http://www.niaid.nih.gov/factsheets/stdpid.htm
TeensHealth: Pelvic Inflammatory Disease
http://www.kidshealth.org/teen/sexual_health/stds/std_pid.html
Vanderbilt Medical Center Adolescent Medicine: Pelvic Inflammatory Disease
http://peds.mc.vanderbilt.edu/vchweb_1/ADOPIDL/pelvinf.htm

SYPHILIS

I. Definition

A. Syphilis is a bacterial STI; when untreated, it progresses through four clinical stages: primary, secondary, latent, and tertiary.

II. Etiology

A. Syphilis is caused by the *Treponema pallidum* spirochete and is contracted through oral, vaginal, or anal sexual activity; transplacentally or perinatally; and by contact with open infected lesions, body fluids, and secretion of infected individuals. It is more prevalent in females than males. The *T. pallidum* spirochete can survive almost anywhere in the body.

III. Characteristics

A. *Incubation period:* approximately 3 weeks with a range of 10-90 days.

B. The majority of cases are asymptomatic.

C. Symptoms:

1. *Primary stage:* Syphilis begins with a painless sore (chancre) at the site of infection, sex organs, or mouth that may be accompanied by regional, swollen glands. The sore appears as a flat ulcer with rolled, raised edges. The sore often is believed to be a cold sore, so treatment is not sought. Untreated chancres can last 2-6 weeks and then disappear.

2. *Secondary stage:* A rash (papular, macular, or annular) may appear anywhere on the body, including the palms, soles of the feet, and mucous tissue. Generalized adenopathy and viral-like symptoms occur. These symptoms last 10-14 days and clear spontaneously without treatment.

3. *Latent stage:* If untreated, no symptoms of the disease exist, but test results will be positive, indicating that the spirochetes are still active in the body.

4. *Tertiary stage:* Onset is usually 5 to 20 years after the primary stage. This stage is rarely seen in adolescents. The spirochetes spread all over the body and affect the skin, subcutaneous tissue, and bone and also can affect the heart, brain, and other vital organs.

IV. Additional Information

A. Treatment is a one-time injection of benzathine penicillin (Bicillin) or 2 weeks of therapy with erythromycin, tetracycline, or doxycycline for the primary stage. Penicillin has remained effective because *T. pallidum* bacteria have not developed resistance. Assessment of the effectiveness of treatment requires blood testing at 3, 6, and 12 months followed by additional therapy if indicated.

    B. During pregnancy, transmission to the fetus approaches 100%. Fetal and perinatal death occur in 40% of cases (Behrman, Klieman, and Jenson, 2000). Early prenatal screening is mandated in all states; some states requiring screening at delivery.

V. Web Sites

    MEDLINEPlus: Syphilis
      http://www.nlm.nih.gov/medlineplus/ency/article/001327.htm
    TeensHealth: Syphilis
      http://www.kidshealth.org/teen/sexual_health/stds/std_syphilis.html
    PBS Frontline: The Lost Children of Rockdale County
      http://www.pbs.org/wgbh/pages/frontline/shows/georgia/
    Campaign for Our Children: Contraceptives: Test Your Knowledge
      http://www.cfoc.org/3_teen/3_test.cfm?test=3
    Epigee.org: Birth Control Guide
      http://www.epigee.org/guide/index.html
    TeensHealth: Sexual Health, Birth Control
      http://www.kidshealth.org/teen/sexual_health/

BREAST AND TESTICULAR SELF-EXAMINATIONS

BREAST SELF-EXAMINATION

Monthly breast self-inspection and palpation of breasts should be done, preferably 7-10 days after the beginning of the menstrual cycle. If cycles are irregular, the breast self-examination (BSE) should be performed on the same day each month and at the same time of day. If any abnormalities are noticed, adolescents should report them to a parent, HCP, or both.

1. Self-inspection:
    • Stand or sit in front of a mirror with arms relaxed at sides.
    • Note size, color, shape, and direction of breasts and nipples; one breast may be slightly larger than the other (this is normal).
    • Examine breasts for dimples or discoloration in the skin, nipple changes, or discharge.
    • Raise arms overhead and examine breasts while turning slowly from side to side.
    • Place hands on hips and, pressing firmly, move shoulders forward, looking at each breast separately.
2. Palpation (examination by feeling):
    • Remain in front of mirror, apply firm pressure with the pads of three middle fingertips. Starting just below the collarbone, make small circles over the breast area in a pattern to cover all of the breast; circular, up and down, or in spokes.
    • Extend the examination to the underarm area.
    • Change hand and complete the BSE on the opposite breast.
    I. Additional Information
      A. Breast cancer is extremely rare in adolescents, but BSE helps them become comfortable and familiar with their breasts and establishes a pattern of preventive care.

Table 8-5 *Contraceptives*

Method	Efficacy of Actual Use (%)	Benefits	Disadvantages
Abstinence	100	Prevents pregnancy and STIs	High motivation by both partners required; peer pressure involved
Condom *Male:* Traps sperm in penile covering *Female:* Single use, inserted into vagina and fits next to cervix	86 79	No prescription needed, easy methods, inexpensive, accessible, decreases STI risk	Must apply correctly, must use consistently, motivation by both partners required, interference with sex
Oral contraceptives Estrogen/progesterone preparation inhibits ovulation	99-95 when used correctly	Nothing required before sex, simple method, decreased dysmenorrhea, and acne	Requires prescription, expensive, requires consistent use, no STI protection, some weight gain
Diaphragm Cervical covering to prevent sperm from entering; use with spermicidal jelly	80	Decreases STI risk, PID, bacterial and viral infection, can use continuously	Increased UTIs; must be used correctly, messy, possible infection; can be placed in vagina up to 1 hr before and stay in place 6 to 8 hr afterward but can leave in for 24 hr; requires cleaning
Spermicides: foam, jelly, creams, suppositories—agents that kill sperm when inserted into vagina; can be used alone or with condom	74	Safe, no prescription needed, inexpensive, and easy to use; do not have to consult partner; effective against bacteria (chlamydia, gonorrhea)	Messy, possible irritation if sensitive to agent, must insert correctly

Method			
Norplant Levonorgestrel released into vascular system over 5 yr; small rods (6) inserted into upper arm; thickens cervical mucosa, inhibits ovulation	99	Nothing required; lasts 5 yr; pregnancy prevention starts within 24 hr after insertion; returns immediately on removal; usually no period; decreased dysmenorrhea and blood loss	No STI protection; expensive, spotting, irregular menses, weight gain significant, minor surgical procedure for insertion and removal
Depo-Provera Progestin prevents ovulation by suppression of hormonal cycle. Injection every 3 mo	99	Nothing required before sex; dose once every 3 mo; decreases in PID, endometriosis	No STI protection; expensive, weight gain significant, breast tenderness, headache, acne, hirsutism; osteoporosis evidence in adolescents; moodiness, depression, decreased libido
Withdrawal	81	Inexpensive, no prescription	Motivation by both partners needed, failure rate; seminal fluid may release before ejaculation and may enter vagina causing pregnancy; no STI protection
Postcoital contraception Oral contraceptive given within 72 hr of unprotected sex and again 12 hr later	75	Useful if method failure or unplanned sexual intercourse	Nausea, vomiting; must take within 72 hr; not for continual use; no STI protection

UTI, Urinary tract infection.

II. Web Sites

National Women's Health Information Center: Breast Self-Exam
http://www.4woman.gov/faq/bsefaq.htm
Women's Information Network: Breast Self-Exam Reminder
http://www.winabc.org/reminder.html
Women's Information Network: Breast Anatomy and Physiology
http://www.winabc.org/yourbody.html

TESTICULAR SELF-EXAMINATION

Testicular self-examination (TSE) is a monthly inspection and palpation of the testes for detection of testicular cancer. TSE should be performed after a warm bath or shower because the heat relaxes the scrotum and increases chances of spotting an abnormality. If any abnormalities are noticed, the adolescent should report them to a parent, HCP, or both.

1. Self-inspection:
   - Stand in front of a mirror and look for any swelling on the skin of the scrotum or any discoloration or changes in the testicle.
   - One testicle may be *slightly* larger than the other, but a significant difference in size should be checked.
   - Look at the entire penis and note bumps or blisters, open sores, warts, or drainage that may be signs of an STI.
2. Palpation (examination by feeling):
   - Stand with the right leg elevated on the toilet or a stool.
   - Support the testicle in the left hand and feel it with the right hand.
   - Gently roll the testicle between the thumb and the fingers.
   - Separate the epididymis (i.e., soft, tubular structure covering the back and bottom of the testicle) from the testicle to palpate the testicle itself.
   - The testicle should be firm and smooth but not hard; no lumps or bumps should be present.
   - No pain should exist.
   - Repeat for the left testicle, elevating the left leg instead.
   I. **Additional Information**
      A. Testicular cancer is one of the most common tumors in males younger than age 40. It usually develops between ages 15 and 34.
   II. **Web Sites**
   Dr.Koop.com
   http://www.drkoop.com/conditions/cancer/page_75_384.asp
   MEDLINEPlus: Testicular Self-Exam
   http://www.nlm.nih.gov/medlineplus/ency/article/003909.htm

BIBLIOGRAPHY

American Dental Association, Division of Communications: Oral piercing and health, *J Am Dent Assoc* 132:127, 2001.
American Medical Association: *Guidelines for adolescent preventive services: recommendations (GAPS),* June 7, 2001, Available online: http://www.ama-assn.org/ama/pub/category/2279.html. Accessed on Oct 10, 2001.
Armstrong ML: You pierced what? *Pediatr Nurs* 222(3):236-238, 1996.

Armstrong ML, Ekmark E, Brooks B: Body piercing: promoting informed decision making, *J School Nurs* 11(2):20-25, 1995.

Ashwill JW, Droske SC, Rader I, editors: *Nursing care of children: principles and practice,* Philadelphia, 1997, WB Saunders.

Benson PL, Galbraith J, Espeland P: *What teens need to succeed: proven, practical ways to shape your own future,* Minneapolis, 1998, Free Spirit Publishing.

Burns CE, Brody MA, Dunn M, et al, editors: *Pediatric primary care: a handbook for nurse practitioners,* ed 2, Philadelphia, 2000, WB Saunders.

Carter R: *Mapping the mind,* Berkeley, 1998, University of California Press.

Centers for Disease Control and Prevention: *Youth risk behavior survey,* Jan 9, 2000, Available online: http://www.cdc.gov/nccdphp/dash/yrbs/. Accessed on Oct 31, 2001.

Freyenberger B: *Tattooing and body piercing: decision making for teens, Iowa Health Book: Dermatology,* Nov 1998, Available online: http://www.vh.org/Patients/IHB/Derm/Tattoo/. Accessed on Oct 10, 2001.

Goldberg L, MacKinnon DP, Elliot DL, et al: The adolescent's training and learning to avoid steroids program: preventing drug use and promoting health behaviors, *Arch Pediatr Adolesc Med* 154:332-338, 2000.

Gottlieb F: *Testicular cancer,* Sept 14, 2001, Available online: http://www.cancer.gov/cancer_information/cancer_type/testicular/. Accessed on Oct 10, 2001.

Gurke B, Armstrong ML: D-tag: erasing the tag of gang membership, *J School Nurs* 13(2):13-17, 1997.

Hofmann A, Greydanus D: *Adolescent medicine,* ed 3, Stamford, Conn, 1997, Appleton & Lange.

Kaplan D: Future doesn't look rosy for some tattoos, *Consultations* 38(11):2592, 1998.

Krowchuk DP, Lucky AW: Managing adolescent acne, *Adolesc Med* 12(2):355-375, 2001.

O'Toole M, editor: *Miller-Keane encyclopedia & dictionary of medicine, nursing, & allied health,* ed 6, Philadelphia, 1997, WB Saunders.

National Institute on Drug Abuse: NIDA initiative targets increasing teen use of anabolic steroids, *NIDA Notes* 15(3):1-6, 2000.

National Institute on Drug Abuse: About anabolic steroid abuse, *NIDA Notes* 15(3):15, 2000.

National Institute on Drug Abuse: Mind over matter, *NIDA Notes* Sept 14, 2001a, Available online: http://www.nida.nih.gov/MOM/MOMIndex.html. Accessed on Oct 10, 2001.

National Institute on Drug Abuse: *Research report: steroid abuse and addiction,* Revision April 2000b, Available online: http://www.nida.nih.gov/ResearchReports/Steroids/AnabolicSteroids.html. Accessed on Oct 10, 2001.

Neinstein L: *Adolescent health care: a practical guide,* ed 3, Philadelphia, 1996, Lippincott Williams & Wilkins.

Parker S, Zuckerman B, editors: *Behavioral and developmental pediatrics: a handbook for primary care,* Boston, 1995, Little, Brown & Co.

Ponton LE: *The romance of risk: why teenagers do the things they do,* New York, 1997, Basic Books.

Schwab N, Gelfman M, editors: *Legal issues in school health services: a resource for school administrators, school attorneys, school nurses,* North Branch, Minn, 2001, Sunrise River Press.

Strasburger V, Brown R: *Adolescent medicine: a practical guide,* ed 2, Philadelphia, 1998, Lippincott-Raven.

U.S. Department of Health and Human Services: *Healthy people 2010,* vol I, Washington, DC, 2000, USDHHS, Available online: http://www.health.gov/healthypeople. Accessed on Oct 11, 2001.

U.S. Department of Health and Human Services: *1998 Guidelines for treatment of sexually transmitted diseases,* Morbidity and Mortality Weekly Report (MMWR), 47(RR-1), Atlanta, 1998, Centers for Disease Control (CDC), Available online: http://www.cdc.gov/mmwr/preview/mmwrhtml/00050909.htm.

U.S. Preventive Service Task Force: *Guide to clinical preventive services,* Baltimore, 1995, Williams & Wilkins. Third edition (2000-2002) available online: http://www.ahcpr.gov/clinic/cps3dix.htm.

Wolfe P: *Brain matters: translating research into classroom practice,* Alexandria, Va, 2001, Association for Supervision and Curriculum Development.

Wong DL, Hockenberry-Eaton M, Wilson D, et al, editors: *Whaley & Wong's nursing care of infants and children,* ed 6, St Louis, 1999, Mosby.

Youngkin E, Davis MS, editors: *Women's health: a primary clinical guide,* Norwalk, Conn, 1998, Appleton & Lange.

CHAPTER 9

Special Education

School nurses, teachers, psychologists, and professional educators face the growing challenge and responsibility of providing exceptional children and young adults with an appropriate education. Individuals with disabilities attend public schools whenever possible, but not too many years ago, they were denied the opportunity of a regular classroom. Support services are available that enhance the chances for students with disabilities to reach their maximum potential. Special education is now a large and integral part of the U.S. educational system as it identifies and meets each student's unique needs.

The primary reason that more than 5.4 million students are receiving special education is passage of Public Law 94-142 and Section 504 and the more current legislation, Public Law 99-457 (1986) and Public Law 105-17 (1987), the revised Individuals with Disabilities Education Act (IDEA). These laws detail educational rights of the disabled and provide funding to help states cover the costs of providing these rights (PMP, 1998). This chapter discusses the changes and the main components of this legislation and cites the 13 handicapping conditions.

As more children and young adults with disabilities are integrated into community life, important implications affect nursing in all fields. An awareness of the effect of the disability on the child, family, and siblings enables the nurse not only to develop a special personal understanding but facilitates the acceptance of the individual into community and school settings.

In addition to discussing legal facets of legislation, this chapter addresses other areas that are useful to the nurse working with special education students, specifically, assessment tools and terminology. As part of a multidisciplinary team, the nurse provides services to special-needs students. As each team member presents the results of personal evaluation, the nurse should understand the use and purpose of assessment tools and educational terminology to obtain a total picture of the student and be an effective and contributing member of the team.

The chapter concludes with specialized health care procedures. Many students, either in the regular classroom or special classes, require specialized procedures. The techniques used in a school setting frequently differ from those used in a hospital. The school nurse now may need to delegate particular health care procedures to licensed and unlicensed personnel and must provide teaching and monitoring for effective management. The needs of these children are complex, requiring multiple treatment modalities and assistance in some form throughout their school career.

THE LAW

The right to a free and appropriate public education (FAPE) for children with disabilities from 5 to 21 years of age was established in 1975 with the enactment of Public Law (PL) 94-142, the Education for All Handicapped Children Act (EHA). This law addressed identification, evaluation, placement, and education of children with disabilities. In 1986, PL 99-457 amended EHA and provided a phase-in mandate for states to provide special education services to children ages 3 to 5 years. EHA provided grants for states to establish programs for children with developmental delay from birth to age 3.

The title of the EHA was changed to Individuals with Disabilities Education Act (IDEA) in 1990, and special education services for 3- to 5-year-olds were mandated in all states. In 1993, Part C of IDEA offered every state the opportunity to apply for federal funding for the implementation of a statewide, comprehensive, coordinated, multidisciplinary, interagency system of early intervention services for infants and toddlers with developmental delay and their families. These early intervention services for children from birth through 2 years of age are provided through various public agencies (e.g., Department of Health, Department of Education), private agencies, or any combination of public and private sources, depending on state laws and the state's lead agency. Presently, states may submit a 3-year application to receive federal funding.

The *first major revision of PL 94-142* occurred in 1997 with passage of PL 105-17, referred to as *IDEA '97*. The 1997 amendments provided a new emphasis on improving educational results for children with disabilities by ensuring they have meaningful access to the general curriculum through improvements in the individualized education program (IEP). A full educational opportunity goal was established to include students with disabilities in the general education reform efforts related to accountability and improvement of teaching and learning.

Major issues addressed by IDEA '97 include the following:
1. Focusing on the IEP as the primary tool for enhancing the child's involvement and progress in the general curriculum. The IEP goals must relate more clearly to the general curriculum that children receive in regular classrooms.
2. Provision of regular progress reports to all parents as often as reports are provided for other children.
3. Inclusion of students in state and district assessments with accommodations and appropriate modifications, if necessary; and establishment of alternate assessments as needed.
4. Inclusion of at least one regular education teacher on the IEP team. Decision regarding participation by the regular education teacher(s) is made on a case-by-case basis.

These changes in IDEA establish high expectations for children with disabilities and exceed merely providing access to an education; they promote an optimal education. Parental involvement at all levels is encouraged, and full inclusion is emphasized.

I. Thirteen Disabling Conditions Defined in IDEA
    A. *Autism* means a developmental disability significantly affecting verbal and nonverbal communication and social interaction, generally evident before age 3, that adversely affects a child's educational performance. Other characteristics often associated with autism are engagement in repetitive activities and stereotyped movements, resis-

tance to environmental change or change in daily routines, and unusual responses to sensory experiences.

   1. The term does not apply if a child's educational performance is adversely affected primarily because the child has an emotional disturbance (see paragraph **D** of this section).

   2. A diagnosis of autism can be made in a child who manifests the characteristics of "autism" after age 3 if the criteria above are satisfied.

B. *Deaf-blindness* indicates concomitant hearing and visual impairments, the combination of which causes such severe communication and other developmental and educational needs that affected children cannot be accommodated in special education programs established solely for children with deafness or children with blindness.

C. *Deafness* is a hearing impairment so severe that the child is impaired in processing linguistic information through hearing, with or without amplification, that adversely affects educational performance.

D. *Emotional disturbance** means a condition exhibiting one or more of the following characteristics over a prolonged period and to a marked degree that adversely affects a child's educational performance.

   1. Inability to learn that cannot be explained by intellectual, sensory, or health factors.

   2. Inability to build or maintain satisfactory interpersonal relationships with peers and teachers.

   3. General pervasive mood of unhappiness or depression.

   4. Tendency to develop physical symptoms or fears associated with personal or school problems.

E. *Hearing impairment* means an impairment in hearing, whether permanent or fluctuating, that adversely affects a child's educational performance but that is not included under the definition of deafness in this section.

F. *Mentally retarded* indicates significantly subaverage general intellectual functioning concurrent with deficits in adaptive behavior and manifested during the developmental period that adversely affects a child's educational performance.

G. *Multiple disabilities* means concomitant impairments (e.g., mental retardation-blindness, mental retardation-orthopedic impairment), the combination of which causes such severe educational problems that the children cannot be accommodated in special education programs set up solely for one of the impairments. The term does not include deaf-blindness.

H. *Orthopedic impairment* means a severe orthopedic impairment that adversely affects a child's educational performance. The term includes impairments caused by congenital anomaly (e.g., club foot, absence of member), impairments caused by disease (e.g., poliomyelitis, bone

---

*The term includes schizophrenia. The term does not apply to children who are socially maladjusted unless they have an emotional disturbance.

tuberculosis), and impairments from other causes (e.g., cerebral palsy, amputations, and fractures or burns that cause contractures).

I. *Other health impairment* means limited strength, vitality, or alertness, including a heightened alertness to environmental stimuli, that results in limited alertness with respect to the educational environment, that meets both of the following conditions.

1. Is related to chronic or acute health problems such as asthma, attention deficit disorder or attention deficit hyperactivity disorder, diabetes, epilepsy, heart condition, hemophilia, lead poisoning, leukemia, nephritis, rheumatic fever, and sickle cell anemia.

2. Adversely affects a child's educational performance.

J. *Specific learning disability* is defined as follows.

1. The term means a disorder in one or more of the basic psychological processes involved in understanding or in using language, spoken or written, that may manifest itself in an imperfect ability to listen, think, speak, read, spell, or to do mathematical calculations, including conditions such as perceptual disabilities, brain injury, minimal brain dysfunction, dyslexia, and developmental aphasia.

2. The term does not include learning problems that primarily result from visual, hearing, or motor disabilities, mental retardation, emotional disturbance, or environmental, cultural, or economic disadvantage.

K. *Speech or language impairment* indicates a communication disorder, such as stuttering, impaired articulation, a language impairment, or a voice impairment, that adversely affects a child's educational performance.

L. *Traumatic brain injury* means an acquired injury to the brain caused by an external physical force resulting in total or partial functional disability or psychosocial impairment, or both, that adversely affects a child's educational performance. The term applies to open or closed head injuries resulting in impairments in one or more areas, such as cognition; language; memory; attention; reasoning; abstract thinking; judgment; problem-solving; sensory, perceptual, and motor abilities; psychosocial behavior; physical functions; information processing; and speech. The term does not apply to brain injuries that are congenital or degenerative or caused by birth trauma.

M. *Visual impairment including blindness* refers to a visual impairment that, even with correction, adversely affects a child's educational performance. The term includes both partial sight and blindness.

II. Components of IDEA

A. *Those served* are from birth through 21 years of age.

B. An effort must be made to *screen and identify all children* who are in need of special educational and related services.

C. The *environment* must be the *least restrictive*. That is, children with disabilities are to be educated with children who are not disabled, and special education classes, separate schooling, or other arrangements that remove children with disabilities from regular education occur only when the disability is so severe that the student cannot be included in regular education when provided with supplementary aids and services. In Part C, for children from birth to age 3, if the children cannot be served in their "natural environment," justification for a restricted placement must be stated on the IFSP. The *natural environment* is defined as any place a typical child of this age may be found (e.g., at home, in day care, Early Head Start, play group).

D. The *program options* within the special education system include the following:
   1. Regular class with supplementary aids and services.
   2. Designated instruction and services.
   3. Resource specialist.
   4. Special day class.
   5. Special schools.
   6. Nonpublic school.
   7. Residential facilities, hospital, home.

E. *Classroom placement* is decided on an individual basis; certain mandated members for the initial placement meeting include the following:
   1. One member of the evaluation team.
   2. A representative of the public agency.
   3. The teacher.
   4. A person knowledgeable about evaluation procedures and results.
   5. One or both parents or representative.
   6. Other people as appropriate.

F. The *Individualized Education Program (IEP)* is a written plan for each student that guarantees appropriate services. Every special education student must have an IEP at least once a year. The IEP is developed by a team composed of the following:
   1. Parent(s) or representative, such as guardian(s) or surrogate parent(s).
   2. One regular education teacher if child is, or may be, participating in a regular education program.
   3. Special education teacher(s).
   4. Administrator or designee.
   5. Individual who may interpret instructional implications of evaluation results.
   6. Other individuals with knowledge or expertise at the parents' or the county or district educational office's discretion.
   7. Child, where appropriate.

G. The *IEP* includes statements of the following:
   1. Present levels of educational performance and how the individual's disability affects progress in the general curriculum.
   2. Measurable annual goals and short-term instructional objectives for meeting the student's needs to enable the student to be involved in and progress in the general curriculum.
   3. Specific special education services, related services, and supplementary aids to be provided for the student; program modifications

or supports to school personnel so the student can participate in regular educational programs and activities as much as possible.

4. An explanation of the extent, if any, to which the child will not participate with nondisabled children in regular education.

5. Modifications needed to participate in statewide and districtwide assessments; if not participating in a particular statewide or districtwide assessment, a statement of why that assessment is not appropriate for the child and how the child will be assessed.

6. Statement of anticipated frequency, location, and duration of services and modifications.

7. Beginning at age 14, a statement of transition service needs for a plan that promotes movement from school to postschool activities.

8. Statement of how student's progress will be measured and how the parent(s) will be regularly informed (e.g., report card).

H. *Student and parent rights* are defined.

1. Parents must receive detailed, written notice in their language whenever the school plans to change or refuses to change the identification, assessment, or educational placement of their child.

2. Parents have a right to an independent educational assessment of their child, to review and inspect all educational records; give written consent to the assessment plan; give written consent before the child is placed; refuse to consent to an assessment.

3. Evaluation and tests must be conducted in the student's own language or mode of communication; a variety of achievement tests and teacher recommendations, as well as physical condition and social or cultural background, are used for placement procedures; an evaluation shall be conducted every 3 years or on request of the parents or teacher.

I. Regarding *confidentiality,* results of assessment data and placement must be kept confidential, and parents or guardians must have access to inspect and obtain copies of information regarding their child. An educational agency receiving federal monies must allow parents to inspect, challenge, and correct their child's records. Students 18 years and older also have the same rights regarding their records. Parents are to be notified when unneeded records are to be destroyed.

J. *Designated Instruction and Services (DIS)* refer to related services as required to help the child with a disability benefit fully from special education. Services are not limited to the following; others may be included, provided they help the child benefit from special education.

1. Speech-language pathology and audiology services.
2. Psychological services.
3. Physical therapy and occupational therapy.
4. Recreation, including therapeutic recreation.
5. Early identification and assessment of disabilities in children.
6. Social work services.
7. School health services.
8. Counseling services, including rehabilitation services.

9. Orientation and mobility services.
10. Medical services for diagnostic and evaluation purposes only.
11. Transportation.
12. Parent counseling and training.
K. *Discipline and safety.*
    1. For the first time, IDEA clarifies how school disciplinary rules apply to children in special education. IDEA specifically states that children who need special education must receive instruction and services to help them follow the rules and behave in school. The law recognizes that if students with disabilities bring illegal drugs or a weapon to school, schools have the right to remove the children to an alternative educational setting for up to 45 days. The law also acknowledges the right of schools to report crimes to law enforcement or judicial authorities. While under suspension or expulsion the student should still receive special education services in an appropriate setting.

SECTION 504 OF REHABILITATION ACT OF 1973

This legislation defines disability more broadly than IDEA, which is limited to 13 categories of eligibility. Children with mental or physical disabilities that affect their ability to care for themselves, perform activities of daily living, or participate in educational activities may not be excluded from general school programs or denied special services because they do not have one of the eligible disabilities. Section 504 does not require a student to be enrolled in special education to receive related services. Accommodations and services must be provided to support the maximum educational opportunities possible (e.g., modifications in student assignments, physical adaptations of the school building, peer assistance).

Students are found eligible for services through an individualized evaluation by a multidisciplinary team. Under Section 504, a "handicapped person" means an individual with a mental or physical impairment that substantially limits one or more major life activities (e.g., self-care, walking, seeing, hearing, speaking, performing manual tasks, learning, breathing). Examples of students who may be eligible for Section 504 include those with attention deficit disorder (ADD), diabetes, alcohol and drug addiction, asthma, obesity, and acquired immunodeficiency syndrome (AIDS).

Section 504 is a civil rights statute that prohibits discrimination on the basis of disability. States must comply with the regulations of Section 504 if they are to continue to receive federal financial assistance, but they do not receive federal funds for services provided under Section 504. The Office of Civil Rights (OCR) is responsible for monitoring compliance with Section 504 regulations.

WEB SITES

IDEA '97
    http://www.ed.gov/offices/OSERS/Policy/IDEA/
Office of Civil Rights
    1-800-421-3481
    http://www.ed.gov/offices/OCR/

Office of Special Education Programs
   http://www.ed.gov/offices/OSERS/OSEP/index.html
National Information Center for Children and Youth with Disabilities
   State Resource Sheets
   http://www.nichcy.org/states.htm

SPECIALIZED HEALTH CARE PROCEDURES AND RELATED ADAPTATIONS

State, county, and district guidelines, procedures, and policies for administering specialized health care procedures (SHCPs) may vary but should include the following components:

1. HCP's authorization for procedure.
2. Parent's written request for the procedure.
3. Waiver signed by parent(s) if procedure is to be performed by nondistrict personnel.
4. Universal precautions.

The *main purpose* of providing SHCPs in the school is to maintain the student in the school environment. Whether the SHCPs are performed in the student's classroom or another location, one *objective* is to minimize disruption in educational programming. Another objective is to address the privacy issues and health needs of the student and their classmates' lack of privacy and social emotional effects surrounding exposure to the procedure executed in the classroom combined with the distraction from classroom work for all students.

When possible the nurse should:

1. Discuss doing procedure before or after school with parent.
2. Provide the procedure at the least disruptive time, if flexible schedule allowed.
3. Minimize the student's time out of classroom.
4. Have necessary equipment ready and medication available.
5. Use the procedure as an opportunity to teach health and secondary prevention.

The SHCP should be included in the student's IFSP, IEP, or Section 504 plan. The plan should reflect information in the SHCP, such as health treatment necessary during school, the frequency, personnel involved, and the educational plan for school participation and optimal health. Include goals and objectives as appropriate.

ALLERGIES
Latex Allergies

Allergic reactions and sensitivity to latex proteins have risen dramatically during the past 15 years. The term *latex* is used here to describe products made from *natural rubber latex, not synthetic* (e.g., latex paint). Children who undergo frequent surgeries or bladder catheterization and individuals who regularly wear latex gloves are at the greatest risk for developing latex allergies. People with allergic rhinitis or other allergies also have a higher risk.

The extensive use of latex gloves to prevent the spread of human immunodeficiency virus (HIV) and hepatitis B virus is believed to have contributed to the increase and awareness of latex sensitivity. This awareness has led to the education of health care providers regarding the potential health hazards and the necessity to minimize latex exposure. Latex sensitivity has decreased recently as a result of this awareness.

Symptoms of latex allergy include flushing of the skin or an itchy skin rash, edema, watery or itchy eyes, hives, and wheezing. Anaphylactic shock also can occur. A more severe reaction is likely when latex contacts moist skin, mucous membranes, the airway, or bloodstream.

Cross-reactivity may occur in individuals with latex sensitivity because they may react to certain foods with a similar protein. This cross-reactivity occurs when the immune system mistakes a similar protein or chemical composition for an allergen. Not all foods containing latexlike proteins affect everyone with latex allergies. An allergist can help identify foods and items that will cause an allergic reaction. Most common manifestations of latex-food syndrome are hives, facial edema, rhinitis, and conjunctivitis.

Prevention is the best treatment; persons who have latex allergy or are at high risk should avoid latex products and foods with latexlike proteins. Those with an allergic reaction to the foods listed in Box 9-1 should discuss a possible latex allergy with their HCP.

I. Procedure
   A. Develop an individualized emergency care plan (IECP) in consultation with the student's parent(s) and HCP.
   B. Educate school staff regarding IECP and have plan readily available.
   C. Indicate latex allergy alert on school records.
   D. Educate staff and student regarding identification of latex products and allergic reaction.
   E. Promote use of personal medical identification (MedicAlert) bracelet.
   F. Discuss availability of injectable epinephrine in all settings (e.g., home, school, car, sports events, day care).

II. Web Sites
American College of Allergy, Asthma & Immunology (ACAAI): About Latex Allergies
http://allergy.mcg.edu/advice/latex.html

Box 9-1   *Foods with Latexlike Proteins*

Bananas*	Pineapples
Avocados*	Tomatoes
Kiwi*	Mangos
Papaya*	Figs
Chestnuts*	Peaches
Passion fruit	Nectarines
Shellfish	Plums
Peanuts	Strawberries
Melons	

*Most common allergies.

Box 9-2   *Items That May Contain Latex*

Adhesive tape	Elastic bandages
Ambu bags	Eye shields/patches
Art supplies (markers, glue, paint)	Foam rubber padding on wheelchairs, lin-
Baby bottle nipples	ing on splints and braces
Balloons	Gloves—examination and sterile
Balls (tennis, bowling, Koosh)	Pacifier
Adhesive bandages (Band-Aids) or similar	Racquet handles
products	Raincoats/gear
Beach toys	Rubber bands
Blood pressure cuffs (bladder and tubing)	Shower cap/swimming cap
Bulb syringes	Stethoscope tubing
Camera eyepiece	Stomach and gastrointestinal tubes
Chewing gum	Swimming fins
Colostomy pouch	Tennis/squash shoes
Condoms and condom urinary collection	Tourniquets
devices	Urinary catheters
Diapers/rubber pants	Underwear
Diaphragm	Wheelchair tires

ELIMINATION
Self-Urinary Catheterization (Clean, Intermittent)

I. Definition

   A. Self-catheterization promotes independence. Self-catheterization is the introduction of a catheter through the urethra into the bladder. This procedure is performed using a clean technique by students with a neurogenic bladder resulting from spinal cord dysfunction or neuromuscular disease.

II. Purpose

   A. The purpose of self-catheterization is to empty the bladder at appropriate intervals for the individual who has no bladder control or the student using a bladder-training program. It relieves bladder distention, which can lead to discomfort, overflow, and dribbling; decreases susceptibility to urinary tract and bladder infection by reducing residual urine, controls odors; and prevents skin breakdown.

III. Equipment

   A. Catheter, as prescribed by HCP.

   B. Mirror for initial female instruction.

   C. Water-soluble lubricant, if ordered.

   D. Cleansing agent, 4 × 4-in gauze squares, cotton balls, alcohol wipes, towelette.

   E. Clean disposable nonlatex gloves when student does not perform procedure.

   F. Container for urine if individual is unable to use toilet.

   G. Storage container for catheter (jar, plastic bags, makeup bag).

NOTE: Facilities often are not available for adequate cleansing of catheter; therefore the individual can carry extra catheters and two containers, one marked "dirty" and one marked "clean."

   H. Storage container for all of the equipment, labeled with student's name.

IV. **Instructions**
   A. Before urinary catheterization:
      1. Wash hands thoroughly.
      2. Place catheter and small amount of lubricant on a paper towel on a clean surface.
      3. Position of student varies according to sex and disability.
      4. Use gloves when nurse or designated individual performs procedure.
      5. Wipe hands with towelettes.
   B. Female student:
      1. The student should lie down or be in sitting position; catheterization may be easier if the student sits facing backward on the toilet or stands with one foot on the toilet edge.
      2. Expose and cleanse urethral area, wiping from front to back.
      3. Identify location of urethral meatus by beginning at clitoris and applying pressure with finger until urethral indentation is felt.
      4. Holding the catheter 3 in (7.5 cm) from tip, insert it through the meatus 1 to 2 inches in a downward and backward direction until urine appears; the other end of the catheter should be placed in collection container or toilet.
      5. When the urine flow stops, advance the catheter slightly. If no more urine is obtained, withdraw the catheter slightly and rotate to ensure drainage of all areas of the bladder.
      6. When the bladder is empty, pinch the catheter and slowly withdraw.
   C. Male student:
      1. Individual should sit on toilet or in chair until technique has been learned.
      2. Hold penis up, at 45- to 90-degree angle; if not circumcised, retract foreskin, and wash glans with soapy cotton balls or with student-specific supplies. Begin at urethral opening and in a circular manner wash away from meatus.
      3. Gently insert the catheter until urine returns; place other end of the catheter in collection container or toilet. If resistance is felt at the external sphincter of the bladder, have student deep breathe or slightly increase the traction on the penis and apply gentle, steady pressure on the catheter; when urine has been obtained, insert the catheter about an additional inch. Rotate the catheter so that the catheter openings have reached all areas of the bladder.
      4. Slowly remove the catheter when urine ceases to flow. When the bladder is emptied, pinch the catheter and withdraw.
   D. After urinary catheterization:
      1. Nurse: remove gloves, wash hands, and reglove.
      2. Wash, rinse, dry, and store catheter.

3. Rinse and dry urine receptacle, if appropriate.
4. Remove gloves and wash hands.
5. Note time, approximate amount of urine, and any signs of infection, such as color, odor, or change in appearance.
6. Help student with any difficult clothing items and transfers if needed.

Other Elimination Adaptations

I. Urinary Diversions

A. Urinary diversion procedures may be used for a neurogenic bladder, urinary strictures, birth defects, damage resulting from trauma, or chronic infections causing ureteral and renal damage. These procedures are used to divert urine from the bladder to another location, most commonly an opening on the skin.

B. *Vesicostomy* is a relatively uncomplicated procedure whereby the bladder is sutured to the abdominal wall and an opening is made through the abdominal wall into the bladder wall, creating a stoma on the outer skin surface for urinary drainage. Diapers are worn high to cover the stoma and must be changed frequently to avoid skin irritation from urinary drainage. A vesicostomy usually is a temporary solution.

C. A recently developed procedure is the *appendicovesicostomy,* which involves using the appendix to join the bladder to the wall of the abdomen. The appendix provides a conduit for catheterization, and a one-way valve is created to prevent urinary leakage. The location of this opening on the abdomen is convenient for catheterization, especially self-catheterization, at routine intervals to maintain continence. In some situations, the bladder is augmented with bowel or stomach tissue to increase bladder size and reduce spasticity. Appendicovesicostomy also is called the *Mitrofanoff catheterizable channel.*

D. Another urinary diversion is a *Kock pouch,* in which an artificial bladder is created surgically from a section of the small intestines. The stoma is located on the skin, which allows for periodic catheterization. This pouch is an adaptation of the one used for bowel continence.

E. Other urinary diversions involve use of a collection bag or pouch. *Urostomy* is the general term used for the surgical technique to divert urine from the bladder. One of the oldest procedures is the *ileal conduit (loop),* which is made by implanting a ureter into a 12-cm loop of ileum or sigmoid colon that is brought out to the abdominal wall for urinary drainage. Urine is collected in an ileostomy bag or pouch. A variety of appliances are available, and most last 3 to 7 days before leaking develops.

II. Bowel Diversions

A. *Colostomy* is the surgical procedure of an opening from the large intestine to the abdomen with a stoma on the skin. The stoma should be shiny and pink to bright red. The colostomy may be temporary or permanent and also is differentiated by the part of the colon brought to the surface of the abdomen. The *sigmoid or descending colostomy* is the most common type, and the stoma is on the lower left side of the abdomen. A *transverse colostomy* results in one or two stomas in the upper, middle, or right side of the abdomen. A *loop colostomy* has two stomas and usually is found in the transverse colon; one stoma is for stool and the other for mucus. A loop colostomy usually is a temporary procedure. Colostomies may be irrigated to establish a regular evacuation pattern.

    B. An *ileostomy* involves bringing the small intestine to the abdomen and creating a stoma that may be temporary or permanent. Contents of the ileum are semiliquid fecal material that seeps continuously; thus routine bowel habits are impossible. Skin care is especially important. Other surgical procedures are used to develop internal pouches that can be drained by a tube or catheter, such as the *ileoanal pouch*.

III. Web Sites

    United Ostomy Association, Inc.

      http://www.uoa.org

Box 9-3   *Urinary and Stool Collection Systems Care*

- Pouching systems attach to the abdomen with an adhesive back and use a bag, which fits over the stoma to collect the diverted output, either urine or stool. The backing may be one-piece (face-plate) or two-piece (flange).
- The bag may be open-ended for required drainage; a closing device such as a clamp, clip, or wire closure is used.
- The sealed type bag is used most commonly for individuals who are undergoing irrigation for control or have a regular elimination pattern.
- Meticulous skin care is needed to prevent peristomal skin breakdown and maintain a good seal.
- Ivory soap removes oils/fats from the skin so that the pouch will adhere better.
- Use of a skin barrier (e.g., tincture of benzoin, Stomahesive, or Stomaguard) helps protect the skin and aids in adhesion. The barrier may be in liquid form or barrier wipes. Some pouches have a built-in skin barrier.
- Skin barrier paste can be used to fill crevices or folds in the skin, thus creating a better seal.
- Special tapes are available to help support the adhesive backing and for waterproofing.

- Ostomy belts that circle the abdomen and attach to the pouch may be used for support or as an alternative to adhesives.
- The bag should be emptied when about one-third full to prevent the weight from pulling it off the skin.
- Most systems will last 3-7 days without leaking.
- Colostomy bags usually are changed every 2-4 days.
- Adhesive remover is useful for removing residue when the system is changed.
- Reusable appliances should be rinsed in warm water and soaked in a 3:1 solution of water and white vinegar or a commercial cleaner for 30 minutes.
- Rinse the appliance with tepid water and dry away from direct sunlight to avoid drying out the material, which may lead to cracking.
- Certain foods (e.g., eggs, cheese, asparagus) give a strong odor to urine.
- Specific foods, such as cabbage, onions, and fish, increase stool odors. Some foods, such as spinach and parsley, help fight odors.
- Some systems have an odor barrier; a liquid deodorizer or a few drops of diluted vinegar may be added to the bag to help fight odors.

FEEDING
Nasogastric Tube Placement

I. **Definition**

A. Nasogastric placement is the insertion of a tube through the nostril into the gastrointestinal tract for feeding. A tube also may be passed through the mouth into the stomach. The tube may be taped and left in place or inserted and removed with each feeding. The HCP's specific order, the type of tube used, or the age of child determines the method. Leaving the tube in place is less traumatic for older students or those with a disability.

II. **Purpose**

A. The nasogastric tube provides an alternate means of delivering nutrients and other essentials into the body because of anomalies of the throat or esophagus, swallowing impairment, and inadequate oral intake.

B. Feeding tubes are made from silicone rubber, polyurethane, polyethylene, and polyvinylchloride. Silicone rubber and polyurethane tubes are more flexible than the others and have a smaller diameter; these may be called *small-bore tubes*.

III. **Equipment**

A. Nasogastric catheter, per student's size and viscosity of the feeding mixture, ordered by HCP.

B. Water-soluble lubricant.

C. Clamp for tube.

D. Emesis basin.

E. Container of water for flushing tube.

F. Stethoscope, large catheter tip syringe for determining tube placement.

G. Nonallergenic tape.

H. Clean disposable nonlatex gloves.

IV. **Instructions**

A. Refer to HCP's prescription for specific recommendations or adaptations to the following procedure.

1. Explain procedure to student according to student's level of understanding. Encourage able student to participate.

2. Position student as follows:

a. *Infant or child*: place in supine position with head and chest slightly elevated.

b. *Infant only,* may hyperextend neck by placing small rolled towel under shoulders.

c. *Older student*: sitting position or high Fowler's position, with neck slightly flexed.

3. Measure tube for correct length for tube insertion and mark with tape. Some controversy exists regarding nasogastric tube measurement, but two techniques currently are used.

a. The distance from the tip of the nose to the earlobe plus the distance to the end of the xiphoid process.

b. From the tip of the nose to the earlobe plus the distance to a point midway between the xiphoid process and the umbilicus.

4. Lubricate the tip of the tubing with water or water-soluble lubricant as ordered to facilitate passage; insert the tube into nares and advance forward and downward until tape mark has been reached.
   a. If coughing, choking, or cyanosis appears, remove tube.
   b. If gagging occurs, let student rest briefly.
   c. If student is able and can tolerate, offer sips of water and advance tube with swallowing.
   d. If student is able and understands, ask student to bend the neck forward, take shallow, rapid breaths, and swallow, which will help advance the tube.
5. After insertion, temporarily secure and check the position of the tube by both methods.
   a. Attach syringe and apply negative pressure; aspiration of stomach contents into syringe may indicate proper placement; however, absence of stomach contents is not always an indication of incorrect placement.
   b. Attach syringe and inject 0.5 to 10 ml of air into the tube, depending on the size of student, while simultaneously listening with stethoscope placed over epigastrium; the nurse should hear sounds of gurgling or growling if the tube has been properly placed. *Be alert* that sounds may be heard when air enters the stomach while the tube is positioned above the gastroesophageal sphincter.
   c. The only accurate method for testing the appropriate tube placement is by radiography and pH testing of aspirated gastric fluid.
6. After tube placement confirmation, securely tape tube in place to maintain proper placement.
   a. Do not disturb vision with placement of tape.
   b. Do not tape to the forehead as this may damage nostril.
7. Clamp off end of tube.
8. Remove gloves and wash hands.
9. Document procedure including the date and time of insertion, type and size of the tube, placement, results of auscultation, tolerance of procedure, and any problems encountered.

Gavage/Nasogastric Feeding

I. Definition
A. Gastric gavage is the process of providing nutrients in a liquid form directly into the stomach by a nasogastric tube. Feeding may be either intermittent or continuous, provided by bolus, gravity, or slow drip. Refer to "Nasogastric Tube Placement" for instruction on proper insertion of the tube.

II. Purpose
A. The purpose of gastric gavage is to administer medication, fluids, and nutrients that the individual is unable to take by mouth because of difficulty swallowing, oral or esophageal disease, trauma, anomalies, malnutrition, or anorexia.

III. Equipment

    A. Large or medium-sized catheter tip syringe, either for small (10 to 20 ml) or for larger amounts (50 ml) of feedings.

    B. Syringe to inject air or aspirate stomach contents to determine tube placement.

    C. Stethoscope to check tube placement.

    D. Formula or feeding solution (room temperature) or medications, measured amount.

    E. Water to flush tube, required amount.

    F. Feeding bag and pump for continuous feed, if ordered.

    G. Wall hook or a stand to suspend the formula during feeding.

    H. Clean, disposable nonlatex gloves.

    I. Nonallergenic or paper tape to reattach tube if necessary.

IV. Instructions

    A. Refer to HCP's prescription for specific recommendations or adaptations to the following procedure.

        1. Position student as follows.

            a. *Infant:* prop on right side for feeding with head and chest elevated; placement in an infant seat is not recommended as pressure on the abdomen may cause reflux.

            b. *Older or larger student*: can be in semi-Fowler's position and propped toward right side.

        2. Wash hands and put on gloves.

        3. Unclamp or remove cap from nasogastric tube.

        4. Check position of tube by using both of the following methods. (See "Nasogastric Tube Placement" for complete position assessment information.)

            a. Attach syringe and apply negative pressure; aspiration of stomach contents (residual) into syringe may indicate proper placement; however, absence of stomach contents does not always indicate incorrect placement.

            b. Attach syringe and inject 0.5 to 10 ml of air into tube, depending on size of student, while simultaneously listening with stethoscope placed over epigastrium; gurgling or growling sounds should be heard if the tube has been placed properly.

        5. Attach syringe barrel to tubing and pour small amount of formula into syringe.

        6. Raise syringe 6 to 8 in and let fluid flow gradually; the flow rate is determined by lowering the syringe or by gravity flow. Continue to add formula without introducing air; when finished, allow formula to drain to bottom of syringe and clamp tube.

        7. Flow rate should be slow, unless instructed to administer formula by bolus method; the average time is 15 to 30 minutes. Feeding too much or too quickly may cause gagging and respiratory distress or vomiting and diarrhea.

        8. Continuous feed.

            a. Not recommended unless continuous supervision is possible to prevent accidental dislodgment and risk of aspiration.

b. Connect feeding tube to tube from feeding bag.

c. Fill feeding bag with appropriate amount of formula; fluids generally should be kept at room temperature to prevent cramping.

d. Adjust flow rate by twisting clamp or programming enteral pump.

9. Avoid bubbles in tubing because they may cause abdominal distention.

10. Follow each feeding with water; 1 to 2 ml for small tubes and 5 to 15 ml or more for larger ones or as prescribed.

11. If tube is to be removed, clamp or pinch and remove gently, but rapidly, to prevent loss of food from tube and decrease risk of aspiration.

12. If tube is to remain in place, clamp before water drains to prevent introduction of air into the stomach with the next feeding or loss of feeding; remove the syringe and insert cap into end of tubing.

13. Remove gloves and wash hands.

14. Have individual remain in semi-Fowler's position or turn to side for 30 to 60 minutes after feeding, or as directed by HCP. Some students tolerate immediate return to activities.

15. Wash catheter-tipped syringe with warm water and mild soap, rinse thoroughly, dry, and store in clean area. May place equipment in zippered plastic bag and refrigerate to inhibit bacterial growth.

16. Document the date and time of procedure, tube placement confirmation methods; color, consistency and amount of residual; type, amount of formula and irrigant used, and student's tolerance of procedure.

Gastrostomy and Jejunostomy Feedings

I. Definition

A. A gastrostomy is an artificial opening through the abdominal wall with a tube extended directly into the stomach; with a jejunostomy, the tube extends directly into the jejunum (i.e., the small intestine between the duodenum and the ileum).

B. Feeding by a *gastrostomy* or *jejunostomy* is performed by passing a nutrient solution, medication, or both through a tube inserted directly into a skin-level device or attached to an external tube at the abdominal site/stoma. Several types of skin-level (button) devices are available.

C. Feeding by a gastrostomy (G) tube may be by bolus (about 15 to 20 minutes), gravity, or slow drip through a pump. The jejunostomy feeding is best tolerated as a continuous slow drip (over hours).

D. The jejunostomy (J) tube may be in a separate stoma. If a student has *both* a *J tube and a G tube*, both tubes may be in the same stoma or one tube (gastrojejunal) with several ports may be used (J port, G port, medication port, or balloon inflation limb). The combination tubes are used for students who require gastric decompression during the J feeding because of an obstruction in the gastric outlet.

II. Purpose

A. Gastrostomy and jejunostomy feedings provide total or supplemental nutritional support, hydration, and administration of medication when the oral route is not feasible or adequate.

III. Equipment

A. Catheter-tipped syringe, 60 ml for irrigation and feeding by gravity or bolus.

B. Feeding bag/bottle for slow drip-feeding.

C. Prescribed formula, medication, or both at room temperature; check expiration date. Opened formula usually is good for 24 hours when refrigerated and 4 hours when not.

D. Water for flushing and hydration, as prescribed.

E. Catheter plug, clamp, or rubber band.

F. Gauze pads (2 × 2 or 3 × 3-in) and scissors.

G. Nonlatex disposable gloves.

H. Extension tube/adapter if skin-level device is being used.

I. Decompression tube needed for some skin-level devices with an antireflux valve/two-way valve to vent when abdominal distention occurs. The decompression tube should be in place no longer than 5-10 minutes; frequent prolonged use may prematurely weaken the valve.

J. Hook on the wall or a stand to suspend the formula for feeding.

K. Feeding pump, if prescribed.

L. Pacifier, for a baby during feeding.

IV. Instructions

A. Refer to HCP's prescription for specific recommendations or adaptations to the following procedure. Students with a feeding tube need written permission from their HCP to be given any oral foods. The order should include texture and amount of oral foods tolerated.

1. The student should be in high Fowler's position, if possible; the back should be well supported. Some students may tolerate feeding while semireclined or lying down; the right side is optimal.

2. Wash hands and glove.

3. With G tube, assess bowel sounds and check abdominal distention before feeding.

4. When tube placement is confirmed, connect the syringe to the external tube or extension tube for skin-level device. Fill extension tube with formula before connecting it to the button.

5. With MIC-KEY (Medical Innovations Corp, Santa Clara, California), line up black lines of the skin-level button and extension tubing, lock into place turning extension tubing a quarter turn clockwise. Do not turn past the stop point because this will break the lock.

6. Pour feeding into tilted syringe, unclamp the filled tubing, and let fluid flow into stomach; tilting of syringe lets air bubbles escape and not enter the stomach.

7. Regulate the flow rate by raising or lowering syringe and tubing.

8. Decompression may be needed before, during, or after feeding to relieve excessive gas.

9. Continuous decompression is provided by using a Y tube (opened) while feeding.

10. For gravity or slow drip feeding, place the bag on a hook at height needed to achieve ordered flow, pour in formula, and allow to fill tubing before attachment to the feeding button. The flow may be 2 to 3 ml/min.
11. After each feeding, flush the tube with 10 to 30 ml of water unless a larger amount is prescribed; clamp or insert plastic stopper before water drains from tubing.
    a. Water will keep the tube clean and prevent clogging;
    b. Air will not enter the stomach with next feeding.
    c. If a clamp is used, a small gauze dressing can be placed over tube opening to keep it clean.
12. Tubing should be secure; an abdominal binder or netting can be used.
13. Wash feeding equipment and store in a clean area. Equipment can be placed in a zippered plastic bag and refrigerated to inhibit bacterial growth.
14. Remove gloves and wash hands.
15. Feed with other students whenever feasible; use of pacifier with infants may provide oral stimulation, improve oral function, and facilitate absorption of nutrients.
16. Refer to general orders for activity level after feeding.
17. Document date and time of procedure, amount and type of formula and irrigant, and tolerance level of procedure.

V. Complications and Treatment for Gastroesophageal Reflux Disease

A. *Gastroesophageal reflux disease (GERD)* occurs when the lower esophageal sphincter is weak or relaxes inappropriately and allows reflux of gastric contents into the esophagus. The exact cause is unknown, but GERD may occur with prematurity, bronchopulmonary dysplasia, neurological disorders, asthma, cerebral palsy, and tube feedings. Reflux may lead to esophagitis, recurrent respiratory infections, aspiration pneumonia, or reflux-associated apnea and bradycardia.

B. *Symptoms of GERD* include restlessness, irritability, spitting up, frequent respiratory tract infections, vomiting, and weight loss.

C. Treatment includes frequent, smaller feedings of thickened liquids/formula. Feeding given with the student in semi-Fowler's position, avoiding slumping, and remaining in semireclining position for 30 minutes after eating may reduce reflux. Medications to improve gastric motility (e.g., metoclopramide [Reglan]) or neutralize gastric acid (e.g., ranitidine hydrochloride [Zantac]) may be prescribed.

VI. Surgical Options for Gastroesophageal Reflux Disease

A. If reflux persists, *fundoplication* surgery is considered. In this procedure the upper portion of the stomach (fundus) is wrapped around the lower part of the esophagus to prevent reflux; it may involve a partial wrap to a full 360-degree wrap. A tight wrap prohibits vomiting and the child may gag or develop respiratory distress when overfed or with intestinal flu. With a gastrostomy a decompression tube can be used to release the gas or stomach contents, thus relieving pressure on the

Box 9-4 *Problems Associated with Enteral Feedings*

Follow specific instructions found in HCP orders, IHCP, and/or state, county, district policies and procedures.

If tube is forcefully pulled out:

1. If bleeding occurs, press on the site with clean gauze pads until bleeding stops.
2. Maintain ostomy by inserting red Robinson or Foley catheter 2-3 in and secure with tape; if Foley catheter is used, inflate balloon and pull Foley catheter back to ensure balloon is inflated adequately.

Follow HCP's instruction for reinsertion if skin-level device is dislodged. Do not attempt replacement unless tube is well established.

3. New gastrostomy tubes (<3 weeks) should be replaced within 3 hours to prevent closure of stoma. Established stomas will remain patent for a longer period and are easier to replace.
4. Jejunostomy tubes must be replaced within 3-4 hours; longer delays may result in tract closure.

If vomiting or diarrhea occur:

1. For formula intolerance, try another formula.
2. Try formulas with texture, more helpful with diarrhea.
3. Dry heaves may occur.
4. Gastrointestinal virus.

If excessive leakage occurs around stoma:

1. Occurs when the tube pulls away from the interior abdominal wall.
2. Occurs when stoma is enlarged so that the button or tube does not fit properly; may need larger button or tube; changes in student's weight (gain or loss) may necessitate adjustment of tube length and space between balloon and fixation device to maintain appropriate tension.
3. Occurs when balloon is not sufficiently inflated to maintain appropriate tension on stoma to prevent leakage (too loose); but may cause necrosis if too tight; tension is appropriate

when tube is flush with the abdomen and the tube fixation device can be easily rotated. Skin-level feeding device should be one-eighth inch above the skin.

4. Is treated with stoma adhesive powder or skin barrier (DuoDerm) cut and placed around stoma.

If peristomal area redness with increased tenderness, swelling, and purulent drainage occur:

1. May result from excessive leakage of caustic gastric juices from stoma.
2. Is cleaned with soap and water and dried thoroughly, check temperature, and notify parent.
3. May have prescribed daily application of antibiotic ointment and placement of gauze dressing around the stoma.
4. May be prevented by keeping peristomal skin dry and rotating button during stoma care to prevent skin breakdown.

If excessive granulation tissue is present:

1. May increase with leakage, although granulation (proud flesh) occurs normally during the healing process of the stoma.
2. May be cauterized with silver nitrate.
3. May decrease in amount or skin may heal with application of moisture barrier (Calmoseptine), sucralfate powder, or foam dressing (Hydrasorb; Kendall).

If tube/button is occluded:

1. May occur after feeding or administration of medication if insufficient irrigation.
2. May be prevented by cleaning inside of feeding button with moist cotton-tipped applicator to help maintain patency.
3. May be irrigated with 2-3 ml of water in a 10-ml syringe while gently trying to dislodged plug. *Do not force.* Notify parent, HCP, or both.

If tube or button must be replaced frequently:

1. May need larger tube or button.

diaphragm and lungs. If fundoplication is performed without a gastrostomy, pressure is relieved by insertion of a nasogastric tube. Over time, the fundoplication may loosen and vomiting is again possible.

B. Newer, less invasive alternatives than fundoplication are available. The Stretta device (Curon Medical, Sunnyvale, California) is inserted by endoscopy. The device coagulates the tissue in the gastroesophageal junction, making it resistant to reflux. Several treatments are required for this procedure, which recently was approved by the Food and Drug Administration (FDA). The EndoCinch (C.R. Bard, Murray Hill, New Jersey) is a tool inserted by endoscopy wherein stitches create a pleat in the sphincter at the gastroesophageal junction, which reduces the backflow of acid from the stomach into the esophagus.

VII. Web Sites

Gastrostomy Support
http://www.g-tube.com/gerd.spml

ORTHOPEDIC

Crutches

I. Definition

A. Crutches are devices used as temporary or permanent aids for walking when the injury or disability is too severe for a cane but not severe enough for a wheelchair. A *crutch gait* is achieved by alternately bearing weight on one or both legs using the crutches. The condition, functional level, and physical abilities of the student determine the gait selected to teach. *Crutch gaits* include two-point, three-point, four-point, swing-through, and swing-to gaits. The term *point* refers to the number of points in contact with the floor during ambulation with crutches.

II. Purpose

A. Crutches are used by students to prevent weight bearing on the affected limb, move gait control to the arms and hands, or support balance while walking with braces. Crutches free the student from dependence on others as much as possible.

III. Equipment

A. A variety of crutch types exist, and the student's specific condition and physical ability determine their use.

1. *Axillary crutches* are the most common for short-term assistance.
2. *Forearm crutches* generally are used when permanent assistance is anticipated. The *Lofstrand crutch* (Lofstrand Labs, Ltd, Gaithersburg, Maryland) has a cuff that fits around the forearm supporting the weight on a hand bar, thus allowing the student to release the hand and grasp objects or a handrail without dropping the crutch.
3. *Trough crutches* allows for body weight to be assumed by the elbow.

IV. Instructions

A. Crutches or any assistive devices (e.g., cane, walker) used by children must be fitted properly to prevent crutch pressure on the axilla, develop a stable and normal gait, maintain safety, and ensure good posture during ambulating. This fitting is commonly done by a physical therapist, whereas the nurse manages the procedure at school and often in the home.

1. When using axillary crutches, the student's weight is on the hands, with crutches pressed against side of chest wall.
2. Crutches should not be pressed into the axilla because pressure can damage the brachial plexus nerves.
3. For a gross check of measurement, have the student stand in good balance with crutches and assess the following points.
   a. Standing base with crutch tips about 4 to 8 inches in front and 4 inches to sides of student; taller individuals need a wider base.
   b. Bend in elbows between 20 and 30 degrees.
   c. Crutch pads 1½ in below axilla.
4. Observe for difficulty in grasping horizontal handpiece.
5. For security, crutch tips should be wide and provide good suction.
6. Check tips and replace worn tips promptly to prevent slipping.
7. Take extra precautions in rainy weather to avoid slipping.
8. Screws and nuts often become loose on mechanical aids; properly maintained equipment increases student's safety.
9. Designate a place in the classroom for crutches to be kept when not in use because they can be a safety hazard to other students; often the custodian is willing to install a hook or other form of crutch holder in a convenient spot.
10. A backpack is useful for students who use crutches or other assistive devices because it allows the student to maintain maximum independence; discuss with student and caregiver the proper packing and distribution of weight and total weight for backpack.
11. Student should wear appropriate nonskid shoes.
12. Consult physical therapist or occupational therapist as needed.

Orthoses

A variety of *orthoses* are available and may be used to prevent deformity, control alignment, increase efficiency of gait, or stabilize weakened or paralyzed extremities.

Orthoses *must be* well fitted and maintained to promote ambulation; if not, they can disturb balance by creating a safety hazard, produce muscle stress, and cause tissue breakdown. If long-term use is determined, ongoing adjustment and replacement by an orthotist is required.

Four common types of lower limb orthoses are used. They are characterized by the joints controlled by the specific device. An *ankle-foot orthosis (AFO)* is used to support the ankle and foot in an appropriate position for standing and walking; prevent footdrop caused by trauma, paralysis of flexor muscles, or bed rest; or prevent heel cord tightening after heel cord–lengthening surgery. AFO devices promote optimal motion and are designed to maintain a rigid ankle but may allow for some flexibility. They are made in distinct lengths for specific ankle-foot conditions and can be ordered in a variety of colors and patterns.

The *knee-ankle-foot orthosis (KAFO)* is used to redistribute weight, control motion at the knees, control functional gait, and improve general safety during ambulation. It is used after paralysis or weakness of the quadriceps muscle or knee extension or to limit weight bearing. The KAFO supports the knee, ankle, and foot and may have locked or unlocked knee joints.

The *hip-knee-ankle-foot orthosis (HKAFO)* is used to provide control of all joints and hip. The hip and knee design may be unlocked, allowing for both sitting and standing, or allow for standing only.

The *reciprocal gait orthosis (RGO)* is similar to the HKAFO but allows paraplegic children to walk in a reciprocal fashion. RGOs are used with children with spina bifida, sacral agenesis, or spinal cord injury.

The *thoracolumbosacral orthosis (TLSO)* is used to prevent the continuation of spinal curvature caused by scoliosis. The device is molded individually to fit snugly around the trunk or body, thus placing pressure on the ribs and back to

---

Box 9-5 *Precautionary Considerations for Skin and Orthoses*

Skin

1. Skin requires meticulous care.
2. Check skin every 4 hours, if decreased sensation in limb occurs or orthosis is new, check more frequently.
3. When placing orthoses, check skin for redness and if clean and dry; greaseless lotions can be used, preferably not before placement of device.
4. Check to ensure orthoses are on correct limbs with proper heel positioning, back and down.
5. Stockinette or sock recommended for wear under device, which allows for skin protection; should be clean, dry, and without wrinkles to prevent skin breakdown.
6. With any redness lasting more than 20 minutes, or if raw or sore spots are present, report to parent and HCP/orthotist.
7. With complaints of burning sensation, check skin, if complaint continues, contact parent and HCP/orthotist.
8. With blister or open skin, cover area with sterile dressing; avoid orthoses until healed.
9. When prolonged healing time occurs, contact parent and HCP/orthotist.

Orthoses

1. Clean plastic area with damp cloth (without soap) and dry thoroughly.
2. Oil (3-in-One Oil; WD-40 Company, San Diego, California) joints of device and periodically check screws for tightness.
3. Clean once a month or more, unscrew joints, clean, oil and reassemble, apply saddle soap to leather.
4. Clean thoracolumbosacral orthosis (TLSO) once a week with soap and water and rinse, must dry completely.
5. Keep away from heat or flame (e.g., hot surfaces, direct sunlight, warm radiator), since usually made of temperature-sensitive material and may melt or lose shape.
6. Misaligned or nonfunctioning brace should be reported immediately to parent and HCP/orthotist.

support the spine in a straight position. The *Boston brace* (Boston Brace, Avon, Massachusetts) is the commonly used brace for scoliosis and is made of polypropylene. It provides the necessary torso support for a paraplegic child and presents fewer difficulties with dressing and is more comfortable than the leather and metal bracing. The *Jewett Hyperextension brace* may be used to provide support to the spine and trunk during ambulation to prevent compression for individuals who have had a spinal column fracture.

Web Sites

Journal of Prosthetics and Orthotics
    http://www.oandp.org/jpo/library
The Medical Center On-Line
    http://www.mccg.org/childrenshealth/ortho/crutch.asp

RESPIRATORY
Postural Drainage and Percussion
  I. Definition
  A. *Postural drainage* is positioning of a student to enhance gravity drainage of secretions from specific segments of the bronchi and major lung segments into the trachea. Coughing generally removes secretions from the trachea. Different positions are required to accomplish complete segmental drainage. The number of positions placed during each session is individualized and depends on the student's age and tolerance level.
  B. *Percussion* is placing the hand in a stiffened, cupped position and striking the student's chest in a rhythmic motion by flexing the wrist. The air pocket enclosed in the cupped hand strikes the chest; a clopping, not a slapping, sound should be heard. Percussion is performed over the rib cage and should be painless.
  C. Newer modes of providing chest percussion therapy (CPT) are available and are effective in clearing mucus. The Vest airway clearance system (Advanced Respiratory, St. Paul, Minnesota) is an inflatable vest with hoses connected to a high-frequency pulse generator. As the air circulates, the vest causes vibrations that loosen secretions. The Flutter mucus clearance mechanism (Scandipharm, Inc., Birmingham, Alabama) and the positive expiratory pressure (PEP) Mask are other methods that allow independent chest percussion therapy, but they are more difficult to perform and require more discipline.
  II. Purpose
  A. Maintains maximum lung capacity by facilitating drainage and expectoration of secretions. Percussion is used in chronic pulmonary conditions that produce thick mucous secretions, such as cystic fibrosis, and paralytic conditions, such as cerebral palsy and muscular dystrophy. It is most effective after other respiratory therapy (e.g., nebulization, bronchodilator therapy) and usually is administered three to four times a day before mealtime.
  III. Equipment
  A. Pillows.
  B. Tissues.

C. Percussion cup, if used.

D. Suction machine and necessary materials, if ordered.

E. Wastebasket with plastic liner.

IV. **Instructions**

A. Refer to HCP prescription for specific recommendations or adaptations.

1. Have all necessary material available before starting.

2. Be alert to the need for suctioning if mucous plug or thick secretions are produced and occlude the airway.

3. If percussion is to be used, percuss 1 to 5 minutes over appropriate lobe; time varies according to student and specific recommendations.

4. Follow HCP prescription or use instructions for drainage and percussion of an infant or young child (Figure 9-1).

5. Use the positions shown in Figure 9-2 for drainage and percussion of students who weigh more than 40 lb; a darkened circle in the figure indicates percussion areas.

B. Figures 9-1 and 9-2 are anatomical, not functional, drawings. These positions promote drainage of secretions in the necessary pulmonary areas.

C. Physician recommendations should be followed and usually are based on radiographic studies. Length of percussion time generally is 5 minutes for each position but varies.

D. The illustrations show approximate percussion points and body positions chosen to cover specific lobes of the lungs while minimizing fatigue or irritability in the infant or young child and diminishing disruptions in the educational programming for older children. Parents and caregivers are more inclined to do postural drainage on a consistent basis when fewer positions are taught yet will provide the necessary action.

Tracheostomy Care

I. **Definition**

A. A tracheostomy is a surgical method of providing an artificial airway through an opening into the trachea. The opening is made between the second and fourth tracheal rings. The inner cannula of the tracheostomy and stoma must be cleaned periodically to maintain a patent airway. The inner cannula is removed and cleaned while the outer cannula remains in place.

B. Plastic inner cannulas are cleaned every 8 hours and as needed. Metal inner cannulas are cleaned every 4 hours and as needed. Many plastic or silicone elastic (silastic) tracheostomy tubes do not have inner cannulas because the tubes resist crusting and do not require daily cleaning.

II. **Purpose**

A. Tracheostomy care helps prevent irritation of the tissue surrounding the tube and skin breakdown around the tracheostomy site to avoid secondary infections, and it removes exudate and secretions to prevent occlusion of the lumen.

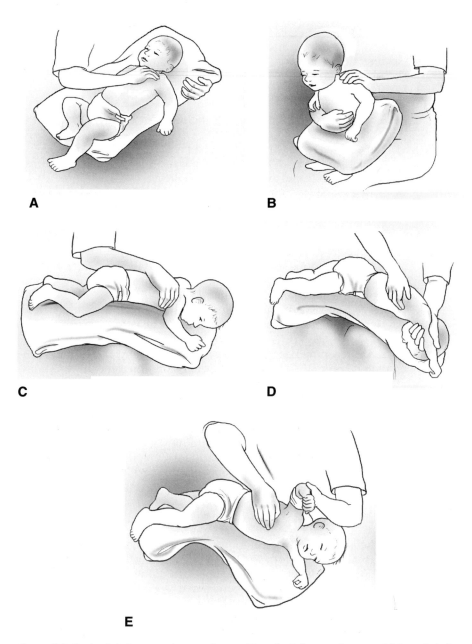

FIGURE 9-1 Postural drainage and percussion positions for infants and young children. **A,** Left upper lobe, apical and anterior segments. Same position, hand moves to right side to percuss right upper lobe, apical and anterior segments. **B,** Left upper lobe, posterior segment. Same position, hand moves to right side to percuss right upper lobe, posterior segment. **C,** Right lower lobe, superior segment and posterior basal segment. Same position, hand moves to left side to percuss left lower lobe, superior segment and posterior basal segment. **D,** Right lower lobe, lateral basal segment. Reverse position and percuss on left for left lower lobe, lateral basal segment. **E,** Right lower lobe, anterior basal segment and right middle lobe. Reverse position and percuss on the left side for left lower lobe, anterior basal and lingular segments.

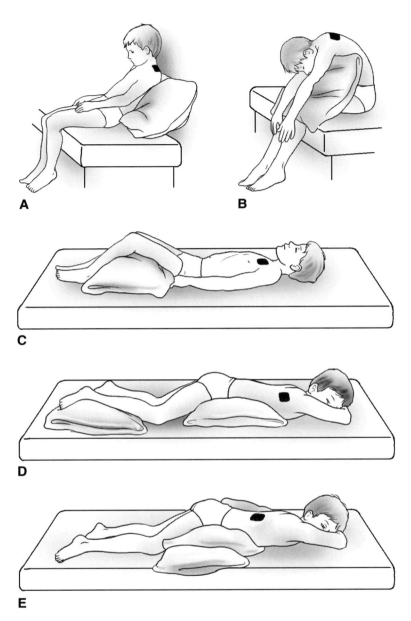

Figure 9-2 Postural drainage and percussion positions for students who weigh more than 40 pounds. **A,** Left and right upper lobes, anterior apical segments. Percuss at shoulders with fingers extending over collarbone in front. Percuss right side and left side. **B,** Right and left upper lobes, posterior apical segments. Percuss with hands on shoulders and fingers extending slightly over the shoulder. Percuss right side and left side. **C,** Right and left upper lobes, anterior segment. Percuss between clavicle and nipple. Percuss right side and left side. **D,** Right and left lower lobes, superior segments. Percuss at lower scapula. Percuss right side and left side. Have student lie flat, with single pillow under stomach and lower legs. **E,** Left and right lower lobes, posterior basal segments. Percuss over lower ribs, avoid kidney area. Percuss right side and left side. Elevate hips 12-16 in.   *Continued*

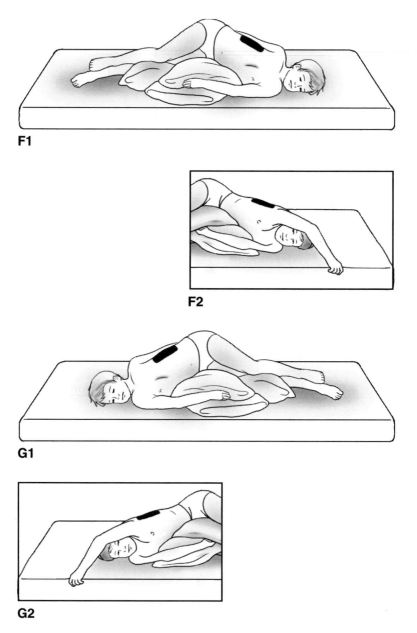

F1

F2

G1

G2

Figure 9-2, cont'd F1, Right middle lobe and lower lobe, anterior basal segment. Elevate hips 12-16 in. With student lying on left side, rotate one quarter turn backward. Percuss over ribs on right side of chest beneath armpit to end of rib cage. **F2,** Right lateral basal lobe. Rotate one quarter turn forward and percuss over ribs beneath armpit to end of rib cage. **G1,** Left lower lobe and lingular segment. Elevate hips 12-16 in. With student lying on left side, rotate one quarter turn backward. Percuss over ribs on left side of chest beneath armpit to end of rib cage. **G2,** Left lateral basal lobe. Rotate one quarter turn forward and percuss over left lower ribs beneath armpit to end of rib cage to drain.

III. Equipment

A. The following materials should be available.

1. Four nonwaxed paper cups.
2. Suction equipment and sterile/clean catheter.
3. Oxygen equipment if needed.
4. Twill tape (½-in wide) or hook-and-loop (Velcro) ties.
5. Six to eight cotton-tipped applicators.
6. Pipe cleaners, doubled for cleaning.
7. Sterile saline solution, water, or both.
8. Hydrogen peroxide (H_2O_2); do not use with sterling silver tracheostomy tube because it may pit the surface.
9. Scissors, if tracheostomy ties are to be changed.
10. Clean disposable nonlatex gloves.
11. Plastic bag for waste.
12. Paper towels.
13. Replacement tracheostomy tube, one size smaller than the one in place, if needed for reintubation.

IV. Instructions

A. Refer to HCP's prescription for specific recommendations or adaptations to the following procedure. Do not leave student unattended during procedure.

1. Explain procedure to student and allow to assist as appropriate.
2. Wash hands.
3. Position student.
   a. *Infant*: place small towel roll under shoulders, since neck is short and this will provide optimal access to trachea. Elbow restraints may be necessary to keep child from reaching for tube, or wrap child in towel or sheet.
   b. *Older child:* position with tracheostomy area exposed; place in Fowler's position, if possible, to prevent any solution from seeping into stoma.
4. Place cotton applicators and pipe cleaners on paper towel.
5. Add four paper cups labeled and filled with the following solutions to paper towel.
   a. Hydrogen peroxide to cover inner cannula.
   b. Sterile saline solution to soak one half of cotton applicators.
   c. Sterile saline solution to soak inner cannula.
   d. Sterile saline solution to rinse inner cannula.
6. Wash hands and don gloves.
7. Perform tracheostomy suctioning as needed (see "Tracheostomy Suctioning").
8. Turn latch that holds inner cannula in place and slowly remove cannula with outward and downward semicircular movement of wrist.
9. If student is receiving mechanical ventilation, use one of the following methods:
   a. Plug tracheostomy opening and encourage student to ventilate by glossopharyngeal breathing.

     b. Attach ambulatory manual breathing unit (ambu bag) to outer cannula and have another person assist by compressing bag.

10. Place inner cannula in cup with hydrogen peroxide and soak 1 to 5 minutes.
11. Roll soaked cotton applicators over skin surrounding stoma:
    a. Use circular motion, cleaning next to stoma first, then work outward to at least 1 in (2.54 cm) beyond outer cannula.
    b. Clean each area of skin only once with each applicator; discard each soiled applicator into waste bag.

NOTE: Normal secretions are clear and white with no odor; odor and green/yellow drainage may indicate infection.

12. Dry skin with dry applicators.
13. Remove inner cannula from hydrogen peroxide and remove secretions with pipe cleaners.
14. Place cannula in cup with saline solution to soak.
15. Remove cannula and pour clean saline solution over and through cannula to rinse thoroughly.
16. Shake excess water from cannula; may dry with clean gauze.
17. Replace inner cannula and secure lock.
18. Pour out solutions and discard cups, pipe cleaners, and so forth.
19. If suction of outer cannula is necessary, complete before replacing inner cannula.
20. Remove gloves and wash hands.
21. Change tape as necessary, using twill or Velcro tapes.
    a. Have another person help keep child still or wrap infant "mummy style."
    b. Keep old ties secured and push to top of holes on tracheostomy flange.
    c. Tie new tapes.
    d. Secure with knot at side of neck (rotate knot occasionally to prevent redness or breakdown of skin).
    e. Tie snugly while neck is flexed but loose enough to allow one or two fingers underneath.
    f. Remove old tapes after new tapes are in place.
    g. Wash hands.
22. Offer student water for hydration.
23. Document procedure, including amount of secretions, color and odor, any complications, and student's tolerance of procedure.
24. Research demonstrates that hydrogen peroxide is cytotoxic and is not recommended as an antiseptic on human tissue (WCIN, 2002).

Tracheostomy Suctioning (Sterile Technique)

I. Definition
    A. Tracheostomy suctioning is the aspiration of excessive secretions from the trachea by insertion of a catheter into the tracheostomy opening.

II. Purpose
    A. Suctioning maintains an open airway and adequate ventilation when the student is unable to cough and clear the airway.

III. Equipment

A. The following materials should be available for suctioning:
1. Suction machine.
2. Sterile suction catheter, no more than half the internal diameter of the tracheostomy tube.
3. Sterile gloves.
4. Sterile normal saline solution.
5. Sterile water.
6. Sterile syringes.
7. Clean paper cup (nonwaxed).
8. Tissues.
9. Plastic bag for contaminated tissues and materials used in suctioning.
10. Replacement tracheostomy tube, one size smaller than tracheostomy tube currently in place.

IV. Instructions

A. Refer to HCP's prescription for specific recommendations or adaptations to the following procedure.
1. Wash hands.
2. On clean paper towel, place paper cup filled with sterile water, sterile syringe filled with sterile saline solution, sterile gloves, and sterile catheter suctioning packages that have been opened carefully so as not to contaminate the contents.
3. Position student.
   a. Position depends on student's condition.
   b. HCP may give specific orders.
   c. *Infants and young children*: place small towel roll under shoulders. (Neck is short, and this will provide optimal access to trachea.)
   d. *Older child*: position with tracheostomy area exposed, and if possible, place in Fowler's position to prevent any solution from seeping into stoma.
4. Wash hands and don sterile gloves. The dominant hand remains sterile, whereas the other hand becomes nonsterile.
5. Remove catheter from opened package with sterile gloved hand, taking precautions to avoid contamination.
6. Hold suction connection tubing in nonsterile hand and connect catheter suction tubing with sterile hand.
7. Turn on suction machine with nonsterile hand.
8. Dip catheter end into cup of sterile water and draw water through briefly.
9. Proceed with suctioning.
   a. Leaving vent of catheter open, gently insert the catheter into the tracheostomy tube just beyond the end of the premeasured tracheostomy tube (usually 4-5 in), then withdraw catheter slightly; use a calibrated catheter—or measure against extra tracheostomy tube—mark with thumb and insert until thumb reaches stoma.
      (1) Depth of suctioning may be specified by physician.
      (2) Tissue damage may occur with suctioning beyond tip of tracheostomy tube.
      (3) Never force catheter.

b. Place thumb of nonsterile hand over vent of catheter intermittently, and with sterile hand, gently rotate catheter between thumb and forefinger while slowly withdrawing from trachea.
c. If student begins to cough, withdraw catheter.
d. Suction intermittently; however, do not suction longer than 5-10 seconds at a time and allow 30 seconds to 1 minute between periods of suctioning.
   (1) *If catheter is not withdrawn intermittently, hypoxia can occur from occlusion of airway.*
   (2) *Prolonged suctioning can precipitate vagal stimulation with cardiac arrest.*

10. If secretions are thick, irrigation with sterile saline solution may be prescribed, but this practice is controversial because it may cause lower airway infections by washing organisms from the tracheostomy tube into the lower airway.
11. Suction water through the catheter between suctionings and when finished to clear.
12. Discard catheter, cup, syringe, gloves, and wash hands.
13. Document procedure, including amount of secretions, color, odor, and any change in secretions. Note tolerance of procedure and complications, if appropriate.

V. Web Sites
   Tracheostomy Care
   http://www.langara.bc.ca/vnc/trach#suctioning

ASSESSMENT TOOLS

ASSESSMENT, EVALUATION, PROGRESS, AND SYSTEMS (AEPS)

I. Use
   A. Assessment and curriculum.
II. Ages
   A. Volume 1: Birth-36 months, but appropriate for ages 3-6.
   B. Volume 3: 3-6 years.

Box 9-6 *Tester Qualification Rating Scale*

A: Completed at least one course in measurement, guidance, or related discipline or has equivalent supervised experience in testing and interpretation.
B: Completed graduate training in measurement, guidance, individual psychological assessment or special training for specific test.
C: Completed recognized graduate training program in psychology and supervised practical experience.

Modified from *Standards for educational and psychological testing,* published by the American Educational Research Association (AERA), the American Psychological Association, and the National Council on Measurement in Education (NCME), 1999.

III. Purpose
  A. Assesses and evaluates child's abilities in familiar environments (home, small group, or center-based program).
IV. Areas Assessed
  A. Six developmental domains: fine motor, gross motor, adaptive, cognitive, social-communication, and social.
V. Additional Information
  A. Generates a comprehensive profile of abilities. Volume 1 and 3 have corresponding volumes, 2 and 4, that provide the necessary curriculum based on the assessment. Can be used to develop goals, objectives, or both for IFSPs or IEPs and monitor progress.
VI. Tester Qualification: B.

ASSESSMENT OF PHONOLOGICAL PROCESSES—REVISED (APP-R)

I. Use
  A. Assessment.
II. Ages
  A. Preschool and school-age children.
III. Purpose
  A. Assesses children with unintelligible speech.
IV. Areas Assessed
  A. Speech sounds and phonological processes.
V. Additional Information
  A. Administration time is 20 minutes. Allows identification of phoneme class deficiency and miscellaneous error patterns. Provides Percentage of Occurrence Average, Phonological Process and Deviancy Scores, and Severity Ratings. Developed by Barbara Hodson; sometimes called *Hodson*.
VI. Tester Qualification: B.

BAYLEY SCALES OF INFANT DEVELOPMENT, SECOND EDITION (BSID-II)

I. Use
  A. Assessment.
II. Ages
  A. 1-42 months.
III. Purpose
  A. Evaluates developmental function, including auditory perception, behavior, motor, and social development.
IV. Areas Assessed
  A. Mental scale:
   1. Sensory perceptual abilities.
   2. Object permanence.
   3. Memory, learning, problem solving.
   4. Emerging language skills.
   5. Emerging abstract and symbolic thinking.
   6. Mental mapping, complex language.
   7. Mathematical concept formation.

B. Psychomotor scale:
1. Degree of body control.
2. Large muscle coordination, fine manipulative motor skills, dynamic movement and praxis, postural imitation, stereognosis.
C. Behavioral rating scale:
1. Attention/arousal.
2. Orientation/engagement.
3. Emotional regulation.
4. Motor quality.
V. **Additional Information**
A. The test assesses the mental areas with a normative standardized test. Data are provided for special-needs students. The second edition contains 100 new items. Results do not correlate well with later intelligence scales. The test takes 25 to 60 minutes to administer, depending on age group.
VI. **Tester Qualification: B**

BECK DEPRESSION INVENTORY-II (BDI-II)

I. **Use**
A. Screening and diagnosis of depression.
II. **Ages**
A. 13-80 years.
III. **Purpose**
A. Measures severity of depression and monitors therapeutic progress.
IV. **Areas Assessed**
A. Twenty-one items that assess the severity of depression.
V. **Additional Information**
A. Items conform to *Diagnostic and Statistical Manual of Mental Disorders, fourth edition (DSM-IV)* criteria; can be administered in 5 minutes. The *BDI-Fast Screen* uses seven self-report items that reflect cognitive and affective symptoms. It provides a fast assessment of depression in those with biological, medical, or substance abuse, or a combination of these problems.
VI. **Tester Qualification: B**

BEHAVIOR ASSESSMENT SYSTEM FOR CHILDREN (BASC)

I. **Use**
A. Evaluation.
II. **Ages**
A. 2.6-19 years.
III. **Purpose**
A. Measures aspects of behavioral and personality, including adaptive, problematic, and attention deficit-hyperactivity disorder (ADHD) behaviors.
IV. **Areas Assessed**
A. The system consists of five dimensions: teacher, parenting, and self-rating scales, student observation system, and structured develop-

mental history. Areas rated include externalizing (aggression, hyperactivity, conduct problems), internalizing (anxiety, depression, somatization), school problems (attention, learning), and adaptive skills (adaptability, leadership, social, study).

V. **Additional Information**
   A. Takes 10 to 45 minutes, depending on scale.

VI. **Tester Qualification:** C

BENDER VISUAL MOTOR GESTALT

I. **Use**
   A. Assessment.

II. **Ages**
   A. 3 years and older.

III. **Purpose**
   A. Measures perceptual motor skills. Assesses visual motor function and identifies developmental problems, regression, and organic brain defects.

IV. **Areas Assessed**
   A. Perceptual maturation and neurological impairment. Nine stimulus cards are shown and the student is asked to draw the figures, one at a time, on a blank sheet of paper. Assesses concepts of form, shape, pattern, and orientation in space.

V. **Additional Information**
   A. Untimed, usually takes about 10 minutes for an individual. Can be administered in a group and takes about 15-25 minutes. It is a nonthreatening test, often used as an introductory test of a larger battery of instruments.

VI. **Tester Qualification:** B

BOEHM TEST OF BASIC CONCEPTS—PRESCHOOL, THIRD EDITION

I. **Use**
   A. Assessment.

II. **Ages**
   A. 3-5 years.

III. **Purpose**
   A. Identifies children who lack understanding of relational concepts to provide early intervention for school success.

IV. **Areas Assessed**
   A. Measures 30 basic concepts.

V. **Additional Information**
   A. Each concept is measured twice to reduce the possibility of guessing. Includes observation and intervention planning tool and modifying and adapting directions for testing differently abled children. Test is normed and standardized on a representative sample. It is available in Spanish and English.

VI. **Tester Qualification:** B

BOEHM TEST OF BASIC CONCEPTS—THIRD EDITION (BOEHM-3)

I. **Use**
   A. Assessment.
II. **Ages**
   A. Kindergarten through second grade.
III. **Purpose**
   A. This test identifies students at risk for learning difficulty and determines need for further testing.
IV. **Areas Assessed**
   A. Measures 50 key concepts occurring in kindergarten, first, and second grades and necessary for achievement during the first years of school. Identifies concepts students know and what they need to know.
V. **Additional Information**
   A. Group administered in the classroom; takes 30-45 minutes. Results of pretest and posttest demonstrate progress as result of intervention/teaching. Spanish version is available.
VI. **Tester Qualification:** B

BRIGANCE INVENTORY OF EARLY DEVELOPMENT—REVISED

I. **Use**
   A. Assessment.
II. **Ages**
   A. Birth to age 7.
III. **Purpose**
   A. Assesses important skills, concepts, and behavior; identifies at-risk infants and preschoolers. Used for diagnostic, record keeping, and intervention purposes.
IV. **Areas Assessed**
   A. Assesses 11 skill areas: motor, self help, speech/language, social, emotional, reading, math, writing, general knowledge, comprehension, and readiness.
V. **Additional Information**
   A. Can be used in preschools and day care centers. Easily administered by aides, volunteers, or tutors. Provides simple progress report. Has optional group developmental records, which helps to monitor class progress. A Brigance Screen is available for three age levels: pre-Kindergarten to grade 1. These screening tools identify children who need immediate referral and take 10 to 15 minutes to administer.
VI. **Tester Qualification:** A

BRIGANCE COMPREHENSIVE INVENTORY OF BASIC SKILLS—REVISED (CIBS-R)

I. **Use**
   A. Assessment.
II. **Ages**
   A. Pre-Kindergarten to 9 years.
III. **Purpose**
   A. Identifies specific areas of need to use for intervention, program planning, and IEP development.

IV. **Areas Assessed**
   A. The 154 assessments of readiness, speech, listening, research and study skills, spelling, writing, reading, and math can be chosen by the teacher according to the student's individual needs.
V. **Additional Information**
   A. Can monitor progress of specific skills; has specific instructions to develop IEP goals and objectives. Options included for group testing and normed and standardized data are available.
VI. **Tester Qualification:** B

BRUININKS-OSERETSKY TEST

I. **Use**
   A. Assessment.
II. **Ages**
   A. 4.6-14.5 years.
III. **Purpose**
   A. Measures fine and gross motor skills.
IV. **Areas Assessed**
   A. Eight subtests include running speed and agility, balance, bilateral coordination, strength, upper limb coordination, response speed, visuomotor control, and upper limb speed and dexterity.
V. **Additional Information**
   A. A short form can be administered in 15 to 20 minutes; the complete battery of tests takes 45 to 60 minutes. The test is used to develop and evaluate motor training programs.
VI. **Tester Qualification:** B

CHILDHOOD AUTISM RATING SCALE (CARS)

I. **Use**
   A. Assessment.
II. **Ages**
   A. 2+ years.
III. **Purpose**
   A. Useful for identification and classification of children with autism.
IV. **Areas Assessed**
   A. Fifteen items measure the student's responses to various activities and situations in relation to people, imitation, emotional response, and body use.
V. **Additional Information**
   A. A score is achieved by using a 7-point scale to indicate the amount of variance from the norm on each item. The total score from all 15 is computed and determines the presence and severity of autism.
VI. **Tester Qualification:** B

CHILDREN'S MEMORY SCALE (CMS)

I. **Use**
   A. Assessment.
II. **Ages**
   A. 5-16 years.

III. **Purpose**
   A. Provides assessment of memory and learning as related directly to IQ.
IV. **Areas Assessed**
   A. Six subtests, including the following dimensions: (1) verbal learning and memory, (2) visual learning and memory, (3) attention/concentration and working memory, (4) general or overall memory, (5) immediate versus delayed memory, and (6) recall versus recognition.
V. **Additional Information**
   A. Memory and learning are compared with ability, achievement, and attention. The test is scored in 20 minutes with a 30-minute delay, followed by 10-15 minutes for testing long-delayed memory. Separate records are used for ages 5-8 and 9-16 years. The scale is standardized and normed on a U.S. representative sample.
VI. **Tester Qualification:** C

CLINICAL EVALUATION OF LANGUAGE FUNDAMENTAL—PRESCHOOL (CELF)

I. **Use**
   A. Assessment.
II. **Ages**
   A. 3-6 years.
III. **Purpose**
   A. Identification, diagnosis, and follow-up of language deficits.
IV. **Areas Assessed**
   A. Language skills, including word meaning, word structure, sentence structure, recall, and retrieval.
V. **Additional Information**
   A. This standardized test provides norm referenced data for each 6-month age level.
VI. **Tester Qualification:** B

CLINICAL EVALUATION OF LANGUAGE FUNDAMENTALS, THIRD EDITION (CELF-3)

I. **Use**
   A. Diagnostic and intervention planning.
II. **Ages**
   A. 3-21 years.
III. **Purpose**
   A. Provides language age and percentiles for processing and production.
IV. **Areas Assessed**
   A. Processing (receptive): sentence structure, semantics relationships, concepts and directions, word classes, listening to paragraphs.
   B. Production (expressive): recalling sentences, word structure, formulated sentences, word associations, sentence assembly.
   C. Optional subtest: rapid, automatic naming.
V. **Additional Information**
   A. The test is standardized, and a Spanish version is available.
VI. **Tester Qualification:** B

COLUMBIA MENTAL MATURITY SCALE (CMMS)

I. Use
   A. Assessment.
II. Ages
   A. 3 years 6 months to 9 years 11 months
III. Purpose
   A. Assesses general reasoning ability.
IV. Areas Assessed
   A. Assesses two categories: discrimination and classification.
V. Additional Information
   A. The test takes 15 to 20 minutes to administer. The test is nonverbal and the student responds by pointing to figures on large cards. This makes the test useful for assessment of students with severely developmental disabilities, particularly those with physical handicaps, such as cerebral palsy.
VI. Tester Qualification: C

DENVER DEVELOPMENTAL SCREENING TOOL-II (DDST-R)

I. Use
   A. Screening.
II. Ages
   A. Birth-6 years.
III. Purpose
   A. Detects infants/children with social, motor, or language delays.
IV. Areas Assessed
   A. Assesses 125 items in the areas of personal-social, fine motor-adaptive, language, and gross motor development.
V. Additional Information
   A. The DDST-R is a nonverbal test and is administered in 15 to 20 minutes. Research is under way; early findings show a high rate of overreferral.
VI. Tester Qualification: B

DETROIT TESTS OF LEARNING APTITUDE (DTLA-4)

I. Use
   A. Assessment.
II. Ages
   A. 6-17 years.
III. Purpose
   A. Isolates intraindividual strengths and weaknesses; identifies students with general deficiency or specific aptitude.
IV. Areas Assessed
   A. Areas assessed are linguistic, cognitive, attention, motor, and visual perception.
V. Additional Information
   A. The test is useful for identifying learning disabilities and mental retardation. It produces a detailed profile of the student's abilities and deficiencies. The test takes 40 minutes to 2 hours to administer.
VI. Tester Qualification: B

DEVELOPMENTAL TEST OF VISUAL-MOTOR INTEGRATION, FOURTH EDITION (VMI; BEERY VMI)

I. Use
   A. Assessment.
II. Ages
   A. 3-18 years.
III. Purpose
   A. The VMI assesses the integration of visual and motor skills and identifies problems that lead to future learning and behavior problems.
IV. Areas Assessed
   A. Visual perception, motor coordination.
V. Additional Information
   A. The test is a developmental sequence of geometric forms that are copied with paper and pencil. A short format is available for ages 3 to 7. It is a standardized test that can be administered to individuals or a group in 10 to 15 minutes. Developed by K.E. Beery.
VI. Test Qualification: B

DRAW A PERSON TEST (DAP)

I. Use
   A. Assessment.
II. Ages
   A. 5-17 years.
III. Purpose
   A. Assesses intellectual maturity based on three drawings: a man, a woman, and the person taking the test.
IV. Areas Assessed
   A. The DAP test has 64 items that are scored for 14 different criteria; areas are ability to perceive, abstract, and generalize.
V. Additional Information
   A. It is standardized, provides an IQ score, and takes about 15 to 30 minutes to administer.
VI. Tester Qualification: B

FAMILY APGAR

I. Use
   A. Questionnaire.
II. Ages
   A. Parents of all ages.
III. Purpose
   A. Provides information about a family member's satisfaction with particular family functions.
IV. Areas Assessed
   A. Five items with three responses (acronym): *a*daptability, *p*artnership, *g*rowth, *a*ffection, and *r*esolve.
V. Additional Information
   A. Scoring includes three choices; scores correlate with highly functional family, moderately functional family, and severely dysfunctional fam-

ily. Each parent answers the five questions, which take only a few minutes.

VI. **Tester Qualification:** B

HAWAII EARLY LEARNING PROFILE (HELP)

I. **Use**
   A. Assessment and intervention.

II. **Ages**
   A. Birth-6 years.

III. **Purpose**
   A. To assess, identify areas of need, monitor progress, and provide sequential developmental activities.

IV. **Areas Assessed**
   A. Six areas are included: cognitive, language, gross and fine motor, social, and self-help.

V. **Additional Information**
   A. Time to administer test depends on number of areas assessed. *Best Beginnings: Helping Parents Make a Difference* is a *HELP* assessment that provides anticipatory guidance for caregivers of children ages birth-3 years.

VI. **Tester Qualification:** B

HOME, EDUCATION, ACTIVITIES, DRUGS, SEX, SUICIDE, AND SAVAGERY (HEADSSS)

I. **Use**
   A. Interview instrument.

II. **Ages**
   A. Adolescents at risk.

III. **Purpose**
   A. Provides information regarding adolescent psychosocial development and facilitates communication.

IV. **Areas Assessed**
   A. Seven areas are assessed (acronym): *h*ome, *e*ducation/vocation, *a*ctivities, *d*rugs, *s*ex, *s*uicide/depression, and *s*avagery.

V. **Additional Information**
   A. Technique may take more than one meeting to complete because it is a comprehensive interview format.

VI. **Tester Qualification:** B

HOME OBSERVATION FOR MEASUREMENT OF THE ENVIRONMENT (HOME)

I. **Use**
   A. Assessment, parental guidance, and intervention.

II. **Ages**
   A. Birth-3 years and 3-6 years.

III. **Purpose**
   A. Sample the quantity and quality of certain social, emotional, and cognitive supports available to the child within the home.

IV. Areas Assessed
   A. Six subscales, birth-3 years: Parental responsiveness, acceptance of child, organization of environment, learning materials, parental involvement, variety in experience.
   B. Eight subscales, 3-6 years: Learning materials, language stimulation, physical environment, parental responsiveness, learning stimulation, modeling of social maturity, variety in experience, acceptance of child.
V. Additional Information
   A. Assesses person-to-person and person-to-object interactions that make up the infant/child's learning environment. Takes 45 to 90 minutes to administer. There are now scales for Middle Childhood (6-10 years) and Early Adolescent (10 to 15 years).
VI. Tester Qualification: B

KAUFMAN ASSESSMENT BATTERY FOR CHILDREN (KABC)

I. Use
   A. Assessment.
II. Ages
   A. 2 years 6 months to 12 years 5 months.
III. Purpose
   A. Establishes cognitive levels and an understanding of the individual's style of solving problems and thought processes. Measures intelligence separately from achievement.
IV. Areas Assessed
   A. There are 16 subtests under 3 scales: sequential processing, simultaneous processing, and achievement scales.
V. Additional Information
   A. Administration time is 35 to 85 minutes; test is standardized.
VI. Tester Qualification: C

KEY MATH—REVISED, NORMATIVE UPDATE (R/NU)

I. Use
   A. Assessment.
II. Ages
   A. Kindergarten through twelfth grade (ages 5-22 years)
III. Purpose
   A. Assesses mathematical skill development.
IV. Areas Assessed
   A. The test consists of 13 subtests in three areas: basic concepts, operations, and applications.
V. Additional Information
   A. The test can be used for program planning and evaluation. It takes 35 to 50 minutes for administration and does not require reading ability. Software is available. Pretest and posttest forms are available.
VI. Tester Qualification: B

LEITER INTERNATIONAL PERFORMANCE SCALE—REVISED (LEITER-R)

I. Use
   A. Screening and assessment.

II. **Ages**
    A. 2-21 years.
III. **Purpose**
    A. Measures fluid intelligence (i.e., intelligence that is not significantly influenced by child's educational, social, and family experience). Provides composite IQ score and scores in each of the 20 subsets and numerous composites.
IV. **Areas Assessed**
    A. Measures visualization and reasoning, attention, and memory. Test has five subsets: IQ screening assessment, learning disability (LD)/ ADHD screening assessment, gifted screening assessment, reasoning and visual battery, and memory and attention battery.
V. **Additional Information**
    A. This nonverbal, standardized test is suitable for persons with speech, hearing, or motor impairments; those was are deaf or cognitively delayed; those with ADHD, autism, those who are disadvantaged, non–English-speaking or use English as a second language, or have sustained traumatic brain injury. The test can be used to determine whether low academic achievement is a result of low IQ or a specific neuropsychological cause such as ADHD.
VI. **Tester Qualification:** B

MCCARTHY SCALES OF CHILDREN'S ABILITIES (MSCA)

I. **Use**
    A. Assessment.
II. **Ages**
    A. 2.5-8.5 years.
III. **Purpose**
    A. Evaluates general intelligence level and strengths and weaknesses in several ability areas.
IV. **Areas Assessed**
    A. Eighteen separate tests and six scales are evaluated: verbal, perceptual performance, quantitative, memory, motor, and general cognitive.
V. **Additional Information**
    A. May identify gifted children. Takes 45 minutes to test children younger than age 5 and 1 hour with older children.
VI. **Tester Qualification:** C

MULLEN SCALES OF EARLY LEARNING

I. **Use**
    A. Assessment.
II. **Ages**
    A. Birth-5.8 years.
III. **Purpose**
    A. Assesses language, motor, and perceptual abilities.
IV. **Areas Assessed**
    A. Consists of five scales: gross motor, visual reception, fine motor, expressive language, and receptive language.

V. Additional Information

    A. Test takes 15 to 60 minutes depending on student's age. It is used to assess school readiness. It provides a baseline for continuum of teaching methods and foundation for interventions; the test is standardized.

VI. Tester Qualification: B

NURSING CHILD ASSESSMENT SATELLITE TRAINING (NCAST)

I. Use

    A. Assessment.

II. Ages

    A. Feeding scale: birth-1 year; teaching scale: birth-3 years.

III. Purpose

    A. Measures caregiver-child interaction during feeding and teaching situations. The scales are designed to assess problems in interaction and communication.

IV. Areas Assessed

    A. The test has two scales: feeding and teaching, with six constructs. Four of the constructs (sensitivity to cues, response to distress, socioemotional growth fostering, and cognitive growth fostering) pertain to the caregiver. Two constructs (clarity of cues and responsiveness to the caregiver) pertain to the child.

V. Additional Information

    A. Significant changes in the scales were made in 1994. Both scales have strong internal consistency and test-retest reliability for the caregiver and child total scores. The caregiver scores have predictive validity for later child cognitive scores; thus the tools can be used to promote early brain development. Positive quality interactions during early childhood promote development of intellectual and language capabilities and bonding with major caregivers.

    B. Another NCAST scale that can be self-taught is the Nursing Child Assessment Sleep/Activity (NCASA). This scale is an established method of helping caregivers record the activities of a child on a 24-hour/ 7-day form. The child's sleep pattern then can be evaluated. The Sleep Activity Manual explains interpretation of the record.

    C. The tests can be administered together or separately. Administration time depends on age of child and instrument used.

VI. Tester Qualification: B

PEABODY INDIVIDUAL ACHIEVEMENT TEST—REVISED-NORMATIVE UPDATE (PIAT-R/NU)

I. Use

    A. Assessment and instructional planning.

II. Ages

    A. 5-22 years.

III. Purpose

    A. This test provides an overview of the student's individual scholastic achievement and identifies possible areas of weakness/learning disabilities.

IV. **Areas Assessed**
   A. Subtests include general information, reading recognition, reading comprehension, written expression, math, and spelling.

V. **Additional Information**
   A. The revised version includes normative update; can be administered in 60 minutes.

VI. **Tester Qualification:** B

PEABODY PICTURE VOCABULARY TEST—THIRD EDITION (PPVT-III)

I. **Use**
   A. Screening.

II. **Ages**
   A. 2.6 years to 90+

III. **Purpose**
   A. Measures receptive vocabulary for standard American English.

IV. **Areas Assessed**
   A. Assesses auditory receptive language skills.

V. **Additional Information**
   A. The test is useful as a pretest and posttest measurement for knowledge of simple words. Can be an initial screening device for bright, low-ability, and language-impaired students. Software is available. Administration takes 10 to 15 minutes.

VI. **Tester Qualification:** B

QUICK NEUROLOGICAL SCREENING TEST (QNST-II)

I. **Use**
   A. Screening.

II. **Ages**
   A. Kindergarten through twelfth grade and adults.

III. **Purpose**
   A. Assesses neurological integration as it relates to learning and identifies those with learning disabilities.

IV. **Areas Assessed**
   A. Motor development, skill in controlling large and small muscles, motor planning and sequencing, sense of rate and rhythm, spatial organization, visual perceptual skills, balance and cerebellovestibular functions, and attention disorders.

V. **Additional Information**
   A. Takes about 20-30 minutes to administer and score. Does not label student as neurological impaired or diagnose brain damage or dysfunction. Includes latest research findings concerning the soft neurological signs associated with learning problems.

VI. **Tester Qualification:** B

RECEPTIVE-EXPRESSIVE EMERGENT LANGUAGE, SECOND EDITION (REEL-2)

I. **Use**
   A. Assessment.

II. Ages
  A. Infants and toddlers.
III. Purpose
  A. Measures development in both receptive and expressive language.
IV. Areas Assessed
  A. Expressive and receptive language.
V. Additional Information
  A. Time of administration varies because it is done interview format. Provides information from child's caregiver. The manual offers interpretation information and reliability and validity data.
VI. Tester Qualification: B

SENSORY PROFILE

I. Use
  A. Assessment.
II. Ages
  A. 3-10 years.
III. Purpose
  A. Measures sensory processing abilities as they relate to functional performance.
IV. Areas Assessed
  A. Long version is 125 items and short is 38 items; three areas included: sensory process modulation, behavioral, and emotional responses. Nine factors: responsiveness to sensory input, sensory seeking, emotional reactivity, endurance/tone, oral-sensory sensitivity, inattention/distractibility, poor registration, sensory sensitivity, sedentary, and fine motor perceptual.
V. Additional Information
  A. Used in combination with other tests because it is judgment based. Results can facilitate diagnosis and intervention planning.
VI. Tester Qualification: B

STANFORD-BINET INTELLIGENCE SCALE

I. Use
  A. Assessment.
II. Ages
  A. 2-23 years and older.
III. Purpose
  A. Assesses general mental ability. Revised edition provides multiple IQ scores rather than a single IQ score.
IV. Areas Assessed
  A. General comprehension; short term memory and concentration; mathematical reasoning; visuomotor ability; vocabulary/verbal fluency; judgment and reasoning.
V. Additional Information
  A. The test is not easy to administer, and many psychologists prefer the Wechsler Intelligence Scale instead. However, this is a highly standardized and reliable tool for measuring a child's intelligence.
VI. Tester Qualification: C

TEST OF ADOLESCENT AND ADULT LANGUAGE, THIRD EDITION (TOAL-3)

I. Use
   A. Assessment.
II. Ages
   A. 12-25 years.
III. Purpose
   A. Identifies students who may need intervention to improve language proficiency; determines language strengths and weaknesses; documents progress resulting from special intervention programs.
IV. Areas Assessed
   A. Eight subtests measure listening, speaking, reading, and writing skills.
V. Additional Information
   A. Six of the eight subtests may be administered in groups; all eight may be administered individually. Administration time is about 1 hour and 45 minutes.
VI. Tester Qualification: B

TEST OF EARLY READING ABILITY, SECOND EDITION (TERA-2)

I. Use
   A. Screening.
II. Ages
   A. 3-10 years.
III. Purpose
   A. Identifies children with reading problems and determines children's progress in learning to read.
IV. Areas Assessed
   A. Construction of meaning, knowledge about the alphabet, and conventions of written language.
V. Additional Information
   A. Two equivalent forms are provided for pretest and posttest. Can be administered in 15-20 minutes.
VI. Tester Qualification: B

TEST OF WRITTEN LANGUAGE, THIRD EDITION (TOWL-3)

I. Use
   A. Assessment.
II. Ages
   A. 7.6-18 years.
III. Purpose
   A. Identifies students who have difficulty in written expression and pinpoints specific areas of deficit.
IV. Areas Assessed
   A. Thematic, vocabulary, handwriting, spelling, word usage, and style.
V. Additional Information
   A. Two equivalent forms are provided to administer the test individually or in small groups. Administration time is 90 minutes.
VI. Tester Qualification: B

THEMATIC APPERCEPTION TEST—CHILDREN AND ADULTS (TAT)

I. Use

A. Assessment.

II. Ages

A. 14 years and older.

III. Purpose

A. Assesses for presence of psychological needs by revealing emotions, sentiments, dominant drives, and conflicts of a personality.

IV. Areas Assessed

A. Emotional and behavioral characteristics. A series of 20 pictures is presented, and the student is asked to tell stories about the pictures.

V. Additional Information

A. Nonstandardized and untimed, but popular in school systems because it provides quality information and is easy to administer as part of a battery of tests. Difficult for nonverbal students; not to be used alone for decision making.

VI. Tester Qualification: C

VINELAND ADAPTIVE BEHAVIOR SCALES

I. Use

A. Assessment.

II. Ages

A. Interview edition: birth through 18 years 11 months and low-functioning adults.

B. Classroom edition: 3 years through 12 years 11 months.

III. Purpose

A. Assesses personal and social skills and responsibility for own needs.

IV. Areas Assessed

A. Four domains are assessed: communication (receptive, written, expressive), daily living skills (personal, domestic, community), socialization (interpersonal relationships, play and leisure time, coping skills), and motor skills (gross, fine).

V. Additional Information

A. Three standardized versions provide flexibility. The Survey Form, which has 297 items, is a caregiver questionnaire that provides a general assessment of adaptive behavior. The Expanded Form has 280 more items and also provides a systematic basis for planning individual, educational, habilitative, or treatment programs. The Classroom Edition, teacher questionnaire, assesses adaptive behavior in the classroom. Administration time is 20-90 minutes, depending on the version used. Available in Spanish.

VI. Tester Qualification: C

VINELAND SOCIAL-EMOTIONAL EARLY CHILDHOOD SCALES (SEEC)

I. Use

A. Assessment.

II. Ages

A. Birth to 5 years 11 months.

III. **Purpose**
  A. Evaluates levels of social-emotional behavior of those with disabilities and how the disabilities affect their daily functioning.
IV. **Areas Assessed**
  A. Social-emotional adjustment.
V. **Additional Information**
  A. Can administer in 14-25 minutes. Sometimes used in conjunction with the Mullen Scales.
VI. **Tester Qualification:** C

WECHSLER INTELLIGENCE SCALE FOR CHILDREN, THIRD EDITION (WISC-III)

I. **Use**
  A. Assessment.
II. **Ages**
  A. 6-17 years.
III. **Purpose**
  A. Provides verbal, performance, and full-scale IQ scores.
IV. **Areas Assessed**
  A. Cognitive ability, distractibility, verbal comprehension, perceptual organization, and processing speed.
V. **Additional Information**
  A. Three scores are obtained: verbal IQ, performance IQ, and full-scale IQ. May be contrasted with results from Wechsler Individual Achievement Test, second edition (WIAT-II) to compare ability with achievement. Core subtests take 50-70 minutes, and supplemental subtests take 10-15 minutes. The two other standardized Wechsler intelligence measures are the Wechsler Adult Intelligence Scale, third edition (WAIS-III) for children older than 16 years, and the Wechsler Preschool and Primary Scale of Intelligence—Revised (WPPSI-R) for children ages 3 through 7.3 years.
VI. **Tester Qualification:** C

WEISS COMPREHENSIVE ARTICULATION TEST (WCAT)

I. **Use**
  A. Testing.
II. **Ages**
  A. All ages.
III. **Purpose**
  A. Provides diagnosis of articulation delays and disorders.
IV. **Areas Assessed**
  A. Assesses articulation and misarticulation patterns.
V. **Additional Information**
  A. Scores obtained include articulation, age-equivalent, intelligibility, and stimulability. Test-retest reliability is available, and normative scores are based on test performance of 4000 children. Administration time is 20 minutes; scoring time is 30 minutes.
VI. **Tester Qualification:** A

WIDE RANGE ACHIEVEMENT TEST 3 (WRAT 3)

I. Use
   A. Assessment.
II. Ages
   A. 5-75 years.
III. Purpose
   A. Identify the need for basic academic skills.
IV. Areas Assessed
   A. Spelling, reading, and arithmetic.
V. Additional Information
   A. Spelling and arithmetic tests may be administered to a group; the reading test is individual only. Takes 15-30 minutes for each form and 5 minutes for scoring. The test is standardized.
VI. Tester Qualification: B

WOODCOCK READING MASTERY TEST—REVISED (WRMT-R)

I. Use
   A. Assessment.
II. Ages
   A. 5 years to 75+.
III. Purpose
   A. Assesses skill development in reading; can be used to plan remedial programs.
IV. Areas Assessed
   A. Visual-auditory learning, letter and word identification, word attack, word and passage comprehension.
V. Additional Information
   A. Normed on a national sampling. Administration time is 10-30 minutes for each cluster of tests.
VI. Tester Qualification: B

THE WORK SAMPLING SYSTEM

I. Use
   A. Assessment.
II. Ages
   A. Preschool-fifth grade.
III. Purpose
   A. Documentation of student's skills, behavior, knowledge, and accomplishments across a variety of curriculum areas on numerous occasions to enhance teaching and learning.
IV. Areas Assessed
   A. Personal and social development, language and literacy, mathematical thinking, scientific thinking, social studies, arts, and physical development.
V. Additional Information
   A. Provides an effective way to record student's progress to share with educators, families, and communities.
VI. Tester Qualification: B

WEB SITES

American Psychological Association (APA): Testing and Assessment
    http://www.apa.org/science/testing.html

GLOSSARY OF SPECIAL EDUCATION TERMS

Adapted physical education   A program of specially designed activities, games, sports, rhythms, and dance for students who demonstrate a developmental delay in motor skills. May be conducted in a special education class or regular classroom.

Affect   Outward manifestation of an individual's emotional tone or feeling in presentation of self.

Agnosia   Inability to process information through any of several major special senses—auditory, visual, olfactory, gustatory, or tactile. May result from organic brain damage and be partial or complete.

Agraphia   Inability to express thoughts in writing.

Anomia   Inability to name objects or recognize names; creates a significant reading and writing problem; a form of aphasia caused by a lesion in the temporal lobe of the brain.

Apgar score   Objective way to assess and describe the extrauterine adaptation by rating five areas—appearance (color), pulse, grimace (response to stimulation), activity (muscle tone), and respiratory effort. Rating is done at 1 and 5 minutes after birth, sometimes at 10 minutes, assigning scores from 0-2 in each area. Named for Virginia Apgar, anesthesiologist. The Apgar score assesses the need for immediate intervention but is a poor predictor of later developmental outcomes.

Aphasia   Disturbance or loss of ability to understand or communicate in spoken or written language or by gesturing. May be complete or partial and most commonly is a mixture of incomplete receptive and expressive aphasia. May be transient or permanent.

Apraxia   Inability to plan and carry out a particular act. Apraxia of speech is caused by brain damage and results in the inability to move speech muscles necessary to produce understandable speech.

Assessment   Multifaceted systematic process of looking at an individual's behaviors and achievements. In the nursing process, assessment includes systematically collecting data on an individual's health status, analyzing the information collected, and determining the information's implications for nursing actions and student learning.

Associated movements (overflow)   Extra motor activity that accompanies a certain motor performance; involuntary movements occurring in one area of the body when a voluntary movement occurs in another part of the body.

Ataxia   Impairment in ability to coordinate voluntary muscular movement. May manifest as a staggering gait or postural imbalance caused by a lesion in the spinal cord or cerebellum.

Auditory association   Ability to draw relationships from what one hears and then respond orally in an appropriate manner.

Auditory closure   Ability to make a word or sound into a whole when parts of the word or sound have been omitted.

Auditory discrimination   Ability to distinguish differences in sounds.

Auditory figure ground   Ability to select relevant sound stimuli from a background of environmental stimuli.

Auditory learner   Individual who acquires knowledge and skills primarily by listening.

Auditory memory   Ability to remember auditory information presented verbally as sounds or in the form of sound symbols.

Auditory reception   Admission of information by auditory avenues; however, this does not necessarily mean that comprehension has been achieved.

Auditory sequential memory   Ability to retain in the correct order a sequence of information presented verbally.

Behavior modification   Method using behavior concepts and laws to produce a positive change in behavior.

Bruxism   Unconscious, compulsive grinding and/or clenching of teeth; bruxism primarily occurs during sleep but also may occur in waking hours reflecting extreme stress or release of tension. May cause headache, muscle spasm, chronic pain in face and jaw, and/or damage to teeth.

Choreiform   Involuntary, irregular, purposeless movements.

Cognitive style   Mode by which the student appears to learn the best; the mode may be visual, auditory, or kinesthetic. See Learning Styles.

Cortical thumb   Fisting with thumb flexed inside the clenched palm. May indicate hypertonicity; neurologically normal up to age 3 months.

Decoding   Process whereby the brain changes symbols into sounds. Examples of such processes are reading, the interpretation of the spoken word, facial expressions, social cues.

Diadochokinesis/diadochokinetic rate   Ability in speech to produce a rapid rate of repetitive oral movements; the rapid production of sounds using different parts of the mouth. Used to assess dyspraxia or dysarthria by noting how quickly the child is able to produce sounds using different parts of the mouth.

Diagnostic tests   Tests that provide a finer analysis than a screening device so that strengths and weaknesses in skill development can be identified more specifically.

Dominance   Tendency to prefer using one side or part of the body over the other.

Dysarthria   Difficulty in articulating words because of impairment in the control of articulation muscles, usually caused by central or peripheral motor system damage; aphasias result from cortical damage.

Dyscalculia   Inability to perform mathematical functions.

Dysgraphia   Inability to produce the motor movements necessary for handwriting; may be part of a language disorder caused by an impairment of the motor system or the parietal lobe.

Dyslexia   An inability to read, spell, or write; can see and identify letters, but may reverse letters and have poor sense of left and right; possible genetic association.

Dyspraxia   Partial loss or failure to develop ability to perform skilled, coordinated movements; not explained by any motor or sensory dysfunction; or mental retardation.

Echolalia   Meaningless repetition of what is heard, both phrases and words. Occurs normally in early language development; seen in Tourette's syndrome, catatonic schizophrenia, and neurological disorders such as transcortical aphasia.

Encoding   Process whereby ideas are changed into symbols for the specific purpose of communication. Such processes include body gestures, sign language, spoken or written words.

Familial   Occurrence in members of the same family more than might be anticipated by chance.

Figure ground disturbance   The inability to distinguish the figure from the background.

Fine motor function   Ability to use small muscle groups efficiently, smoothly, and quickly; usually parallels gross motor development.

Form constancy   Ability to perceive words or objects as basically the same; unaware of the differences in their presentation or occurrence.

Glossopharyngeal breathing   Method of forcing air into lungs with the pharynx and tongue. May be used by individuals dependent on mechanical ventilation to maintain adequate oxygenation during suctioning.

Graphesthesia   Ability to discriminate shapes, symbols, words, numbers, or letters drawn on the skin, particularly the palm of the hand, when the eyes are closed. Believed to have a relationship with intersensory integration.

Gross motor function   Ability to move large muscles in a coordinated and efficient manner.

Gustatory   Pertaining to sense of taste.

Hyperactivity   Excessive activity or restless motor movement, impulsivity, or both. It is an atypical behavior beyond the ability of the student to regulate well.

Impulsivity   Tendency to act without considering the consequences.

Intonation   Rise and fall in the pitch of the voice during speech.

Kinesthetic   Sense by which the individual is aware of the position, weight, and movement of various body parts in space.

Language   Communication of ideas through symbols that are used according to grammatical and semantic rules.

Laterality   The superior development of one side of the brain or body; use of one hand in preference over the other. Often referred to as preferential use; dominance or mixed preference, such as left-eyed, right-handed, right-legged.

Lateralization   The ability of one section of the brain to take the lead in organizing and processing a certain behavior or mental process; functional specialization of the brain occurring mainly in the right hemisphere, such as the perception of spatial and visual relationships.

Learning disability   A disorder manifest by significant difficulties in learning, speaking, reasoning, reading, writing, or doing mathematical calculations. Often occurs in an individual with normal or above-average intelligence. May result from psychological or organic causes. Specific testing is used to identify.

Learning styles/intelligence factor   Eight intelligence/learning styles have been theorized, including visuospatial, verbal/linguistic, logical/mathematical, bodily/kinesthetic, musical/rhythmic, interpersonal, intrapersonal, and naturalistic (Gardner, 1998). Emotional intelligence is another theoretical concept.

Mirror movements   Phenomenon in which associated movements occur on the opposite side.

Neurodevelopmental examination   Assessment of the student's nervous system's maturation level and developmental status in a variety of areas, including fine and gross motor function, visual perceptual function, and auditory language ability.

Nonacademic services   Extracurricular services for students with disabilities (e.g., clubs, athletics, recreational activities, transportation).

Obturator   A device used to guide tracheostomy tube or gastrostomy button into position without causing trauma to tissue. The obturator is removed once the tracheostomy tube or gastrostomy button is in place.

Occupational therapist   Registered professional who evaluates and treats those who have difficulty with activities of daily living, play, fine motor skills, oral motor function, and other activities. Services include design and fabrication of adaptive equipment, assessment and treatment of sensory integration problems, adaptation of physical environment for the disabled, consultation to classroom teacher/staff, and prevocational evaluation. Licensed in some states.

Orthosis   A special brace or device to correct, control, or compensate for muscle or bone deformities.

Orthotics   The design and manufacture of external devices used to promote a specific motion, correct a deformity, or support a paralyzed limb.

Parent   Natural or adoptive parent; person acting in place of a parent, for example, grandparent or stepparent with whom the child lives or a person legally responsible for the child's welfare; and in certain circumstances, a foster parent or surrogate parent unless prohibited by state law.

Perception   Recognition and appropriate interpretation of stimuli received in the brain.

Percutaneous endoscopic gastrostomy   Percutaneous endoscopic gastrostomy (PEG) is placement of a gastrostomy tube into the stomach from the abdomen with the guidance of the endoscope. A small incision is made, usually with the patient under light sedation or local anesthetic. Generally heals quickly.

Peristomal   Area of skin around a stoma.

Perseveration   Continuation of an activity, response, or reply after the causative stimuli has ceased. A student may continue with one activity long after offered a new task.

Phonation   Controlling the breath flow to produce the sounds of speech.

Phoneme   Smallest sound units in a language. The English language designates 44 different phonemes. Phonemes vary from language to language.

Phonetics   Study of speech sounds.

Physical therapist   Licensed professional who evaluates, plans, and implements a therapy program that promotes self-sufficiency. Assesses abilities in gross motor skills, motor planning, balance and equilibrium, postural tone, gait, and kinesthesia. Designs and develops adaptive equipment and provides assistance and information on the use of mechanical aids (e.g., wheelchairs and braces).

Praxis   The ability of the brain to process, organize, and perform unfamiliar actions. Children who have difficulty planning and carrying out motor activities are said to be *apraxic* or *dyspraxic*.

Projective test   Standardized assessment performed to elicit information concerning an individual's personality, subconscious feelings, and sources of conflicts; testing protocols may include the Thematic Apperception Test (TAT) or Rorschach or ink blot test.

Related services   Defined in IDEA as transportation and developmental, corrective, and other supportive services required to assist a child with a disability to benefit from special education.

School psychologist   Licensed professional who uses the science of psychometrics to evaluate student's need for special services and assess the student's educational progress. A school psychologist interprets interpersonal behavior, assists students in coping with their environment, and helps teachers and staff in behavior management techniques.

School social worker   Licensed professional who is a member of the multidisciplinary team providing counseling to students, consultation to teachers, and liaison to the families of students in the educational setting. They network with community agencies and social support systems that can advance students' educational achievement and psychosocial functioning.

Screening   Identifying potential deviance (e.g., vision and hearing screenings). When indicated, assessment, diagnosis, and then treatment follow screening.

Self-esteem   The personal estimation or evaluation that the student has about himself or herself; includes emotional and value-based assessments. Self-esteem has variations and is on a continuum of strong or weak, low or high, and worthy or unworthy.

Semantics   Study of language regarding the meanings of words or symbols and rules for use.

Soft neurological signs   Slight or mild neurological abnormalities that are difficult to detect or interpret and may indicate immature or ineffective function of the central nervous system.

Sound blending   Ability to combine separate parts of a word and produce the complete word.

Spatial relationships   Ability to determine size, right and left, distance, and how one object is related to another.

Speech and language pathologist/speech therapist   Licensed professional who screens, evaluates, diagnoses, and treats those with communication disorders.

Stimulus   Anything that incites the individual to function, become active, or respond; stimuli may be physical, chemical, biological, or social.

Stoma   A surgically created opening of an internal organ on the surface of the body, (e.g., ileostomy, colostomy, gastrostomy, vesicostomy, tracheostomy).

Supplementary aids and services   As defined in IDEA, includes instructional assistants, services, and other supports that are provided in regular education classes or other education-related settings to enable children with disabilities to be educated with nondisabled children to the maximum extent appropriate.

Syntax/grammar   How words are put together in sentences according to established rules.

Tactile   Pertaining to sense of touch.

Testing   Presentation of a collection of predetermined tasks or questions to which predetermined responses exist.

Travel training   As defined in IDEA, providing instruction to children with significant cognitive or other disabilities to enable them to develop an awareness of the environment in which they live; and teaching the skills necessary to move effectively and safely within that environment (e.g., in school, at home, in the community).

Visual aphasia   Inability to comprehend written language; caused by a lesion in the left visual cortex and the connection between the right visual cortex and the left hemisphere.

Visual association   Ability to see the relationship between various visual symbols.

Visual closure   Recognition of shapes, objects, or words when the visual presentation is incomplete.

Visual discrimination   Detection of differences in letters, forms, objects, or words.

Visual figure ground   Ability to separate a figure or object from its background.

Visual learner   Individual who acquires knowledge and skills primarily through vision.

Visual reception   Ability to look at symbols (words, letters, and so forth) and interpret their meaning.

Visual sequential memory   Ability to store, retrieve, and reproduce visual information from memory.

Visuomotor function   Ability to coordinate vision with movements of the body or body parts.

Visuoperceptual disability   Difficulty in organizing and interpreting visual sensory stimuli.

ACRONYMS USED IN SPECIAL EDUCATION

ADD Attention deficit disorder
ADHD Attention deficit hyperactivity disorder
APE Adapted physical education
AT Assistive technology
CEC Council for Exceptional Children
CH Communicatively handicapped
CLD Council for Learning Disabilities
CSPD Comprehensive system of personnel development
DB Deaf-blind
DHH Deaf and hard of hearing

DIS Designated instruction and services
EHA Education of the Handicapped Act
EPSDT Early periodic screening, diagnosis, and treatment
ESA Educational Service Agency
ESL English as a second language
FAPE Free and appropriate public education
FERP Family Educational Rights and Privacy Act
HCP Health care provider
HI Hearing impaired
ICC Interagency Coordinating Council
IDEA Individuals with Disabilities Education Act
IEE Independent educational evaluation
IEP Individualized education program
IFSP Individualized family service plan
ILS Integrated life skills
LD Learning disabled
LEA Local Education Agency
LEP Limited English proficiency
LRE Least restrictive environment
MIC-KEY Skin-level gastrostomy button that turns and locks into place
MR Mentally retarded
NICHCY The National Information Center for Children and Youth with Disabilities; previously known as National Information Center for Handicapped Children and Youth.
NPRM Notice of proposed rulemaking
O&M Orientation and mobility
OH Orthopedically handicapped
OHI Other health-impaired
OMB Office of Management and Budget
OSEP Office of Special Education Programs
OSERS Office of Special Education and Rehabilitative Services
OT Occupational therapy
PE Physical education
PH Physically handicapped
PT Physical therapy
RSP Resource specialist program
SEA State educational agency
SH Severely handicapped
TDD Telecommunications device for the deaf
TPA Total parenteral alimentation
TPN Total parenteral nutrition
VH Visually handicapped
VI Visually impaired

WEB SITES

National Information Center for Children and Youth with Disabilities (NICHCY)
    1-800-695-0285
    http://www.nichcy.org
National Organization for Rare Disorders
    1-800-999-6673
    http://www.rarediseases.org

BIBLIOGRAPHY

American Guidance Service: *AGS products A to Z,* Available online: http://www.agsnet. com/azproducts.asp. Accessed on April 8, 2001.

Anderson K, editor: *Mosby's medical, nursing, & allied health dictionary,* ed 6, St Louis, 2001, Mosby.

Arnold MJ, Silkworth CK, editors: *The school nurse's source book of individualized healthcare plans,* vol 2, North Branch, Minn, Sunrise River Press.

Ashwill JW, Droske SC, Rader I, editors: *Nursing care of children: principles and practice,* Philadelphia, 1997, WB Saunders.

Bowden VR, Dickey SB, Greenberg CS: *Children and their families: the continuum of care,* Philadelphia, 1968, WB Saunders.

Council of Educators for Students with Disabilities (CESD): *Special education laws,* Oct 2, 2001, Available online: http://www.504idea.org/. Accessed Oct 16, 2001.

Gardner H: *Frames of mind: the theory of multiple intelligences,* New York, 1983, Basic Books.

Gardner H: A multiplicity of intelligences, *Sci Am* 9(4):18-23, 1998.

Haas M, editor: *The school nurse's source book of individualized healthcare plans,* vol 1, North Branch, Minn, 1994, Sunrise River Press.

O'Toole M, editor: *Miller-Keane encyclopedia & dictionary of medicine, nursing, & allied health.* Philadelphia, 1999, WB Saunders.

Pierangelo R, Giuliani G: *Special educator's complete guide to 109 diagnostic tests,* West Nyack, 1998, The Center for Applied Research Education.

Policymaker Partnership (PMP) for Implementing IDEA: *Regulations & law & reports,* 1998, Updated 2002, Available online: http://www.ideapolicy.org/Relaunch/rr.htm. Accessed April 19, 2002.

Porter S, Ahynie M, Bierle T, editor: *Children and youth assisted by medical technology in educational settings: guidelines for care,* Baltimore, 1997, Brookes Publishing.

Psychological Corporation: *2001 Psychological Corporation catalog listing,* April 8, 2001, Available online: http://www.psychcorp.com/catalogs/tpc_catlist.htm. Accessed Sept 18, 2001.

Schwab N, Gelfman M, editors: *Legal issues in school health services: a resource for school administrators, school attorneys, school nurses,* North Branch, Minn, 2001, Sunrise River Press.

U.S. Department of Education: *Discover IDEA* (CD-ROM), 2001, Office of Special Education Programs, Available online: http://www.ideapractices.org.

Wound Care Information Network: *Summary of the Agency for Health Care Policy and Research (AHCPR) clinical practice guidelines 1995-2002,* Available online: http://www.medicaledu.com/ahcpr.htm. Accessed April 19, 2002.

CHAPTER 10

Twenty-first Century Health Challenges

*E*merging incidences and prevalence of certain developmental variations and behavioral disorders are becoming more common in the school setting. This chapter includes frequently discussed and documented occurrences by school nurses and other staff on elementary and secondary school campuses. These issues affect the health and learning ability of students at all ages.

The conditions in this chapter are presented in two different formats. "Backpack Syndrome" and "Computer Ergonomics" are presented in the manual's traditional outline format. The other health-related issues are in paragraph format with the nursing management processes listed for quick access. These issues, some of which are new, are current health challenges for the nurse in the school setting and include computer-related exploitation, commercialism of public schools, schools as community health centers, home schooling/alternative education, youth gambling, precocious puberty, bipolar disorder, obsessive compulsive disorder, and terrorism, including domestic homeland terrorism and bioterrorism: anthrax and other threats.

BACKPACK SYNDROME

I. **Definition**
   A. Backpacks used by the school-age student to carry school books and supplies, other articles, and equipment. Students often carry between 10 and 40+ lb on their back to and from school and between classes.

II. **Etiology**
   A. Backpacks can be a threat to the health of the student when they are too heavy, are packed, lifted, or worn improperly, or if these factors are combined. Human beings have used their backs for centuries to carry heavy loads, including infants and babies on their mothers' backs. The school student carry their backpacks in a variety of positions that can adversely affect them physically and affect the spinal column and other bone structures that are not fully developed.

   B. Wearing backpacks alters the mobility of the spine, leading to passive movement (involuntary movement from an outside force), which is a risk factor for back pain (Vacheron et al, 1999). Low back pain during the adolescent years can result in low back pain in adults (Salminen et al, 1999). No studies on the effects of long-term use of heavy and chronic backpack use have been conducted, but research suggests that it may trigger adult back pain and disability in individuals with genetic predisposition or biological disease process.

III. **Characteristics**
   A. Poor posture.
   B. Headache, fatigue, or both.
   C. Low back pain that may become chronic.

    D. Discomfort, pain, or both in the neck and shoulders.

    E. Muscle spasms of neck and shoulders.

    F. Pressure sores or blisters on the back or shoulders from straps or inappropriately packed objects.

IV. **Health Concerns/Emergencies**

    A. Heavy backpacks.

        1. May cause long-term health problems resulting from neck, shoulder and back pain, soreness, and fatigue.

        2. May contribute to or accelerate progression of scoliosis.

V. **Effects on Individual**

    A. Poor posture and pain resulting from leaning forward with neck thrust forward.

    B. Shoulder and arm strain from dragging backpack.

    C. Strain and stress on one side of the body caused by using only one shoulder strap.

    D. Headaches, neck and low back pain, numbness, and tingling in the upper arm area.

    E. Fatigue.

VI. **Management/Treatment**

    A. Teach the proper techniques of packing, lifting, and carrying backpacks and health concerns regarding their improper use.

    B. Teach back-strengthening exercises.

    C. Encourage weighing the pack and contents, limiting the contents to 10% to 15% of body weight to prevent neck and back strain.

NOTE: Percentage of pack weight to body weight varies because no definitive studies are available.

    D. *Backpack specifications and proper use.*

        1. The pack should not be longer than the distance between the shoulders and hips and not wider than the rib cage. Shoulder straps should be wide and padded to avoid shoulder pressure and possible nerve damage. A waist or hip belt provides good support and may help with weight distribution and stabilization.

        2. Sling-style packs worn over one shoulder are available.

        3. Briefcases and backpacks on wheels are recommended by many health professionals and are being used.

        4. The pack should be worn high up on the back, not low near the hips, because it shifts posture forward, producing back and neck strain.

        5. The weight should be distributed evenly to ease carrying and prevent injury and strain.

        6. Pack heaviest items close to the body with lighter items farther away or in small sections.

        7. Avoid carrying bulky or pointed objects next to the back, which creates an uneven surface and causes painful blisters from repeated rubbing.

        8. When lifting a pack, squat using the knees and legs. If the pack is very heavy, it should be placed on a desk or table before pulling it onto the back.

VII. **Additional Information**
   A. Several conditions have arisen that cause this syndrome:
      1. Students are multitasking from early morning until late evening, causing them to carry not only their classroom needs but also items ranging from food to sports equipment.
      2. The short time intervals between classes do not permit them to go to their lockers.
      3. Some schools have eliminated lockers because of security, safety, and budget controls.
   B. Occasionally students may need special accommodations to leave class early to go to their lockers, assistance with carrying supplies, or a second set of books because of individualized needs. Some schools require that backpacks be made of see-through vinyl or mesh to discourage the transport of weapons, alcohol, or drugs. This demand seems to forgo the adolescent's need for privacy.
   C. New technology may eliminate the need to carry heavy books between classes and to and from home. Small technological devices are available that can scan the written work or page and transfer the data to a home computer. Computerized textbooks are being developed for use on a lightweight device similar to a laptop computer, allowing students to highlight and take notes as they would a textbook.

VIII. **Web Sites**
   BackCare
   http://www.backpain.org/index.htm
   American Academy of Pediatrics
   http://www.aap.org
   Backpack Safety America
   1-800-775-2225
   http://www.backpacksafe.com

COMPUTER ERGONOMICS

   I. **Definition**
      A. The computer video display terminal (VDT) and workstation are used for academic learning and entertainment. Workstations can be cluttered with keyboard, monitor, mouse, files, books, notes, pens and pencils, and other school materials and supplies.

   II. **Etiology**
      A. Using a computer workstation poses a threat to the individual's health because of repetitive stress and fatigue from inappropriate body positioning, work environment, and repetitive activity. Health hazards from inappropriate or cumulative use of computers include carpal tunnel syndrome, back and neck pain, and computer visual syndrome (CVS). VDT symptoms occur as a result of a variety of factors: glare or reflections, failure to blink frequently enough to maintain moisture on the surface of the eyes (decreased blinking and increased tear evaporation), corrective lenses that are inappropriate for the individual's distance and position from screen, minor visual

defects that manifest by intense computer use, and poor body positioning in relationship to the computer and workstation.

III. **Characteristics**

    A. Visual symptoms include the following:

        1. Temporary myopia.

        2. Eye fatigue and strain.

        3. Blurry vision at near and far distance.

        4. Dry, watery, or irritated eyes.

        5. Oversensitivity to light.

        6. Neck aches, backaches, muscle spasms.

        7. Headaches.

        8. Carpal tunnel syndrome with chronic use (development of this type of injury may take 5 to 10 years).

IV. **Health Concerns/Emergencies**

    A. Delayed socialization can result from computer use beginning at an early age. Supervision and support by an adult is especially critical for children younger than age 7. Software is now available for infants younger than 1 year.

    B. Temporary or possible permanent damage to vision or upper body muscles, nerves, or tendons.

    C. No *current data* suggest permanent visual damage.

    D. No *current* evidence that VDTs emit hazardous radiation (ultraviolet or ionizing radiation) or data suggestive of a health risk from exposure to electromagnetic fields associated with monitor use exist.

V. **Effects on Individual**

    A. Complaints of aching or pain, tenderness, swelling, cracking, numbness or tingling, loss of strength, decreased coordination in the injured area or loss of joint movement of the fingers, shoulders, back or neck, but most commonly in the hand, wrist, or arm. These complaints usually are called *repetitive strain injuries (RSIs)* (see "Additional Information").

    B. In young children, excessive computer use impedes the development of critical skills, such as creativity, imagination, and attention span, and decreases pretending skills, motivation, and desire to persevere. Select high-quality developmental software versus rote learning or drill and practice software.

VI. **Management/Treatment**

    A. For home or school:

        1. All students should wear corrective eyeglasses (if prescribed). Computer glasses may be ideal when computer use involves several hours per day.

        2. Determine computer use during vision screening.

        3. Check display screen position for viewing without neck tilted either backward or forward. If screen position is too high, the individual will tip the neck backward, and if the screen is too low, the individual will bend forward for easier viewing (see Figure 10-1).

        4. Maintain glare-free screen and reposition computer screen. It should be at a right angle to windows, or awning or blinds can be

used to decrease glare. Check for glare by turning the screen off and observing any reflection of lights or lightly colored objects that are seen on the screen. Adjust the brightness of room lighting or use an American Optometry Association (AOA)–approved antiglare filter or three-sided computer hood. Clean the screen often with antistatic cloth.

5. Use a document holder. Place the text document or book in holder and move as close to the screen as possible. Maintain sufficient light on any paper documents by using a freestanding, adjustable brightness task light. The light in the work area should be approximately the same as the background illumination of the screen.

6. Ensure that appropriate workstation equipment and furniture is used. Use a height-adjustable chair with good back support. The work surface should be stable. Use a negative-slope/tilt-down keyboard system for a height-adjustable mouse/keyboard platform. The keyboard and mouse should be appropriate for the child's or adult's hand size (e.g., small hands use a smaller keyboard [LittleFingers keyboard; Datadesk Technologies, Bainbridge Island, Washington]).

7. Schedule timely work breaks because postural problems associated with computer use depend on the length of continual use time. Breaks every 20 to 30 minutes are ideal for younger students. Software can be programmed to remind the user to take a break by providing on-screen alerts; many provide guidance on simple exercises (e.g., ErgoPal software; Magnitude Information Systems, Inc., Chester, New Jersey). Adolescents can focus on distant object for about 2 minutes. Frequent blinking of the eyes also is necessary. Saline solution eye drops may reduce irritation and dryness. Computer users should stretch frequently; stretching exercises can relieve tension in the neck and back.

8. Apply ergonomic guidelines for computer use. The neutral work posture applies to children, adolescents, and adults. It ensures comfortable and ergonomically correct computer use. Applying principles of ergonomics (i.e., fitting the workspace to the individual's body) can alleviate many of the health risks associated with computer use.

B. Problem postures and keyboard positions.

1. An upward-sloping keyboard increases muscle loads in upper arms, shoulders, and neck. Positioning the keyboard on the desk makes maintenance of neutral position difficult because the forearms tire and sag, placing the wrists into greater wrist extension and elbows usually flexed, which compresses the median and ulna nerves at the elbow, thus restricting blood flow to the hands.

VII. **Additional Information**

A. Ergonomics is a science that uses current knowledge of human abilities and limitations to design or organize systems, products, machines, or tools for efficient, comfortable, and safe use by human

---

Box 10-1 *Upper Body Support*

1. Back supported by chair; sit with back into chair.
2. Chair seat should not apply pressure behind knees.
3. Place feet on a flat surface for support—either floor or footrest.
4. Head should be in balanced medial position, not tilted backward or too far forward.
5. Monitor should be below eye level so that eyes are directed at a 10- to 20-degree declination from straight-ahead gaze.

6. Popliteal angle should be greater than 90 degrees; angle behind knees should be open.
7. Upper arms should be relaxed and close to body (not flexed forward or abducted to the side).
8. The elbow angle should be greater than 90 degrees with the forearm below horizontal.
9. The wrist should be in a neutral position, less than 15 degrees; hand/wrist should be level with forearm.

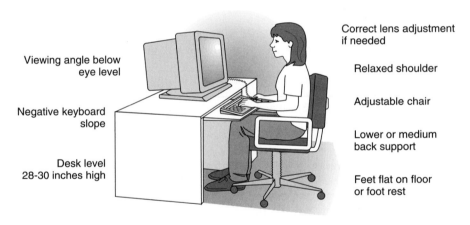

Viewing angle below eye level

Negative keyboard slope

Desk level 28-30 inches high

Correct lens adjustment if needed

Relaxed shoulder

Adjustable chair

Lower or medium back support

Feet flat on floor or foot rest

Figure 10-1 Suggested computer workstation positioning.

beings. Research is limited, and little is known of the effects of computer use on infants and young children.

B. RSIs involve muscles, tendons, and nerves that are overused or misused. The damage is caused by repetitive tasks, forceful movements, awkward or fixed postures, or insufficient relaxation time between activity. RSIs may include carpal tunnel syndrome, ganglionic cysts, tendinitis, tenosynovitis and epicondylitis (tennis elbow), trigger finger, thoracic outlet syndrome, De Quervain's disease, and possibly computer vision syndrome.

VIII. Web Sites
Cornell University Ergonomics Web
http://ergo.human.cornell.edu
Massachusetts Institute of Technology
http://web.mit.edu/atic/www/rsi/mitrsi.htm
Cergo S: Computer Ergonomics for Elementary Students
http://www.orosha.org/cergos

SCHOOL TRENDS AND PHENOMENA

COMPUTER-RELATED CHILD EXPLOITATION

Computers are a common, contemporary, and almost mandated educational modality in all schools throughout the country. Students in early elementary grades are trained to use the Internet, e-mail, and chat rooms for educational and entertainment pursuits. Preschool programs even have cyberspace access for the youngest of our citizens, with software produced for infants as young as 9 months. Internet connection makes every American youth a world citizen and world traveler to all the commercial, educational, and entertainment sites available to adults throughout the world.

Like other technology developed in the twentieth century, such as the telephone, television, cellular phones, video games, and handheld devices, the computer is a wonderful and novel communication tool for children. As with all technology, cyberspace has a "down" side or an antisocial, destructive potential in its application. Conscientious parents, health providers, and political leaders increasingly are sounding the alarm about exploitation of children by pornographers, predators, and peddlers who place them at risk for abuse, disease, and disorders that can end tragically in death (Lukefahr, 1999). A national survey of 1500 youngsters conducted by the National Center for Missing and Exploited Children (2000) reported that 1 in 5 received unwanted sexual overtures on the World Wide Web.

Internet exploitation of children and youth is becoming a national public health problem. Examples include the solicitation of expensive products for sale, display of soft and hard-core pornography, invitation to associate with sexual predators and criminals, and the access to antisocial peer group norms by way of chat rooms. E-mail provides unlimited and diverse communication with people whose belief systems and values may conflict with those of family, character-building organizations, and religious affiliation. The outcome is purveying prejudicial and discriminatory ideologies that can lead to hate crimes.

Continued, excessive, and even compulsive use of the Internet by children has been documented by clinicians and educators to have a deleterious effect on personality development and mastery of age-appropriate social skills. These effects can lead to symptoms of depression, fears and strong anxiety reactions, traumatic memories, and schizoid behavior. Some clinical studies have documented sexual addictions resulting from habitual use of pornographic cyberspace sites, especially for late adolescents. Chronic use of the computer has been reported to be a disincentive to reading children's literature and a contributor to academic underachievement when children do not use it for studying educationally assigned material. Physical health and well-being can be compromised by poor posture, visual strain, muscle fatigue, and excessive weight as a result of inactivity (see "Computer Ergonomics"). Finally, children lose the opportunity for family togetherness, friendships, and peer group leisure activities.

Recommendations for nurses and other educational leaders for safe, secure, and healthy Internet use by children and youth include the following:
1. Closer adult monitoring and supervision of Internet use in the home.
2. Closer adult monitoring and supervision of Internet use in school and all community organization access (i.e., libraries).
3. Safety through commercial software that restricts violence, pornography, nudity, and other sexually exploited images.
4. Availability for students of video games depicting common approaches to child abduction.
5. Use of a home page with links to only child-friendly Web pages.
6. Training of children and youth for safe communication, such as not providing personal identification information, not sending photographs, and not agreeing to meet people on the Internet without parental consent.
7. Support of and membership in national cyberspace child/youth protective organizations.

COMMERCIALISM OF PUBLIC SCHOOLS

Over the last two decades, corporate businesses have contracted with local school boards or school educational groups to provide services and products for the benefit of the students. In exchange for promoting services and products, schools receive monetary contributions toward operating budgets, equipment, and supplies.

The most documented and widespread agreements are with Channel One (Primedia Inc., Los Angeles, California). By contrast, Channel One offers a daily in-school news and advertising program to 8 million students in 12,000 schools—40% of America's middle school and high school students. Students are obligated to watch television every day. In exchange, Channel One provides the school with a satellite dish, videocassette recorders (VCR), and television sets. The daily television viewing includes 10 minutes of fast-paced, flashy infotainment and 2 minutes of advertisements by companies such as Pepsi, McDonald's, and Nintendo. These companies pay Channel One $195,000 for a single 30-second advertisement, which represents a larger amount of money than that received by some high-end, prime-time television networks (Center for Commercial-Free Public Education, 2000).

Opposition by parents and educators to the commercialization of the schools by Channel One is growing. Three studies conclude that continuation of these contracts is not in the best interest of the students, educators, or school districts. An extensive study by Consumers Union Education Services (1995) revealed that 80% of the information on the daily television feed is biased and incorrect. The second study (Hoynes, Pesnick, and Miller, 1997), by a team of researchers from Vassar College, Johns Hopkins University, and the Center for Media Education, revealed that only 20% of the channel air time is spent covering stories and 80% is advertising and infotainment (i.e., sports, weather, natural disasters, and features). The study concluded that the "news" program serves as a filler between profitable advertisements. The third study, conducted by the University of Massachusetts at Amherst (1998), disclosed that Channel One serves more than twice as many low-income community classrooms as high-income community schools. Obviously, low-income schools are a target for commercialism of products and services that do not promote responsible student health or good education.

Another major corporate commercial contract with schools across the country is with soft-drink beverage companies, Coca-Cola and Pepsi. These commercial giants offer cash to the schools in exchange for vending and advertising rights. Schools receive a percentage of the sales for consumption of the beverages, prompting administrators to encourage students to purchase them. These companies have exclusive, noncompetitive contracts with schools for the sale of their product. For years public health researchers have documented that carbonated beverages and soft drinks are detrimental to bone growth in active girls and promote overweight and tooth decay as a result of the high caloric and sugar content. Caffeine-containing beverages are replacing the consumption of water and healthy fruit juices (Wyshak, 2000). Confronted with opposition from national education organizations and state legislatures, these commercial giants are directing local bottlers to withdraw soda from the schools and to replace them with water, fruit juice, and other nutritious drinks.

Other commercial and advertising enterprises related to public schools include school bus advertisements, book covers with ad displays for name-brand products, sponsorship of high school assemblies by drug companies related to the National Depression Screening Day, and the use of brand-name pizza companies in math classes as a way to teach students to count using an ingredient (e.g., pepperoni) (Center for Commercial-Free Public Education, 2000).

As an advocate for health promotion and wellness, it is imperative that the nurse:
1. Stress the importance of providing healthy food and fitness products at schools.
2. Lead in educating school administrators regarding unhealthy life styles resulting from particular school commercialism products.
3. Promote and support legislation for responsible consumerism at school sites by contacting legislators, local newspapers, and trade journals as appropriate.
4. Distribute educational literature to the students, their families, and faculty.

Web Sites

Center for Commercial-Free Public Education
    1-800-867-5841
    http://www.commercialfree.org
Center for Media Education
    202-331-7833
    http://www.cme.org

SCHOOLS AS COMMUNITY HEALTH CENTERS

Although public schools are not designed primarily to provide health services, for many years the movement to identify the school as a health center has been advocated by parent organizations, educators, health and mental health associations, and political parties. Recently the Department of Health and Human Services, The National Association of School Nurses, and other prominent health care organizations have issued policy statements promoting expansion of school-based and school-linked health centers into community-based health care systems.

In January 2001 the American Academy of Pediatrics (AAP) issued the School Health Centers and Other Integrated Health Services policy statement. The objectives of the AAP are to enhance accessibility, provide quality health care, link children to a medical home, be financially sustainable, and address both long- and short-term wellness needs of children and adolescents. In other words, the school reform movement in the area of health and human services would provide a seamless web of services from the school to the home for all children and their families.

The school as a community health care facility has been a long-standing operational reality throughout the country, but no uniform model of the ideal health service system exists in any local school district. Many school districts do not offer conventional health services, such as school nursing, immunization clinics, or preventive screening programs. More innovative and progressive school districts offer greater comprehensive services, such as school-based clinics, home health education, and collaboration with hospitals and community clinics.

School nursing practice will expand and become more challenging in the twenty-first century, given the community collaboration and centralization of health care services at the school site. Thus school nurses:

1. Must assume a strategic role in influencing and shaping the medical ecology of school staff, students, and families.
2. Need to expand their job description to include increased case management, networking, monitoring, evaluation, and research to keep pace with the partnership of community health care providers (HCPs) and systems.
3. Must present greater visibility, since they are required to be in the community and away from the school campus as representatives of the educational sector of services.
4. Be innovative and progressive in determining the "right size" of comprehensive services, such as school-based clinics, home health education, and collaboration with hospitals and community clinics. A "one size fits all" approach to a school health care delivery system is not possible.
5. Increase proficiency in information and communication technology (e.g., computer, Internet, e-mail).
6. Ensure provision of adequate funding for these services.

Web Sites

The Center for Health and Health Care in Schools
    202-466-3396
    http://www.healthinschools.org/home.asp
National Assembly on School-Based Health Care
    1-888-286-8727
    http://www.nasbhc.org
Bureau of Primary Health Care's Healthy Schools, Healthy Communities
    http://www.bphc.hrsa.gov/HSHC

Center for Studying Health System Change
202-484-5261
http://www.hschange.com

HOME SCHOOLING/ALTERNATIVE EDUCATION

The societal phenomenon of educating children and youth at home with the parents as the exclusive, if not the primary educators, is a cherished tradition in the United States. In the 1980s and 1990s, the home was promoted and advocated as an alternative to both public and parochial schools. Since 1993, home schooling is legal in all 50 states, and reports indicate the number of students in home schooling has almost tripled since then. Various state and national studies estimate that 1.7 million children are being taught by their parents; this number represents a small percentage of the country's 47 million students.

Public policy debate among educators and politicians is ongoing regarding the benefits and detriments of this societal trend. However, parents of all socioeconomic and ethnic groups continue to assert their prerogative and exercise more control over their children's education and socialization. Home schooling is more popular with and provided more often by white, middle-class, and traditional two-parent families.

The reported reasons for the tremendous growth of home schooling in the past and its continuing increase in all socioeconomic and ethnic groups include: (1) transmission of a distinct belief system and values to children, (2) stronger filial bonds for nurturing and socialization, (3) controlled and positive peer interactions, (4) personal instruction and quality learning of academics, (5) education of gifted children and those with special needs, and (6) safety from antisocial influences (e.g., bullying, aggression, substance abuse, sexual harassment/assault). With recent research documenting higher academic achievement and strong prosocial character development of children who are home schooled, parents have added motivation to keep their children at home despite the personal sacrifices and financial limitations associated with home schooling.

No epidemiological studies have implicated the home school movement in inadequate medical care or at-risk health status of the children. These children and youth receive home health care and community services from public health agencies, clinics, and hospitals funded by private and public insurance.

Recommendations for nurses include the following:
1. Identify students receiving in-home schooling.
2. Assume a strategic role in providing required health screening to home-schooled students of all ages.
3. Be innovative and collaborative in determining approaches to provision of health-related education and collaboration with the student, parents, or both parties (i.e., on school site, by e-mail, one-on-one meeting, home visits).
4. Data gathering for research is necessary and valuable for this population of students.

Web Sites

Homeschool Central
http://www.homeschoolcentral.com/index.htm
National Association of Catholic Home Educators
540-349-4314
http://www.nache.org
National Home Education Research Institute
503-364-1490
http://www.nheri.org
National Home Education Network
http://www.nhen.org/

SCHOOL SOCIAL PROBLEMS

YOUTH GAMBLING

The generation born in the 1990s is the first in modern American history to grow up with gambling considered legal and culturally acceptable. With gambling more widespread throughout the United States by state lotteries, at Native American gaming casinos, and on the Internet, more adults are gambling than ever before. This increase has been accompanied by more prevalent problem gambling and pathological gambling among the adult population. Youth practices follow those of the adult population with social behavior such as smoking, alcohol use, drug abuse, and games of chance.

Only in the last 10 years have systematic and reliable studies on youth gambling been conducted. According to researchers at the Harvard Medical School in Children's Hospital Boston, between 76% and 91% of all teenagers have gambled by their senior year of high school. Approximately 4% to 6% of youth ages 12 to 17 are pathological gamblers, whereas 1% to 3% of adults are problem gamblers according to a recent study (1998) by the American Psychological Association. A meta-analysis study of youth gambling in North America by the Center for Addictive Studies at Harvard Medical School found that the rate of problem gambling ranged between 9.9% and 14.2%; the number of youth exhibiting compulsive gambling ranged from 4.4% to 7.4% (Shaffer and Hall, 1996).

The National Council on Problem Gambling issued a summary of several studies that revealed adolescent pathological gambling to be associated with low grades, truancy, alcohol and drug abuse, problematic parent gamblers, and involvement in unlawful activities to finance their gambling (NGISC, 1999). Studies cite the reasons for problematic gambling as enjoyment, excitement, and motivation to win money. Pathological gamblers cite enjoyment and excitement but also want to escape, relieve depression, and cope with loneliness without winning money as the key motivator. Among youth gamblers, males gamble three to four times more than females, and high school students gamble more than junior high school students. Furthermore, male high school students prefer sports gambling, whereas female high school students prefer gambling with lottery tickets and bingo.

Youth in America have traditionally engaged in social and informal gambling such as sports lottery tickets and bingo. Recently youth have increased gambling through unlawful access to casinos and the Internet. The most illegal gambling for American youth occurs through the Internet, done anonymously or by deceptive practices posing as adults. Studies have revealed that gambling addiction is growing fastest among high school and college-age youth than any other age group in the year 2001. The trend in youth gambling is toward more widespread occurrence throughout the United States in urban and rural areas and all socioeconomic and ethnic groups. Estimates predict that gambling addiction will increase steadily in the next decade, as will youth crime (i.e., burglary, illicit drug use), which usually occurs with gambling.

Educational and school health implications vary. Youths who gamble are involved in illegal and unlawful behavior and bring such activity to the school site. This practice contributes to an antisocial culture and environment that requires more adult supervision, school security surveillance, and administrative discipline. Gambling youth tend to lose interest in academic and regular study to achieve passing grades. The lure of "quick and easy" money is a disincentive for youth to invest in educational approaches to later vocational and career opportunities as an adult. Truancy and school dropout are more likely with gambling youth in pursuit of more pleasurable activity. Often the associated personality and behavior disorders are untreated and therefore create complicated health and mental health problems (e.g., depression, conduct disorders, obsessive compulsive disorders).

Action plans for the school nurse and other staff include the following:
1. Work together to develop a uniform and integrated gambling prevention strategy.
2. Develop a positive discipline code and an array of corrective and remedial services that can be implemented throughout the school district.
3. Recommend detection and profiling of high-risk youth as for other youth.
4. High-risk youth should be given more targeted services for recovery and resiliency.
5. Serve as advocate for more community, statewide, and national remedies to prevent youth access to adult gambling sources.

PRECOCIOUS PUBERTY

Precocious puberty is the development of secondary sexual characteristics before age 8 in girls and age 9 in boys. This atypical variation has been reported in girls as young as 3 years. Development of breasts and growth of axillary and pubic hair in 5- to 8-year-old children are not isolated phenomena or statistical outliers but actual concerns of parents, nurses, HCPs, and other school professionals. Other characteristics include accelerated development of external genitalia and changes in behavior. Girls experienced increased moodiness and irritability, whereas boys may develop a sex drive and become more aggressive and hyperactive than their peers. Boys develop more body mass, body hair, and have deeper voices.

Precocious puberty may occur as a result of an underlying condition, such as a hypothalamic tumor or disorder of the adrenal glands, but the cause generally is unknown. The recent increase in idiopathic precocious puberty causes alarming concerns for physical, psychological, and social effects in the child because all developmental stages take an upward spiral from the norm. The increase is so new that etiological research lags, although several theories exist. These theories include better nutrition; an association between weight gain and early development; the presence of hormones found in milk and meat; exposure to dichlorodiphenyldichloroethylene (DDE), a by-product of the chemical dichlorodiphenyltrichloroethane (DDT), banned in 1972, or polychlorinated biphenyls (PCBs), which are chemicals used in electrical equipment as a flame retardant; or contact with phthalates, chemicals found in certain plastics.

Regardless of the cause, evaluation of precocious puberty for possible treatment is necessary. When no underlying cause is found, assessment of bone age determines the need for treatment. Children with precocious puberty with advanced bone age experience early rapid growth that plateaus in adolescence. If untreated, males typically do not exceed 5 feet 2 inches as an adult and females usually are only about 5 ft tall.

In middle elementary students, precocious puberty is an antecedent to a host of psychosocial and relational issues affecting age-appropriate self-care, mastery of social skills, moral conduct, and peer group acceptance. These issues have been documented in the health literature as it relates to females, including reference to negative body images, engaging in sexual activity and acting out behavior, negative mood and depression, and a greater risk for eating disorders. Precocious female development differs by racial group; white adolescents experience a greater decrease in self-worth than African-American females (Rosenthal, Lewis, and Biro, 2000).

Precocious puberty for both male and female students increases their risk for early sexual activity, sexual harassment, transmission of sexually transmitted diseases, and childhood pregnancy risk. Marginal peer relationships and exposure to older adolescent and adult relationships also contribute to confusing sex, romance, intimacy, and love issues. Males face issues of masculine identity, whereas both sexes face premature readiness for exclusive dating and committed relationships with the opposite sex and the prospect of assuming parenting obligations before attaining necessary personal, educational, and economic resources.

School nurse practice focuses on supporting and providing health care and knowledge to students with advanced psychosexual development. Services provided to the students include the following:

1. Education about sexual hygiene and self-care according to student's developmental age, not grade level.
2. Monitoring of growth anthropometry.
3. Provision for "safe sex" for youth if and when sexual experimentation and activity occur.
4. Sensitization of school staff to the implications and consequences of precocious puberty.
5. Prevention and intervention for sexual harassment with or without peer group verbal and social discriminatory behaviors.
6. Provision of adult guidance to student related to precocious puberty.
7. Referral of the student to social, family counseling, and mental health services as needed.

Web Sites

The Magic Foundation for Children's Growth
    708-383-0808
    http://www.magicfoundation.org/cpp.html

PHYSICAL AND MENTAL HEALTH

Bipolar disorder (BPD), or manic depression, and obsessive compulsive disorder (OCD) are common disorders diagnosed in adults. However, the related behaviors of these disorders are observed and diagnosed in very young children and students in elementary school, secondary school, and high school.

For early identification and treatment and a clearer prognosis, nurses can do the following:

1. Increase their knowledge and be alert to signs, symptoms, and treatment regimens unique to schools.
2. Provide leadership in educating school faculty, administrators, and other involved staff.
3. Increase understanding of the disorder and continue support to the student and the family.

BIPOLAR DISORDER OR MANIC-DEPRESSIVE DISORDER

Children with BPD are characterized by increased self-esteem and inflated personal worth, decreased sleep, talkativeness or rapid speech, excessive motor activity or overactivity, and distractibility with periods of low mood, introspection, loneliness, social withdrawal, and generally sad affect.

BPD usually is diagnosed in adults, and in the past rarely was diagnosed in children and adolescents, especially before age 13. Recent clinical and epidemiological research has documented an increasing prevalence of BPD in late adolescence. Studies by researchers at the National Institute of Mental Health cite that BPD affects 1 in 1000 children and increases in frequency during late adolescence and young adulthood to a rate of 1 in 100 adults (Swedo and Leonard, 1999).

Cyclothymic disorder often is a precursor to the mood disorder and is more common during adolescence, especially in girls. Dysthymia, another mood disorder, also is increasingly diagnosed in children and adolescents. Both cyclothymic and dysthymic disorders can be easily misdiagnosed for bipolar disorder, especially with concurrent hyperactivity.

OBSESSIVE COMPULSIVE DISORDER

OCD is a biologically based mental disorder among children who have a pattern of obsessions or worrisome thoughts and compulsions or consuming rituals. These children and adolescents are bothered with bad thoughts related to dirt, germs, and other contaminants, as well as ideas of harm, violence, and moral wrongdoing. Therefore they have feelings of inadequacy and worthlessness and self-condemning thoughts. The repetitive rituals are performed or enacted by the child to relieve the anxiety and fears caused by the obsessions. These rituals include handwashing, cleaning, checking, counting, and confessing on a repetitive basis.

OCD is more common in adolescence and can be a precursor to a diagnosis of obsessive compulsive personality in adults, as with cyclothymia and bipolar disorder. Children, especially young children, generally do not have an awareness of the disorder as do adults. Furthermore, the association of the obsession with the compulsions in childhood OCD is less clear than for adults. Most children in elementary years are aware of their obsessive thinking and view it as "stupid or dumb," causing them embarrassment and discomfort in social situations. Younger children usually are less secretive about their compulsions and more overt in their expressions. Children express their compulsions with more irritability and moodiness than adolescents or adults. They also have more mental rituals (i.e., cognitive repetitions in their mind that are not visible to an adult or peers, such as counting exercises, reciting of phrases). Some children have vocal tics similar to Tourette's syndrome. Many clinicians conceptualize that OCD is related to trichotillomania and Tourette's syndrome. Tics and obsessive compulsive symptoms occur together in a majority of children; more than two thirds of children with OCD have tics, and 50% to 75% of children with Tourette's disorder have obsessive compulsive symptoms (Swedo and Leonard, 1999).

Web Sites

The Obsessive Compulsive Foundation
>203-315-2190
>http://www.ocfoundation.org/index.html

Madison Institute of Medicine
>http://www.miminc.org/index.html

National Depressive and Manic-Depressive Association
>1-800-826-3632
>http://www.ndmda.org/index.html

TERRORISM

DOMESTIC HOMELAND TERRORISM

Given the threat of domestic terrorism in the United States, the school nurse must be a resource to the school population, both students and staff, for preventive and triage health services. When terrorists attack the school site, community, or other regions of the country, the physical safety, emotional well-being, and moral integrity of the school population is at risk. As a member of the crisis response team at the school and in the community, the school nurse should be prepared to implement public health services. A central focus of this service includes first aid and crisis management for the psychosocial trauma that results from the act of terrorism. Every county and district school office currently is organizing systemwide responses to acts of terrorism, and the school nurse can be involved as a policy maker and health care practitioner in this organized endeavor.

An adequate trauma response by the school nurse includes the following measures:

1. Provide realistic, yet reassuring, information about the terrorism that is reliable and up-to-date.
2. Focus on provision of calm and caring for the fears and the grief of students and staff.
3. Promote dialogue about the morality of terrorism and its implications for trust, meaning in life, and personal security in a time of threat and violence.
4. Facilitate peer support, family care, and neighborhood goodwill for a functional and practical sense of safety and security.

5. Educate on the consequences of horrific and tragic life experiences as related to acute stress disorder (ASD), posttraumatic stress syndrome (PTSS), and other mental health disorders.
6. Understand that some fear is good. Fear is an evolutionary survival mechanism, but fear that is not remedied by environmental relief or physical actions can lead to detrimental changes to the brain and mental disorganization, leading to dysfunction in the school setting and learning.
7. Advocate for useful research, relevant technology, and effective national or community response to future terrorism.

BIOTERRORISM: ANTHRAX AND OTHER BIOTERRORISM THREATS

I. **Definition**
 A. Anthrax is an acute infectious disease that can be manifest in three forms: inhalational, cutaneous, and gastrointestinal. Exposure means an individual has come into contact with spores, and infection means that the spores are multiplying in the body. Spores may reside on the skin, in the alveoli of the lungs, or in the gastrointestinal tract.

II. **Etiology**
 A. Anthrax is caused by bacterium *Bacillus anthracis*. It is spread by inhalation of the bacterium, handling infected animals or their products, or eating infected meat. The bacteria can be found naturally in the soil and forms a protective coat called *spores*. The spores can remain viable for years and can be stored and transported easily.

III. **Health Concerns/Emergencies**
 A. Difficulty in recognition and diagnosis.
 B. Delay in treating pulmonary/inhalation anthrax usually leads to death.

IV. **Management/Treatment**
 A. Obtain history to differentiate exposure to flu versus anthrax exposure.
 B. Observe for skin lesions with painless black scab bordered by vesicles.
 C. Be aware of flu symptoms and respiratory symptoms without rhinitis, chest pain, seizures without a prior history; shock may indicate inhalational anthrax.
 D. Be aware of pain with swallowing, vomiting, diarrhea.
 E. If any suspicion call parent(s) and refer to HCP.
 F. Treatment is symptomatic.
 G. Standard/universal precautions should be used in the care of students with suspected infection.
 H. Prophylaxis and treatment regimens are the same for all type exposures and for all ages of individuals. Prophylaxis is given after confirmed exposure.
 I. Pediatric treatment initially is the same medication and can be given intravenously or orally. The treatment of choice is ciprofloxacin (Cipro) every 12 hours and doxycycline (Vibramycin) two times a day, both for 60 days.
 J. Treatment is administered for 60 days to eradicate spores.

Table 10-1 *Characteristics of Anthrax*

Anthrax Type	Incubation Period	Transmission	Symptoms	Complications	Mortality Rate
Inhalational Most severe form	2-7 days; may be up to 60 days	By inhalation of aerosolized or airborne spores Not known to be spread from person to person	Prodromal: brief, flulike respiratory symptoms, cough, fatigue, muscle aches (runny nose or discharge is rare), vomiting, possible chest pain, followed by development of dyspnea, low blood pressure, shock	Sepsis or meningitis	High—90% Death can follow within 36 hr after occurrence of respiratory distress
Cutaneous	1-12 days	Through cut or opening in skin Not known to be spread from person to person	Evolves from papule, to vesicle, to depressed eschar (black scab) Usually painless Other symptoms include fever, malaise, headache, and regional adenopathy Usually 3-7 days for eschar to develop	Can lead to sepsis, meningitis, thrombocytopenia, and anemia, severe edema (head and neck), secondary bacterial infection causing cellulitis and lymphadenitis	20% without treatment and less than 1% with antibiotic treatment
Gastrointestinal	1-7 days	Eating raw or undercooked contaminated meat or drinking contaminated water Not known to be spread from person to person	Overall symptoms: severe abdominal pain, fever, signs of septicemia Oral pharyngeal forms: lesions at base of tongue, dysphagia, fever, regional lymphadenopathy Abdominal form: nausea, loss of appetite, fever, abdominal pain, hematemesis, bloody diarrhea	Systemic toxicity, sepsis, shock, and meningitis	Estimated 25% to 60% Early antibiotic effectiveness unknown

K. A vaccine is available; not known to be effective against inhalational anthrax. The vaccine is not recommended for the general public and is given to at-risk populations (e.g., military personnel, veterinarians, laboratory workers). A new vaccine is being developed.

L. Anthrax is a reportable disease.

M. Local health departments can provide information regarding the disease, who should receive antibiotics, and when.

V. **Additional Information**

A. Future development of an alarm system that will sound when the air-handling system is contaminated or when a biological agent is released into a public space is being explored.

B. *Centers for Disease Control and Prevention (CDC)* recommendations for letter or package suspected of biological contamination:

1. *For closed contamination, powder:*

   a. Do not shake or empty contents.

   b. Place in plastic bag to prevent leaking or spreading or cover with clothing, trash can, or available object.

   c. Leave room, close door, and restrict others from area.

   d. Wash hands.

   e. Report to building supervisor, principal, custodian, and local police.

   f. List all people who were in the room or may have been exposed; make list available to law enforcement and public health officials.

2. *For powder spread:*

   a. If powder leaks, cover it immediately, do not attempt to clean up.

   b. Leave room, close door, and restrict others from area.

   c. Wash hands.

   d. Report to building supervisor, principal, custodian, and local police.

   e. Remove contaminated clothing and place in a plastic bag and seal; make available to emergency responders for proper handling.

   f. Shower with soap and water as soon as possible.

   g. List all people who were in the room or may have been exposed; make list available to law enforcement and public health officials.

VI. **Web Sites**

Centers for Disease Control and Prevention
http://www.cdc.gov

Federal Emergency Management Agency—Fact Sheet
http://www.fema.gov/library/terrorf.htm

Kaiser Permanente Medical Group
http://www.kp.org/members/bioterrorism.html

Terrorism and Children—Purdue Extension
http://www.ces.purdue.edu/terrorism/children/

Terrorism Research Center
http://www.terrorism.com/index.shtml

Table 10-2			Other Bioterrorism Diseases and Clinical Data		
Disease	Etiology Incubation Period	Transmission	Symptoms and Complications	Treatment	Mortality Rate
Smallpox	Variola virus 7-17 days; virus is fragile and inactivated in 1-2 days Prior infection provides lifelong immunity	By infected saliva, from handling infected clothing, or bedding; it can be airborne Most infectious first week after rash appears, risk of transmission lasts until all scabs are off	High fever, headache and backaches, malaise; flat lesions become pustules on face and/or torso; scabs develop and fall off in 3-4 weeks; delirium and abdominal pain In early stages may be misdiagnosed as chickenpox Smallpox rash erupts quickly beginning in mouth/throat, progressing downward, occurs on palms and soles of feet	Vaccination up to 4 days after exposure, no available pharmaceutical treatment New vaccine being developed	30%
Botulism	Clostridium botulinum bacillus Symptoms start 12-36 hr after exposure, can be several days Inhalation is 24-72 hr	Ingestion of improperly prepared or canned food; not spread person to person, found in human feces	Early signs are double or blurred vision, slurred speech, and muscle weakness; progressive limb paralysis and respiratory failure, normal mental status Symptoms may be similar to food-borne exposure, vomiting, constipation, or diarrhea	Equine antitoxins can stop progression; ventilator for respiratory failure; a vaccine is being researched	5%-8%

Disease	Agent	Transmission	Symptoms	Treatment	Mortality
Hemorrhagic fevers	Various viruses	Some spread by arthropods, others by infected humans or animals	Vary according to virus; can include coma, bleeding, and shock	No treatment for Ebola virus; antiviral ribavirin often helpful with other viruses. Ebola vaccine being researched	Varies
Pneumonic plague	*Yersinia pestis* bacillus. Pulmonary exposure symptoms occur 1-3 days, flea-borne 2-8 days	Spread by respiratory droplets; person-to-person; known to be spread from infected rodents to humans by infected fleas	Headache, malaise, weakness, productive cough, chest pain, fever, chills progressing to pneumonia in 2-4 days; septic shock, death; early treatment critical	*Antibiotics:* streptomycin, tetracycline (Achromycin), chloramphenicol (Chloromycetin) and doxycycline (Vibramycin). Prophylactic antibiotics for 7 days to protect those exposed. New vaccine being developed	50%-90%, if untreated, 15% with diagnosis and treatment
Tularemia	*Francisella tularensis* bacillus. One of the most infectious pathogenic bacteria. Incubation 1-14 days	Bite of infective arthropod, handling infected animal tissues or fluids, direct contact with/or ingestion of contaminated food, water, or soil, and inhalation of infective aerosols. Acquired through skin, mucous membranes, lungs, and gastrointestinal tract	Fever, fatigue, chills, headache, sore throat, weakness, and weight loss; pharyngitis, bronchitis, and pneumonia	*Antibiotics:* streptomycin, gentamicin (Garamycin), doxycycline, (Vibramycin) ciprofloxacin (Cipro). Vaccine under review by FDA	30%-60% for untreated inhalational; less than 2% when treated

Data from Centers for Disease Control, Public Health Emergency Preparedness and Response, Fact Sheets; Kaiser Permanente Medical Group: *Anthrax guidelines update #12*, October 31, 2001.
When bacterial or viral diseases are used for bioterrorism, they may be aerosolized or spread in water.

BIBLIOGRAPHY

American Academy of Pediatrics, Committee on School Health: Qualifications and utilization of nursing personnel delivering health services in schools, *Pediatrics* 79(4):647-648, 1987.

American Academy of Pediatrics: *Children, bioterrorism, and disaster,* Nov 20, 2001, Available online: http://www.aap.org/advocacy/releases/cad.htm. Accessed on Dec 2, 2001.

Anshel J: *Smart medicine for your eyes,* Garden City Park, NY, 1999, Avery.

Behrman RE, Shields MK: Children and computer technology: analysis and recommendations, *The Future of Children* 10(2):4-30, 2000.

Center for Commercial-Free Public Education: *Commercialism in the schools,* Feb 2000, Available online: http://www.commercialfree.org. Accessed on Jun 10, 2001.

Center for Health and Health Care in Schools: *1999-2000 Survey of school-based health care in schools,* Mar 14, 2001, Available online: http://www.healthinschools.org/sbhcs/sbhcs_table.htm. Accessed on Aug 5, 2001.

Centers for Disease Control and Prevention: *Public health emergency preparedness and response,* Oct 25, 2001, Available online: http://www.bt.cdc.gov. Accessed Dec 2, 2001.

Cergo S: *Computer ergonomics for elementary school,* Mar 14, 2000, Department of Consumer and Business Services, Oregon OSHA, Available online: http://www.orosha.org/cergos. Accessed on Oct 1, 2000.

Consumers Union Education Services: *Captive kids,* Yonkers, NY, 1995, Consumers Union Education Services.

CUErgo: *Children's backpack design,* March 2000, Cornell University Ergonomics Web, Available online: http://ergo.human.cornell.edu/backpacks/cubackpacks.html. Accessed on Nov 18, 2000.

CUErgo: *Workstation ergonomics guidelines for computer use by children,* Aug 5, 2000, Cornell University Ergonomics Web, Available online: http://ergo.human.cornell.edu. Accessed on Nov 6, 2000.

Dennis DT, Inglesby TV, Henderson DA, et al: Tularemia as a biological weapon: medical and public health management, *JAMA* 285:2763-2774, 2001.

Department of Health and Human Services: *Report of the surgeon general's conference on children's mental health: a national action agenda,* Jul 24, 2001, Available online: http://www.surgeongeneral.gov/cmh/.

Dryfoos JG: *Full-service schools: a revolution in health and social services for children, youth, and families,* San Francisco, 1994, Jossey-Bass.

Franklin C, Streeter CL: School reform: linking public schools with human services, *Social Work* 40:773-782, 1995.

Grimmer K, Gill T, Williams M: University of South Australia Centre for Allied Health Research, Nov 11, 1999, *High school students and backpacks: a cross sectional study,* Available online: http://www.unisa.edu.au/AlliedHealth/report1998.html. Accessed on Nov 18, 2000.

Grimmer KA, Williams MT, Gill TK: The association between adolescent head-on-neck posture, backpack weight, and anthropometric features, *Spine* 24(21):2262-2267, 1999.

Guilday P: School nursing practice today: implications for the future, *J School Nurs* 16(5):25-31, 2000.

Gurwitch RH, Silovsky JF, Schultz S, et al: *Reactions and guidelines for children following trauma/disaster,* American Psychological Association, Nov 12, 2001, Available online: http://helping.apa. org/daily/ptguidelines.html.

Henderson DA, Inglesby TV, Bartlett JG, et al: Smallpox as a biological weapon: medical and public health management. Working Group on Civilian Biodefense, *JAMA* 281:2127-2137, 1999.

Hoynes W, Pesnick S, Miller MC: *Channel One online: advertising, not educating,* Washington, DC, 1997, Center for Media Education.

Igoe J, Giardano B: *Expanding school health services to serve families in the 21st century,* Washington, DC, 1992, American Nurses Association.

Inglesby TV, Henderson DA, Bartlett JG, et al: Anthrax as a biological weapon: medical and public health management. Working Group on Civilian Biodefense, *JAMA* 281:1735-1745, 1999.

Kaiser Permanente Medical Group: *Anthrax guidelines update #12,* Oct 31, 2001, Available online: http://www.kpcmi.org/guideline_anthrax_mas.pdf.

Kelly K: Why computers fail as teachers: too much screen time can harm your child's development, *U.S. News & World Report* 12(129):48-55, 2000.

Lukefahr JL: Eluding pornographers, predators, and peddlers: Internet safety for children, *Contemp Pediatr* 16(11):141-156, 1999.

Marx E, Wooley S, Northup D: *Health is academic: a guide to coordinated school health programs,* New York, 1998, Teachers College Press.

Meyers-Walls J: *Terrorism and children,* Purdue Extension, Sep 2001, Available online: http://www.ces.purdue.edu/terrorism/children/terrorism.html. Accessed on Nov 12, 2001.

Nader PR, editor: *School health: policy and practice,* Elk Grove Village, Ill, 1997, American Academy of Pediatrics.

National Center for Missing and Exploited Children: *Internet-related child exploitation,* 2000, Available online: http://www.missingkids.com. Accessed on Jul 14, 2001.

National Center for Posttraumatic Distress Syndrome: *Terrorism and children: a National Center for PTSD fact sheet,* Sep 26, 2001, Available online: http://www.ncptsd.org/facts/disasters/fs_children_disaster.html. Accessed on Nov 12, 2001.

National Gambling Impact Study Commission: *Final report,* Aug 3, 1999, Available online: http://govinfo.library.unt.edu/ngisc/index.html. Accessed on Jun 11, 2001.

National Institute of Mental Health: *Bipolar disorder research fact sheet,* 2000, Available online: http://www.nimh.nih.gov/publicat/bipolarresfact.cfm. Accessed on Jul 22, 2001.

Olsen T, Anderson RL, Dearwater SR, et al: The epidemiology of low back pain in an adolescent population, *Am J Public Health* 82(4):606-608, 1992.

Ray B: *Home schoolers across America: academic achievement, family characteristics, and longitudinal traits,* Salem, Ore, 1997, National Home Education Research Institute.

Rosenthal S, Lewis L, Biro F: Psychosexual development. In Coupey SM, editor: *Primary care of adolescent girls,* Philadelphia, 2000, Hanley & Belfus.

Salminen J, Erkintalo MO, Pentti J, et al: Recurrent low back pain and early disc degeneration in the young, *Spine* 24(13):1316-1321, 1999.

Schwab N, Gelfman M, editors: *Legal issues in school health services: a resource for school administrators, school attorneys, school nurses,* North Branch, Minn, 2001, Sunrise River Press.

Shaffer H, Hall M: Estimating the prevalence of adolescent gambling disorders: a quantitative synthesis and guide toward standard gambling nomenclature, *J Gambl Stud* 12(2):193-196, 1996.

Stanhope M, Lancaster J: *Community health nursing: promoting health aggregates, families, and individuals,* ed 4, St Louis, 1996, Mosby.

Swedo S, Leonard H: *Is this just a phase?* New York, 1999, Golden Books.

Tsubota K, Nakamori K: Dry eyes and video display terminals, *N Engl J Med* 328(8):584, 1993 (letter).

Vacheron JJ, Poumarat G, Chandezon R, et al: Changes of contour of the spine caused by load carrying, *Surg Radiol Anat* 21(2):109-113, 1999.

Walker PH, Martinez RJ: *Excellence in mental health: a school health curriculum. A training manual for practicing school nurses and educators,* 2001, Available online: http://www.uchsc.edu/schoolhealth.

Weist MD: Expanded school mental health services: a national movement in progress. In Ollendick TH, Prinz RJ, editors: *Advances in clinical child psychology,* vol 19, New York, 1997, Plenum Press.

Wyshak G: Teenaged girls, carbonated beverage consumption, and bone fractures, *Arch Pediatr Adolesc Med* 154(6):610-613, 2000.

CHAPTER 11

Emergency Disaster Preparedness and First Aid

When student illness or emergencies occur in the school setting, the school nurse generally is called on to provide guidance. The school nurse must be knowledgeable to provide necessary care and direct others in providing first aid for both daily individual care and in emergency disaster situations. A school emergency plan for all students and staff should be in place. Individual plans should be available for specific medically involved students. These plans allow the nurse to be free from all tasks except caring for the involved student while others are helping with the necessary telephone calls and other duties. Documentation must follow all incidences regardless of severity.

This chapter provides basic information for emergency preparedness and basic first aid for many common emergency situations. When a nurse cannot be at the school site when an emergency arises, teachers or other school personnel must know how to handle such situations. The nurse can use this chapter as a teaching tool for training school staff, thereby ensuring provision of appropriate medical care and sound advice. Nurse practice acts vary by each state, county office of education, and school district; the nurse must be aware of and compliant with their individual policies and procedures.

The following are used by nurse practitioners or with physician's order and parent's signature:

1. Autoinjector with epinephrine (EpiPen; Dey Laboratories, Napa, California).
2. Diphenhydramine (Benadryl).
3. Epinephrine.
4. Acetaminophen.
5. Syrup of ipecac (in consultation with poison control).

The nurse must check individual state/county/school policies allowing particular medication items.

EMERGENCY AND DISASTER PREPAREDNESS

ORGANIZATIONAL PERSONNEL

I. Incident Commander: Head Administrator on Site
   A. Coordinates and manages all other teams in the event of an emergency.
   B. Controls internal and external communications.
   C. Accounts for the presence of all students and staff.

II. Student Management (Usually Teachers)
   A. Takes attendance and reports missing students on teacher report form.

III. First-Aid and Health Team (School Nurse and Trained Staff Members)
   A. Under supervision of school nurse and team leaders, provides first aid according to triage procedures and manages acute and chronic health problems.

471

| **Box 11-1** | *Nurse's Health Office Supplies* |

The Following Items Are Listed by A or B When Useful for the Following Kits:

A First-aid kit for classroom
B First-aid kit for field trips

First-aid manual, for classroom/field trip instructional information (A, B)
Vinyl gloves (A, B)
Mild soap
Antiseptic solution
Hydrogen peroxide
Sodium bicarbonate
Hypoallergenic adhesive tape, several sizes (B)
Elastic (Ace) wraps, 2- and 4-in (B)
Gauze rolls, stretch (B)
Gauze squares, different sizes
Triangular bandage
Adhesive bandages (Band-Aids), various sizes; Steri-Strips, butterfly bandages (A, B)
Cotton balls (A, B)
Cotton applicators
Tongue blades (A)
Combine dressings (ABD pads) for heavy bleeding (B)
Topical skin powders/adhesives for lacerations or wounds (B)

Splints, small, medium, and large
Tweezers
Cold packs, instant
Moistened towelettes
Antibacterial hand soap (B)
Sunscreen (B)
Eye cup
Eye pads
Bottle of eye irrigation solution
Contact lens case (B)
Paper cups
Red plastic bags
Small plastic bags, resealable plastic bag (A, B)
Scissors (A, B)
Thermometer
Matches
Penlight (B)
Blanket, lightweight, washable
Bleach
Sanitary napkins
Disposable protective gown and or apron
Protective eyeglasses
Mouth-to-mouth resuscitator (one-way valve) (A, B)

    B. Documents treatment and disposition of students and staff on nurse's emergency forms.
IV. Security Team (Usually Custodians)
    A. Secures and patrols all entrances to the site.
    B. Shuts off gas, water, and electricity.
    C. Prevents community members from entering site without permission.
    D. Directs emergency vehicles and directs parents to reunion gate.
V. Search and Rescue Teams (Can Be Teachers or as Assigned)
    A. Rescue the injured.
    B. Check for and control dangerous situations resulting from the disaster.
VI. Reunion Team (Usually Clerical Staff)
    A. Reunites students with parents and documents all releases.
VII. Public Information Officer (Usually Assistant Principal or Administrator)
    A. Collects all communication for incident commander.
    B. Signs in media personnel.

FORMS AND PROCEDURES

I. **Emergency Health Cards for Students and Staff, Including Health Information and Contact Numbers**
II. **Documentation Forms**
   A. Teacher report forms.
   B. Nurse's emergency forms.
   C. Release forms—to whom and where.
III. **School Site Map with Locations Marked as Listed Below**
   A. Emergency operations center.
   B. Emergency assembly areas (students).
   C. First-aid area.
   D. Reunion gate.
   E. Morgue.
   F. Location of emergency equipment and shut-off valves for gas, water, electricity.

STAFF RESPONSIBILITIES

Prior arrangements should be made for family members in case of emergency. Students may need to remain on the school site for up to 72 hours. State laws vary. The nurse should maintain personal supplies in a classroom or another designated area, such as car (except medications). The following items should be available.
   1. Change of clothing, sturdy shoes, and warm jacket
   2. Blanket
   3. Water and food supplies
   4. Heavy gloves
   5. Flashlight/batteries
   6. Glasses and/or materials to care for contact lenses
   7. Medications
I. **Water Purification Methods**
   A. Empty bleach bottles—add water without rinsing; expires in 1 year.
   B. Water purification tablets—follow directions (available at sporting goods stores and drug stores).
   C. Unscented bleach—add 16 drops per gallon or 1 tsp per 5 gallons of water.
   D. Rolling boil for 10 minutes.
II. **Student Comfort Packs**
   A. Request comfort pack from parents for each child at beginning of school year. Can send home a gallon zippered plastic bag with list of suggested items to include: food options (high-protein foods, small hard candies, avoid salty snacks), pictures of family members, favorite book, small package of facial tissue, and so forth, plus small comfort note written by parent if elementary or younger student. Include note from parent indicating any allergies and regular medications taken at home. A 3-day supply of medications should be kept in the nurse's office. The comfort bag and medications should be returned home at the end of the school year. Comfort packs are kept in classroom emergency supply container.

Box 11-2   *Emergency Equipment*

Job description clipboards for teams
Vests to identify teams
Stretchers: 1 for every 150 persons
Two-way radios to search area
System to mark areas that have been
  searched (e.g., red tape on doorknob)
Tables and chairs for emergency opera-
  tions center and reunification teams
Marking pens, paper, pencils
Leather gloves
Crowbar (full-size)
Shovel
Short-handled axe
Short-handled sledge hammer
Set of screwdrivers
Pipe wrench, 14-in
12-hour snap light (friction)
One 5.5-lb fire extinguisher
Gray tape, duct tape
Whistle, bullhorn
Box safety matches in waterproof
  container
Small votive candles

Multipurpose pocket knife (e.g., Swiss
  army knife)
Can opener
AM/FM portable radio and batteries
50 ft of nylon cord (braided)
Individual handheld personal warmth
  packets (HotHands; Heatmax, Inc.,
  Dalton, Georgia); shake to activate
1 pair protective glasses
Ground cover/tarps
Portable toilets: 1 per 150 persons,
  21 bags, 10 rolls of toilet tissue
or
Deluxe water sanitation kit. Toileting
  supplies includes emergency bucket,
  deodorant, plastic bags, toilet paper,
  and adhesive tape sealer.
Water supplies: 1 gallon per day per
  person—2 quarts for drinking and
  2 quarts for sanitation and food
  preparation. 50-gallon drums of water
  are available for purchase.

III. First-Aid Supplies*
   A. 4 × 4-in compresses: 1000 per 500 students
   B. 8 × 10-in compresses: 150 per 500 students
   C. Sponge wound dressing (Kerlix; Kendall Products, Mansfield, Massa-
      chusetts) or bandaging: 12 per 500 students
   D. Elastic (Ace) wrap bandage: 2-in: 12 per 500 students; 4-in: 12 per 500
      students
   E. Triangular bandage: 24 per 500 students
   F. Cardboard splints: 24 each—small, medium, large
   G. Cardiopulmonary resuscitation (CPR) pocket masks, deluxe
   H. Ice packs: instant
   I. Tapes: 1-in cloth: 50 rolls per 1000 students; 2-in cloth: 24 per 1000
      students
   J. Wound closure strips (Steri-Strips; 3M, Minneapolis, Minnesota) or
      butterfly bandages: 50 per 500 students.
   K. Triple-antibiotic ointment (Neosporin): 144 squeeze packs per 1000
      students
   L. Hydrogen peroxide: 10 pints per 500 students
   M. Antiseptic
   N. Towelettes

---

*First-aid supplies must follow the laws related to the delivery of nursing care in each state.

Box 11-3	*Rapid Triage Treatment for Injured*

Tag system for injured and triage conditions

Tag guidelines: Can be seen from a distance and cannot be damaged by liquids

Red: Immediate Care

Delayed capillary refill (greater than 2 sec)

Unable to follow simple commands

Respirations present only after opening airway; or greater than 30/minute

Major lacerations with extensive hemorrhage

Open fractures of major bones

Critical injuries to respiratory tract or central nervous system (CNS)

Severe burns

Ionizing radiation

Yellow: Delayed Care

Any living injured person not fitting into red or green categories

Fractures or minor burns

Major lacerations without extensive hemorrhage

Green: Walking Wounded

All injured persons not requiring hospital intervention

Black: Dead and Nonsavable

No respirations present even after attempting to reposition the airway

State law may require that a body not be removed, searched, or undressed until released by the coroner, unless it presents a hazard or hinders care of others.

Modified from *START simple triage and rapid treatment: a race with time,* Newport Beach, Calif, 1994, Hoag Hospital and Newport Beach Fire and Marine.

    O. Waterless antibacterial hand wash
    P. Unscented bleach, 1 bottle
    Q. Paramedic scissors (for cutting through heavy materials): 4 per campus
    R. Tweezers: 3 assorted per campus
    S. Triage tags: 50 per 500 students
    T. Oval eye patch: 50 per 1000 students
    U. Dust masks: 25 per 100 students
    V. First-aid books: 2 standard and 2 advanced per campus
    W. Vinyl gloves: 100 per 500 students
    X. Heavy duty rubber gloves, 4 pairs
NOTE: To disinfect rubber gloves, use 1 part bleach per 10 parts of water.
  IV. **Individual Classroom Supplies (keep in clean trash cans with lids)**
    A. Current list of classroom students.
    B. Permanent marker and note pads.
    C. Masking tape to put name on each student.
    D. Package hard candy (1-2 lb).
    E. Flashlight and batteries.
    F. Paper cups.
    G. Leather gloves: 1 pair.
    H. Vinyl gloves.
    I. Sunscreen SPF 15 or higher.
    J. Supplies for maintenance of body heat for each person (thermal blanket, aluminum or large garbage bags to wrap up in).
    K. Diapers and special feeding supplies for very young or disabled students.

L. Large card identifying teacher, grade, and room number for display to facilitate reunification.

NOTE: The nurse should be included in the preparation of all school emergency planning. Provision of disaster supplies must be coordinated between the nurse and school staff.

During emergency drills, check expiration date of supplies.

ABDOMINAL PAIN

I. **Immediate First Aid**
   A. Have the student lie down; keep student warm and quiet.
   B. Obtain appropriate history regarding onset, circumstances, and duration of pain; note presence of fever, nausea, vomiting, guarding, abdominal rigidity, constipation, or diarrhea.
   C. Determine type of pain: dull, diffuse, sharp, localized, continuous, or intermittent.
   D. Do not give student anything to eat or drink.
   E. Notify parent and urge parent to seek immediate medical care if pain is severe, persistent, or if history indicates a pathological condition.

BEE, WASP, YELLOW JACKET, AND HORNET STINGS

Any stings by bees, wasps, yellow jackets, or hornets can present a life-threatening emergency; therefore special precautions are necessary when administering first aid. If a child is known to be sensitive or allergic to bee stings, keep an *emergency bee sting kit* at the school site and take it on all field trips. More than one individual, including the student, should be trained in the proper administration of the injection. After the injection is given, call 911.

I. **Immediate First Aid**
   A. Remove stinger as soon as possible, keeping it intact by brushing it out as gently as possible with hand or piece of cardboard if available. Speed is essential. Do not delay removal to hunt for material; use thumb and forefinger to pull the stinger directly out if necessary.
   B. Pinching or use of tweezers; may inject venom.
   C. Wash with soap and water.
   D. Apply ice, ice water, cold wash cloth, or paste of sodium bicarbonate (baking soda).
   E. Notify parent(s).
II. **Symptoms of Allergic Systemic Reaction**
   A. Flushed skin.
   B. Puffy face, mouth, or eyelids.
NOTE: At this time administer medication to anyone with known sensitivity; often symptoms do not appear in any given order.
   C. Hives or extensive skin rash.
   D. Difficulty breathing or swallowing or hoarseness.
   E. Sneezing or coughing.
   F. Asthmalike wheezing.
   G. Generalized swelling.
   H. Gastrointestinal complaints, dizziness, confusion, or weakness.

III. **Procedure for Allergic Reaction Action Depends on Severity of Distress**
   A. Give antihistamine, if not contraindicated on student health record; some states/school districts/counties require medical order (either generic or child-specific).
   B. If student is in respiratory distress, has compromised breathing episodes, or other severe symptoms, see **B, D, F,** and **H** in previous list; call 911.
   C. Notify parent(s).

WARM-BLOODED ANIMAL BITES

I. **Immediate First Aid**
   A. Capture animal if it can be done safely; if not, have someone follow animal so that authorities can capture it later. The animal must be kept under observation for 14 days to rule out rabies.
   B. Rinse wound immediately under running water; scrub wound thoroughly with soap and water; repeat procedure three to four times. Cleaning of the bite is important to remove animal's saliva.
   C. Notify parent(s); inform them of importance of consulting their local physician.
   D. Report the bite to state or county health department and follow their instructions (*incubation period* in humans for rabies can range from 10 days to 1 year).

HUMAN BITES

Wounds caused by human bites, especially if they are deep and penetrating, are extremely dangerous because they can infect a person with bacteria.

I. **Immediate First Aid**
   A. If wound is bleeding freely, allow bleeding for 3 to 4 seconds, then irrigate wound under running water.
   B. Wash wound with soap and water (preferably antiseptic soap).
   C. Let wound dry and apply sterile dressing.
   D. Further treatment depends on hepatitis B immunization information regarding both individuals.
   E. Human immunodeficiency virus (HIV) transfer is a threat, and victim, perpetrator, or both may need testing depending on county/district/school policy.
   F. Notify parents and urge them to contact their physician; alert parents to signs of possible infection.

INSECT BITES

Bites from insects such as mosquitoes, fleas, and chiggers can cause swelling, irritation, and redness. Impetigo can occur as a result of scratching the bites.

I. **Immediate First Aid**
   A. Wash with soap and water.
   B. If the bite is swollen or inflamed, cover it with ice pack or cool compress.

C. Chiggers are tiny red mites usually found on legs and around the belt line; itching lasts 5 to 6 days but can persist for months (chiggers can live in tall grass and weeds).

D. If no systemic allergic reaction occurs, follow procedures for bee and wasp stings.

E. Notify parent(s).

TICK BITES

Ticks can transmit bacteria of several diseases, including Lyme disease (diagnosed in almost every state) and Rocky Mountain spotted fever, which occurs in temperate zones. Ticks are found in shrubs, grasses, vines, and brush and attach themselves to humans and animals. They adhere tenaciously to the skin or scalp. All parts of the tick must be removed. If mouth fragments or proboscis is left in the skin, local symptoms will develop. Ticks are small, brown blood-sucking mites (arachnids). Evidence suggests that the longer the infected tick remains attached, the greater the chance of disease transmission.

I. **Immediate First Aid**

A. Carefully and quickly remove tick with tweezers or gloved fingers in one motion grasping close to the skin, being careful to remove all parts of the insect. Save tick for identification of possible serious disease transmission.

B. Gently scrub area from which tick was found to remove any bacteria present on skin.

C. Do not apply heat (lighted match or cigarette) to tick's body or cover with any type of oil, alcohol, or other such liquids. These methods may leave tick parts in the wound, injure the victim's skin, or cause more complications.

D. If student must stay in school and tick has not been removed, cover it with a dressing. The tick should be removed as soon as possible. The risk of infection increases between 24 to 72 hours after the tick attaches to the skin.

E. Notify parent(s) and educate them regarding disease transmission and signs of infection.

BLEEDING

I. **Immediate First Aid**

A. Place thick sterile gauze pad directly over wound (if sterile material is not available, use cleanest cloth or material available and use gloved hands).

B. If bleeding is severe and continuous, apply pressure directly over the wound until bleeding stops; elevate above victim's heart level, if feasible.

C. Never remove initial dressing; if additional dressings are needed, place them over the old dressing; continue direct hand pressure even more firmly if bleeding persists.

D. Notify parents of injury; recommendations to parents depend on the extent of injury (e.g., immediate care for suturing or observation for infection).

BLISTERS
I. Immediate First Aid
A. If blister has not ruptured and surrounding area is clean, apply only sterile gauze dressing; do not attempt to open blister.
B. If area is dirty, clean blister and surrounding area with soap and water, rinse and apply sterile dressing.
C. If blister is open, clean surrounding area with soap and water, rinse and cover with sterile dressing.
D. Notify parent(s).

BRUISES
I. Immediate First Aid
A. Immediately apply cold compresses or ice bag to reduce swelling and relieve pain; elevate bruised part if possible.
B. Notify parent(s).

BURNS
First-degree burns are superficial and cause the skin to turn red (e.g., sunburn, scalding). Such burns may cause pain and mild swelling and blanch with pressure but are not a major medical problem because they heal rapidly, affecting only the epidermis. Individuals with severe sunburn should receive medical care as soon as possible.

Second-degree burns are deeper than first-degree burns, painful, and split or blister the skin layers and cause swelling. The skin is red or mottled and blanches with pressure. The skin also may appear wet because of the loss of plasma through the damaged layers of skin. Second-degree burns affect the epidermis and dermis.

Third-degree burns destroy all layers of the skin and extend into deeper tissues. They are painless because nerve endings have been destroyed. These burns appear white and charred, swollen but dry, and do not blanch to touch.
I. Immediate First Aid
A. First degree, superficial burn:
1. Remove rings, bracelets, or any constricting jewelry before swelling occurs. Place burned area under cold running water or put ice packs or cold compresses on area (cover them before placing on skin).
2. Repeat step 2 until pain stops.
3. Cover burn with sterile gauze or clean dressing.
4. Do not apply any ointments.
5. Notify parent(s).

B. Second-degree, partial-thickness burn.
1. Remove rings, bracelets, or any constricting jewelry before swelling occurs.
2. Run cool running water over burned area or put cold compresses on area until the pain subsides (but *not* directly on skin).
3. Cover with sterile gauze or clean dressing.
4. If arms or legs are burned, elevate them above victim's heart level.
5. Do not apply ointments or attempt to break blisters or remove tissue.
6. Notify parent(s) and recommend that the student be seen by primary care provider.
C. Third-degree, full-thickness burn.
1. Activate emergency medical services (EMS) and notify parent(s).
2. Remove rings, bracelets, or any constricting jewelry before swelling occurs.
3. Do not attempt to remove garments that are clinging to area; cut around them.
4. Do not apply cold water, cold compresses, ice packs, or ointments.
5. Cover area with sterile gauze or clean cloth.
6. If legs or arms are burned, elevate them above victim's heart level if possible.
7. Keep student warm, calm, and reassured.
8. If necessary, treat student for shock or administer CPR.
9. Check immunization records for current tetanus vaccine.

CHEMICAL BURNS

Chemical burns in schools can occur in chemistry, shop, photography, or automobile classes.
  I. Immediate First Aid
A. Activate EMS and notify parent(s).
B. If possible, immediately remove all contaminated clothing.
C. Run water over area for at least 15 minutes.
D. Cover burn area with sterile dressing.

CHEMICAL BURNS OF THE EYE

  I. Immediate First Aid
A. Flush eye with tap water for 15 minutes. While flushing the eye, notify parent(s) and arrange transportation of student to hospital emergency department.
B. If person is lying down, turn head to side and pour water into eye, from inner corner of eye outward; hold eye open and do not wash chemical toward other eye.
C. Immobilize eye by covering it with dry dressing.
D. If possible, cover both eyes.
E. Alkali burns of the eye can be caused by drain cleaner, laundry and dishwasher detergent, or other cleansing agents; an eye may appear

only slightly injured but later may become deeply inflamed and develop tissue damage with possible loss of sight.

DISLODGED CONTACT LENS

I. Immediate First Aid
   A. Gently push on eyelid to manipulate lens into proper position.
   B. If necessary, use eye irrigation solution or sterile saline solution to facilitate free movement of the lens.

DIABETES MELLITUS

A child with diabetes may face two serious emergencies: *insulin reaction (hypoglycemia)* or *diabetic coma (hyperglycemia)*. Insulin reaction has a *rapid* onset, usually within minutes or a few hours; diabetic coma (acidosis) develops *gradually* over a few hours or days. Insulin reaction is the usual school emergency because of the sudden onset of symptoms. The two conditions must be distinguished because two separate procedures should be followed. If in doubt regarding the condition, give glucagon because it will not be harmful if not needed.

Insulin reaction is caused by too much insulin, not eating enough food, unusual amount of exercise, or a delayed meal. Diabetic coma is caused by too little insulin, failure to follow diet, infection, fever, or emotional stress. Symptoms vary with individual students.

I. Signs of Insulin Reaction (Rapid Onset)
   A. Excessive sweating or faintness.
   B. Headache.
   C. Hunger.
   D. Pounding of heart; trembling; impaired vision.
   E. Irritability.
   F. Personality change.
   G. Inability to waken.

II. Immediate First Aid for Insulin Reaction
   A. Give sugar or any food containing sugar (e.g., juice, candy); follow with protein source such as cheese.
   B. Do not give student insulin.
   C. Give glucagon (as per individual student's instructions, standing orders, or nurse practice act/state educational requirements) if student loses consciousness (do not give foods or fluids by mouth).
   D. Call parent(s).

III. Signs of Diabetic Coma (Slow Onset)
   A. Increased thirst and urination.
   B. Weakness; abdominal pains; centralized aches.
   C. Loss of appetite; nausea and vomiting.
   D. Large amount of sugar and ketones in urine when urine is tested.
   E. Sweet-smelling breath.

IV. Immediate First Aid for Diabetic Coma
   A. Activate EMS and notify parent(s).

FOREIGN BODY IN EAR

I. **Immediate First Aid**
  A. Notify parents and urge treatment.
  B. Do not attempt to remove object, rinse or flush ear, or put anything into ear.

EAR LACERATION/INJURY

I. **Immediate First Aid**
  A. Lacerations.
    1. Save any torn or detached part of ear.
    2. Raise victim's head.
    3. Apply dressing.
    4. Place tissue in plastic bag and put bag in ice.
    5. Notify parents and call EMS.
  B. Perforation of eardrum.
    1. Drainage of ear generally accompanies perforation.
    2. Notify parents and urge medical care.
    3. Do not insert instruments, medication, or any kind of liquid into ear canal.

EYE INJURY

I. **Immediate First Aid**
  A. When an eye sustains a severe blow, cut, or perforating wound, do not attempt to open eye; put eye pad on affected eye and notify parents for immediate care.
  B. If student is cooperative, patch both eyes to restrict movement.
  C. Do not apply pressure.
  D. Treat bruises immediately with cold applications.

FOREIGN BODY IN EYE

I. **Immediate First Aid**
  A. Flush eye several times with warm water. Tilt head so that water runs from inner to outer aspect of eye.
  B. If flushing does not remove foreign body, close eye, apply eye pad, and notify parents; advise immediate medical care.
  C. If student will tolerate, patch both eyes to control eye movement.

FAINTING

I. **Immediate First Aid**
  A. Have student lie on back with feet slightly raised.
  B. Notify parent(s).
  C. To prevent fainting, student who feels weak or dizzy should lie down.

SEVERE FALL

I. Immediate First Aid
  A. Keep student lying down, warm, and quiet.
  B. Do not move child if any of the following signs are present.
    1. Severe headache.
    2. Inability to move extremities.
    3. Inability to perceive another's touch in any extremity.
    4. Severe neck or back pain.
    5. Altered mental status.
    6. If such signs are present, activate EMS and notify parents.

FLESH WOUNDS/LACERATIONS

Flesh wounds are minor, major, or puncture. Minor flesh wounds include minor cuts, scratches, abrasions, and rug burns. Punctures can be serious because of the danger of tetanus.
  I. Immediate First Aid
    A. Minor wounds.
      1. Gently cleanse wound with mild soap solution using applicator, cotton ball, or gauze.
      2. Rinse wound well, let dry, and then apply sterile gauze dressing only.
    B. Major wounds.
      1. Stop bleeding with pressure (see "Bleeding" section) and protect wound from further contamination.
      2. Notify parent(s) and advise immediate care.
      3. *Punctures:* Let wound bleed freely for several seconds to wash wound; then wash area around wound with mild soap solution and rinse well.
      4. Flush wound itself with *running* water; let wound dry and then cover it with sterile dressing.
      5. Notify parent(s) and remind them that tetanus booster or antitoxin may be needed (parents should discuss this with their primary care provider).
      6. Check school immunization record for date of last tetanus immunization (effective for 5 years).

FRACTURES

Simple fractures (unopen wounds) are more common than compound fractures (open wounds); generally an x-ray is needed for accurate diagnosis. The following signs indicate a possible fracture:
    1. Edema, swelling.
    2. Discoloration.
    3. Pain.
    4. Tenderness to the touch.
    5. Deformity and possible shortening of limb.
    6. Inability to bear weight or inability to move. Even if doubt exists as to the presence of a fracture, provide first-aid measures for fracture to prevent aggravation of existing injuries.

I. Immediate First Aid

A. Keep student quiet and, if indicated, treat for shock (see later "Shock" section).

B. Notify parent(s) and activate EMS.

C. If paramedics or ambulance can arrive within short time, do not attempt to move victim unless in danger of fire, drowning, and so forth. Do not attempt to set fracture or push back protruding bone.

D. If paramedic or ambulance service is not available and student must be moved, apply splint and then elevate limb slightly. If student is unconscious, always lift and move as though neck or spine is injured.

   1. Make emergency splints from newspapers, rolled blankets, pillows, sticks, or boards. Splints should extend beyond the joint at either end of the suspected fracture.

   2. Another immobilization method involves tying or taping the injured leg to the uninjured leg or securing an injured arm to the chest or side. When possible, place padding between the legs or affected arm and body and immobilize joints above and below possible fracture.

   3. Always check pulses distal to injury before and after splinting.

   4. Loosen ties or tape if swelling, cyanosis, or numbness occurs, if student complains of tingling sensation, or is unable to move toes or fingers.

   5. If someone with suspected neck or spinal injury must be moved, use three or four persons to lift victim with all moving in unison and providing rigid support; place the injured person on a firm and level surface (e.g., blackboard or other similar surface); do not use blanket for lifting and carrying because such support is not adequately firm.

E. Do not let person's head move with possible neck or spine injury.

F. For compound fracture, use the following measures:

   1. Cut away clothing to prevent injured part from moving.

   2. Control hemorrhage by applying pressure with sterile or clean dressing over wound.

   3. Do not wash, probe, or insert fingers into wound.

   4. If bone is protruding, cover wound with sterile or clean bandage, compress, or pads.

   5. Do not attempt to replace bone fragments.

   6. Notify parent(s) and call EMS.

HEADACHE

A headache may represent the onset of illness, stress, vision concerns, exposure to toxins, classroom avoidance, or be idiopathic. The nurse should determine the onset, location, type of pain (sharp, dull, pulsating), duration, frequency (continuous or intermittent), time of day, and associated symptoms or factors. If fever or other symptoms are identified, contact parent. If child is known for chronic visits with the same symptoms, further investigation is needed. If headache is described as the "worst pain ever," is accompanied by behavioral changes, altered mental status, or a combination of these symptoms, call 911.

HEAD INJURY

I. **Symptoms of Possible Head Injury**
   A. Excessive drowsiness.
   B. Nausea, persistent vomiting.
   C. Unequal pupils.
   D. Slurred speech or loss of speech.
   E. Severe headache.
   F. Double vision.
   G. Seizures.
   H. Unsteady gait, dizziness.
   I. Uncoordination of arms or legs.
   J. Paresthesia (numbness, tingling).
   K. Behavioral changes with or without altered mental status.

II. **Immediate First Aid**
   A. Keep student quiet and lying down; conduct initial assessment and call EMS if any of the above symptoms are present.
   B. Keep student quiet and maintain in cervical spine stabilization. Log roll if need to eliminate vomit or saliva.
   C. Never position student so that head is lower than rest of body.
   D. Do not give fluids by mouth.
   E. Do not attempt to clean scalp wound because cleaning may cause more bleeding or cerebral infection if a fracture is present.
   F. Control bleeding with sterile dressing bandage.
   G. Notify parent(s).

EPISTAXIS (NOSEBLEED)

I. **Immediate First Aid**
   A. Have student sit with head erect, leaning forward, if possible, to avoid drainage of blood into airway or esophagus.
   B. With gloved fingers, apply firm but gentle pressure over bleeding nostril for at least 10 minutes.
   C. Apply cold compresses.
   D. If bleeding does not stop within about 15 minutes, notify parent(s) and urge care; deter student from blowing or picking at nose.

FOREIGN BODY IN NOSE

I. **Immediate First Aid**
   A. Do not attempt to remove object from nostril.
   B. Try to keep student from sniffing; may instruct blowing of nose to dislodge object.
   C. Notify parent(s) and refer for care.

HEAT CRAMPS

Heat cramps are caused by sodium depletion after prolonged or excessive exercise during periods of high temperature and low humidity.

I. Symptoms of Heat Cramps
A. Profuse sweating.
B. Severe muscle cramps.
C. Blood pressure and pulse usually normal.
D. Normal or slightly elevated temperature.
E. Alert and oriented.

II. Immediate First Aid
A. Provide fluids containing salt (e.g., any drink containing high levels of sodium or solution of 1 teaspoon of salt in 500 ml [two 8-oz glasses] of water).
B. Rest in cool place.

HEAT EXHAUSTION

Heat exhaustion is caused by heat exposure and excessive sweating without necessary fluid replacement. The student may have water and/or salt depletion. First-aid measures are directed toward removal from heat source and replenishment of fluids.

I. Symptoms of Heat Exhaustion
A. Normal body temperature.
B. Pale and clammy skin.
C. Profuse perspiration.
D. Anxiety, tiredness, and weakness.
E. Headache.
F. Cramps and muscle spasms.
G. Nausea, dizziness, and possibly fainting.

II. Immediate First Aid
A. Take student to a cool, shaded, and well-ventilated room.
B. Remove or loosen clothing as much as possible, and have student lie down with feet elevated.
C. Apply cool, wet cloths and fan student, or remove student to air-conditioned room.
D. If student is conscious, give sips of water with or without salt (e.g., any drink containing high levels of sodium or solution of 1 teaspoon of salt in 500 ml [two-8-oz. glasses] of water). If student vomits, do not give more fluids; activate EMS if no response to first-aid measures.
E. Notify parent(s).

HEATSTROKE/SUNSTROKE

Heatstroke or sunstroke occurs when body systems are overwhelmed by heat and are unable to compensate. Heatstroke or sunstroke can be immediate and life-threatening. First aid is directed toward immediate measures to cool the body quickly.

I. Symptoms of Heatstroke/Sunstroke
A. High body temperature (105 degrees F or higher).
B. Hot, red, and dry skin.
C. No sweating.
D. Rapid and strong pulse.

E. Anorexia, nausea, and vomiting.

F. Headache and fatigue.

G. Confusion and disorientation.

H. Can progress to coma and seizures.

II. **Immediate First Aid**

A. Call 911 or emergency medical help.

B. Take student into shade or cool room indoors and sponge with cool water or wrap in wet, cold sheets, or use ice packs.

C. Notify parent(s).

SHOCK

Determine the cause of symptoms.

I. **Symptoms of Shock**

A. Weakness.

B. Moist, clammy, and pale skin.

C. Rapid and weak pulse.

D. Increased rate of breathing, which may be shallow, labored, irregular, or a combination of these rates.

E. Dilated pupils.

F. Possible anxiety and disorientation that later may progress to unresponsiveness and loss of consciousness.

II. **Immediate First Aid**

A. Activate EMS and notify parent(s).

B. Elevate feet 6 to 12 in, unless injury contradicts position; if so, keep student lying flat and quiet, loosen tight clothing.

C. Keep student warm.

D. Give nothing by mouth.

E. Activate EMS and notify parent(s).

SPLINTERS

I. **Immediate First Aid**

A. If splinter is large and deeply embedded, leave it alone and notify parent.

B. If splinter is near surface and protruding, cleanse area thoroughly with mild soap solution (taking care to not break splinter) and gently remove splinter with tweezers.

C. Apply light sterile dressing.

SPRAINS

In a sprain, ligaments, muscles, tendons, and blood vessels are stretched or torn. Differentiation of a sprain from a closed fracture usually is impossible without radiography; treat the injury as a possible fracture (see "Fracture" section).

I. **Symptoms of Sprain**

A. Swelling.

B. Tenderness.

C. Pain with motion.

D. Discoloration.

II. Immediate First Aid
    A. If possible, elevate injured part and apply cold compresses or ice pack.
    B. Always place thin towel or cloth between skin and application of any cold treatment.
    C. Notify parent(s) immediately.

TOOTH INJURIES

I. Immediate First Aid
    A. Notify parent(s) and urge immediate dental care.
    B. If permanent tooth has been avulsed as a result of trauma, it probably can be saved if it is kept moist and promptly replaced.
        1. Gently wash dirt and debris from tooth; avoid touching or disturbing the root.
        2. If possible, place tooth into its socket if no risk to student.
    C. If replacement is impossible, place tooth in student's or parent's mouth *or* place in milk or normal saline solution.
    D. If tooth is transported in saline solution, it must be replanted within 1 hour; if left dry, tooth must be replanted within 30 minutes. Special containers are available to transport avulsed teeth.

WEB SITES

American Red Cross
    http://www.redcross.org
Federal Emergency Management Agency (FEMA)
    http://www.fema.gov
U.S. Department of Health and Human Services, Office of Emergency Preparedness (OEP)
    http://ndms.dhhs.gov/

BIBLIOGRAPHY

Bethel School District: *Bethel school district: site emergency planning guidelines,* Spanaway, Wash, 1998, Bethel School District.

Doyle J: Personal communication, February 1, 2001.

Emergency Management Institute: *Multi-hazard program for schools,* Emmitsburg, Md, 2000, The Institute.

The Nemours Foundation: *Kids health,* February 11, 2001, Available online: http://kidshealth.org/parent/firstaid_safe/. Accessed on Feb 11, 2001.

Schwab N, Gelfman M, editors: *Legal issues in school health services: a resource for school administrators, school attorneys, school nurses,* North Branch, Minn, 2001, Sunrise River Press.

GLOSSARY

Acanthosis nigricans A velvety hyperpigmentation found on the neck, axillae, and groin that is probably the skin manifestation of severe and chronic hyperinsulinemia. Associated with obesity and type 2 diabetes.

Agonist Any agent with a certain cellular affinity that produces a predictable response.

Agranulocytosis An acute febrile condition in which production of white blood cells is severely depressed. Symptoms include chills, swollen neck, sore throat, and prostration; sometimes with local ulceration of rectum, mouth, and vagina. May be side effects of certain medications or to radiation therapy. Also known as *granulocytopenia*.

Amenorrheic Not having menstruation.

Amygdala A nucleus of tissue found at the base of the temporal lobe, which is one of several structures of the limbic system and regulates aspects of emotional behavior.

Anovulatory Inability of the ovaries to produce, mature, or release eggs.

Antagonists Any agent that competes or exerts a negative action to that of a receptor site or another action.

Anthropometry Science of measuring the height, weight, and size of various parts of the human body, such as skinfolds. Ability to compare proportions for normal and atypical findings.

Antibody Develops in reaction to bacteria, virus, and to other antigenic (foreign to the body) substances. An antibody is specific to an antigen.

Asthenia Loss of strength and energy; weakness.

Atopy Genetic predisposition for development of an IgE (immunoglobulin E)-mediated response to common allergens. Determined by a skin test.

Autoimmunity Abnormal condition in which one's body acts against its own tissue constituents.

Autosomal dominant disorder If one parent is a carrier and the other is normal, there is a 50% chance a child will inherit the trait.

Autosomal recessive disorder Both parents must be carriers for their child to have the disease; if their child inherits the gene from only one parent, he or she will be a carrier. If the child inherits the gene from both parents, he or she will have the disease.

Bacteria Simple one-celled organism and the most plentiful of pathogens. Most bacteria do not cause disease.

Beta-blockers Drugs that block the response to epinephrine/norepinephrine, slowing the heart rate and decreasing cardiac output; they cause bronchoconstriction, thus increasing airway resistance in asthmatics.

Bioavailability The level of activity or quantity of administered drug or other substance that becomes available for use by the targeted cells.

Blepharitis An inflammatory condition of the lash follicles and glands of the eyelids, characterized by redness, swelling, and crusting of dried mucus. Ulcerative blepharitis is caused by bacteria, and nonulcerative blepharitis is caused by seborrhea, psoriasis, or an allergic response.

Bolus feeding   A concentrated mass of food or pharmaceutical preparation given by mouth, nasogastric tube, or gastrostomy feeding methods over a short period.

Celiac sprue/celiac disease   An inborn error of metabolism that affects the ability to hydrolyze peptides contained in gluten. Gluten is found in barley, wheat, and oats. Gluten-free substitutes are rice and corn; vitamin or mineral deficiencies can be fulfilled with oral preparations.

Chelation therapy   Using a chelating agent to bind with a metal in the body so that the metal loses its toxic effect. Procedure used in lead poisoning.

Cholelithiasis   Formation or presence of calculi (gallstones) in the gallbladder. Factors that increase the probability of gallstones include female gender, increased age, obesity, and a positive family history.

Chorionic villus sampling   Chorionic villus sampling (CVS) is a procedure used for prenatal diagnosis in the first trimester of pregnancy by withdrawing a chorionic villi sample from the fetal membranes. CVS tests for similar range of abnormalities as an amniocentesis. The advantage of CVS is that the results are obtained much earlier in pregnancy (8 to 12 weeks). CVS carries a risk of complications, as does amniocentesis.

Chromatin-positive nuclei   Description of the nuclei of cells that have characteristics of the normal female but also may be present in some chromosomal abnormalities (e.g., Klinefelter's syndrome).

Chromosomal analysis   An analysis of the chromosome, which is the threadlike structure in the nucleus of the cell that functions as the transmission of genetic information.

Clinodactyly   A congenital anomaly of the hand marked by lateral or medial bending of one or more fingers or toes.

Coarctation of the aorta   A congenital anomaly in which there is localized narrowing of the aorta. Symptoms include headaches, dizziness, fainting, nosebleeds, and muscle cramps during exercise secondary to tissue anoxia. Murmur may or may not be present. Surgical correction is recommended for even a minor defect.

Computed tomography   In computed tomography (CT), the CT scan functions as a diagnostic tool; also known as *computed axial tomography* or *CAT scan*. A rotating camera is used to film the head or other body parts, taking images from numerous x-ray beams going through the body and converting the information into a three-dimensional picture of the body part. The x-ray image is defined by various shades of gray delineated by the tissue density.

Congenital adrenogenital hyperplasia   Congenital adrenogenital hyperplasia (CAH) is a category of autosomal recessive disorders that results in virilization of female fetuses.

Convolutions   Rolled or twisted together, with one part over the other.

Cortex   The outer layer of a structure or other body organ as identified from the internal matter. In the brain, the gray matter of the cerebellum and cerebral hemispheres is where most neurons are found. Cortic means "cortex" or "bark."

Coryza   An acute inflammation of the nasal mucous membrane with a profuse discharge from the nostrils.

Cyclothymic disorder   Cycle of moods from hypomania to depression, but not severe enough to meet the criteria for major depressive disorder. Must be of at least 1 year duration in children and adolescents.

Cytotoxic   Describes a drug or agent that damages or destroys tissue cells.

Demineralization   The process of removing minerals, in the form of mineral ions, from dental enamel. Precursor of caries. It is another term for dissolving of the enamel.

Desquamation   A normal process of shedding of epithelium elements, mainly the skin, in fine sheets or scales; peeling.

Dopamine   Primarily an inhibitory catecholamine. An important part of the brain's reward and pleasure system, causing feelings of euphoria. Roles includes regulation of conscious movement and mood and effects management of hormonal balance and the immune system via the pituitary gland.

Dysfluency   Disruption of the normal pattern of speech for the individual's developmental age (e.g., stuttering, prolonged sounds, word substitution).

Dyspareunia   Unusual pain during sexual intercourse.

Ectoderm, mesoderm, and endoderm   The three *embryonic germ layers:* the *ectoderm,* or outer layer, which gives rise to the nervous system (brain and spinal cord) and epidermis; the *mesoderm,* or middle layer, which gives rise to the connective tissue, muscle, skeleton, and other structures; and the *endoderm,* or inner layer, which is the source of the epithelium of the digestive tract and its derivatives.

Effusion   The escape of fluid, usually into a body cavity. In the middle ear, the disorder otitis media, an accumulation of fluid present in the middle ear space, decreases the mobility of the eardrum.

Electromyogram   The electromyogram (EMG) measures electrical activity in a skeletal muscle by putting on surface electrodes or inserting electrode needles into the muscle and displaying the activity on an oscilloscope.

Endoscopy   Visualization of the interior organs and cavities of the gastrointestinal tract with a flexible instrument called an *endoscope.*

Epiphyseal   The enlarged distal and proximal ends of a large bone.

Functional magnetic resonance imaging   Functional magnetic resonance imaging (fMRI) is a diagnostic tool that uses the same technology as an MRI by adding to the basic anatomical picture. It measures the areas with the highest oxygen level in the brain that indicate the part of the brain as the individual does different tasks or reacts to different stimuli. Particular areas of brain activity use larger concentrations of oxygen, which correspond to brighter areas in the color image created by this technique.

Fungus   Single or multicelled organism that reproduces by spores present in soil, air, or water.

Gamma aminobutyric acid   Gamma aminobutyric acid (GABA) is an inhibitor. Aggression and violence are associated with low levels of GABA, together with low levels of serotonin. Passive behavior is associated with high levels of GABA and serotonin.

Genital tubercle   A small eminence or nodule on the skin that is larger than a papule.

Glia/glial   A neural cell that provides support and nutrition. It is a non-neuron because it is not involved in the networking process. The Greek translation for glia is "glue."

Gonad   A sex gland; the ovary in the female and the testis in the male.

Health care provider   A health care provider (HCP) is any health care professional who has the ability to assess and diagnosis health, provide treatment, and prescribe medication.

Helminthic   Referring to a parasitic worm.

Hydronephrosis   Distension of the kidney secondary to structural or functional changes in the urinary tract that obstruct normal urine flow, sometimes leading to renal dysfunction (obstructive nephropathy). May be due to kidney stone in ureter, tumor, or edema from urinary tract infection.

Hyperconvex fingernails   Nails that have an extreme curve outward.

Hypogonadism   Insufficiency in the secretory activity of the ovary or testes. May be primary or secondary (e.g., caused by a hypothalamus-pituitary disorder).

Hypopituitarism   Decreased activity of the pituitary gland, resulting in excessive deposits of fat and persistence of adolescent characteristics.

Icteric phase   A jaundice phase caused by an abnormal amount of bilirubin in the blood.

Ig   Abbreviation for *immunoglobulin*. Antibodies in the serum and external secretions of the body. They are formed in the spleen, bone marrow, and all lymphoid tissues, except the thymus, in response to a specific antigen. IgA, IgD, IgE, IgG, and IgM are all abbreviations for their respective immunoglobulin letters, and IGF is an abbreviation for insulin-like growth factors.

Interphalangeal   Situated or occurring between the phalanges (the bones of the fingers or toes); relating to an interphalangeal joint.

Keratin   A constituent of the epidermis, hair, nails, horny tissues, and enamel of the teeth.

Keratitis   An inflammation of the cornea.

Laparotomy   A surgical incision into the peritoneal cavity under general or regional anesthesia, usually for exploration.

Leptin   A protein hormone that provides the body with an indication of nutritional status and helps regulate body weight, metabolism, and reproductive function. Leptin's effects on body weight occur through effects on hypothalamic centers that control feeding behavior and hunger, body temperature, and energy expenditure.

Leukopenia   Abnormal decrease in white blood cells to below 5000 per cubic millimeter.

Limbic system   Term that refers to subcortical and cortical structures of the brain that are associated with emotions and feelings, such as sadness, anger, fear, and sexual arousal; structures of the limbic system include the cingulate gyrus, hippocampal gyrus, uncus, and amygdala.

Live-attenuated   Decreasing the virulence of a pathogenic microorganism for its host by increasing virulence for a new host; a basis for live vaccine development.

Lordosis   An abnormal anterior concavity of the lumbar spine.

Macule   A small flat discoloration or blemish that is skin level (e.g. freckle, certain rashes).

Maculopapular   A rash consisting of both macules and papules.

Magnetic resonance imaging   Magnetic resonance imaging (MRI) is a diagnostic tool sometimes called *nuclear magnetic resonance imaging (NMR)*. It creates a magnetic field around the brain by using a large magnet and radio waves. A three-dimensional computer image of the brain/body part results as the cells respond to the radio waves. The image is made when the tissues with high concentrations of water (such as fat) appear light and bone (with less water) appears dark. A high-level software system, computerized tomography (CT) converts the image data into a 3-D picture.

Melatonin   A hormone secreted by the pineal gland, especially in response to darkness, that has been linked to the regulation of diurnal rhythms. An over-the-counter supplement is often taken to regulate sleep patterns and is claimed to have antiaging properties.

Micrognathia   Small, underdeveloped jaw, especially the mandible.

Myalgias   Pain in one or more muscles, usually diffuse.

Myelin   A fatty substance that forms a covering around some axons, is composed mainly of protein and phospholipids, and acts like an electrical insulator by helping to speed the conduction of nerve impulses.

Myelination   The production of myelin surrounding an axon; also called the *myelin sheath*.

Neocortex   The six-layered cortex that covers most of the cerebral hemispheres in the brain.

Neuraxis   The spinal cord and brain, central nervous system, and a point of reference for given directions within the nervous system.

Neuron   The basic nerve cell of the nervous system. Neurons are identified by the direction in which they send impulses. *Sensory neurons* send information towards the spinal cord and the brain, whereas *motor neurons* send information from the brain and spinal cord toward muscles and glandular tissue. Each neuron has one axon and one or more dendrites.

Neurotransmitter   A chemical involved in the transmission of nerve impulses between synapses. *Excitatory impulses* decrease the negativity potential, thus increasing transmission of impulses between synapses. *Inhibitory impulses* increase the negativity potential, thus decreasing neural transmission.

Noradrenergic   Released by the sympathetic nervous system and not subject to voluntary control. A vasoconstrictor relaxes the muscle wall, raises blood pressure, dilates eyes, and initiates the fight-or-flight response.

Nucleus accumbens   A structure in the middle of the brain.

Oligohydramnios   An abnormal condition in which there is a very small amount or an absence of amniotic fluid.

Orthostatic blood pressure   Measurement of blood pressure while in a standing position.

Papillae   A small nipple projection or extension from tissue or fibers.

Papilledema   Swelling of the optic disc caused by increased intracranial pressure. Vision is usually normal.

Papule   A solid raised skin lesion that is 1 cm or less in diameter (e.g., non-pustular acne/pimple).

Parasite   Multicellular animal that attacks specific tissues or organs and competes with host for nutrients.

Paresthesias   Feelings of numbness or tingling that are subjective and may change with posture, edema, rest, activity, or an underlying disorder. Sometimes called *acroparesthesia* when felt in the extremities.

Parotitis   Inflammation of one or both of the parotid salivary glands. Infectious or epidemic parotitis is known as *mumps.*

Pectus excavatum   An abnormal formation of the chest in which the sternum is depressed. Also called *funnel chest.* Surgical correction may be necessary if the pectus excavatum interferes with breathing and is often sought for cosmetic reasons.

Philtrum   The natural groove of the upper lip, extending to the nose. The groove is usually smooth or nonexistent in persons with fetal alcohol syndrome.

Photophobia   Atypical sensitivity to light, especially by the eyes; is found in certain conditions (albinism) and a symptom of various diseases and disorders (e.g., measles, encephalitis, Reiter's syndrome).

Pilosebaceous units   Well-developed sebaceous glands with miniature hairs.

Polyhydramnios   Excess amount of amniotic fluid, indicating a problem in the pregnancy. Also called *hydramnios.* See oligohydramnios.

Positron emission tomography   Positron emission tomography (PET) functions as a research tool more than as a diagnostic one. A radioactive chemical compound marker is injected into the blood stream. The compound attaches to glucose molecules, giving off gamma rays, which translate as color images onto a computer screen. PET produces a clear picture of the brain areas working the hardest; however, it does not have the same fine resolution as a fMRI.

Primordial   The most primitive or underdeveloped state, such as those cells formed during the early stages of embryonic development.

Prepuce   A fold of skin that forms a retractable sheath; foreskin of the penis or the fold around the clitoris.

Prognathia   One or both jaws, mandible and maxilla, project forward.

Pyoderma   A purulent skin disease (e.g., impetigo).

Serotonin   Primarily an inhibitory monoamine. Plays a role in the regulation of mood, control of eating, arousal, perception of pain, and in sleep. It appears to be related to dreaming.

Sinovaginal bulbs   Endodermal outgrowths that fuse to become the opening of the vagina.

Spermatogenesis   Process of development of spermatozoa.

Stridor   A harsh, shrill sound usually heard on inspiration in laryngeal obstruction.

Subacute   A disease in which clinical symptoms are not apparent.

Subluxation   An incomplete separation of the articular surfaces of a joint.

Superior colliculus   A nucleus in the midbrain that controls saccadic eye movement. The superior colliculus is also responsible for turning the head and eyes to see a stimulus that is heard or felt.

Synapse   The space between two neurons across which nerve impulses that either *inhibit* or *continue* the impulse are transmitted.

Synovial membrane   The connective-tissue membrane lining the articular capsules that surround freely moving joints. It secretes thick synovial fluid that normally lubricates the joint, but when an injury occurs, an excess amount may accumulate, causing pain.

Temporomandibular joint   The temporomandibular joint (TMJ) is the joint between the temporal bone of the skull and the mandible of the jaw that includes the condyloid process and allows for the opening, closing, protrusion, retraction, and lateral movement of the mandible.

Tenesmus   Persistent ineffectual spasms of the bladder or rectum accompanied by a desire to empty the bladder or bowel.

Torticollis   An abnormal tipping of the head to one side caused by muscle contractures on that side of the neck. May be congenital or acquired. Treatment depends on the cause and includes physical therapy, heat, immobilization, or surgery.

Toxigenicity   There are differences in virulence because of growth rate differences and the ability to produce the toxin. When the organism reproduces at an increased rate, it may be able to probe further into its host, producing still greater amounts of the toxin.

Trichotillomania   Repetitive behaviors to the body, such as pulling out hair, scratching, and drawing blood to the skin.

Tricyclic antidepressants   Tricyclic antidepressants (TCAs) are a group of drugs that are useful in a wide range of disorders, including enuresis, panic disorder, social phobia, bulimia, narcolepsy, attention deficit disorder (ADD) with or without hyperactivity, and migraine headaches.

Ultrasonography   Assessment of the deep structures within the body by measuring and recording the reflection of pulsed sound waves.

Vasculitis   An inflammatory condition of the blood vessels characteristic of particular systemic diseases.

Velopharyngeal insufficiency   Incomplete closure of the oral cavity beneath the nasal passages, as found in cleft palate, allowing regurgitation of food through the nose. It impairs speech and is usually corrected with surgery.

Vesicles   A small sac that contains liquid, such as a blister.

Virilization   Masculinization.

Virus   The smallest form of organism causing disease; also the toughest.

X-linked recessive   Inheritance in which an abnormal recessive gene on the X chromosome results in a carrier state in females and characteristics of the condition in males.

APPENDIX CONTENTS

RESOURCES USED FOR APPENDIX

Bowden VR, Dickey SB, Greenberg CS: *Children and their families: the continuum of care,* Philadelphia, 1998, WB Saunders.

Mosby's medical, nursing, & allied health dictionary, ed 6, St Louis, 2002, Mosby.

National Information Center for Children and Youth with Disabilities (NICHCY): *National resources 2002,* Available online: http://www.nichcy.org/database/orgsrch.htm.

O'Toole M, editor: *Miller-Keane encyclopedia dictionary of medicine, nursing, & allied health,* Philadelphia, 1997, WB Saunders.

Siberry GK, Iannone R: *The Harriet Lane handbook,* ed 5, St Louis, 2000, Mosby.

APPENDIX A

Growth Measurements (Anthropometry)

BODY MASS INDEX

Body mass index (BMI) is a convenient standard for estimating body fat. The World Health Organization (WHO) and the National Institutes of Health (NIH) have adopted standards for overweight and obese *adults* based on BMI standards. If BMI is more than 25, that individual is considered *overweight* and *obese* if it is 30 or more. In children, the U.S. Centers for Disease Control and Prevention (CDC) published revised growth charts in 2000.

The International Task Force on Obesity has suggested new worldwide *pediatric standards* for overweight and obesity based on BMI. Data for the new study were collected globally using survey results from various countries, including the United States, Singapore, Brazil, Hong Kong, Great Britain, and the Netherlands, thus making the school nurse's weight monitoring of *children* from diverse cultures standardized.

BODY MASS INDEX FORMULAS

English Formula:

Weight in pounds ÷ Height in inches ÷ Height in inches × 703 = BMI

Metric Formula:

Weight in kilograms ÷ Height in meters ÷ Height in meters = BMI

For adults: BMI classification for an adult is read as calculated.

For children: BMI classification has a broad range of healthy weights and uses population norms. For children, BMI is calculated and plotted by age and sex. The BMIs by age that increase concern in the 2 to 20-year-old age range are:

Underweight	BMI-for-age <5th percentile
At risk of overweight	BMI-for-age ≥85th percentile
Overweight	BMI-for-age ≥95th percentile

See p 508 and p 516 for BMI charts for children ages 2 to 20. Additional charts and a conversion calculator can be found at http://www/cdc.gov/nccdphp/dnpa/bmi/bmi-for-age.htm.

BOYS
Birth to 36 months
Weight-for-age percentiles

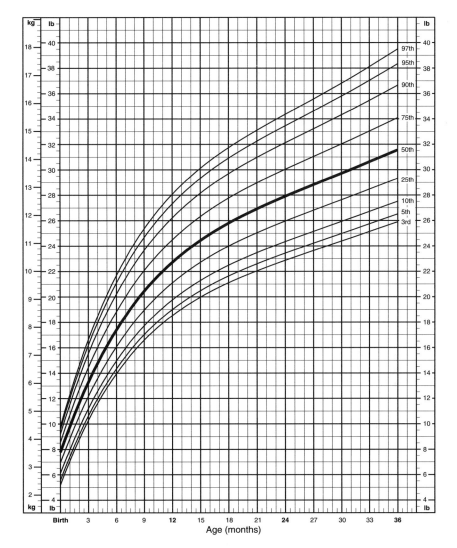

FIGURE A-1 From Centers for Disease Control and Prevention, 2000, Available online: http://www.cdc.gov/nchs/about/major/nhanes/growthcharts/charts.htm.

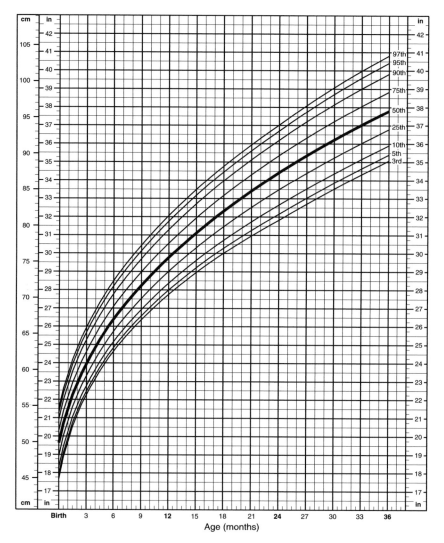

BOYS
Birth to 36 months
Length-for-age percentiles

Figure A-2 From Centers for Disease Control and Prevention, 2000, Available online: http://www.cdc.gov/nchs/about/major/nhanes/growthcharts/charts.htm.

BOYS
Birth to 36 months
Weight-for-length percentiles

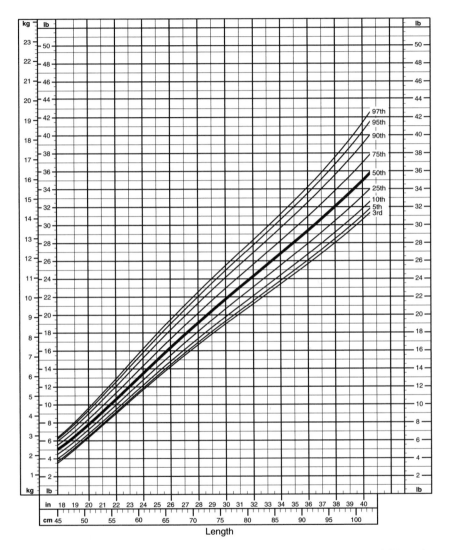

FIGURE A-3 From Centers for Disease Control and Prevention, 2000, Available online: http://www.cdc.gov/nchs/about/major/nhanes/growthcharts/charts.htm.

BOYS
Birth to 36 months
Head circumference-for-age percentiles

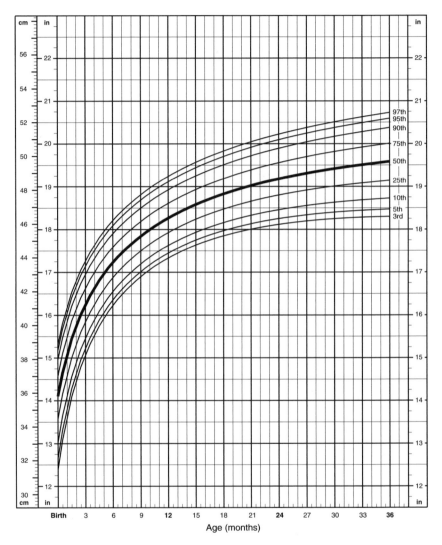

Figure A-4 From Centers for Disease Control and Prevention, 2000, Available online: http://www.cdc.gov/nchs/about/major/nhanes/growthcharts/charts.htm.

BOYS
2 to 20 years
Weight-for-age percentiles

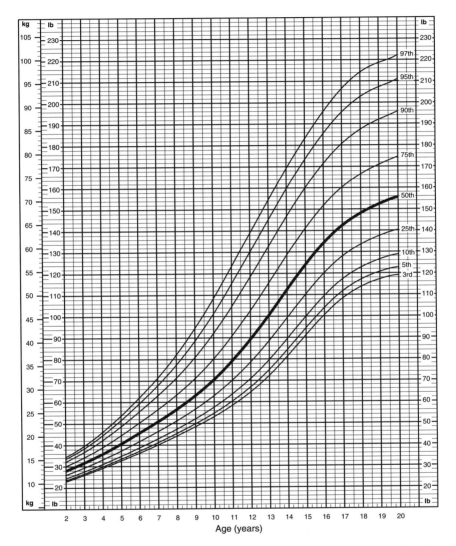

FIGURE A-5 From Centers for Disease Control and Prevention, 2000, Available online: http://www.cdc.gov/nchs/about/major/nhanes/growthcharts/charts.htm.

BOYS
2 to 20 years
Stature-for-age percentiles

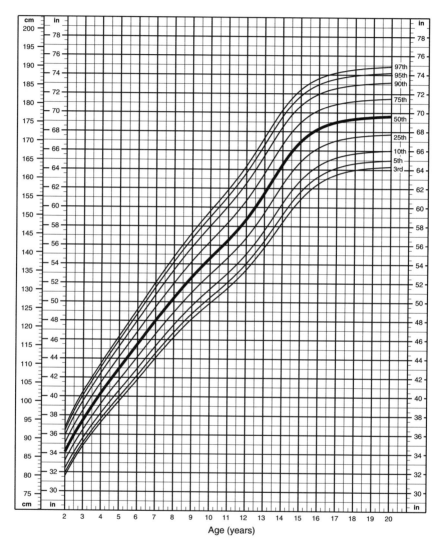

Figure A-6 From Centers for Disease Control and Prevention, 2000, Available online: http://www.cdc.gov/nchs/about/major/nhanes/growthcharts/charts.htm.

BOYS
2 to 20 years
Weight-for-stature percentiles

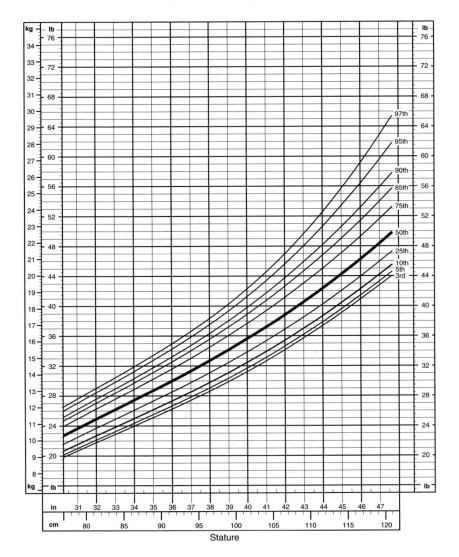

FIGURE A-7 From Centers for Disease Control and Prevention, 2000, Available online: http://www.cdc.gov/nchs/about/major/nhanes/growthcharts/charts.htm.

BOYS
2 to 20 years
Body mass index-for-age percentiles

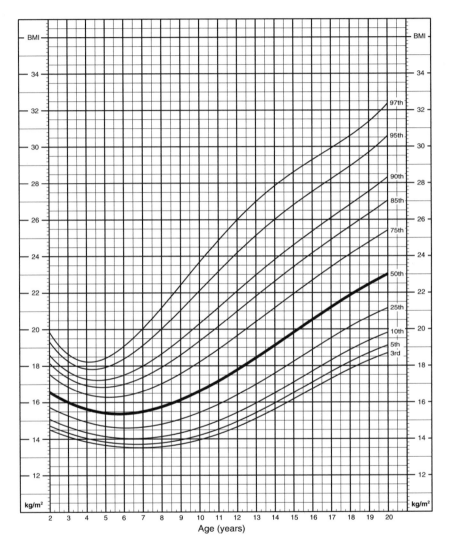

FIGURE A-8 From Centers for Disease Control and Prevention, 2000, Available online: http://www.cdc.gov/nchs/about/major/nhanes/growthcharts/charts.htm.

GIRLS
Birth to 36 months
Weight-for-age percentiles

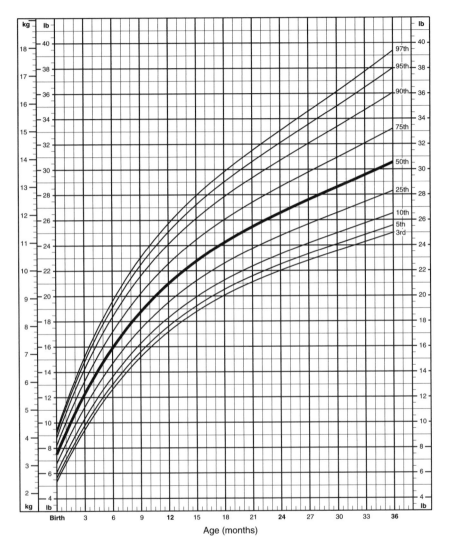

FIGURE A-9 From Centers for Disease Control and Prevention, 2000, Available online: http://www.cdc.gov/nchs/about/major/nhanes/growthcharts/charts.htm.

GIRLS
Birth to 36 months
Length-for-age percentiles

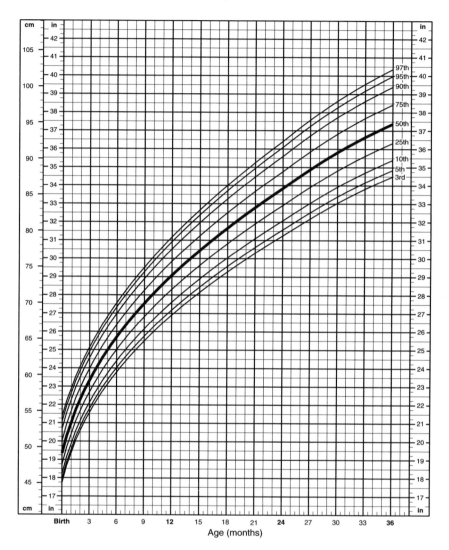

FIGURE A-10 From Centers for Disease Control and Prevention, 2000, Available online: http://www.cdc.gov/nchs/about/major/nhanes/growthcharts/charts.htm.

GIRLS
Birth to 36 months
Weight-for-length percentiles

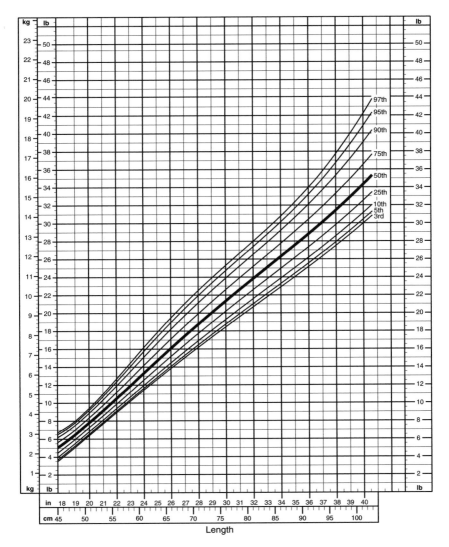

Figure A-11 From Centers for Disease Control and Prevention, 2000, Available online: http://www.cdc.gov/nchs/about/major/nhanes/growthcharts/charts.htm.

GIRLS
Birth to 36 months
Head circumference-for-age percentiles

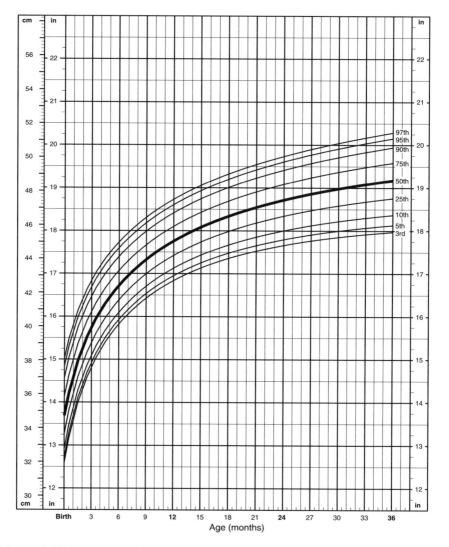

FIGURE A-12 From Centers for Disease Control and Prevention, 2000, Available online: http://www.cdc.gov/nchs/about/major/nhanes/growthcharts/charts.htm.

GIRLS
2 to 20 years
Weight-for-age percentiles

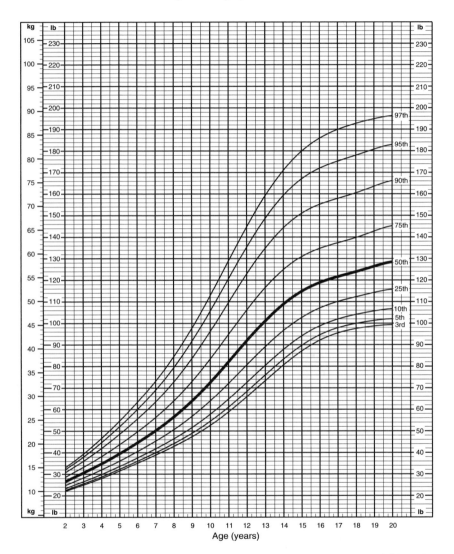

FIGURE A-13 From Centers for Disease Control and Prevention, 2000, Available online: http://www.cdc.gov/nchs/about/major/nhanes/growthcharts/charts.htm.

GIRLS
2 to 20 years
Stature-for-age percentiles

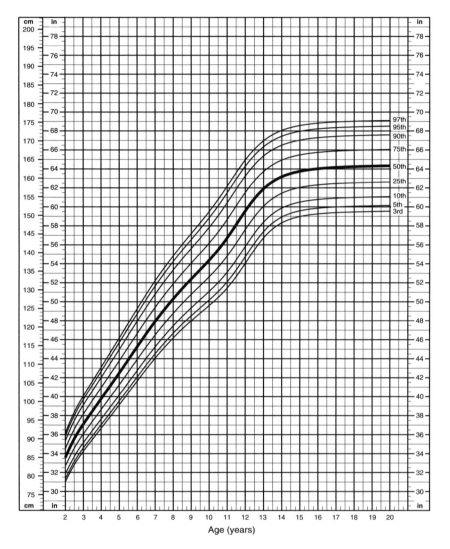

Figure A-14 From Centers for Disease Control and Prevention, 2000, Available online: http://www.cdc.gov/nchs/about/major/nhanes/growthcharts/charts.htm.

GIRLS
2 to 20 years
Weight-for-stature percentiles

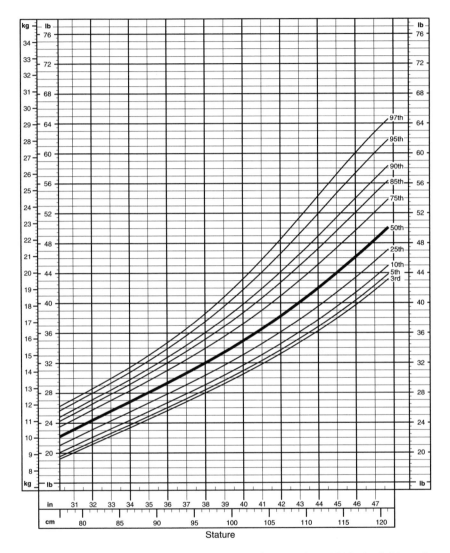

FIGURE A-15 From Centers for Disease Control and Prevention, 2000, Available online: http://www.cdc.gov/nchs/about/major/nhanes/growthcharts/charts.htm.

GIRLS
2 to 20 years
Body mass index-for-age percentiles

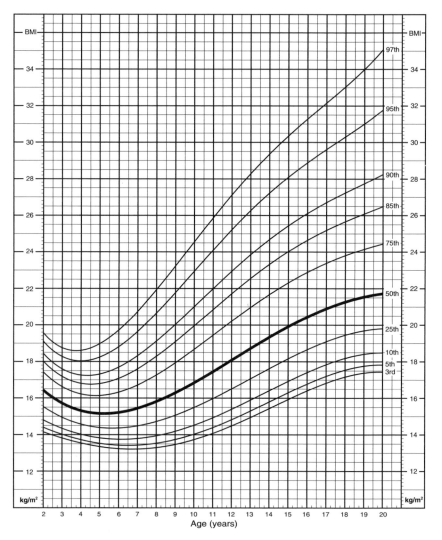

FIGURE A-16 From Centers for Disease Control and Prevention, 2000, Available online: http://www.cdc.gov/nchs/about/major/nhanes/growthcharts/charts.htm.

ACHONDROPLASIA
Height for boys with achondroplasia from birth to 18 years

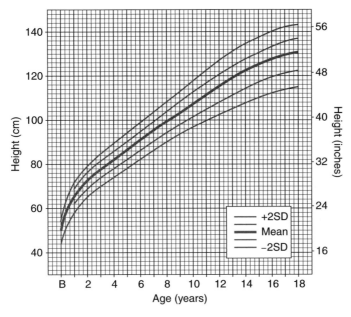

FIGURE A-17 From Horton WA, Rotter JI, Rimoin DL, et al: *J Pediatr* 93:435-438, 1978.

ACHONDROPLASIA
Head circumference for boys with achondroplasia from birth to 18 years

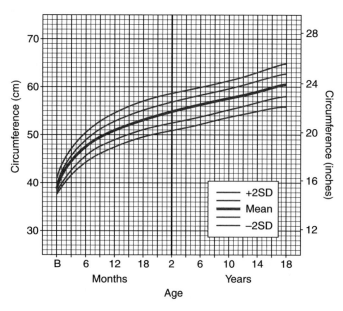

FIGURE A-18 From Horton WA, Rotter JI, Rimoin DL, et al: *J Pediatr* 93:435-438, 1978.

ACHONDROPLASIA
Height for girls with achondroplasia from birth to 18 years

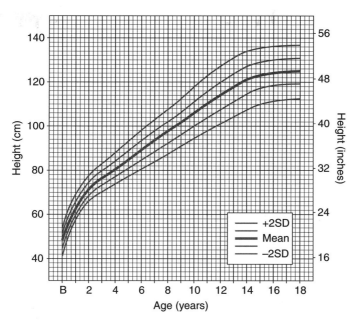

FIGURE A-19 From Horton WA, Rotter JI, Rimoin DL, et al: *J Pediatr* 93:435-438, 1978.

ACHONDROPLASIA
Head circumference for girls with achondroplasia from birth to 18 years

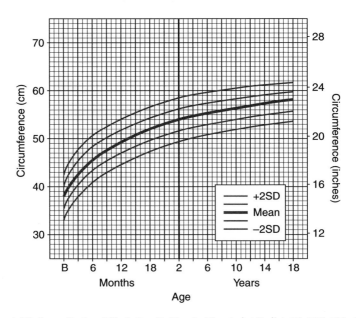

FIGURE A-20 From Horton WA, Rotter JI, Rimoin DL, et al: *J Pediatr* 93:435-438, 1978.

DOWN SYNDROME
Length and weight for boys with Down syndrome from birth to 36 months

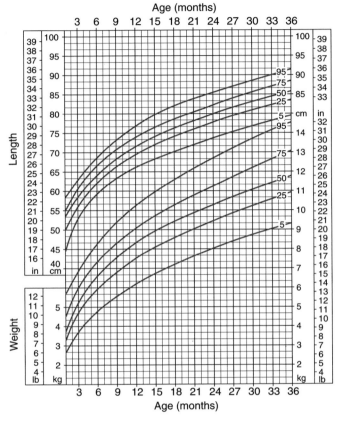

FIGURE A-21 Modified from Cronk C, Crocker AC, Pueschel SM, et al: *Pediatrics* 81:102-110, 1988.

DOWN SYNDROME
Stature and weight for boys with Down syndrome from 2 to 18 years

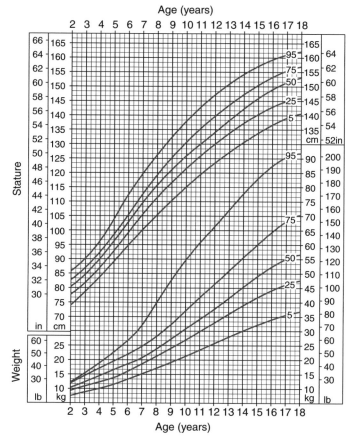

FIGURE A-22 Modified from Cronk C, Crocker AC, Pueschel SM, et al: *Pediatrics* 81:102-110, 1988.

DOWN SYNDROME

Length and weight for girls with Down syndrome from birth to 36 months

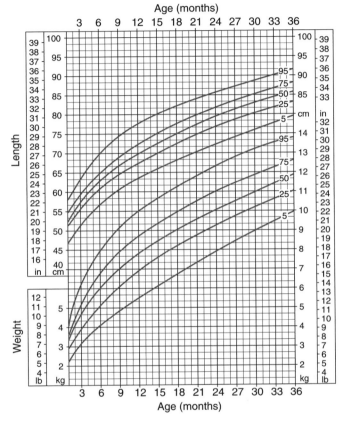

FIGURE A-23 Modified from Cronk C, Crocker AC, Pueschel SM, et al: *Pediatrics* 81:102-110, 1988.

DOWN SYNDROME
Stature and weight for girls with Down syndrome from 2 to 18 years

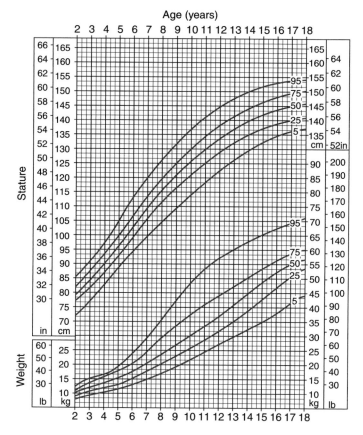

FIGURE A-24 Modified from Cronk C, Crocker AC, Pueschel SM, et al: *Pediatrics* 81:102-110, 1988.

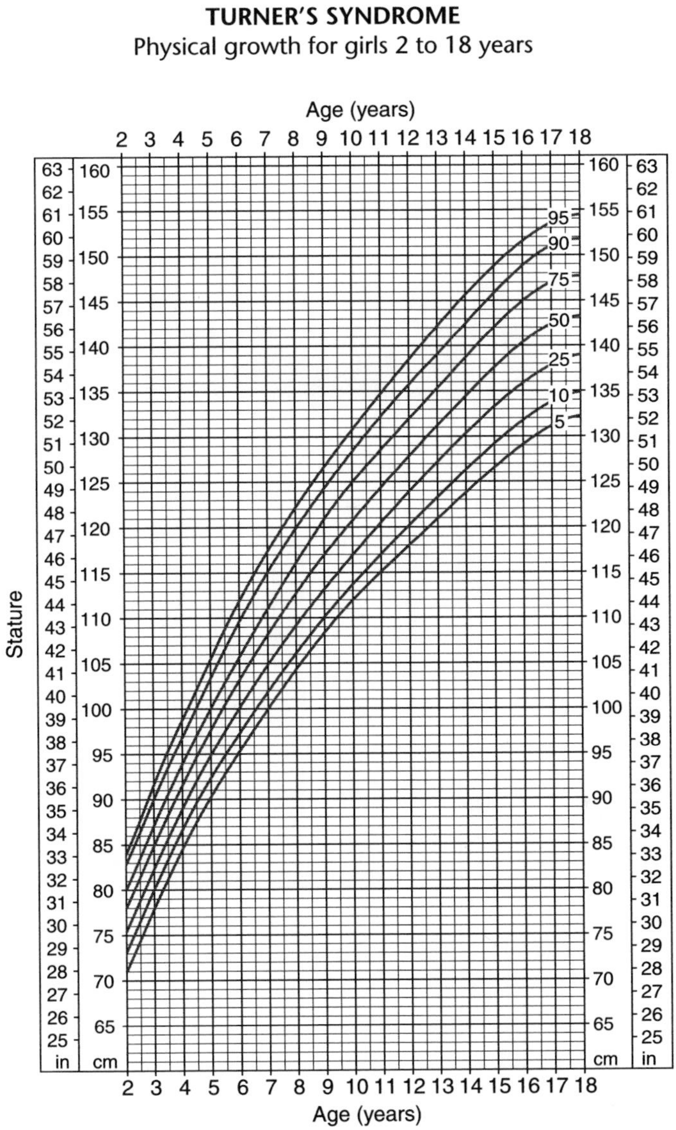
TURNER'S SYNDROME
Physical growth for girls 2 to 18 years
Age (years)
2 3 4 5 6 7 8 9 10 11 12 13 14 15 16 17 18
Stature
in
cm
95
90
75
50
25
10
5

FIGURE A-25 From Lyon AJ, Preece MA, Grant DB: *Arch Dis Child* 60:932-935, 1985. Courtesy Genentech, Inc., 1987.

APPENDIX B

Immunizations

Recommended Childhood Immunization Schedule
United States, 2002

Legend: range of recommended ages | catch-up vaccination | preadolescent assessment

Vaccine ▼ / Age ►	Birth	1 mo	2 mos	4 mos	6 mos	12 mos	15 mos	18 mos	24 mos	4-6 yrs	11-12 yrs	13-18 yrs
Hepatitis B[1]	Hep B #1	Hep B #2 (only if mother HBsAg(-))	Hep B #2		Hep B #3						Hep B series	
Diphtheria, Tetanus, Pertussis[2]			DTaP	DTaP	DTaP		DTaP			DTaP	Td	
Haemophilus influenzae Type b[3]			Hib	Hib	Hib	Hib						
Inactivated Polio[4]			IPV	IPV		IPV				IPV		
Measles, Mumps, Rubella[5]						MMR #1				MMR #2		MMR #2
Varicella[6]						Varicella				Varicella		
Pneumococcal[7]			PCV	PCV	PCV	PCV			PCV	PPV		
Hepatitis A[8]										Hepatitis A series		
Influenza[9]						Influenza (yearly)						

Vaccines below this line are for selected populations

This schedule indicates the recommended ages for routine administration of currently licensed childhood vaccines, as of December 1, 2001, for children through age 18 years. Any dose not given at the recommended age should be given at any subsequent visit when indicated and feasible. ▨ Indicates age groups that warrant special effort to administer those vaccines not previously given. Additional vaccines may be licensed and recommended during the year. Licensed combination vaccines may be used whenever any components of the combination are indicated and the vaccine's other components are not contraindicated. Providers should consult the manufacturers' package inserts for detailed recommendations.

Approved by the **Advisory Committee on Immunization Practices** (www.cdc.gov/nip/acip) the **American Academy of Pediatrics** (www.aap.org), and the **American Academy of Family Physicians** (www.aafp.org).

Footnotes: Recommended Childhood Immunization Schedule United States, 2002

1. Hepatitis B vaccine (Hep B). All infants should receive the first dose of hepatitis B vaccine soon after birth and before hospital discharge; the first dose may also be given by age 2 months if the infant's mother is HBsAg-negative. Only monovalent hepatitis B vaccine can be used for the birth dose. Monovalent or combination vaccine containing Hep B may be used to complete the series; four doses of vaccine may be administered if combination vaccine is used. The second dose should be given at least 4 weeks after the first dose, except for Hib-containing vaccine which cannot be administered before age 6 weeks. The third dose should be given at least 16 weeks after the first dose and at least 8 weeks after the second dose. The last dose in the vaccination series (third or fourth dose) should not be administered before age 6 months.

Infants born to HBsAg-positive mothers should receive hepatitis B vaccine and 0.5 mL hepatitis B immune globulin (HBIG) within 12 hours of birth at separate sites. The second dose is recommended at age 1-2 months and the vaccination series should be completed (third or fourth dose) at age 6 months.

Infants born to mothers whose HBsAg status is unknown should receive the first dose of the hepatitis B vaccine series within 12 hours of birth. Maternal blood should be drawn at the time of delivery to determine the mother's HBsAg status; if the HBsAg test is positive, the infant should receive HBIG as soon as possible (no later than age 1 week).

2. Diphtheria and tetanus toxoids and acellular pertussis vaccine (DTaP). The fourth dose of DTaP may be administered as early as age 12 months, provided 6 months have elapsed since the third dose and the child is unlikely to return at age 15-18 months. **Tetanus and diphtheria toxoids (Td)** is recommended at age 11-12 years if at least 5 years have elapsed since the last dose of tetanus and diphtheria toxoid-containing vaccine. Subsequent routine Td boosters are recommended every 10 years.

3. *Haemophilus influenzae* type b (Hib) conjugate vaccine. Three Hib conjugate vaccines are licensed for infant use. If PRP-OMP (PedvaxHIB® or ComVax® [Merck]) is administered at ages 2 and 4 months, a dose at age 6 months is not required. DTaP/Hib combination products should not be used for primary immunization in infants at age 2, 4 or 6 months, but can be used as boosters following any Hib vaccine.

4. Inactivated poliovirus vaccine (IPV). An all-IPV schedule is recommended for routine childhood poliovirus vaccination in the United States. All children should receive four doses of IPV at age 2 months, 4 months, 6-18 months, and 4-6 years.

5. Measles, mumps, and rubella vaccine (MMR). The second dose of MMR is recommended routinely at age 4-6 years but may be administered during any visit, provided at least 4 weeks have elapsed since the first dose and that both doses are administered beginning at or after age 12 months. Those who have not previously received the second dose should complete the schedule by the visit at age 11-12 years.

6. Varicella vaccine. Varicella vaccine is recommended at any visit at or after age 12 months for susceptible children (i.e. those who lack a reliable history of chickenpox). Susceptible persons aged ≥ 13 years should receive two doses, given at least 4 weeks apart.

7. Pneumococcal vaccine. The heptavalent **pneumococcal conjugate vaccine (PCV)** is recommended for all children aged 2-23 months and for certain children aged 24-59 months. **Pneumococcal polysaccharide vaccine (PPV)** is recommended in addition to PCV for certain high-risk groups. See *MMWR* 2000;49(RR-9);1-37.

8. Hepatitis A vaccine. Hepatitis A vaccine is recommended for use in selected states and regions, and for certain high-risk groups; consult your local public health authority. See *MMWR* 1999;48(RR-12);1-37.

9. Influenza vaccine. Influenza vaccine is recommended annually for children age ≥ 6 months with certain risk factors (including but not limited to asthma, cardiac disease, sickle cell disease, HIV and diabetes; see *MMWR* 2001;50(RR-4);1-44), and can be administered to all others wishing to obtain immunity. Children aged ≤12 years should receive vaccine in a dosage appropriate for their age (0.25 mL if age 6-35 months or 0.5 mL if aged ≥ 3 years). Children aged ≤ 8 years who are receiving influenza vaccine for the first time should receive two doses separated by at least 4 weeks.

Additional information about vaccines, vaccine supply, and contraindications for immunization, is available at www.cdc.gov/nip or at the National Immunization Hotline, 800-232-2522 (English) or 800-232-0233 (Spanish).

FIGURE B-1 Recommended Childhood Immunization Schedule, United States, 2002.

Table B-1	Adolescent Immunization Schedule
Vaccine	**Timing of Immunizations**
Hepatitis A*	First dose (for international travelers at least 4 wk before departure)
	Second dose: 6-12 mo after first dose
Hepatitis B†	First dose
	Second dose: 1-2 mo after first dose
	Third dose: 4-6 mo after second dose
Influenza*	One dose given annually, usually September through December, to adolescents with chronic illness/at high risk
Measles, mumps, rubella (MMR)‡	First dose
	Second dose: 28 days or more after first dose
Meningococcal*	One dose
Pneumococcal*	First dose given to persons 2-64 yr old with chronic illness/at high risk
	One-time revaccination recommended 5 yr after first dose
Tetanus, diphtheria (Td)	Three-dose initial series (if not given in childhood): first dose, second dose (1-2 mo after first dose), third dose (6-12 mo after second dose)
	Booster series: every 10 yr thereafter
Varicella§	First dose
	Second dose: 1-2 mo after first dose

Based on the recommendations of the Advisory Committee on Immunization Practices (ACIP), Centers for Disease Control and Prevention.
Refer to ACIP guidelines for specific vaccine recommendations.
*Consult your doctor to determine your level of risk.
†Some adolescents may be eligible for an alternate two-dose hepatitis B vaccination series. See ACIP recommendations.
‡Should not be given to pregnant women; pregnancy should be avoided for 3 months after MMR vaccine.
§Should not be given to pregnant women; pregnancy should be avoided for 1 month after varicella vaccine. Susceptible individuals include adolescents who have not been immunized previously and who do not have a reliable history of chickenpox.

Dental Development

UPPER DECIDUOUS		Erupt (months)	Shed (years)
	Central incisor	6 to 8	6 to 7
	Lateral incisor	8 to 11	8 to 9
	Canine (cuspid)	16 to 20	11 to 12
	First molar	10 to 16	10 to 11
	Second molar	20 to 30	10 to 12
LOWER DECIDUOUS			
	Second molar	20 to 30	11 to 13
	First molar	10 to 16	10 to 12
	Canine	16 to 20	9 to 11
	Lateral incisor	7 to 10	7 to 8
	Central incisor	5 to 7	5 to 6

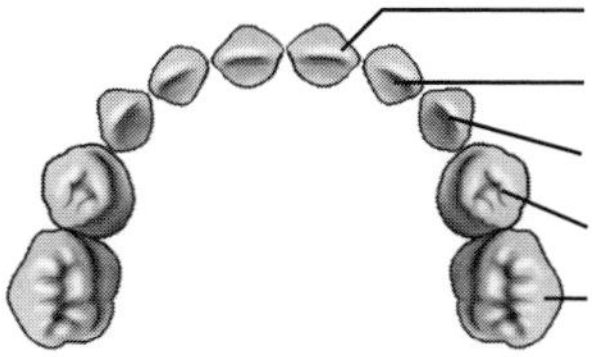

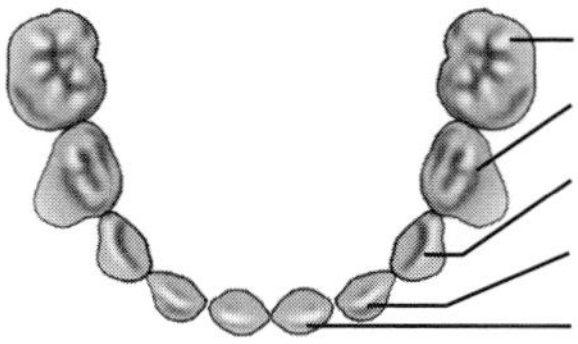

UPPER PERMANENT		Erupt (years)
	Central incisor	7 to 8
	Lateral incisor	8 to 9
	Canine (cuspid)	11 to 12
	First premolar	10 to 11
	Second premolar	10 to 12
	First molar	6 to 7
	Second molar	12 to 13
	Third molar	17 to 25
LOWER PERMANENT		
	Third molar	17 to 25
	Second molar	12 to 13
	First molar	6 to 7
	Second premolar	11 to 13
	First premolar	10 to 12
	Canine	9 to 11
	Lateral incisor	7 to 8
	Central incisor	6 to 7

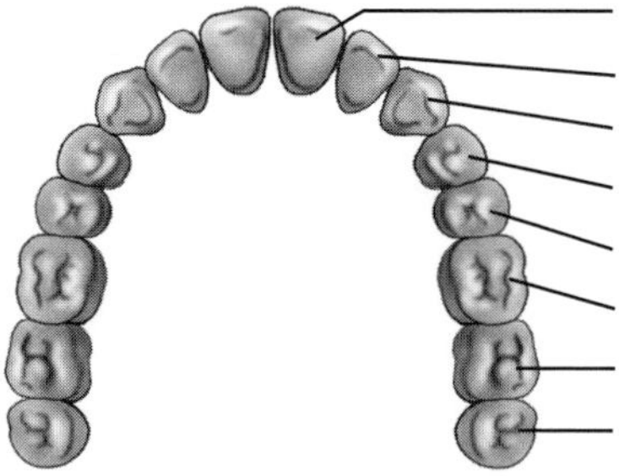

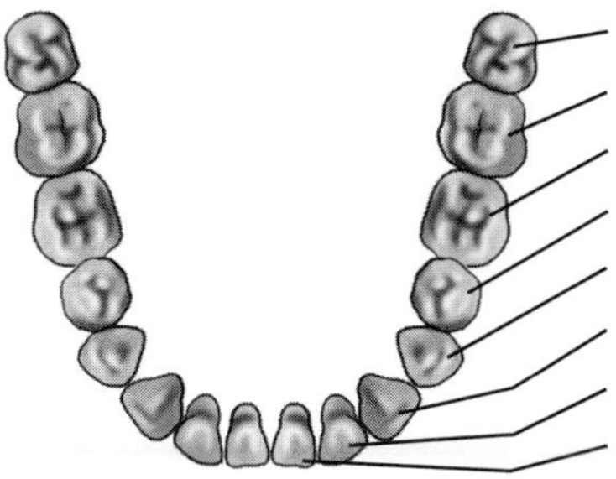

FIGURE C-1 Upper and lower deciduous and permanent teeth.

APPENDIX D

Tanner Stages of Development

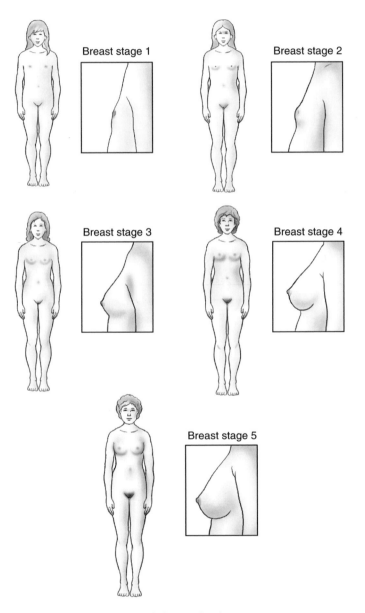

FIGURE D-1 Female breast development stages.

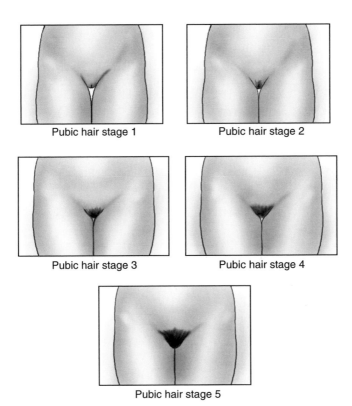

Pubic hair stage 1

Pubic hair stage 2

Pubic hair stage 3

Pubic hair stage 4

Pubic hair stage 5

FIGURE D-2 Female pubic hair stages.

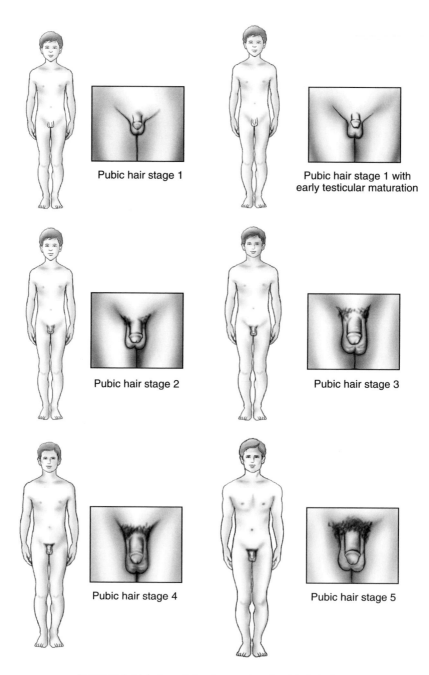

Pubic hair stage 1

Pubic hair stage 1 with early testicular maturation

Pubic hair stage 2

Pubic hair stage 3

Pubic hair stage 4

Pubic hair stage 5

FIGURE D-3 Male breast development and pubic hair stages.

APPENDIX E

Conversion Tables, Formulas, and Biostatistics

Table E-1 Temperature Equivalents Table Celsius (Centigrade): Fahrenheit Scale

CELSIUS : FAHRENHEIT
$$°F = (°C \times \tfrac{9}{5}) + 32$$

°C	°F	°C	°F
−50	−58.0	49	120.2
−40	−40.0	50	122.0
−35	−31.0	51	123.8
−30	−22.0	52	125.6
−25	−13.0	53	127.4
−20	−4.0	54	129.2
−15	+5.0	55	131.0
−10	14.0	56	132.8
−5	23.0	57	134.6
0	32.0	58	136.4
+1	33.8	59	138.2
2	35.6	60	140.0
3	37.4	61	141.8
4	39.2	62	143.6
5	41.0	63	145.4
6	42.8	64	147.2
7	44.6	65	149.0
8	46.4	66	150.8
9	48.2	67	152.6
10	50.0	68	154.4
11	51.8	69	156.2
12	53.6	70	158.0
13	55.4	71	159.8
14	57.2	72	161.6
15	59.0	73	163.4
16	60.8	74	165.2
17	62.6	75	167.0

FAHRENHEIT : CELSIUS
$$°C = (°F - 32) \times \tfrac{5}{9}$$

°F	°C	°F	°C	°F	°C
−50	−46.7	99	37.2	157	69.4
−40	−40.0	100	37.7	158	70.0
−35	−37.2	101	38.3	159	70.5
−30	−34.4	102	38.8	160	71.1
−25	−31.7	103	39.4	161	71.6
−20	−28.9	104	40.0	162	72.2
−15	−26.6	105	40.5	163	72.7
−10	−23.3	106	41.1	164	73.3
−5	−20.6	107	41.6	165	73.8
0	−17.7	108	42.2	166	74.4
+1	−17.2	109	42.7	167	75.0
5	−15.0	110	43.3	168	75.5
10	−12.2	111	43.8	169	76.1
15	−9.4	112	44.4	170	76.6
20	−6.6	113	45.0	171	77.2
25	−3.8	114	45.5	172	77.7
30	−1.1	115	46.1	173	78.3
31	−0.5	116	46.6	174	78.8
32	0	117	47.2	175	79.4
33	+0.5	118	47.7	176	80.0
34	1.1	119	48.3	177	80.5
35	1.6	120	48.8	178	81.1
36	2.2	121	49.4	179	81.6
37	2.7	122	50.0	180	82.2
38	3.3	123	50.5	181	82.7
39	3.8	124	51.1	182	83.3
40	4.4	125	51.6	183	83.8

18	64.4	76	168.8	41	5.0	126	52.2	184	84.4
19	66.2	77	170.6	42	5.5	127	52.7	185	85.0
20	68.0	78	172.4	43	6.1	128	53.3	186	85.5
21	69.8	79	174.2	44	6.6	129	53.8	187	86.1
22	71.6	80	176.0	45	7.2	130	54.4	188	86.6
23	73.4	81	177.8	46	7.7	131	55.0	189	87.2
24	75.2	82	179.6	47	8.3	132	55.5	190	87.7
25	77.0	83	181.4	48	8.8	133	56.1	191	88.3
26	78.8	84	183.2	49	9.4	134	56.6	192	88.8
27	80.6	85	185.0	50	10.0	135	57.2	193	89.4
28	82.4	86	186.8	55	12.7	136	57.7	194	90.0
29	84.2	87	188.6	60	15.5	137	58.3	195	90.5
30	86.0	88	190.4	65	18.3	138	58.8	196	91.1
31	87.8	89	192.2	70	21.1	139	59.4	197	91.6
32	89.6	90	194.0	75	23.8	140	60.0	198	92.2
33	91.4	91	195.8	80	26.6	141	60.5	199	92.7
34	93.2	92	197.6	85	29.4	142	61.1	200	93.3
35	95.0	93	199.4	86	30.0	143	61.6	201	93.8
36	96.8	94	201.2	87	30.5	144	62.2	202	94.4
37	98.6	95	203.0	88	31.0	145	62.7	203	95.0
38	100.4	96	204.8	89	31.6	146	63.3	204	95.5
39	102.2	97	206.6	90	32.2	147	63.8	205	96.1
40	104.0	98	208.4	91	32.7	148	64.4	206	96.6
41	105.8	99	210.2	92	33.3	149	65.0	207	97.2
42	107.6	100	212.0	93	33.8	150	65.5	208	97.7
43	109.4	101	213.8	94	34.4	151	66.1	209	98.3
44	111.2	102	215.6	95	35.0	152	66.6	210	98.8
45	113.0	103	217.4	96	35.5	153	67.2	211	99.4
46	114.8	104	219.2	97	36.1	154	67.7	212	100.0
47	116.6	105	221.0	98	36.6	155	68.3	213	100.5
48	118.4	106	222.8	98.6	37.0	156	68.8	214	101.1

Table E-2	Weight Conversion Table							
Ounces	1 lb	2 lb	3 lb	4 lb	5 lb	6 lb	7 lb	8 lb
0	454 g	907	1361	1814	2268	2722	3175	3629
1	482	936	1389	1843	2296	2750	3204	3657
2	510	964	1418	1871	2325	2778	3232	3686
3	539	992	1446	1899	2353	2807	3260	3714
4	567	1021	1474	1928	2381	2835	3289	3742
5	595	1049	1503	1956	2410	2863	3317	3771
6	624	1077	1531	1985	2438	2892	3345	3799
7	652	1106	1559	2013	2466	2920	3374	3827
8	680	1134	1588	2041	2495	2948	3402	3856
9	709	1162	1616	2070	2523	2977	3430	3884
10	737	1191	1644	2098	2552	3005	3459	3912
11	765	1219	1673	2126	2580	3033	3487	3941
12	794	1247	1701	2155	2608	3062	3515	3969
13	822	1276	1729	2183	2637	3090	3544	3997
14	851	1304	1758	2211	2665	3119	3572	4026
15	879	1332	1786	2240	2693	3147	3600	4054

1 lb = 16 oz = 454 g; 1 kg = 2.2 lb. To convert pounds to grams, multiply by 454. To convert kilograms to pounds, multiply by 2.2.

Length and Weight Calculations
1. Length: To convert inches to centimeters, multiply by 2.54.
2. Weight (Table E-2): To convert pounds to kilograms, divide by 2.2.

Table E-3 Conversion of Pounds and Ounces to Grams for Newborn Weights*

| | **Ounces** | | | | | | | | | | | | | | | |
Pounds	0	1	2	3	4	5	6	7	8	9	10	11	12	13	14	15
0	—	28	57	85	113	142	170	198	227	255	283	312	340	369	397	425
1	454	482	510	539	567	595	624	652	680	709	737	765	794	822	850	879
2	907	936	964	992	1021	1049	1077	1106	1134	1162	1191	1219	1247	1276	1304	1332
3	1361	1389	1417	1446	1474	1503	1531	1559	1588	1616	1644	1673	1701	1729	1758	1786
4	1814	1843	1871	1899	1928	1956	1984	2013	2041	2070	2098	2126	2155	2183	2211	2240
5	2268	2296	2325	2353	2381	2410	2438	2466	2495	2523	2551	2580	2608	2637	2665	2693
6	2722	2750	2778	2807	2835	2863	2892	2920	2948	2977	3005	3033	3062	3090	3118	3147
7	3175	3203	3232	3260	3289	3317	3345	3374	3402	3430	3459	3487	3515	3544	3572	3600
8	3629	3657	3685	3714	3742	3770	3799	3827	3856	3884	3912	3941	3969	3997	4026	4054
9	4082	4111	4139	4167	4196	4224	4252	4281	4309	4337	4366	4394	4423	4451	4479	4508
10	4536	4564	4593	4621	4649	4678	4706	4734	4763	4791	4819	4848	4876	4904	4933	4961
11	4990	5018	5046	5075	5103	5131	5160	5188	5216	5245	5273	5301	5330	5358	5386	5415
12	5443	5471	5500	5528	5557	5585	5613	5642	5670	5698	5727	5755	5783	5812	5840	5868
13	5897	5925	5953	5982	6010	6038	6067	6095	6123	6152	6180	6209	6237	6265	6294	6322
14	6350	6379	6407	6435	6464	6492	6520	6549	6577	6605	6634	6662	6690	6719	6747	6776
15	6804	6832	6860	6889	6917	6945	6973	7002	7030	7059	7087	7115	7144	7172	7201	7228
Pounds	0	1	2	3	4	5	6	7	8	9	10	11	12	13	14	15
	Ounces															

*To convert pounds and ounces to grams, multiply the pounds by 453.6 and the ounces by 28.35; add the totals.
To convert grams into pounds and decimals of a pound, multiply the grams by 0.0022.
To convert grams into ounces, divide the grams by 28.35 (16 oz = 1 lb).

APPENDIX F

Nutritional Allowances and Supplements

| Table F-1 | *Recommended Energy Intake for Age* | | |

Age (yr)	REE (kcal/kg/day)	AVERAGE ENERGY NEEDS (kcal/kg/day)	(kcal/day)
Infants			
0.0-0.5	53	108	650
0.5-1.0	56	98	850
Children			
1-3	57	102	1300
4-6	48	90	1800
7-10	40	70	2000
Males			
11-14	32	55	2500
15-18	27	45	3000
Females			
11-14	28	47	2200
15-18	25	40	2200
Pregnancy			
1st trimester			+0
2nd and 3rd trimesters			+300
Lactation			
			+500

Modified from Food Nutrition Board, National Research Council: *Recommended dietary allowances,* ed 10, Washington, DC, 1989, National Academy Press.
REE, Resting energy expenditure (based on Food and Agricultural Organization [FAO] equations).

Table F-2. Recommended Dietary Allowances*—Minerals

Age (yr)	Weight† (kg)	Weight† (lb)	Height† (cm)	Height† (in)	Calcium (mg)	Phosphorus (mg)	Magnesium (mg)	Iron (mg)	Zinc (mg)	Iodine (µg)	Selenium (µg)
Infants											
0.0-0.5	6	13	60	24	400	300	40	6	5	40	10
0.5-1.0	9	20	71	28	600	500	60	10	5	50	15
Children											
1-3	13	29	90	35	800	800	80	10	10	70	20
4-6	20	44	112	44	800	800	120	10	10	90	20
7-10	28	62	132	52	800	800	170	10	10	120	30
Males											
11-14	45	99	157	62	1200	1200	270	12	15	150	40
15-18	66	145	176	69	1200	1200	400	12	15	150	50
19-24	72	160	177	70	1200	1200	350	10	15	150	70
Females											
11-14	46	101	157	62	1200	1200	280	15	12	150	45
15-18	55	120	163	64	1200	1200	300	15	12	150	50
19-24	58	128	164	65	1200	1200	280	15	12	150	55
Pregnant					1200	1200	320	30	15	175	65
Lactating											
1st 6 mo					1200	1200	355	15	19	200	75
2nd 6 mo					1200	1200	340	15	16	200	75

Modified from the Food Nutrition Board, National Research Council: *Recommended dietary allowances*, ed 10, Washington, DC, 1989, National Academy Press.

*The allowances, expressed as daily intakes over time, are intended to provide for individual variations among most normal persons as they live in the United States under usual environmental stresses. Diets should be based on a variety of common foods in order to provide other nutrients for which human requirements have been less well defined.

†Weights and heights of Reference Adults are based on actual medians for the United States population of the designated age, as reported by NHANE. II. The median weights and heights of those under 19 years of age are from Hamill.[4] The use of these figures does not imply that the height-to-weight ratios are ideal.

Table F-3 *Recommended Dietary Allowances*—Vitamins*

Age (yr)	Weight† (kg)	Weight† (lb)	Height† (cm)	Height† (in)	Protein (g)	Fat-Soluble Vitamins Vitamin A (IU)‡	Vitamin D (IU)§	Vitamin E (IU)‖	Vitamin K (μg)	Vitamin C (mg)	Thiamin (mg)	Riboflavin (mg)	Water-Soluble Vitamins Niacin (mgNE)¶	Vitamin B$_6$ (mg)	Folate (μg)	B$_{12}$ (μg)
Infants																
0.0-0.5	6	13	60	24	13	1250	300	3	5	30	0.3	0.4	5	0.3	25	0.3
0.5-1.0	9	20	71	28	14	1250	400	4	10	35	0.4	0.5	6	0.6	35	0.5
Children																
1-3	13	29	90	35	16	1333	400	6	15	40	0.7	0.8	9	1.0	50	0.7
4-6	20	44	112	44	24	1667	400	7	20	45	0.9	1.1	12	1.1	75	1.0
7-10	28	62	132	52	28	2333	400	7	30	45	1.0	1.2	13	1.4	100	1.4
Males																
11-14	45	99	157	62	45	3333	400	10	45	50	1.3	1.5	17	1.7	150	2.0
15-18	66	145	176	69	59	3333	400	10	65	60	1.5	1.8	20	2.0	200	2.0
19-24	72	160	177	70	58	3333	400	10	70	60	1.5	1.7	19	2.0	200	2.0

Females																
11-14	46	101	157	62	46	2667	400	8	45	50	1.1	1.3	15	1.4	150	2.0
15-18	55	120	163	64	44	2667	400	8	55	60	1.1	1.3	15	1.5	180	2.0
19-24	58	128	164	65	46	2667	400	8	60	60	1.1	1.3	15	1.6	180	2.0
Pregnant					60	2667	400	10	65	70	1.5	1.6	17	2.2	400	2.2
Lactating																
1st 6 mo					65	4333	400	12	65	95	1.6	1.8	20	2.1	280	2.6
2nd 6 mo					62	4000	400	11	65	90	1.6	1.7	20	2.1	260	2.6

Modified from the Food Nutrition Board, National Research Council: *Recommended dietary allowances*, ed 10, Washington, DC, 1989, National Academy Press.

*,†See footnotes in Table F-2.

Conversion factors for international unit (IU):

‡Vitamin A: µg RE/0.3 = IU, where RE is retinol equivalent.

§Vitamin D: 40 × mcg cholecalciferol = IU.

||Vitamin E: as RRR-α-tocopherol.

¶Niacin equivalent (NE) is equal to 1 mg niacin or 60 mg dietary tryptophan.

APPENDIX G

Vital Signs for Normal Values

Table G-1	*Blood Pressure Levels by Percentiles of Height, Boys, 1 to 17 Years*

| | | SYSTOLIC BP (mmHg) BY PERCENTILE OF HEIGHT | | | | | | |
Percentiles Age (yr)	Height*→ BP†↓	5%	10%	25%	50%	75%	90%	95%
1	90th	94	95	97	98	100	102	102
	95th	98	99	101	102	104	106	106
2	90th	98	99	100	102	104	105	106
	95th	101	102	104	106	108	109	110
3	90th	100	101	103	105	107	108	109
	95th	104	105	107	109	111	112	113
4	90th	102	103	105	107	109	110	111
	95th	106	107	109	111	113	114	115
5	90th	104	105	106	108	110	112	112
	95th	108	109	110	112	114	115	116
6	90th	105	106	108	110	111	113	114
	95th	109	110	112	114	115	117	117
7	90th	106	107	109	111	113	114	115
	95th	110	111	113	115	116	118	119
8	90th	107	108	110	112	114	115	116
	95th	111	112	114	116	118	119	120
9	90th	109	110	112	113	115	117	117
	95th	113	114	116	117	119	121	121
10	90th	110	112	113	115	117	118	119
	95th	114	115	117	119	121	122	123
11	90th	112	113	115	117	119	120	121
	95th	116	117	119	121	123	124	125
12	90th	115	116	117	119	121	123	123
	95th	119	120	121	123	125	126	127
13	90th	117	118	120	122	124	125	126
	95th	121	122	124	126	128	129	130
14	90th	120	121	123	125	126	128	128
	95th	124	125	127	128	130	132	132
15	90th	123	124	125	127	129	131	131
	95th	127	128	129	131	133	134	135
16	90th	125	126	128	130	132	133	134
	95th	129	130	132	134	136	137	138
17	90th	128	129	131	133	134	136	136
	95th	132	133	135	136	138	140	140

BP, Blood pressure.
*Height percentile determined by standard growth curves.
†Blood pressure percentile determined by a single measurement.

Diastolic BP (DBP) (mmHg) by Percentile of Height

5%	10%	25%	50%	75%	90%	95%
50	51	52	53	54	54	55
55	55	56	57	58	59	59
55	55	56	57	58	59	59
59	59	60	61	62	63	63
59	59	60	61	62	63	63
63	63	64	65	66	67	67
62	62	63	64	65	66	66
66	67	67	68	69	70	71
65	65	66	67	68	69	69
69	70	70	71	72	73	74
67	68	69	70	70	71	72
72	72	73	74	75	76	76
69	70	71	72	72	73	74
74	74	75	76	77	78	78
71	71	72	73	74	75	75
75	76	76	77	78	79	80
72	73	73	74	75	76	77
76	77	78	79	80	80	81
73	74	74	75	76	77	78
77	78	79	80	80	81	82
74	74	75	76	77	78	78
78	79	79	80	81	82	83
75	75	76	77	78	78	79
79	79	80	81	82	83	83
75	76	76	77	78	79	80
79	80	81	82	83	83	84
76	76	77	78	79	80	80
80	81	81	82	83	84	85
77	77	78	79	80	81	81
81	82	83	83	84	85	86
79	79	80	81	82	82	83
83	83	84	85	86	87	87
81	81	82	83	84	85	85
85	85	86	87	88	89	89

Table G-2 *Blood Pressure Levels by Percentiles of Height, Girls, 1 to 17 Years*

Percentiles Age (yr)	Height*→ BP†↓	Systolic BP (mmHg) by Percentile of Height							Diastolic BP (DBP) (mmHg) by Percentile of Height						
		5%	10%	25%	50%	75%	90%	95%	5%	10%	25%	50%	75%	90%	95%
1	90th	97	98	99	100	102	103	104	53	53	53	54	55	56	56
	95th	101	102	103	104	105	107	107	57	57	57	58	59	60	60
2	90th	99	99	100	102	103	104	105	57	57	58	58	59	60	61
	95th	102	103	104	105	107	108	109	61	61	62	62	63	64	65
3	90th	100	100	102	103	104	105	106	61	61	61	62	63	63	64
	95th	104	104	105	107	108	109	110	65	65	65	66	67	67	68
4	90th	101	102	103	104	106	107	108	63	63	64	65	65	66	67
	95th	105	106	107	108	109	111	111	67	67	68	69	69	70	71
5	90th	103	103	104	106	107	108	109	65	66	66	67	68	68	69
	95th	107	107	108	110	111	112	113	69	70	70	71	72	72	73
6	90th	104	105	106	107	109	110	111	67	67	68	69	69	70	71
	95th	108	109	110	111	112	114	114	71	71	72	73	73	74	75

Age	BP† Percentile	Systolic BP (mm Hg) by Height Percentile*							Diastolic BP (mm Hg) by Height Percentile*						
7	90th	106	107	108	109	110	112	112	69	69	69	70	71	72	72
	95th	110	110	112	113	114	115	116	73	73	73	74	75	76	76
8	90th	108	109	110	111	112	113	114	70	70	71	71	72	73	74
	95th	112	112	113	115	116	117	118	74	74	75	75	76	77	78
9	90th	110	110	112	113	114	115	116	71	72	72	73	74	74	75
	95th	114	114	115	117	118	119	120	75	76	77	78	78	78	79
10	90th	112	112	114	115	116	117	118	73	73	73	74	75	76	76
	95th	116	116	117	119	120	121	122	77	77	77	78	79	80	80
11	90th	114	114	116	117	118	119	120	74	74	75	75	76	77	77
	95th	118	118	119	121	122	123	124	78	78	79	79	80	81	81
12	90th	116	116	118	119	120	121	122	75	75	76	76	77	78	78
	95th	120	120	121	123	124	125	126	79	79	80	80	81	82	82
13	90th	118	118	119	121	122	123	124	76	76	77	78	78	79	80
	95th	121	122	123	125	126	127	128	80	80	81	82	82	83	84
14	90th	119	120	121	122	124	125	126	77	77	78	79	79	80	81
	95th	123	124	125	126	128	129	130	81	81	82	83	83	84	85
15	90th	121	121	122	124	125	126	127	78	78	79	79	80	81	82
	95th	124	125	126	128	129	130	131	82	82	83	83	84	85	86
16	90th	122	122	123	125	126	127	128	79	79	79	80	81	82	82
	95th	125	126	127	128	130	131	132	83	83	83	84	85	86	86
17	90th	122	123	124	125	126	128	128	79	79	79	80	81	82	82
	95th	126	126	127	129	130	131	132	83	83	83	84	85	86	86

BP, Blood pressure.
*Height percentile determined by standard growth curves.
†Blood pressure percentile determined by a single measurement.

Table G-3 · Age-Specific Heart Rates, Birth to 15 Years

Age	2%	Mean	98%
<1 day	93	123	154
1-2 days	91	123	159
3-6 days	91	129	166
1-3 wk	107	148	182
1-2 mo	121	149	179
3-5 mo	106	141	186
6-11 mo	109	134	169
1-2 yr	89	119	151
3-4 yr	73	108	137
5-7 yr	65	100	133
8-11 yr	62	91	130
12-15 yr	60	85	119

Table G-4 · Age-Specific Respiratory Rates, Birth to 18 years

Age (yr)	Boys	Girls	Age (yr)	Boys	Girls
0-1	31 ± 8	30 ± 6	9-10	19 ± 2	19 ± 2
1-2	26 ± 4	27 ± 4	10-11	19 ± 2	19 ± 2
2-3	25 ± 4	25 ± 3	11-12	19 ± 3	19 ± 3
3-4	24 ± 3	24 ± 3	12-13	19 ± 3	19 ± 2
4-5	23 ± 2	22 ± 2	13-14	19 ± 2	18 ± 2
5-6	22 ± 2	21 ± 2	14-15	18 ± 2	18 ± 3
6-7	21 ± 3	21 ± 3	15-16	17 ± 3	18 ± 3
7-8	20 ± 3	20 ± 2	16-17	17 ± 2	17 ± 3
8-9	20 ± 2	20 ± 2	17-18	16 ± 3	17 ± 3

From Illif A, Lee V: *Child Dev* 23:240, 1952.

APPENDIX H

Reference Ranges for Laboratory Tests

Table H-1	Prefixes Denoting Decimal Factors

Prefix	Symbol
mega	M
kilo	k
hecto	h
deka	da
deci	d
centi	c
milli	m
micro	μ
nano	n
pico	p
femto	f

Table H-2	Abbreviations

Ab	absorbance
AI	angiotensin I
AU	arbitrary unit
cAMP	cyclic adenosine 3',5' monophosphate
cap	capillary
CH^{50}	dilution required to lyse 50% of indicator RBC; indicates complement activity
CHF	congestive heart failure
CKBB	brain isoenzyme of creatine kinase
CKMB	heart isoenzyme of creatine kinase
CNS	central nervous system
conc.	concentration
Cr.	creatinine
d	diem, day, days
F	female
g	gram
hr	hour, hours
Hb	hemoglobin
HbCO	carboxyhemoglobin

Continued

Table H-2	*Abbreviations—cont'd*
Hgb	hemoglobin
hpf	high-power field
HPLC	high-performance liquid chromatography
IFA	indirect fluorescent antibody
IU	International Unit of hormone activity
L	liter
M	male
MCV	mean corpuscular volume
mEq/L	milliequivalents per liter
min	minute, minutes
mm^3	cubic millimeter; equivalent to microliter (μl)
mm Hg	millimeters of mercury
mo	month, months
mol	mole
mOsm	milliosmole
MW	relative molecular weight
Na	sodium
nm	nanometer (wavelength)
Pa	pascal
pc	postprandial
RBC	red blood cell(s); erythrocyte(s)
RIA	radioimmunoassay
RID	radial immunodiffusion
RT	room temperature
s	second, seconds
SD	standard deviation
std.	standard
therap.	therapeutic
U	International Unit of enzyme activity
V	volume
WBC	white blood cell(s)
WHO	World Health Organization
wk	week, weeks
yr	year, years

Table H-3	**Abbreviations for Specimens**
S	serum
P	plasma
(H)	heparin
(LiH)	lithium heparin
(E)	EDTA
(C)	citrate
(O)	oxalate
W	whole blood
U	urine
F	feces
CSF	cerebrospinal fluid
AF	amniotic fluid
(NaC)	sodium citrate
(NH_4H)	ammonium heparinate

Table H-4	**Symbols**
$>$	greater than
$\geq$	greater than or equal to
$<$	less than
$\leq$	less than or equal to
$\pm$	plus/minus
$\cong$	approximately equal to

Table H-5	Reference Ranges for Laboratory Tests	
	Conventional Units	**SI Units**

Acid Phosphatase
(Major sources: prostate and erythrocytes[1])

Newborn	7.4-19.4 U/L	7.4-19.4 U/L
2-13 yr	6.4-15.2 U/L	6.4-15.2 U/L
Adult male	0.5-11.0 U/L	0.5-11.0 U/L
Adult female	0.2-9.5 U/L	0.2-9.5 U/L

Alanine Aminotransferase (ALT)
(Major sources: liver, skeletal muscle, and myocardium[1])

Infant	<54 U/L	<54 U/L
Child/adult	1-30 U/L	1-30 U/L

Aldolase
(Major sources: skeletal muscle and myocardium[1])

Newborn	<32 U/L	<32 U/L
Child	<16 U/L	<8 U/L
Adult	<8 U/L	<8 U/L

Alkaline Phosphatase
(Major sources: liver, bone, intestinal mucosa, placenta, and kidney[1])

Infant	150-420 U/L	150-140 U/L
2-10 yr	100-320 U/L	100-320 U/L
11-18-yr-old boy	100-390 U/L	100-390 U/L
11-18-yr-old girl	100-320 U/L	100-320 U/L
Adult	30-120 U/L	30-100 U/L

α_1-**Antitrypsin**	93-224 mg/dL	0.93-2.24 g/L

α-Fetoprotein

>1 yr-adult	<30 ng/mL	<30 µg/L
Tumor marker	0-10 mg/mL	

Ammonia (heparinized venous specimen on ice analyzed within 30 min)

Newborn	90-150 µg/dL	64-107 µmol/L
0-2 wk	79-129 µg/dL	56-92 µmol/L
>1 mo	29-70 µg/dL	21-50 µmol/L
Adult	0-50 µg/dL	0-35.7 µmol/L

Amylase
(Major sources: pancreas, salivary glands, and ovaries[1])

Newborn	0-44 U/L	5-65 U/L
Adult	0-88 U/L	0-130 U/L

Antihyaluronidase Antibody

	<1:256	

Table H-5 | *Reference Ranges for Laboratory Tests—cont'd*

	Conventional Units	SI Units

Antinuclear Antibody (ANA)

Not significant	<1:80	
Likely significant	>1:320	
Patterns with clinical correlation		
Centromere—CREST		
Nucleolar—Scleroderma		
Homogeneous—nDNA, antihistone Ab		

Antistreptolysin O Titer (4× rise in paired serial specimens is significant)

Preschool	<1:85	
School age	<1:170	
Older adult	<1:85	

Note: Alternatively, values up to 200 Todd units are normal.

Arsenic

Normal	<3 μg/dL	<0.39 μmol/L
Acute poisoning	60-930 μg/dL	7.98-124 μmol/L
Chronic poisoning	10-50 μg/dL	1.33-6.65 μmol/L

Aspartate Aminotransferase (AST)

(Major sources: liver, skeletal muscle, kidney, myocardium, and erythrocytes[1])

Newborn/infant	20-65 U/L	20-65 U/L
Child/adult	0-35 U/L	0-4350 U/L

Bicarbonate

Preterm	18-26 mEq/L	18-26 mmol/L
Full term	20-25 mEq/L	20-25 mmol/L
>2 yr	22-26 mEq/L	22-26 mmol/L

Bilirubin (Total)

Cord	Preterm	<2 mg/dL	<34 μmol/L
	Term	<2 mg/dL	<34 μmol/L
0-1 day	Preterm	<8 mg/dL	<137 μmol/L
	Term	<6 mg/dL	<103 μmol/L
1-2 day	Preterm	<12 mg/dL	<205 μmol/L
	Term	<8 mg/dL	<137 μmol/L
3-5 day	Preterm	<16 mg/dL	<274 μmol/L
	Term	<12 mg/dL	<205 μmol/L
Thereafter	Preterm	<2 mg/dL	<34 μmol/L
	Term	<1 mg/dL	<17 μmol/L
Adult		0.1-1.2 mg/dL	1.7-20.5 μmol/L

Bilirubin (Conjugated)		0-0.4 mg/dL	0-8 μmol/L

Continued

Table H-5 — Reference Ranges for Laboratory Tests—cont'd

	Conventional Units	SI Units
Calcium (Total)		
Preterm <1 wk	6-10 mg/dL	1.5-2.5 mmol/L
Full term <1 wk	7.0-12.0 mg/dL	1.75-3.0 mmol/L
Child	8.0-10.5 mg/dL	2-2.6 mmol/L
Adult	8.5-10.5 mg/dL	2.1-2.6 mmol/L
Calcium (Ionized)		
Newborn <48 hr	4.0-4.7 mg/dL	1.00-1.18 mmol/L
Adult	4.52-5.28 mg/dL	1.13-1.32 mmol/L
Carbon Dioxide (CO$_2$ Content)		
Cord blood	14-22 mEq/L	14-22 mmol/L
Infant/child	20-24 mEq/L	20-24 mmol/L
Adult	24-30 mEq/L	24-30 mmol/L
Carbon Monoxide (Carboxyhemoglobin)		
Nonsmoker	0%-2% of total hemoglobin	
Smoker	2%-10% of total hemoglobin	
Toxic	20%-60% of total hemoglobin	
Lethal	>60% of total hemoglobin	
Carotenoids (Carotenes)		
Infant	20-70 µg/dL	0.37-1.30 µmol/L
Child	40-130 µg/dL	0.74-2.42 µmol/L
Adult	50-250 µg/dL	0.95-4.69 µmol/L
Ceruloplasmin	21-53 mg/dL	210-530 mg/L
Chloride (Serum)		
Pediatric	99-111 mEq/L	99-111 mmol/L
Adult	96-109 mEq/L	96-109 mmol/L
Cholesterol (see Lipids)		
Copper		
0-6 mo	20-70 µg/dL	3.1-11 µmol/L
6 yr	90-190 µg/dL	14-30 µmol/L
12 yr	80-160 µg/dL	12.6-25 µmol/L
Adult male	70-140 µg/dL	11-22 µmol/L
Adult female	80-155 µg/dL	12.6-24.3 µmol/L
C-Reactive Protein	0-0.5 mg/dL	

(Other laboratories may have different reference values)

Table H-5   *Reference Ranges for Laboratory Tests—cont'd*

	Conventional Units	SI Units
Creatine Kinase (Creatine Phosphokinase)		
(Major sources: myocardium, skeletal muscle, smooth muscle, and brain[1])		
Newborn	10-200 U/L	10-200 U/L
Man	12-80 U/L	12-80 U/L
Woman	10-55 U/L	10-55 U/L
Creatinine (Serum)		
Cord	0.6-1.2 mg/dL	53-106 μmol/L
Newborn	0.3-1.0 mg/dL	27-88 μmol/L
Infant	0.2-0.4 mg/dL	18-35 μmol/L
Child	0.3-0.7 mg/dL	27-62 μmol/L
Adolescent	0.5-1.0 mg/dL	44-88 μmol/L
Man	0.6-1.3 mg/dL	53-115 μmol/L
Woman	0.5-1.2 mg/dL	44-106 μmol/L
ESR		
Ferritin		
Newborn	25-200 ng/mL	25-200 μg/L
1 mo	200-600 ng/mL	200-600 μg/L
6 mo	50-200 ng/mL	50-200 μg/L
6 mo-15 yr	7-140 ng/mL	7-140 μg/L
Adult male	15-200 ng/mL	15-200 μg/L
Adult female	12-150 ng/mL	12-150 μg/L
Fibrinogen	200-400 mg/dL	2-4 g/L
Folic Acid (Folate)	3-17.5 ng/mL	4.0-20.0 nmol/L
Folic Acid (RBCs)	153-605 μg/mL RBCs	
Galactose		
Newborn	0-20 mg/dL	0-1.11 mmol/L
Thereafter	<5 mg/dL	<0.28 mmol/L
γ-Glutamyl Transferase (GGT)		
(Major sources: liver [biliary tree] and kidney[1])		
Cord	19-270 U/L	19-270 U/L
Preterm	56-233 U/L	56-233 U/L
0-3 wk	0-130 U/L	0-130 U/L
3 wk-3 mo	4-120 U/L	4-120 U/L
>3 mo boy	5-65 U/L	5-65 U/L
>3 mo girl	5-35 U/L	5-35 U/L
1-15 yr	0-23 U/L	0-23 U/L
Adult male	11-50 U/L	11-50 U/L
Adult female	7-32 U/L	7-32 U/L

Continued

Table H-5 Reference Ranges for Laboratory Tests—cont'd

	Conventional Units	SI Units
Gastrin	<100 pg/mL	<100 ng/L
Glucose (Serum)		
Preterm	45-100 mg/dL	1.1-3.6 mmol/L
Full term	45-120 mg/dL	1.1-6.4 mmol/L
1 wk-16 yr	60-105 mg/dL	3.3-5.8 mmol/L
>16 yr	70-115 mg/dL	3.9-6.4 mmol/L
Iron		
Newborn	100-250 µg/dL	18-45 µmol/L
Infant	40-100 µg/dL	7-18 µmol/L
Child	50-120 µg/dL	9-22 µmol/L
Adult male	65-170 µg/dL	12-30 µmol/L
Adult female	50-170 µg/dL	9-30 µmol/L
Ketones (Serum)		
Qualitative	Negative	
Quantitative	0.5-3.0 mg/dL	5-30 mg/L
Lactate		
Capillary blood		
Newborn	<27 mg/dL	0.0-3.0 mmol/L
Child	5-20 mg/dL	0.56-2.25 mmol/L
Venous	5-20 mg/dL	0.5-2.2 mmol/L
Arterial	5-14 mg/dL	0.5-1.6 mmol/L

Lactate Dehydrogenase (at 37° C)

(Major sources: myocardium, liver, skeletal muscle, erythrocytes, platelets, and lymph nodes[1])		
Neonate	160-1500 U/L	160-1500 U/L
Infant	150-360 U/L	150-360 U/L
Child	150-300 U/L	150-300 U/L
Adult	0-220 U/L	0-220 U/L

Lactate Dehydrogenase Isoenzymes (% total)

LD_1 heart	24%-34%	
LD_2 heart, erythrocytes	35%-45%	
LD_3 muscle	15%-25%	
LD_4 liver, trace muscle	4%-10%	
LD_5 liver, muscle	1%-9%	
Lead		
Child	<10 µg/dL	<48 µmol/L
Lipase	4-24 U/dL	

Table H-5 *Reference Ranges for Laboratory Tests—cont'd*

	Conventional Units	SI Units

Lipids²

	Cholesterol (mg/dL) Desirable Borderline High			LDL (mg/dL) Desirable Borderline High		
Child/adolescent	<170	170-199	≥200	<110	110-129	≥130
Adult	<200	200-239	≥240	<130	130-159	≥160
HDL	>45					

	Conventional Units	SI Units
Magnesium	1.3-2.0 mEq/L	0.65-1.0 mmol/L
Manganese (Blood)		
Newborn	2.4-9.6 µg/dL	0.44-1.75 µmol/L
2-18 yr	0.8-2.1 µg/dL	0.15-0.38 µmol/L
Methemoglobin	0%-1.3% total Hgb	
Osmolality	285-295 mOsmol/kg	285-295 mmol/kg
Phenylalanine		
Preterm	2.0-7.5 mg/dL	0.12-0.45 mmol/L
Newborn	1.2-3.4 mg/dL	0.07-0.21 mmol/L
Adult	0.8-1.8 mg/dL	0.05-0.11 mmol/L
Phosphorus		
Newborn	4.2-9.0 mg/dL	1.36-2.91 mmol/L
0-15 yr	3.2-6.3 mg/dL	1.03-2.1 mmol/L
Adult	2.7-4.5 mg/dL	0.87-1.45 mmol/L
Porcelain³	0.52-1.94 mg/dL	0.32-9.93 mmol/L
Potassium		
<10dy of age	4.0-6.0 mEq/L	4.0-6.0 mmol/L
>10dy of age	3.5-5.0 mEq/L	3.5-5.0 mmol/L
Prealbumin		
Newborn-6 wk	4-36 mg/dL	
6 wk-16 yr	13-27 mg/dL	
Adult	18-45 mg/dL	

Proteins

Protein electrophoresis (g/dL)

Age	TP	Albumin	α-1	α-2	β	γ
Cord	4.8-8.0	2.2-4.0	0.3-0.7	0.4-0.9	0.4-1.6	0.8-1.6
Newborn	4.4-7.6	3.2-4.8	0.1-0.3	0.2-0.3	0.3-0.6	0.6-1.2
1 day-1 mo	4.4-7.6	2.5-5.5	0.1-0.3	0.3-1.0	0.2-1.1	0.4-1.3
1-3 mo	3.6-7.4	2.1-4.8	0.1-0.4	0.3-1.1	0.3-1.1	0.2-1.1
4-6 mo	4.2-7.4	2.8-5.0	0.1-0.4	0.3-0.8	0.3-0.8	0.1-0.9
7-12 mo	5.1-7.5	3.2-5.7	0.1-0.6	0.3-1.5	0.4-1.0	0.2-1.2
13-24 mo	3.7-7.5	1.9-5.0	0.1-0.6	0.4-1.4	0.4-1.4	0.4-1.6
25-36 mo	5.3-8.1	3.3-5.8	0.1-0.3	0.4-1.1	0.3-1.2	0.4-1.5

Continued

Table H-5   *Reference Ranges for Laboratory Tests—cont'd*

	Conventional Units					SI Units	

Proteins—cont'd

3-5 yr	4.9-8.1	2.9-5.8	0.1-0.4	0.4-1.0	0.5-1.0	0.4-1.7	
6-8 yr	6.0-7.9	3.3-5.0	0.1-0.5	0.5-0.8	0.5-0.9	0.7-2.0	
9-11 yr	6.0-7.9	3.2-5.0	0.1-0.4	0.7-0.9	0.6-1.0	0.8-2.0	
12-16 yr	6.0-7.9	3.2-5.1	0.1-0.4	0.5-1.1	0.5-1.1	0.6-2.0	
Adult	6.0-8.0	3.1-5.4	0.1-0.4	0.4-1.1	0.5-1.2	0.7-1.7	

Pyruvate   0.3-0.9 mg/dL   0.03-0.10 mmol/L

Rheumatoid Factor   <20

Rheumaton Titer (modified Waaler-Rose slide test)
          <10

Sodium

Preterm	130-140 mEq/L	130-140 mmol/L
Older	135-148 mEq/L	135-148 mmol/L

Transaminase (SGOT) (see Aspartate aminotransferase [AST])

Transaminase (SGPT) (see Alanine aminotransferase [ALT])

Transferrin

Newborn	130-275 mg/dL	1.3-2.7 g/L
Adult	200-400 mg/dL	2.0-4.0 g/L

Triglycerides (fasting)[4]

	Male (mg/dL)	Female (mg/dL)	Male (g/L)	Female (g/L)
Cord blood	10-98	10-98	0.10-0.98	0.10-0.98
0-5 yr	30-86	32-99	0.30-0.86	0.32-0.99
6-11 yr	31-108	35-114	0.31-1.08	0.35-1.14
12-15 yr	36-138	41-138	0.36-1.38	0.41-1.38
16-19 yr	40-163	40-128	0.40-1.63	0.40-1.28
20-29 yr	44-185	40-128	0.44-1.85	0.40-1.28
Adults	40-160	35-135	0.40-1.60	0.35-1.35

Troponin   0.03-0.15 ng/mL

Urea Nitrogen   7-22 mg/dL   2.5-7.9 mmol/L

Uric Acid

0-2 yr	2.4-6.4 mg/dL	0.14-0.38 mmol/L
2-12 yr	2.4-5.9 mg/dL	0.14-0.35 mmol/L
12-14 yr	2.4-6.4 mg/dL	0.14-0.38 mmol/L
Adult male	3.5-7.2 mg/dL	0.20-0.43 mmol/L
Adult female	2.4-6.4 mg/dL	0.14-0.38 mmol/L

Table H-5   *Reference Ranges for Laboratory Tests—cont'd*

	Conventional Units	SI Units
Vitamin A (retinol)		
Newborn	35-75 μg/dL	1.22-2.62 μmol/L
Child	30-80 μg/dL	1.05-2.79 μmol/L
Adult	30-65 μg/dL	1.05-2.27 μmol/L
Vitamin B$_1$ (thiamine)	5.3-7.9 μg/dL	0.16-0.23 μmol/L
Vitamin B$_2$ (riboflavin)	3.7-13.7 μg/dL	98-262 μmol/L
Vitamin B$_{12}$ (cobalamin)	130-785 pg/mL	96-579 pmol/L
Vitamin C (ascorbic acid)	0.2-2.0 mg/dL	11.4-113.6 μmol/L
Vitamin D$_3$ (1,25-dihydroxy-vitamin D)		
	25-45 pg/mL	60-108 pmol/L
Vitamin E	5-20 mg/dL	11.6-46.4 μmol/L
Zinc	70-150 μg/dL	10.7-22.9 μmol/L

1. Burtis CA, Ashwood ER: *Tietz textbook of clinical chemistry,* ed 2, Philadelphia, 1994, WB Saunders.
2. Summary of the NCEP Adult Treatment Panel II Report: HIghlights of the report of the Expert Panel on Blood & Cholesterol Levels in Children and Adolescents, 1991, U.S. Department of Health and Human Services, *JAMA* 269:1993.
3. Iannone P, Reddy U, Siberry V, et al: *Surviving pediatric chief residency at Hopkins: patient and virtue,* Baltimore and Wilmington, Del, 1998-1999, Johns Hopkins.
4. Behrman RE, Kliegman RM, Arvin AM: *Nelson textbook of pediatrics,* ed 15, Philadelphia, 1996, WB Saunders.

APPENDIX I

Weights and Measures

Table I-1   Measures of Capacity: Apothecaries' (Wine) Measures

Minims	Fluid Drams	Fluid Ounces	Gills	Pints
1	0.0166	0.002	0.005	0.0013
60	1	0.125	0.0312	0.0078
480	8	1	0.25	0.0625
1920	32	4	1	0.25
7680	128	16	4	1
15360	256	32	8	2
61440	1024	128	32	8

Table I-2   Measures of Capacity: Metric Measure

Microliter	Milliliter	Centiliter	Deciliter	Liter
1	—	—	—	—
10^3	1	—	—	—
10^4	10	1	—	—
10^5	100	10	1	—
10^6	10^3	100	10	1
10^7	10^4	10^3	100	10
10^8	10^5	10^4	10^3	100
10^9	10^6	10^5	10^4	10^3
10^{12}	10^9	10^8	10^7	10^6

1 liter = 2.113363738 pints (Apothecaries').

Quarts	Gallons	Cubic Inches	Milliliters	Cubic Centimeters
			Equivalents	
—	—	0.00376	0.06161	0.06161
0.0039	—	0.22558	3.6967	3.6967
0.0312	0.0078	1.80468	29.5737	29.5737
0.125	0.0312	7.21875	118.2948	118.2948
0.5	0.125	28.875	473.179	473.179
1	0.25	57.75	946.358	946.358
4	1	231	3785.434	3785.434

Dekaliter	Hectoliter	Kiloliter	Megaliter	Equivalents (Apothecaries' Fluid)
—	—	—	—	0.01623108 min
—	—	—	—	16.23 min
—	—	—	—	2.7 fl dr
—	—	—	—	3.38 fl oz
—	—	—	—	2.11 pts
1	—	—	—	2.64 gal
10	1	—	—	26.418 gals
100	10	1	—	264.18 gals
10^5	10^4	10^3	1	26418 gals

Table I-3   Measures of Length: Metric Measure

Micrometer	Millimeter	Centimeter	Decimeter	Meter	Dekameter	Hectometer	Kilometer	Megameter	Equivalents
1	0.001	10^{-4}	—	—	—	—	—	—	0.000039 in
10^3	1	10^{-1}	—	—	—	—	—	—	0.03937 in
10^4	10	1	—	—	—	—	—	—	0.3937 in
10^5	100	10	1	—	—	—	—	—	3.937 in
10^6	1000	100	10	1	—	—	—	—	39.37 in
10^7	10^4	1000	100	10	1	—	—	—	10.9361 yd
10^8	10^5	10^4	1000	100	10	1	—	—	109.3612 yd
10^9	10^6	10^5	10^4	1000	100	10	1	—	1093.6121 yd
10^{10}	10^7	10^6	10^5	10^4	1000	100	10	—	6.2137 m
10^{12}	10^9	10^8	10^7	10^6	10^5	10^4	1000	1	621.370 m

Table I-4   *Conversion Tables: Avoirdupois—Metric Weight*

Ounces	Grams	Ounces	Grams	Pounds	Grams	Kilograms
1/16	1.772	7	198.447	1 (16 oz)	453.59	
1/8	3.544	8	226.796	2	907.18	
1/4	7.088	9	255.146	3	1360.78	1.36
1/2	14.175	10	283.495	4	1814.37	1.81
1	28.350	11	311.845	5	2267.96	2.27
2	56.699	12	340.194	6	2721.55	2.72
3	85.049	13	368.544	7	3175.15	3.18
4	113.398	14	396.893	8	3628.74	3.63
5	141.748	15	425.243	9	4082.33	4.08
6	170.097	16 (1 lb)	453.59	10	4535.92	4.54

Table I-5   *Conversion Tables: Metric—Avoirdupois Weight*

Grams	Ounces	Grams	Ounces	Grams	Pounds
0.001 (1 mg)	0.000035274	1	0.035274	1000 (1 kg)	2.2046

Table I-6   *Conversion Tables: Apothecaries'—Metric Weight*

Grains	Grams	Grains	Grams	Scruples	Grams
1/150	0.0004	2/5	0.03	1	1.296 (1.3)
1/120	0.0005	1/2	0.032	2	2.592 (2.6)
1/100	0.0006	3/5	0.04	3 (1ʒ)	3.888 (3.9)
1/90	0.0007	2/3	0.043		
1/80	0.0008	3/4	0.0	**Drams**	**Grams**
1/64	0.001	7/8	0.057		
1/60	0.0011	1	0.065	1	3.888
1/50	0.0013	1 1/2	0.097 (0.1)	2	7.776
1/48	0.0014	2	0.12	3	11.664
1/40	0.0016	3	0.20	4	15.552
1/36	0.0018	4	0.24	5	19.440
1/32	0.002	5	0.30	6	23.328
1/30	0.0022	6	0.40	7	27.216
1/25	0.0026	7	0.45	8 (1ℨ)	31.103
1/20	0.003	8	0.50		
1/16	0.004	9	0.60	**Ounces**	**Grams**
1/12	0.005	10	0.65		
1/10	0.006	15	1.00	1	31.103
1/9	0.007	20 (1ℨ)	1.30	2	62.207
1/8	0.008	30	2.00	3	93.310
1/7	0.009			4	124.414
1/6	0.01			5	155.517
1/5	0.013			6	186.621
1/4	0.016			7	217.724
1/3	0.02			8	248.828
				9	279.931
				10	311.035
				11	342.138
				12 (1 ℔)	373.242

Table I-7			*Conversion Tables: Metric—Apothecaries' Weight*		
Milligrams	**Grains**	**Grams**	**Grains**	**Grams**	**Equivalents**
1	0.015432	0.1	1.5432	10	2.572 drams
2	0.030864	0.2	3.0864	15	3.858 "
3	0.046296	0.3	4.6296	20	5.144 "
4	0.061728	0.4	6.1728	25	6.430 "
5	0.077160	0.5	7.7160	30	7.716 "
6	0.092592	0.6	9.2592	40	1.286 oz
7	0.108024	0.7	10.8024	45	1.447 "
8	0.123456	0.8	12.3456	50	1.607 "
9	0.138888	0.9	13.8888	100	3.215 "
10	0.154320	1.0	15.4320	200	6.430 "
15	0.231480	1.5	23.1480	300	9.644 "
20	0.308640	2.0	30.8640	400	12.859 "
25	0.385800	2.5	38.5800	500	1.34 lb
30	0.462960	3.0	46.2960	600	1.61 "
35	0.540120	3.5	54.0120	700	1.88 "
40	0.617280	4.0	61.728	800	2.14 "
45	0.694440	4.5	69.444	900	2.41 "
50	0.771600	5.0	77.162	1000	2.68 "
100	1.543240	10.0	154.3240		

Table I-8			*Conversion Tables: Apothecaries'—Metric Liquid Measure*		
Minims	**Milliliters**	**Fluid Drams**	**Milliliters**	**Fluid Ounces**	**Milliliters**
1	0.06	1	3.70	1	29.57
2	0.12	2	7.39	2	59.15
3	0.19	3	11.09	3	88.72
4	0.25	4	14.79	4	118.29
5	0.31	5	18.48	5	147.87
10	0.62	6	22.18	6	177.44
15	0.92	7	25.88	7	207.01
20	1.23	8 (1 fl oz)	29.57	8	236.58
25	1.54			9	266.16
30	1.85			10	295.73
35	2.16			11	325.30
40	2.46			12	354.88
45	2.77			13	384.45
50	3.08			14	414.02
55	3.39			15	443.59
60 (1 fl dr)	3.70			16 (1 pt)	473.17
				32 (1 qt)	946.33
				128 (1 gal)	3785.32

Table I-9	Conversion Tables: Metric—Apothecaries' Liquid Measure				
Milliliters	Minims	Milliliters	Fluid Drams	Milliliters	Fluid Ounces
1	16.231	5	1.35	30	1.01
2	32.5	10	2.71	40	1.35
3	48.7	15	4.06	50	1.69
4	64.9	20	5.4	500	16.91
5	81.1	25	6.76	1000 (1 L)	33.815
		30	7.1		

Table I-10	Conversion Tables: U.S. and British—Metric Length		
Inches	Millimeters	Centimeters	Meters
1/25	1.00	0.1	0.001
1/8	3.18	0.318	0.00318
1/4	6.35	0.635	0.00635
1/2	12.70	1.27	0.00127
1	25.40	2.54	0.0254
12 (1 foot)	304.80	30.48	0.3048

APPROXIMATE APOTHECARY EQUIVALENTS

These *approximate* dose equivalents represent the quantities usually prescribed, under identical conditions, by physicians using, respectively, the metric system or the apothecary system of weights and measures. In labeling dosage forms in both the metric and the apothecary systems, if one is the approximate equivalent of the other, the approximate figure shall be enclosed in parentheses.

When prepared dosage forms such as tablets, capsules, and pills are prescribed in the metric system, the pharmacist may dispense the corresponding *approximate* equivalent in the apothecary system, and vice versa, as indicated in the following table.

For the conversion of specific quantities in converting pharmaceutical formulas, equivalents must be used. In the compounding of prescriptions, the exact equivalents, rounded to three significant figures, should be used.

Table I-11 — Liquid Measure

Metric	Approximate Apothecary Equivalents	Metric	Approximate Apothecary Equivalents
1000 ml	1 quart	3 ml	45 minims
750 ml	1 1/2 pints	2 ml	30 minims
500 ml	1 pint	1 ml	15 minims
250 ml	8 fluid ounces	0.75 ml	12 minims
200 ml	7 fluid ounces	0.6 ml	10 minims
100 ml	1 1/2 fluid ounces	0.5 ml	8 minims
50 ml	1 3/4 fluid ounces	0.3 ml	5 minims
30 ml	1 fluid ounce	0.25 ml	4 minims
15 ml	4 fluid drams	0.2 ml	3 minims
10 ml	2 1/2 fluid drams	0.1 ml	1 1/2 minims
8 ml	2 fluid drams	0.06 ml	1 minims
5 ml	1 1/4 fluid drams	0.05 ml	3/4 minim
4 ml	1 fluid drams	0.03 ml	1/2 minim

Table I-12 — Weight

Metric	Approximate Apothecary Equivalents	Metric	Approximate Apothecary Equivalents
30 g	1 ounce	30 mg	1/2 grain
15 g	4 drams	25 mg	3/8 grain
10 g	2 1/2 drams	20 mg	1/3 grain
7.5 g	2 drams	15 mg	1/4 grain
6 g	90 grains	12 mg	1/5 grain
5 g	75 grains	10 mg	1/6 grain
4 g	60 grains (1 dram)	8 mg	1/8 grain
3 g	45 grains	6 mg	1/10 grain
2 g	30 grains (1/2 dram)	5 mg	1/12 grain
1.5 g	22 grains	4 mg	1/15 grain
1 g	15 grains	3 mg	1/20 grain
750 mg	12 grains	2 mg	1/30 grain
600 mg	10 grains	1.5 mg	1/40 grain
500 mg	7 1/2 grains	1.2 mg	1/50 grain
400 mg	6 grains	1 mg	1/60 grain
300 mg	5 grains	800 μg	1/80 grain
250 mg	4 grains	600 μg	1/100 grain
200 mg	3 grains	500 μg	1/120 grain
150 mg	2 1/2 grains	400 μg	1/150 grain
125 mg	2 grains	300 μg	1/200 grain
100 mg	1 1/2 grains	250 μg	1/250 grain
75 mg	1 1/4 grains	200 μg	1/300 grain
60 mg	1 grain	150 μg	1/400 grain
50 mg	3/4 grain	120 μg	1/500 grain
40 mg	2/3 grain	100 μg	1/600 grain

The above *approximate* dose equivalents have been adopted by the *United States Pharmacopeia* and the *National Formulary,* and these dose equivalents have the approval of the federal Food and Drug Administration.

National Health and Educational Resources

The Web sites listed here do not imply endorsement. An attempt has been made to list important and informative health resources, but as with any electronic site, locations may change; therefore data needs to be reviewed for correctness and the date the data were updated.

CLEARINGHOUSES

ERIC Clearinghouse on Disabilities and Gifted Education
Council for Exceptional Children (CEC)
800-328-0272
Web site: www.ericec.org

Healthfinder—Your Guide to Reliable Health Information—US DHHS
Web site: www.healthfinder.gov/

Health Resources and Services Administration Information Center—US DHH
888-275-4772
Web site: www.ask.hrsa.gov/

Links to State Education Agencies
202-408-5505
Web site: www.ccsso.org/seamenu.html

National Clearinghouse for Alcohol and Drug Information (NCADI)
800-729-6686; 301-468-2345
Web site: www.health.org

National Clearinghouse on Child Abuse and Neglect Information
800-394-3366; 703-385-7565
Web site: www.calib.com/nccanch/index.cfm

National Council of State Boards of Nursing, Inc.
State Boards of Nursing: Contacts and Web Sites
Web site: www.ncsbn.org/public/regulation/boards_of_nursing_board.htm

National Diabetes Information Clearinghouse (NDIC)
301-654-3327
Web site: www.niddk.nih.gov/health/diabetes/ndic.htm

National Health Information Center (NHIC)
800-336-4797; 301-565-4167
Web site: www.health.gov/nhic/

National Heart, Lung, and Blood Institute Information Center (NHLBI)
800-575-9355; 301-592-8573
Web site: www.nhlbi.nih.gov

National Information Center for Children and Youth with Disabilities (NICHCY)
800-695-0285; 202-884-8200
Web site: www.nichcy.org

National Institute of Arthritis and Musculoskeletal and Skin Diseases Information Clearinghouse (NIAMS)
>877-226-4267; 301-495-4484
>Web site: www.nih.gov/niams

National Institute on Deafness and Other Communication Disorders Clearinghouse (NIDCD)
>800-241-1044
>Web site: www.nidcd.nih.gov

National Kidney and Urologic Diseases Information Clearinghouse (NKUDIC)
>301-654-3327
>Web site: www.niddk.nih.gov/health/kidney/nkudic.htm

National Lead Information Center
>800-424-5323
>Web site: www.epa.gov/lead/nlic.htm

National Organization for Rare Disorders (NORD)
>800-999-6673; 203-746-6518
>Web site: www.rarediseases.org

ORGANIZATIONS

Alexander Graham Bell Association for the Deaf and Hard of Hearing (AGBELL)
>202-337-5220
>Web site: www.agbell.org

Alliance for Technology Access (ATA)
>800-455-7970; 415-455-4575
>Web site: www.ataccess.org

American Academy of Allergy, Asthma, & Immunology (AAAAI)
>Web site: www.aaaai.org/

American Academy of Pediatrics (AAP)
>847-434-4000
>Web site: www.aap.org

American Brain Tumor Association (ABTA)
>847-827-9910
>Web site: www.abta.org/

American Diabetes Association
>800-342-2383; 703-549-1500
>Web site: www.diabetes.org

American Foundation for the Blind (AFB)
>800-232-5463
>Web site: www.afb.org

American Heart Association—National Center (AHA)
>800-242-8721; 214-373-6300
>Web site: www.americanheart.org

American Lung Association (ALA)
>800-586-4872; 212-315-8700
>Web site: www.lungusa.org/

American Occupational Therapy Association (AOTA)
>301-652-2682
>Web site: www.aota.org

American Physical Therapy Association (APTA)
>800-999-2782; 703-684-2782
>Web site: www.apta.org

American Psychological Association (APA)
800-374-2721; 202-336-5510
Web site: www.apa.org

American School Health Association (ASHA)
330-678-1601
Web site: www.ashaweb.org

American Speech-Language-Hearing Association (ASHA)
800-498-2071
Web site: www.asha.org

Angelman Syndrome Foundation
800-432-6435; 630-734-9267
Web site: www.angelman.org

Anxiety Disorders Association of America (ADAA)
301-231-9350
Web site: www.adaa.org

Aplastic Anemia & MDS International Foundation, Inc.
800-747-2820; 410-867-0242
Web site: www.aamds.org

Autism Society of America
800-328-8476; 301-657-0881
Web site: www.autism-society.org

Brain Injury Association (BIA)
800-444-6443; 703-236-6000
Web site: www.biausa.org

Center for Health and Health Care in Schools
202-466-3396
Web site: www.healthinschools.org/home.asp

Center for Mental Health Services (CMHS)
800-789-2647
Web site: www.mentalhealth.org

Centers for Disease Control (CDC)
Web site: www.cdc.gov

Childhood Apraxia of Speech Association of North America (CASANA)
412-767-6589
Web site: www.apraxia.org

Children and Adults with Attention-Deficit/Hyperactivity Disorder (CHADD)
800-233-4050; 301-306-7070
Web site: www.chadd.org

Children's Environmental Health Network (CEHN)
202-543-4033
Web site: www.cehn.org/

Chronic Fatigue and Immune Dysfunction Syndrome Association (CFIDS)
800-442-3437; 704-365-2343
Web site: www.cfids.org/youth/

Cleft Palate Foundation (CPF)
800-242-5338; 919-933-9044
Web site: www.cleftline.org

Closing the Gap, Inc.
(for information on computer technology in special education and rehabilitation)
507-248-3294
Web site: www.closingthegap.com

Council for Exceptional Children (CEC)
    703-620-3660
    Web site: www.cec.sped.org/
Cross Cultural Health Care Program (CCHCP)
    206-621-4161
    Web site: www.xculture.org/
Easter Seals—National Office
    800-221-6827; 312-726-6200
    Web site: www.easter-seals.org
Epilepsy Foundation—National Office
    800-332-1000; 301-459-3700
    Web site: www.efa.org
FACES: The National Craniofacial Association
    800-332-2372; 423-266-1632
    Web site: www.faces-cranio.org
**Family Voices (a national coalition speaking for children with special
health care needs)**
    888-835-5669
    Web site: www.familyvoices.org
Father's Network
    425-747-4004, ext. 218
    Web site: www.fathersnetwork.org
Food Allergy & Anaphylaxis Network (FAAN)
    800-929-4040
    Web site: www.foodallergy.org/
Foundation for Ichthyosis and Related Skin Types (FIRST)
    215-631-1411
    Web site: www.scalyskin.org
**Future of Children—publication of The David and Lucile Hewlett Packard
Foundation**
    650-917-7110
    Web site: www.futureofchildren.org
Global SchoolNet Foundation
    760-635-0001; 619-475-4852
    Web site: www.globalschoolnet.org/index.html
Head Start Bureau
    202-205-8572
    Web site: www.acf.dhhs.gov/programs/hsb/
Healthy People 2010
    Web site: www.health.gov/healthypeople/
Hydrocephalus Association
    415-732-7040
    Web site: www.hydroassoc.org
Immunization Action Coalition (IAC)
    651-647-9009
    Web site: www.immunize.org/
Kids Count
    410-547-6600
    Web site: www.aecf.org/kidscount/
International Dyslexia Association (IDA)
    800-222-3123; 410-296-0232
    Web site: www.interdys.org

Learning Disabilities Association of America (LDA)
888-300-6710; 412-341-1515
Web site: www.ldanatl.org
Leukemia & Lymphoma Society (formerly Leukemia Society of America)
800-955-4572; 212-573-8484
Web site: www.leukemia-lymphoma.org
Little People of America—National Headquarters (LPA)
888-572-2001
Web site: www.lpaonline.org
March of Dimes Birth Defects Foundation (MOD)
914-428-7100; 888- 663-4637
Web site: www.modimes.org
Muscular Dystrophy Association (MDA)
800-572-1717; 520-529-2000
Web site: www.mdausa.org
National Alliance for the Mentally Ill (NAMI)
800-950-6264; 703-524-7600
Web site: www.nami.org
National Association of Pediatric Nurse Practitioners (NAPNAP)
877-662-7627; 856-667-1773
Web site: www.napnap.org
National Association of School Nurses (NASN)
877-627-6476; 207-883-2117
Web site: www.nasn.org
National Attention Deficit Disorder Association (ADDA)
847-432-2332
Web site: www.add.org
National Brain Tumor Foundation (NBTF)
800-934-2873; 510-839-9777
Web site: www.braintumor.org
National Center for Education Statistics (NCES)
202-502-7300
Web site: www.nces.ed.gov/
National Center for Health Statistics (NCHS)
301-458-4636
Web site: www.cdc.gov/nchs/
National Down Syndrome Congress (NDSC)
800-221-4602; 212-460-9330
Web site: www.ndsc.center.org
National Eating Disorders Association
206-382-3587
Web site: www.nationaleatingdisorders.org
National Federation for the Blind (NFB)
410-659-9314
Web site: www.nfb.org
National Fragile X Foundation (FXF)
800-688-8765; 303-333-6155
Web site: www.nfxf.org
National Institutes of Health (NIH)
Web site: www.nih.gov/
National Library of Medicine (NLM)
Web site: www.nlm.nih.gov/

National Mental Health Association (NHMA)
　　800-969-6642; 703-684-7722
　　Web site: www.nmha.org
National Neurofibromatosis Foundation (NF)
　　800-323-7938; 212-344-6633
　　Web site: www.nf.org
National Organization for Albinism and Hypopigmentation (NOAH)
　　800-473-2310; 603-887-2310
　　Web site: www.albinism.org
National Organization on Fetal Alcohol Syndrome (NOFAS)
　　800-666-6327; 202-785-4585
　　Web site: www.nofas.org
National Reye's Syndrome Foundation (NRSF)
　　800-233-7393; 419-636-2679
　　Web site: www.reyessyndrome.org
National Resource Center for Paraprofessionals in Education and Related Services (NRCP)
　　435-797-7272
　　Web site: www.nrcpara.org
National Sleep Foundation (NSF)
　　202-347-3471
　　Web site: www.sleepfoundation.org
Obsessive Compulsive Foundation, Inc. (OCF)
　　203-315-2190
　　Web site: www.ocfoundation.org
Occupational Safety and Health Association (OSHA)
　　800-321-6742
　　Web site: www.osha.gov/
Osteogenesis Imperfecta Foundation (OI Foundation)
　　800-981-2663; 301-947-0083
　　Web site: www.oif.org
Parents Helping Parents (PHP)
　　408-727-5775
　　Web site: www.php.com
Prader-Willi Syndrome Association (PWSA)
　　800-926-4797; 941-312-0400
　　Web site: www.pwsausa.org
Schwab Foundation for Learning
　　Web site: www.schwablearning.org
Society for Adolescent Medicine (SAM)
　　816-224-8010
　　Web site: www.adolescenthealth.org
Special Olympics International
　　202-628-3630
　　Web site: www.specialolympics.org/
Spina Bifida Association of America (SBAA)
　　800-621-3141; 202-944-3285
　　Web site: www.sbaa.org
Stuttering Foundation of America
　　800-992-9392
　　Web site: www.stutterhelp.org

Tourette's Syndrome Association (TSA)
    800-237-0717; 718-224-2999
    Web site: www.tsa-usa.org
Tuberous Sclerosis Alliance
    800-225-6872
    Web site: www.tsalliance.org/
United Cerebral Palsy Association, Inc. (UCP)
    202-776-0406; 800-872-5827
    Web site: www.ucpa.org
U.S. Department of Education (DOE)
    800-872-5327
    Web site: www.ed.gov/index.jsp
U.S. Department of Health and Human Services (DHHS)
    877-696-6775; 202-619-0257
    Web site: www.os.dhhs.gov/
U.S. Food and Drug Administration (FDA)
    888-463-6332
    Web site: www.fda.gov
Vestibular Disorders Association (VEDA)
    800-837-8428; 503-229-7705
    Web site: www.vestibular.org
Williams Syndrome Association, Inc. (WSA)
    248-541-3630
    Web site: www.williams-syndrome.org
World Health Organization (WHO)
    (+00 41 22) 791 21 11
    Web site: www.who.int/home-page/

English-Spanish Equivalents of Commonly Used Health Terms and Phrases

English	Spanish
General Phrases	
What is your name?	¿Cómo se llama usted? (¿Cuál es su nombre?)
Where do you work?	¿Dónde trabaja? (Cuál es su profesión o trabajo?) (¿Qué hace usted?)
How are you feeling? Where does it hurt?	¿Cómo se siente? ¿Dónde le duele?
Do you feel better today?	¿Se siente mejor hoy?
Are you sleepy?	¿Tiene usted sueño?
You may take a bath.	Puede bañarse.
You may take a shower.	Puede tomar una ducha.
Have you noticed any bleeding?	¿Ha notado alguna hemorragia?
Do you still have any numbness?	¿Todavía siente adormecimiento?
Do you have any drug allergies?	¿Es usted alérgico(a) algún médicamento?
I need to change your dressing.	Necesito cambiar su vendaje.
What medications are you taking now?	¿Qué médicamentos está tomando ahora?
Do you take any medications?	¿Toma usted algunas medicinas?
Do you have a history of:	¿Padece:
heart disease?	del corazón?
diabetes?	de diabetes?
epilepsy?	de epilepsia?
bronchitis?	de bronquitis?
asthma?	de asma?
Relax. Try to sleep.	Relájese. Trate de dormir.
Please turn on your side.	Favor de ponerse de lado.
Do you have to urinate?	¿Tiene que orinar?
Have you had any sickness from any medicine?	¿Le ha caido mal alguna medicina?
Are you allergic to anything? Medicines, drugs, foods, insect bites?	¿Es usted alergico(a) a algo? ¿Medicinas, drogas, alimentos, picaduras de insectos?
Do you use contact lenses? Do you have any loose teeth or any prosthesis?	¿Usa usted lentes de contacto? ¿Tiene dientes flojos o cualquier prostesis?

From *Mosby's medical, nursing, and allied health dictionary,* ed 6, St Louis, 2002, Mosby.

Continued

English	Spanish
Assessment	
General	
I am _____.	Soy _____.
I would like to examine you now. Please take off your clothes, except for your underwear (and bra), and put on this gown.	Quisiera examinarlo(a) ahora. Por favor, quítese la ropa menos la ropa interior (y el sostén), y póngase este camisón.
I am going to take your temperature now. Open your mouth.	Le voy a tomar la temperatura ahora. Abra la boca.
I am going to take your blood pressure now.	Le voy a tomar la presión ahora.
Your blood pressure is low.	Su presión es baja.
Your blood pressure is too high.	Su presión es demasiado alta.
Here is a prescription to reduce your blood pressure.	Aquí tiene una receta para bajar la presión de sangre.
You must follow a diet to lose weight.	Debe seguir una dieta para perder peso.
Bend your elbow.	Doble el codo.
Make a fist.	Haga un puño.
I am going to give you an injection.	Le voy a poner una inyección.
Breathe normally.	Respire normalmente.
Cough.	Tosa.
Squeeze my hand.	Apriete mi mano.
You have a slight fever.	Ud. tiene un poco de fiebre.
Hold your leg up.	Levante la pierna.
Stand up and walk.	Parese y camine.
Straighten your leg.	Enderece la pierna.
Bend your knee.	Doble la rodilla.
Push/pull.	Empuje/jale.
Up/down.	Arriba/abajo.
In/out.	Adentro/afuera.
Slow/fast.	Despacio/aprisa.
Rest.	Descanse.
Kneel.	Arrodíllese.
Ambulation history	
Do you use equipment (canes, crutches, braces)?	¿Usa equipo (bastones, muletals, abrazaderas)?
Do you use a wheelchair?	¿Usa usted una silla de ruedas?
Do you drive a car?	¿Maneja usted un carro?
Can you climb stairs?	¿Puede usted subir las escaleras?
Cardiology	
Have you ever had chest pain? Where?	¿Ha tenido alguna vez dolor de pecho? ¿Dónde?
Do you notice any irregularity of heart beat or any palpitations?	¿Nota cualquier latido o palpitación irregular?
Do you get short of breath? When?	¿Tiene falta de aire? Cuándo?
Do you take medicine for your heart? How often?	¿Toma medicina para el corazón? ¿Con qué frecuencia?

From *Mosby's medical, nursing, and allied health dictionary,* ed 6, St Louis, 2002, Mosby.

English	Spanish
Cardiology—cont'd	
Do you know if you have high blood pressure?	¿Sabe usted si tiene la presión alta?
Is there a history of hypertension in your family?	¿Hay historia de hipertensión en su familia?
You have had a heart attack.	Ha tenido un ataque al corazón.
Diabetes	
You have diabetes.	Usted tiene diabetes.
Drug-related problems	
What drugs do you use? heroin? cocaine? uppers? downers? barbiturates? speed?	¿Cuáles drogas usa usted? ¿heroína? ¿cocaína? ¿estimulantes? ¿abajos? ¿diablitos o barbitúricos? ¿blancas?
Where do you shoot the drugs?	¿Dónde se pone usted las drogas?
Have you ever been through a detoxification program before?	¿Ha participado alguna vez en un programa de desintoxicación?
Have you ever overdosed on drugs?	¿Alguna vez se ha sobredrogado?
Ears, nose, and throat	
Do you have any hearing problems?	¿Tiene Ud. problemas de oir?
Do you use a hearing aid?	¿Usa Ud. un audífono?
Do your ears ring?	¿Siente un tintineo o silbido en los oídos?
Do you have allergies?	¿Tiene alergias?
Do you have a cold?	¿Tiene usted un resfriado/resfrío?
Do you have sore throats frequently?	¿Le duele la garganta con frecuencia?
Have you ever had strep throat?	¿Ha tenido alguna vez (infección de la garganta)?
I want to take a throat culture. Open your mouth. This will not hurt.	Quiero hacer un cultivo de la garganta. Abra la boca. Esto no le va a doler.
Endocrinology	
Have you ever had problems with your thyroid?	¿Ha tenido alguna vez problemas con la tiroides?
Have you noted any significant weight gain or loss? What is your usual weight?	¿Ha notado pérdida o aumento de peso? ¿Cuál es su peso usual?
How is your appetite?	¿Qué tal su apetito?
(Women) How old were you when your periods started? How many days between periods? Have you ever been pregnant? How many children do you have?	¿Cuántos años tenía cuando tuvo la primera regla? ¿Cuántos días entre las reglas? ¿Ha estado embarazada? ¿Cuántos hijos tiene?
Gastrointestinal	
What foods disagree with you?	¿Qué alimentos le caen mal?
Do you get heartburn?	¿Suele tener ardor en el pecho?

Continued

English	Spanish
Gastrointestinal—cont'd	
Do you have indigestion often?	¿Tiene indigestión con frecuencia?
Are you going to vomit?	¿Va a vomitar (arrojar)?
Do you have blood in your vomit?	¿Tiene usted vómitos con sangre?
Headaches/head	
Do you have headaches?	¿Tiene Ud. dolores de cabeza (jaquecas)?
Do you have migraines?	¿Tiene Ud. migrañas (jaquecas)?
Where is the pain exactly?	¿Dónde le duele, exactamente?
What causes the headaches?	¿Qué la causa los dolores de cabeza?
Are there any changes in your vision?	¿Hay algunos cambios en su vista?
Neurology	
Have you ever had a head injury?	¿Ha tenido alguna vez daño a la cabeza?
Have you ever had a sports injury?/ motorcycle accident?	¿Ha tenido alguna vez un daño deportivo?/(accidente en su motocicleta?)
Do you have convulsions?	¿Tiene convulsiones?
Do you see double?	¿Ve usted doble?
Do you have tingling sensations?	¿Tiene hormigueos?
Do you have numbness in your hands, arms, or feet?	¿Siente entumecidos las manos, los brazos, o los pies?
Have you ever lost consciousness? For how long?	¿Perdió alguna vez el sentido? ¿Por cuánto tiempo?
How frequently does this happen?	¿Con qué frecuencia ocurre esto?
Is this hot or cold?	¿Está frío o caliente esto?
Obstetrics and gynecology	
How often do you get your periods?	¿Cada cuándo le viene la regla?
When was your last menstrual period?	¿Cuándo fue su última regla?
When was your last Pap smear?	¿Cuándo fue su última prueba de Papanicolado?
Would you like information on birth control methods?	¿Quiere usted. información sobre los métodos del control de la natalidad? (los métodos anticonceptivos)?
Do you have an IUD in place?	¿Le han puesto un aparato intrauterino?
Do you have a lot of pain?	¿Tiene usted mucho dolor?
Ophthalmology	
Have you had pain in your eyes?	¿Ha tenido dolor en los ojos?
Do you wear glasses?	¿Usa usted anteojos/gafas/lentes/ espejuelos?
Were you exposed to anything that could have injured your eye?	¿Fue expuesto a cualquier cosa que pudiera haberle dañado el ojo?
Do your eyes water much?	¿Le lagrimean mucho los ojos?
I am going to put drops in your eyes in order to examine them. This medicine may burn at first.	Le voy a poner gotas en los ojos para examinarlos. Esta medicina puede arderle al principio.
Please look into this apparatus.	Favor de mirar dentro de este aparato.

From *Mosby's medical, nursing, and allied health dictionary,* ed 6, St Louis, 2002, Mosby.

English	Spanish

Orthopedics

English	Spanish
You have broken (a bone).	Usted se ha quebrado/roto (un hueso).
You have dislocated (a joint).	Usted se ha dislocado (una coyuntura).
You have pulled (a muscle).	Usted se ha distendido (un músculo).
You have sprained (a muscle)/ (a ligament).	Usted se ha torcido (un músculo)/ (un ligamento).
Do you feel pain when you stand?	¿Siente dolor al pararse?
Do you feel pain when you bend?	¿Siente dolor al doblarse?

Pain

English	Spanish
What were you doing when the pain started?	¿Qué hacía usted cuando le comenzó el dolor?
Where is the pain?	¿Dónde está el dolor?
How severe is the pain? Mild, moderate, sharp, or severe?	¿Qué tan fuerte es el dolor? ¿Ligero, moderado, agudo, severo?
Have you ever had this pain before?	¿Ha tenido este dolor antes? ¿Ha sido siempre así?
Does it hurt when I press here? How did the accident happen?	¿Le duele cuando le aprieto aquí? ¿Cómo sucedió el accidente?
How did this happen? How long ago?	¿Cómo sucedío esto? ¿Cuanto tiempo hace?

Poison control (telephone information)

English	Spanish
What was swallowed?	¿Qué se tragó?
Please spell the name of the product for me.	¿Favor de deletrear el nombre del producto?
How old is the person who swallowed this?	¿Cuántos años tiene la persona que se tragó esto?
How much does the person weigh?	¿Cuánto pesa?
Is the person breathing all right?	¿Está respirando bien?
Is the person complaining of any pain or other difficulty?	¿Se queja de algún dolor, o de otra dificultad?
How long ago did the person swallow the product?	¿Cuánto hace que esta persona se tragó el producto?

Pulmonary/respiratory

English	Spanish
Do you smoke? How many packs a day?	¿Fuma usted? ¿Cuántos paquentes al día?
How long have you been coughing?	¿Desde cúando tiene tos?
Does it hurt when you cough?	¿Le duele cuando tose?
Do you cough up phlegm?	¿Al toser, escupe usted flema(s)?
Do you cough up blood?	¿Al toser, arroja usted sangre?
Do you wheeze?	¿Le silba a usted el pecho?
Have you ever had asthma?	¿Ha tenido asma alguna vez?
Have you ever had: tuberculosis? pneumonia? emphysema? bronchitis?	¿Ha tenido alguna vez: tuberculosis? pulmonía? enfisema? bronquitis?
Breathe deeply.	Aspire profundamente. (Respire profundo.)

Continued

English	Spanish

Sexually transmitted diseases

English	Spanish
Do you have urethral discharge?	¿Tiene descho de la uretra?
Do you have burning with urination?	¿Tiene ardor al orinar?
Do you have a vaginal discharge?	¿Tiene descho vaginales?
Do you have abdominal pain?	¿Tiene dolor en el abdomen?
When did you last have intercourse?	¿Cuándo fue la última vez que tuvo relaciones sexuales?

Unconscious patient

English	Spanish
What happened to him/her?	¿Que le pasó? (Que le sucedío?)
Has he vomited?	¿Ha vomitado?
Is she pregnant?	¿Está embarazada?

Patient Instructions
General

English	Spanish
Roll over and sit up over the edge of the bed.	Voltéese y siéntese sobre el borde de la cama.
Stand up slowly. Put weight only on your right/left foot.	Párese despacio. Ponga peso sólo en la pierna derecha/izquierda.
Lift your head up.	Levante la cabeza.
Take a step to the side.	Dé un paso al lado.
Turn to your left/right.	Doble a la izquierda/derecha.

Drugs

English	Spanish
I want you to take your medicine.	Quiero que tome su medicina.
Let it dissolve in your mouth.	Que se le disuelva en la boca.
Apply _____ to the affected part.	Aplique _____ en la parte afectada.
Cool in the refrigerator.	Enfrie en el refrigerador.
Here is some medication for _____.Take _____ tablets every _____ hours as needed.	Aquí tiene la medicina para _____. Tome _____ tabletas cada _____ horas según la necesite.
These pills are vitamins.	Estas pastillas son vitaminas.
These pills are for pain.	Estas pastillas son para dolor.
Take _____ of these pills each day.	Tome _____ de estas pastillas cada día.
Here is enough medicine for _____ days.	Aquí tiene suficiente medicina para _____ días.
Take one of these pills every _____ hours.	Tome una de estas pastillas cada _____ horas.
Take one pill daily for _____ days.	Tome una pastilla por _____ días.
But no more than _____ a day maximum.	Pero no más de _____ en total cada día.
Fill the medicine dropper to this line and mix with a glass of water, juice, or milk.	Llene el gotero hasta esta linea y mezcle con un vaso de agua, jugo, o leche.

From *Mosby's medical, nursing, and allied health dictionary,* ed 6, St Louis, 2002, Mosby.

English	Spanish
Drugs—cont'd	
It is important for you to eat/drink liquids.	Es importante que usted coma/beba o tome líquidos.
Vocabulary	
Anatomy	
abdomen	el abdomen
ankle	el tobillo
anus	el ano
appendix	el apéndice
arm	el brazo
back	la espalda
lower back	la cintura
bladder	la vejiga
blood	la sangre
body	el cuerpo
bone	el hueso
bowels	los intestinos, las entrañas
brain	el cerebro
breasts	el pecho, los senos
buttocks	las nalgas, las posaderas, las sentaderas
calf	la pantorrilla, el chamorro
chest	el pecho
coccyx	la cóccix
collarbone	la clavícula
ear (inner)	el oído
ear (outer)	la oreja
eardrum	el tímpano
ears	las orejas
elbow	el codo
eye	el ojo
face	la cara
fallopian tube	el tubo falopio
finger	el dedo
foot	el pie
genitals	los genitales
hair (of the head)	el pelo, el cabello
hand	la mano
head	la cabeza
heart	el corazón
heart valve	la válvula del corazón
hip	la cadera
hormone	la hormona
intestines	los intestinos
jaw	la quijada
joint	la coyuntura, la articulación
kidney	el riñón
knee	la rodilla
leg	la pierna
ligament	el ligamento

Continued

English	Spanish
Vocabulary—cont'd	
Anatomy—cont'd	
lip	el labio
liver	el hígado
lung	el pulmón
mouth	la boca
muscle	el músculo
neck	el cuello
nerve	el nervio
nose	la naríz
ovary	el ovario
pelvis	la cadera, la pelvis
penis	el pene, el miembro
pulse	el pulso
pupil	la niña del ojo, la pupila
rib	la costilla
saliva	la saliva
shoulder	el hombro
sinus	el seno
skin	la piel
skin (of the face)	el cutis
skull	el cráneo
spine	el espinazo, la columna vertebral
stomach	el estómago, la panza, la barriga
tendon	el tendón
thigh	el muslo
toe	el dedo del pie
tongue	la lengua
tonsils	las angínas, las amígdalas
tooth, molar	el diente, la muela
trachea	la tráquea
urine	la orina
uterus	el útero, la matríz
vagina	la vagina
vein	la vena
wrist	la muñeca
Common medical problems	
abortion	el aborto
abscess	el absceso
appendicitis	la apendicitis
arthritis	la artritis
asthma	el asma
backache	el dolor de espalda
blindness	la ceguera
bronchitis	la bronquitis
bruise	moretón, magulladura
burn (first, second, or third degree)	la quemadura (de primer, segundo o tercer grado)

From *Mosby's medical, nursing, and allied health dictionary,* ed 6, St Louis, 2002, Mosby.

English	Spanish
Common medical problems—cont'd	
cancer	el cáncer
chickenpox	la varicela
chills	los escalofrios
cold	el catarro, el resfriado
constipation	la constipación
convulsion	la convulsión
cough	la tos
cramps	los calambres
cut	cortada, cortadura
deafness	la sordera
diabetes	la diabetes
diarrhea	la diarrea
dizziness	el vértigo, el mareo
epilepsy	la epilepsia
fainting spell	el desmayo
fatigue	la fatiga
fever	la fiebre
flu	la influenza, la gripe
food poisoning	el envenamiento por comestibles
fracture	la fractura
gall stone	el cálculo biliar
gastric ulcer	la úlcera gástrica
hallucination	la alucinación
handicap	el impedimento
headache	el dolor de cabeza
heart attack	el ataque al corazón
heartbeat	el latido-el palpito
heart disease	la enfermedad del corazón
heart murmur	el soplo del corazón
hemorrhage	la hemorragia
hemorrhoids	la almorranas, hemorroides
hernia	la hernia
herpes	el herpes
high blood pressure	la presión alta
hives	la urticaria
illness	la enfermedad
immunization	la inmunización
infection	la infección
inflammation	la inflamación
injury	la herida, el daño
itch	la picazón-la comezón
laryngitis	la laringitis
lice	los piojos
malignant	maligno(a)
malnutrition	la desnutrición
measles	el sarampión
meningitis	la meningitis
miscarriage	un malparto, un aborto, una pérdida
mononucleosis	la mononucleosis infecciosa

Continued

English	Spanish
Common medical problems—cont'd	
multiple sclerosis	la esclerosis múltiple
mumps	las paperas
muscular dystrophy	la distrofía muscular
mute	mudo(a)
obese	obeso(a)
obstruction	la obstrucción
overdose	la sobredosis
overweight	el sobrepeso
pain	el dolor
palsy, cerebral	la parálisis cerebral
paralysis	la parálisis
pneumonia	la pulmonía
poison ivy/oak	la hiedra venenosa
polio	la poliomielitis
rabies	la rabia
rash	la roncha, el salpullido, la erupción
redness	enrojecimiento o inflamación
relapse	la recaída
scar	la cicatriz
shock	el choque
sore	la llaga
spasm	el espasmo
spider bite	la picadura de araña
sprain	la torcedura
stomachache	el dolor de estómago
sunstroke	la insolación
swelling	la hinchazón
tetanus	el tétano(s)
tonsillitis	amigdalitis
toothache	el dolor de muela
trauma	el trauma
tuberculosis	la tuberculosis
tumor	el tumor
unconsciousness	la insensibilidad
venereal disease	la enfermedad venérea
virus	el virus
vomit	el vómito, los vómitos
weakness	la debilidad
welt	roncha, verdugón
whiplash	concusión de la espina cervical, lastimado del cuello
Equipment and supplies	
bandage	la venda
bed	la cama
blanket	cobija
catheter	el cateter
crutches	las muletas

From *Mosby's medical, nursing, and allied health dictionary,* ed 6, St Louis, 2002, Mosby.

English	Spanish

Equipment and supplies—cont'd

pillow	la almohada
shower	la ducha
soap	el jabón
stethoscope	el estetoscopio
stretcher	la camilla
syringe	la jeringa
thermometer	el termometro
toilet	el excusado
tongue depressor	el pisalengua
toothbrush	el cepillo de dientes
wheelchair	la silla de ruedas

Medications and related supplies

alcohol	alcohol
amphetamine	anfetamina
antibiotic	antibiótico
application	aplicación
artifical limb	el miembro artificial
aspirin (for children)	aspirina (para niños)
Band-Aid	la curita
barbiturate	barbitúrico
birth control pill	la píldora anticonceptiva
booster shot	la inyección secundaria
brace	el braguero
calcium	calcio
capsule	cápsula
cocaine	cocaína
codeine	codeína
cold pack	el emplasto frío
compress (hot)	la compresa (caliente)
condom	goma, condón
contact lens	lentes de contacto
contraceptive pills	pastillas anticonceptivas
cotton	algodón
cough syrup	jarabe para la tos
diuretic	diurético
dose	dosis
dressing	vendaje
dropper	el gotero
drops	gotas
enema	enema
gauze	gasa
glucose	glucosa
hearing aid	el aparato para la sordera
heroin	heroína
ice	hielo
ice pack	la bolsa de hielo
insulin	insulina
intrauterine device (IUD)	el dispositivio intrauterino

Continued

English	Spanish
laxative	laxante, purgante, purga
lotion	loción
narcotic	narcótico
needle	aguja
Novocaine	novocaína
ointment	ungüento
pacemaker	el marcapaso
penicillin	penicilina
pill	píldora, pastilla
prosthesis	miembro artificial (prótesis)
sedative	sedante, calmante
sling	el cabestrillo
smelling salts	sales aromáticas
splint	la tablilla
support	el apoyo
suppository	supositorio
syrup of ipecac	jarabe de ipecacuana
vitamin	vitamina

Medication instructions

English	Spanish
right	derecho(a)
left	izquierdo(a)
tablespoonful	cucharada
teaspoonful	cucharadita
one-half teaspoonful	media cucharadita
bid	dos veces al d;0;0>a
tid	tres veces al d;0;0>a
qid	cuatro veces al d;0;0>a
every hour	cada hora
each day, daily	cada d;0;0>a, diariamente
every other day	cada otro d;0;0>a (cada tercer d;0;0>a)
till gone	hasta terminar (acabar)
Let it dissolve in your mouth.	Que se le disuelva en la boca.
as needed for pain	cuando la necesite para el dolor
symptoms	sintomas
insert	inserte
when you get up in the morning	al levantarse
apply	aplique
one-half hour after meals	una hora antes de comidas
now (stat)	ahora (ahora mismo)
before bedtime	antes de acostarse
before you exercise	antes de hacer ejercicios
chew	mastique
mix	mezcle
dissolved in	disuelto en
Shake well.	Agite bien.
as directed	de acuerdo con las instrucciones
by mouth	por la boca
rub	frote

From *Mosby's medical, nursing, and allied health dictionary,* ed 6, St Louis, 2002, Mosby.

English	Spanish

Medication instructions—cont'd

gargle	haga gargaras
soak	remoje, empape

Tests and procedures

allergy test	prueba para alergias
analysis	análisis
blood count	recuento (conteo) globular
blood transfusion	la transfusion de sangre
cardiogram	cardiograma
checkup, medical	reconocimiento (chequeo) médico
culture (throat)	cultivo de la garganta
electrocardiogram	electrocardiograma
electroencephalogram	electroencefalograma
enema	la enema
eye test	examen de la vista (de los ojos)
injection	la inyección
laboratory	laboratorio
massage	el masaje
pregnancy test	prueba de embarazo
specimen	muestra (espécimen)
traction	la traccion
urinalysis	análisis de orina
vaccination	la vacuna
x-rays	radiografias (rayos equis)

INDEX

Page numbers followed by *f* indicate figures; by *t,* tables; and by *b,* boxes.